T0317728

THE WORKS OF WILLIAM HARVEY

THE WORKS OF
WILLIAM
HARVEY

Translated by
Robert Willis, M.D.

Introduction by
Arthur C. Guyton, M.D.

upp

University of Pennsylvania Press
Philadelphia

UNIVERSITY OF PENNSYLVANIA PRESS
CLASSICS IN
MEDICINE AND BIOLOGY SERIES
Edited by
ALFRED P. FISHMAN, M.D.
William Maul Measey Professor of Medicine
University of Pennsylvania

Library of Congress Cataloging-in-Publication Data
Harvey, William, 1578–1657.
[Works. 1989]
The works of William Harvey / translated by Robert Willis;
introduction by Arthur C. Guyton.
  p. cm.—(University of Pennsylvania Press classics in
medicine and biology series)
Reprint. Originally published: New York : Johnson Reprint Corp.,
1965.
Bibliography: p.
ISBN 0-8122-8166-7
1. Physiology—Early works to 1800. 2. Blood—Circulation—Early
works to 1800. 3. Embryology—Early works to 1800. I. Willis,
Robert, 1799–1878. II. Title. III. Series.
QP29.H37A2 1989
612—dc19   88–28081
                                                    CIP

INTRODUCTION

WILLIAM HARVEY, HIS TIMES, AND HIS ACHIEVEMENTS*

ARTHUR C. GUYTON, M.D.

William Harvey's book on the circulation, published in 1628, demonstrated clearly that the heart pumps blood in a circle through the body. Strange as it seems to us today, this concept was so revolutionary to Harvey's contemporaries that the world's basic understanding of how the body functions was thrown into turmoil. Only after another half century did the immediate aftershocks clear, leaving a legacy that affected forever all of medical science. This book, written in Latin, was entitled *Exercitatio Anatomica de Motu Cordis et Sanguinis in Animalibus*, and commonly referred to as *de Motu Cordis*. Its English translation is *Anatomical Studies on the Motion of the Heart and Blood in Animals*. Probably no other scientific work in history so changed the fundamental knowledge of physiology, changing also the essential bases of medical practice.

Yet, Harvey's life goals were even loftier than merely to revise circulatory physiology, for during the last two-thirds of his career an inner fire drove him incessantly to explain the origin of life itself; what could be more gratifying to one's intellect, even to one's soul? His eventual book on this subject, entitled *Anatomical Exercises on the Generation of Animals*, was published in 1851.

Reprinted in this volume are these two monumental works, along with various letters and sundry other writings that tell much about Harvey as a man. Harvey wrote both his books in

Latin, and there is no evidence that he personally ever translated them into English. The first English translation of his book on the circulation was not published until 1653, twenty-five years after the Latin version. The translator is unknown, but subsequent scholars have found this early translation to be so inadequate that it is rarely if ever quoted or reproduced. Since that time there have been at least five other English translations. The translation most often reprinted, the one reprinted here as well, is that of Robert Willis, M.D. Willis also translated the other writings of Harvey that are reprinted here. These translations were completed in 1847, as a work of love on the part of Willis, but also for the specific purpose of publication in the Sydenham Society of London's scientific historical series entitled *The Sources of Science*.

There are many reasons for this new reprinting of Harvey's works, but they are especially to keep before all of us the historical perspective of Harvey's revolutionary achievements—especially to let everyone remember that only a short while ago our knowledge of the circulatory system, indeed of the whole body, was based more on whimsical fancy than on truth. And equally important, we again remind ourselves how difficult it is to remold the thinking of even the most astute scientist when doctrines from the past are so often repeated that they achieve the infinite authority of age.

Harvey's greatness in history rests almost exclusively on his discovery of the circulation. However, it could have rested equally securely on his work and discoveries on the generation of life, had he lived but a few years later when the necessary scientific tools, especially the microscope, had become available. Harvey's book on this subject displays the same genius that was the basis of his success in studying the circulation, though it did not have the same fortune.

Harvey almost certainly was not the only person of his times who contemplated the circulation of the blood. In particular, some historians interpret the fifteenth-century writings of Caesalpinus to have postulated in general terms not only a pulmonary circulation but a peripheral circulation as well, even suggesting the presence of anastomoses between the arteries and the veins, *vasa in capillamenta resoluta*. Therefore, it is clear that at least a few others besides Harvey were beginning to understand that the newer knowledge of the heart and blood vessels was incompatible with older concepts.

However, the difference between Harvey and these others was that Harvey marshaled a vast amount of experimental evidence, accurately observed and forcefully presented, which painted a composite picture of a heart pumping large quantities of arterial blood continuously throughout the entire body, thence back by way of the veins to the right heart and lungs and around the circulation again. Only this concept could fit the large amounts of evidence that Harvey amassed.

The fact that blood flows in a circuitous route through the body is so much second nature to us now, and seems to be so elementary, that it is very difficult to conceive of anything different. Yet, less than 400 years ago, a few years *after* the first European settlement of America, it was still almost inviolate doctrine that blood did not flow in a circuit through the body; instead, it ebbed to and fro in the arteries from the heart to the tissues, and in the veins from the liver to the tissues. The purpose of the heart was more to warm the blood and to add "vital spirits" than to pump the blood, if indeed it pumped blood at all.

Where did these previous concepts come from? The answer: most of them went all the way back to Galen in the second century A.D., perpetuating fourteen centuries of dogma repeated from generation to generation. In turn, a few of Galen's own concepts came from Aristotle, and even from Hippocrates and Plato five centuries earlier in the fourth century B.C. Thus, the science of the circulation had been almost static for nearly 2,000 years.

Harvey's Times

Harvey was born in 1578 during the latter part of the Renaissance. In England the revival of literature, philosophy, public discussion, and free thought had already been underway for over a hundred years, brought about partly through mass dissemination of knowledge as an aftermath of the invention of the printing press in 1439. Medical knowledge, however, lagged generations behind, partly because medical learning was strongly dominated by a fanatic, almost religious devotion to the teachings of Galen that had been made almost sacred by the strictures on free thought during medieval times. Also, the force of the Inquisition still remained in many areas of Europe, insuring that new writings be consistent with the doctrine of truth as held by the church from antiquity. The goal of the medieval scholar was mainly to perpetuate this truth, not to inquire into its validity.

Under Greek and Roman cultures, from the time of Aristotle (384–322 B.C.) through the life of Galen, a period of over five centuries, thought and scientific inquiry had enjoyed a period of relative freedom. An understanding of the anatomical structure of the body took form, and beginning theories of bodily function were born, finding their greatest flowering in the hands of Galen (131–201). Galen was an exceptional talent among the Graeco-Roman physicians. He summarized in prolific writings virtually all the physiological knowledge gained from the early Greek and Alexandrian sources, as well as greatly expanding this with numerous personal anatomical dissections and physiological experiments. Galen's observational methods included vivisection, from which he studied the motions of living internal organs, including the heart and arteries. But, wherever his observational knowledge ended, he had few qualms about supplementing it with vivid imagination. Thus, he was able to provide detailed treatises on the function of almost any part of the body, including exact accounts of the roles of the heart and vascular structures in the life of the body.

Though Galen was often seriously wrong, especially so in his description of the function of the heart and blood vessels, his advances were still monumental. Not long after Galen's time, church doctrinairism began to shroud free thought and inquiry. Therefore, it is no wonder that Galen's physiological teachings, by far the greatest that had yet been achieved, should become enshrined as the ultimate of medical knowledge. And as long as the oppressive rule of the medieval times held sway, so also did Galen remain the supreme physiological authority of western culture, spanning a period of fourteen centuries.

Beginning in the 1400s the Renaissance of literature, philosophy, and public debate led the way out of the medieval strait jacket. In England, King Henry VIII (1491–1547), who lived almost a century before Harvey, blazed the way in breaking with supreme ecclesiastical authority, and in 1558, only eleven years after the end of Henry VIII's reign, Elizabeth I (1533–1603) came to the throne. Her rule, coupled after 1603 with that of her successor James I (1566–1625), provided three-quarters of a century of dynamic progress in British life, leading to the world exploits of Sir Francis Drake (1540?–1596), the literary works of Shakespeare (1564–1616), and the philosophy of Sir Francis Bacon (1561–1626). But after Charles I (1600–1649) came to power in 1625, a turbulent period of public activism began, characterized by religious conflicts pitting Roman Catholics against Protestants, and by political conflicts between opposing advocates of divine right of the king and parliamentary rule. These conflicts eventuated in England's First Civil War from 1642 to 1646, in which Harvey, as personal physician to the king, was deeply involved. At the beginning of this war, Harvey was already 64 years old, and the havoc of the war years followed by their aftermath of Cromwellian reforms plus several other smaller wars trod heavily on his life, as we shall see.

The world of science during the 1500s likewise saw a dawn of dramatic changes, but certain scientific discoveries also became the cause of serious religious backlash, delaying development in at least some areas of science until several generations after literature and philosophy had already reached full flowering. Especially revolutionary were the studies of Copernicus (1473–1543), a Prussian astronomer who lived a century before Harvey. He succeeded in mapping the motions of the planets with respect to the earth and sun and stars, and came to the inescapable conclusion that earth and the other planets move in orbits around the sun, a direct contradiction to strict literal interpretation of the Bible that ascribed to earth the central position. Then, during Harvey's lifetime, Kepler (1571–1630) added mathematical precision to the Copernican system of planetary motion, and Galileo (1564–1642), from his study of the heavens with his telescope, gave undeniable experimental proof to the theories of both Copernicus and Kepler.

Galileo was a teacher of mathematics at Padua, Italy, where Harvey studied medicine from the years 1600 to 1602. Though evidence is lacking that Harvey had significant direct contact with Galileo, nevertheless, the climate of changing thought was everywhere about Harvey. Yet, restrictions were also still alive.

This was emphasized by the Inquisitional trial of Galileo in 1633, followed by enforced suppression of many of his ideas, as well as by house imprisonment for the last eight years of his life.

It was in this same period of time that M. Servetus (1509–1553) provided the first written description (1553) of blood flow through the lungs. Servetus was burned at the stake at the instigation of Calvin, a strict Protestant reformer, only a few months thereafter, not specifically for his description of blood flow in the lungs but for a totality of heretical thinking.

Thus, Harvey was born into a time of blossoming yet restricted thought, with science still under many restrictions of medieval doctrine. He was born into a landed family of moderate to well-to-do means near Folkestone, England, in 1578. His father was later mayor of Folkestone on four separate occasions. Otherwise, not much is known about Harvey's early life except that his pre-university education was in a private school of good repute and that he entered Cambridge University at the age of 15. Four years later, in 1597, he received a B.A. degree from Cambridge, but remained there another two years studying mainly pre-medical subjects. In early 1600 he traveled to Padua, Italy, to study medicine at the greatest scientific university of the day. He received his medical certificate with at least some level of honors in 1602.

On returning to London after his medical schooling in Padua, he began the practice of medicine in 1603; he rose rapidly in the medical world, helped at least partly by his marriage to Elizabeth Browne, the daughter of Dr. Lancelot Browne, Physician to Queen Elizabeth and later to King James. By the year 1607 Harvey had been admitted to the Royal College of Physicians, but only after a series of four stiff examinations. In 1615 he was given a lifetime appointment by the Royal College of Physicians as Lumleian Lecturer, and in 1616 he was appointed as Physician to St. Bartholomew's Hospital, which made him chief of the medical program of that hospital as well, a position he held until 1646.

It was in his inaugural series of Lumleian lectures in 1616 that he first described the circulation of the blood in many of the same terms that he later used in his book. Yet, it was another twelve years before he collected all his arguments and experimental evidence, and published these in his book *de Motu Cor-*

dis as undeniable bases for believing that the blood does indeed circulate.

Throughout his professional life, Harvey had close associations with royalty, beginning in 1616 in the footsteps of his father-in-law as a Physician to King James I and his court and eventually serving in the special position of Principal Physician to Charles I. He continued in this capacity through England's Civil War (1642–1646) and, though less actively so, even until Charles was hanged in 1649.

Harvey had real personal affection for Charles. In turn Charles was clearly a personal friend and patron of Harvey's scientific inquiry. Both James and Charles, especially the latter, observed some of Harvey's experiments and were keenly interested in Harvey's scholarship and philosophy. In fact, Charles participated actively in some of Harvey's experiments. When Charles was deposed in 1646, imprisoned in 1647, and hanged in 1649 as an aftermath of the Civil War, Harvey indeed lost a great supporter, and he retreated into melancholic solace among his thoughts and work for the remaining eight years of his life, dying at the age of 79 in 1657.

To understand fully how Harvey was affected by these times, it is worth reading carefully his own feelings as expressed in 1650 to his friend George Ent: "And truly, did I not find solace in my studies, and a balm for my spirit in the memory of my observations of former years, I should feel little desire for longer life."

Because of Harvey's loyalty to Charles through and after the Civil War (1642–1646), he was fined 2000 pounds. Also, he was legally banished for two years from within twenty miles of London, though in reality he remained in the homes of his brothers only a few miles from London.

The Scientific Background for Harvey's Discoveries

On graduating in medicine in 1602, Harvey inherited a fourteen-century-old legacy of almost sacred anatomical and physiological truth as originally expressed by Galen. Medical science even in the seventeenth century was still fearful of challenging this truth. Harvey reflected this fear at several points in *de Motu*

Cordis, but he also pleaded for open minds. He did not blame Galen for this state of medical science; the blame was on the nature of man himself. In fact, Harvey revered Galen for his achievements, especially for the fact that Galen, like himself, contributed to medical science through experiments and observation. The genius of both these men was that they trusted their senses of observation and contrived new and novel ways to demonstrate observational truth rather than accepting hearsay from the past as ultimate authority.

Yet, with all that Galen had accomplished, the unknowns in medical science remained vast. Unfortunately, as we noted above, many of Galen's more speculative theses on the mysteries of the body had been repeated so often over the centuries that they had become almost inviolable truth.

The mysteries of the circulatory system, as formulated in Galen's teachings and still so interpreted at the time of Harvey, were that the blood did not circulate through the body at all but instead was formed centrally and carried peripherally to the outlying tissues by both the arteries and the veins. There, great portions of the blood were eventually consumed. The teachings were basically the following.

An initial portion of the blood came from the stomach where "raw aliment" was concocted from the food. The stomach refined this aliment to form "chyle" that went by way of the portal vein to the liver. In the liver, the chyle was freed of impurities and further concocted to form venous blood. In turn, the venous blood was considered to be the "natural spirit" that provided the body's nourishment. From the liver a portion of the venous blood went by way of the vena cava to the right heart and lungs, giving nourishment to both of these. A small amount of this blood passed from the right ventricle through "porosities" in the interventricular septum into the left ventricle. In the meantime, air was pulled by respiration into the lungs. This air contained "pneuma," another basic necessity of life. From the lungs, pneuma entered the pulmonary veins and, after passing through the left atrium, entered the left ventricle. Here pneuma and venous blood were mixed, and the heart itself added heat to this mixture, providing an ultimate concoction containing "vital spirits." The vital spirits in turn were carried in the arteries to all parts of the body. Pulsation in the arteries was believed to be the result of ebbing of blood forward and backward, carrying vital spirits to all the body's tissues and then returning "fuliginous vapors" from the tissues back to the heart and lungs to be breathed out into the air.

The remaining venous blood from the liver flowed to the tissues in the reverse direction through the veins, directly providing nourishment, the "natural spirits," in addition to the "vital spirits" provided by the arteries. Some believed that the venous blood traveled only in the outward direction to the tissues, though other variations of the theory had blood ebbing to and fro in the veins in a manner similar to that in the arteries.

Thus, the Galenic system provided for transfer of nourishment, heat, and "pneuma" to the tissues, so that most of the mystery of how food and air sustained the living body was resolved. Galen had come to these conclusions because he could not demonstrate direct connections between the arteries and the veins either in the lungs or in the peripheral tissues. Yet, strangely, his thesis required blood to flow from the right ventricle to the left ventricle through porosities in the interventricular septum of the heart. He thought that he had observed such porosities, though perhaps what he saw were instead the non-penetrating spaces among the intraventricular trabeculae.

Thus, the science of the circulatory system was a morass of almost mystical musings. Even so, it is not correct to believe that before Harvey there were no significant changes in medical science affecting this area. Many anatomists, in particular, were adding intricate structural detail to our knowledge of gross anatomy, and writing books and publishing anatomical drawings that made this detail available to all. The most famous of these anatomists was Vesalius (1514–1564) who preceded Harvey by three-quarters of a century. Equally learned and adding much more to Vesalius's anatomy was his pupil Fabricus (1536–1619). Fabricus was one of Harvey's teachers at Padua, and probably the person who had the single greatest influence on Harvey's subsequent career. Even Leonardo da Vinci (1452–1519), the great scientist-artist of the fifteenth and early sixteenth centuries, who preceded Vesalius by two generations and Harvey by a full century, had left intricate drawings of many structures of the body, including very detailed drawings of the heart valves.

Yet, despite all the advances in the study of anatomy, most

scholars adapted their anatomical thought to fit with Galen's explanation of the physiology of the heart and blood vessels. Still, a few chinks in the Galenic armour were beginning to appear. For instance, Vesalius stated that he had not been able to find the Galen-postulated "porosities" in the interventricular septum of the heart. But he was careful not to state that they did not exist, thus not challenging directly the Galenic scheme. In addition, when Fabricus described the venous valves, he fitted their function to Galenic principles by stating that their purpose was only to delay the peripheral flow of blood in the veins, not to prevent it. In other words, Fabricus's idea of the venous valves was simply that they provided resistance to peripherally-directed flow of venous blood, thereby promoting more appropriate distribution of blood to the different tissues.

A few anatomists were more adventurous and were willing to state flatly that there were no interventricular porosities between the right and left ventricles through which blood could flow. The only other way in which blood could pass from the right ventricle to the left heart and aorta would therefore have to be by way of the lungs. This idea was first expressed in writing by M. Servetus in 1553, but was embedded in a fanatical religious treatise that in its entirety was found by the Calvinist church to be heretical. As a result, only a few months after the printing of his book, Servetus was burned at the stake along with all the copies of the book that could be found. At about the same time, Realdus Columbus (1516–1559) was beginning also to state definitively the non-existence of porosities in the interventricular septum, and he proposed that blood flowed from the right heart through a pulmonary circulation and thence into the left heart (published posthumously in 1560). A pupil-colleague of Columbus, Andreas Caesalpinus (1524–1603), further popularized the discoveries and thoughts of Columbus and added others of his own during the 44 years that he lived after the death of Columbus.

The evidence for blood flow through the pulmonary circulation, though expressed by these authors in different ways, was mainly threefold. (1) There were no openings through the interventricular septum by which blood could go directly from the right ventricle into the left ventricle. (2) The pulmonary artery was filled with blood and not with air, and the pulmonary venous blood also had characteristics different from the blood in the vena cava because of addition of air in the lungs, not in the heart. (3) The mitral valve allowed blood to flow only unidirectionally from the lungs into the left ventricle without any flow in the backward direction to deliver to the lungs the arterial "fuliginous vapors" of Galen. Thus, the arguments of all these anatomists served rather to prove the lack of logic of the Galenic scheme than to give positive proof of blood flow through the lungs. Some of the other very famous anatomists of the day, including especially Fallopius (1523–1562), for whom the fallopian tubes are named, continued to ridicule the idea of blood flowing from the right heart to the left heart by way of the lungs. Thus was the state of knowledge of the circulation when Harvey studied medicine, and thus it remained for another quarter century until Harvey published *de Motu Cordis* in 1628.

Harvey's Achievement

I do not wish to detract from Harvey's achievement by pretelling the arguments, experiments, and observations presented in his book. Mainly, I will allow the reader to judge these for him- or herself from Harvey's own writing. However, the essence of Harvey's achievement was that he brought forth in one book massive amounts of experimental evidence, including human clinical observation, observation on multiple forms of lower animals, and for the first time significant advances in quantitative thinking, logic, and even physiological measurement, all this evidence supporting from multiple different directions the inescapable conclusion that the heart is basically a muscular pump, pumping large quantities of blood in only one direction in a continuous circuit again and again around the vascular system. Some of the special points of his argument included:

(1) absolute denial of any porosities through the interventricular septum between the right ventricle and the left ventricle;

(2) demonstration of total competence of the heart valves, so that any compressive action of the heart whatsoever would of necessity cause the blood to flow only in the forward direction as dictated by the valves;

(3) quantitative calculations, based on heart rate and degree of ventricular wall excursion, of the minimum amount of blood pumped by the heart, showing this minimum to be so vast that it could not possibly be contributed by continuous liver concoction of new blood as required by the Galenic scheme;

(4) demonstration of total competence of the venous valves, denying that these could function merely as resistances in the Fabricus sense to delay peripherally-directed blood flow in the veins;

(5) demonstration that when a vein is squeezed empty and then compressed peripherally but not centrally, the emptied vein will not fill from its central connection because valves block any backflow; yet, when the peripheral compression is released the vein fills instantly because the peripheral valves open in the central direction; furthermore the rapidity with which the vein fills attests to a rate of blood flow several hundred times as great as the dribbling flow allowed by the Galenic schemes;

(6) observation that when an animal is bled to death by opening an artery, not only are the left heart and arteries emptied of blood but also the veins as well;

(7) likewise, when an animal is bled to death by opening a vein, the left heart and all the arteries are emptied of blood, the same as occurs when bleeding to death through the arteries;

(8) when a vein is severed but is occluded peripherally, the animal bleeds hardly at all; when the severed vein is occluded centrally but not peripherally, blood loss is rapid and can readily lead to death;

(9) when the root of the aorta is clamped in a living open-chested animal, all chambers of the heart fill within seconds to the bursting point—quantitatively, this effect could occur only with extremely rapid unidirectional flow of blood into the heart chambers from the venous reservoirs, the only direction allowed by the venous valves and heart valves; and

(10) if a small puncture wound is made in the left ventricle, blood is ejected under great force from the wound with each beat of the heart.

Again and again, quantification played a major role in Harvey's thinking. And Harvey was exceedingly inventive in devising new experiments and searching for new observations that would tell the truth about blood flow in the circulatory system. Often, this truth could not be observed in studies on human beings nor even by vivisection in large mammals. Therefore, he learned still much in addition from observations in lower forms of animals, a scientific habit inherited partly from his teacher Fabricus, who was also an outstanding comparative anatomist. To give an example, Harvey observed carefully the beating hearts of cold blooded animals in which the heart rate was slow enough that the sequence of contraction, beginning in the atria and followed by contraction of the ventricles, was unmistakable—in contrast, this sequence was not easily apparent from observing the dog's heart, which beat too rapidly for one to separate the sequential events. Also, using a magnifying glass, Harvey even studied a type of transparent shrimp that he found in the Thames estuary, observing the beating heart without disturbing its natural function. Finally, he observed wounded or sick human beings and larger mammals in the last throes of life when the heart beat slowed enough that the pumping action was then unmistakable.

Thus, from almost every direction imaginable within the limits of the scientific technology of the day, Harvey marshaled his arguments. Regardless whence the arguments stemmed, all of them led to the undeniable conclusion not only that blood circulates from arteries to veins throughout the body, but also that the quantity circulating each hour and each day is enormous in comparison with that previously believed.

It is true, as many historians have pointed out, that Harvey's estimates of the cardiac output were much lower than present-day measurements. Yet, if one will study carefully Harvey's own words, it will be evident that he took great pains to impress upon the reader that he was using absolute minimum estimations. He did this so that there could be no room for doubt that the amount of blood flowing in the circulation had to be far greater than could possibly be accounted for by the oozing amounts of flow allowed in the Galenic scheme.

One final word on Harvey's achievement. Certainly, at least some other persons of Harvey's time and before had considered the concept that blood flows in a circuit through the body. In fact, the writings of Hippocrates, Plato, and Aristotle all speak of a circular flow of blood, though never explained in the sense meant by Harvey; even Shakespeare, writing decades before Harvey's book, referred to "rivers of flowing blood" in the body. Furthermore, it is almost inconceivable that Servetus, Columbus, and Caesalpinus, when they proposed the flow of blood through the pulmonary circulation, would not also have at least imagined a generalized scheme of blood flow by way of a circuit throughout the entire body. Even John Hunter, the great English surgeon of the 1700s, pointed out that, once Realdus Columbus and the others a half century before Harvey had proposed blood flow through the lungs, it was but a small step to complete the circuit concept of flow throughout the entire body.

Thus, it was not Harvey's discovery of the circuit flow of blood that was so remarkable, for undoubtedly others were considering this at least as a possibility. Harvey's achievement, instead, was the vast amount of solid quantitative evidence that he collected into one living treatise, evidence so thorough and convincing that the conclusions were inescapable—evidence so compelling that it literally demolished within one generation fourteen centuries of Galenic thought.

When Harvey had completed his reconstruction of the circulatory scheme, virtually all the elements of modern circulatory physiology were present, for he spoke of the pumping volume of the heart (cardiac output); the force, the impelling power, the turgor associated with heart contraction and arterial pulsations (pressure); and the resistance to the movement of blood in the vessels and especially through the tissues. He spoke of selective ventricular hypertrophy under the respective loads of the two sides of the heart, and thickening of the arterial walls in comparison to the veins because of the greater force that they must endure. He recounted the control capabilities of the circulation, that the cardiac output varies according to the needs of the body—according to temperament, age, sleep, rest, and food—and that exercise and even affections of the mind can greatly increase the cardiac output. And he noted that following the onset of hemorrhage one sees immediate control reactions that limit the degree of hemorrhage, as well as other reactions occurring within minutes to give "vitality" back to the pumping action of the heart and flow of blood. He even recognized the concept of *vis a tergo*, a concept not too easily grasped by most modern circulatory physiologists, when he wrote that in the veins "the blood is thus more disposed to move from the circumference to the centre," and therefore an impeller (the heart) is required to return it continually to the periphery.

How much more have we added to this scheme in the three and a half centuries since Harvey's time?

The Missing Link in Harvey's Scheme of the Circulation

The great missing link in Harvey's scheme of the circulation was lack of visual proof that either blood capillaries or any other connections exist between the arteries and the veins. In reality, this was not a serious detriment to Harvey's arguments, for he pointed out very rightly that water percolates through the earth even though one cannot see the channels, that urine flows through the kidneys without channels, and absorbates from the gut pass through the liver. Furthermore, his description of blood flow patterns in the body provided such firm evidence of functional flow from the arteries to the veins that no other conclusion could be reached except that blood in some way percolates through the tissues, either through minute vessels or through open channels or pores too small to be seen.

Yet the logical mind always wishes to close the last missing link. Therefore, absence of anatomical proof of blood capillaries or other channels from the arteries to the veins gave solace for several more decades to many anatomists and physiologists who still wished to adhere to the Galenic scheme of blood distribution.

Available to Harvey was a magnifying glass, but not a microscope that would allow him to see the capillaries. Yet, in 1661, only four years after Harvey's death, Marcello Malpighi (1628–1694), one of the earliest to use the microscope to study tissues, published two letters describing anatomically the capillaries of the lung as well as visual observation of blood flow in these capillaries. Indeed, it was Malpighi's desire to affirm Harvey's scheme of blood flow that led him to his studies. This was 45 years after Harvey first proposed the circulation of blood in his

Lumleian lectures in 1616, and 33 years after publication of his book in 1628. The missing link had been demonstrated.

The Period of Controversy Surrounding Harvey's Concepts, and the Test of His Spirit

When Harvey published *de Motu Cordis* in 1628, he knew in advance that his new ideas on the circular motion of blood in the body would cause consternation. In his book he expressed this fear by stating that the concept "is of so novel and unheard-of character, that I fear not only injury to myself from the envy of a few, but I tremble lest I have mankind at large as enemies, so much doth wont and custom, that become as another nature, and doctrine once sown and that hath struck deep root, and respect for antiquity influence all men."

True enough, Harvey did have his detractors, some of whom rose to the attack almost immediately. In fact, soon after Harvey's book was published, James Primrose wrote an entire book specifically to attack Harvey's ideas, stating that his own book had taken only "fourteen days" to write. It is clear that this attack was one of emotion, based exactly on Harvey's own observation that "respect for antiquity" influences all men.

But Harvey had also written in his book, "My hope is in the love of truth and in the integrity of intelligence."

Harvey's main response to his critics was silence, except that he did continue teaching without apology the circular motion of the blood in his oft-repeated anatomical lectures at the Royal College of Physicians. In addition, he demonstrated experiments on multiple occasions, sometimes even to King Charles and others of the court. In fact, Charles himself once joined Harvey in investigating the motion of the human heart through a chronic open wound in a man's chest into which Harvey and Charles could pass their fingers and actually feel the heart beating.

Even so, many of the prominent anatomists of the day, principally those on the Continent but even some who were closely associated with Harvey personally, simply ignored Harvey's teachings. For instance, in the anatomy books of two fellow Englishmen—Thomas Winston, whose book was published in 1659, 31 years after Harvey's book on the circulation, and Alexander Reed, whose book was published in multiple editions between 1634 and 1658—Harvey's concept of the circular motion of blood through the body was not given credence.

To only one critic did Harvey ever make a major response: in 1649, 21 years after his book was published, he wrote two long letters which are reprinted in this volume to Jean Riolan, a Regius Professor in Paris and Dean of the Faculty of Medicine. Riolan had written a book in 1648, in which he criticized several aspects of Harvey's concepts. Riolan accepted circular motion of blood in the major arteries and veins but not in some of the smaller vessels, especially in the portal system, still arguing for the older concept of back and forth blood movement in these vessels to transfer nutrients in the peripheral direction and tissue waste in the central direction. In Harvey's first letter he merely countered Riolan's own arguments with experimental observations that he, Harvey, had made during his life's work. In his second letter, he added new thoughts and experiments that gave new substance to the original observations in his book. But, most important, Harvey lectured Riolan on the importance of experimental observation in contrast to repetition of unproved theory.

Yet, despite Harvey's usual avoidance of open controversy, the turmoil caused by his concepts was a trial to him for the remainder of his life. The depths of his concern are best understood by reading Harvey's own words in the preamble of his second letter to Riolan:

It is now many years, most learned Riolanus, since, with the aid of the press, I published a portion of my work. But scarce a day, scarce an hour, has passed since the birth-day of the Circulation of the blood, that I have not heard something for good or for evil said of this my discovery. Some abuse it as a feeble infant, and yet unworthy to have seen the light; others, again, think the bantling deserves to be cherished and cared for; these oppose it with much ado, those patronize it with abundant commendation; one party holds that I have completely demonstrated the circulation of the blood by experiment, observation, and ocular inspection, against all force and array of argument; another thinks it scarcely yet sufficiently illustrated—not yet cleared of all objections. There are some, too, who say that I have shown a vainglorious love of vivisections, and who scoff at and deride the introduction of frogs and serpents, flies, and others of the lower animals upon the scene, as a piece of puerile levity, not even refraining from opprobrious epithets.

To return evil speaking with evil speaking, however, I hold to be unworthy in a philosopher and searcher after truth; I believe that I shall do better and more advisedly if I meet so many indications of ill breeding with the light of faithful and conclusive observation. It cannot be helped that dogs bark and vomit their foul stomachs, or that cynics should be numbered among philosophers; but care can be taken that they do not bite or inoculate their mad humours, or with their dogs' teeth gnaw the bones and foundations of truth.

Again, in 1650 when Harvey's friend George Ent urged him to publish his quarter-of-a-century work on the *Generation of Animals*, Harvey at first demurred and gave as his reasons:

And would you be the man who should recommend me to quit the peaceful haven, where I now pass my life, and launch again upon the faithless sea? You know full well what a storm my former lucubrations raised. Much better is it oftentimes to grow wise at home and in private, than by publishing what you have amassed with infinite labour, to stir up tempests that may rob you of peace and quiet for the rest of your days.

These reactions of the medical world in Harvey's day are not very surprising, for modern day medical scientists have changed very little. Suppose, for instance, that you, a prominent physician or anatomist, have spent your life studying a medical subject, and at last have become thoroughly satisfied that you know all there is to know in your field; then someone comes along with a completely new view that explodes your lifetime's work. Imagine your emotions. Those were the reactions of many of Harvey's contemporaries; the medical scientists who did in fact know the current doctrines most thoroughly were Harvey's greatest critics. Indeed, it was said that Harvey failed to convince any medical scientist who was already past the age of 40. But others who knew little were often ready to accept Harvey's views with only mild convincing, including even his special benefactor Charles I. The same psychology of acceptance or rejection of revolutionary thoughts is true today. Those who have much to lose quite understandably vent their emotions; those who can look more impartially from a distance with a fresh point of view are often much more susceptible to new arguments.

Yet, one cannot totally deprecate the human mind's natural resistance to change, for we in science all experience vast numbers of exorbitant claims that later prove to be totally invalid.

Therefore, it is almost second nature to resist new and disturbing concepts.

I must confess that I, personally, have had many occasions to wish for much more open-mindedness among my scientific peers even though I respect and understand resistance to new ideas. Once, early in my career, I proposed that many of the slowly cycling waves in blood pressure recordings were caused by oscillation of the baroreceptor pressure control mechanism. I felt that I had marshaled enough arguments to prove this beyond doubt; indeed, subsequent evidence from many corners of the world now seems to have established the concept as truth. But the editorial reviewer of my paper used the expression "poppycock" to describe what he thought of the idea, which was truly devastating to a young researcher. I wondered whether physiological research was a field worth my life's work.

In subsequent years, I and my colleagues have collected what we considered to be strong evidence for other new concepts some of which require significant changes in quantitative understanding of circulatory physiology. Among these have been: (1) a concept that, except when the heart fails, the long-term cardiac output is controlled almost entirely by the summation of local blood flow controls in the tissues and not by the heart itself; and (2) a concept that long-term arterial pressure control is quite different from short-term control, that long-term control is based almost entirely on the body's salt and water balance and the role of the kidneys in this.

Each of these concepts has trod heavily on long-time, deeply held beliefs, such beliefs as, "It is the heart that pumps the blood; therefore, it is clear that the heart and nervous control of heart activity together are the principal controllers of cardiac output," and, "Virtually all persons who have hypertension have high total peripheral resistance; therefore, it is fundamental that arterial pressure is controlled by blood vessels that alter total peripheral resistance, not by the kidneys and salt and water balance."

These types of elemental and historical thinking are powerful adversaries. Therefore, it is not surprising that concepts which are new or different, but which each of us might construe to be our most important achievements, virtually always evoke the same counter-responses as those experienced by Harvey: the highest of praise from some, but the ultimate of deprecation from others. And, most chilling of all is the interminable slowness of acceptance of new ideas even when unopposed. Thus, it is easy to understand why a scientist often experiences melancholy, as did Harvey, for want of open minds.

Harvey's Luck of the Genius

There are many geniuses in science who never have the luck to make a great discovery. And many other scientists have luck but unfortunately do not have the genius to succeed. In Harvey's studies of the circulation, the two were juxtaposed. From what little evidence is available, Harvey's intellect already clearly showed even during his period of education, especially so in his medical education in Padua, Italy, where he completed the entire medical course in only two years despite stringencies of learning a new language, yet graduating with honors. As further evidence of his scholarship, his published writings are punctuated with abundant references to the world of the then-current medical literature as well as to the work of the ancients, displaying an especially profound knowledge of the works of Aristotle and Galen. Thus, his was a prepared mind.

And, too, Harvey was born not in the city but in a farming community where it is to be expected that he would know the ways of nature.

Then, there was the luck to be born in a family never to be wanting in the necessities of life, with fully adequate means to provide all the education that Harvey required. Perhaps it was also luck that he married the daughter of a very prominent physician, a physician to both Elizabeth and James. Indeed, his father-in-law did attempt to promote Harvey's medical career, though it is equally true that there is no evidence that this help mattered. Then there was another element of chance—perhaps this time it was negative luck—for his marriage was barren of children, and Harvey spoke of "solace in his work," suggesting that his work was truly his life.

But undoubtedly his greatest luck of all was the special juncture in history in which he found himself. The most important of all concepts of the circulation was still to be discovered and proved, the circulation of the blood itself. The needed methodology and background information were at precisely that time beginning to coalesce so that someone somewhere with appropriate genius and love of truth and time to give to the work should be bound to make the great discovery that was Harvey's.

If Harvey had had only his genius and not his luck as well, would his greatness have been the same that we acclaim today? Let us answer this indirectly. Most of us forget that Harvey had other scientific interests besides the circulation of the blood. In fact, his most prodigious work was not his book on the circulation but instead his book on reproduction entitled *Exercitationes de Generatione Animalium*, first published in 1651 and also reprinted in its English translation in this volume. Into this book went as much genius as into *de Motu Cordis*. Indeed, it was a much longer book, developed from notes and research that spanned a quarter of a century. Harvey's great purpose in this book was to explain the origin of life itself, which was an even more laudable goal than his earlier goal to prove the circulation of the blood. But all the elements required for great success did not come together for these studies. Most importantly, the technology was not available to discover the initial stages of conception, which was the crucial question to be answered. Therefore, the basic explanation of the generation of life escaped Harvey. By the time of publication of this book, Harvey was 73 years old. The earliest microscope had been invented 50 years before that time, but had rarely as yet been used in medicine, and there is no evidence that Harvey had become familiar with its use. Furthermore, the mammalian ovum, because it is only a speck in a wide expanse of uterine fluid, has always been very elusive and difficult to find even with the microscope. Therefore, it was not until 200 years later that the ovum released from the ovary was eventually discovered to be the focal point for the origin of the fetus. Thus, for this prodigious work of Harvey's, his genius was as much at work as it had been for *de Motu Cordis*, but the luck of coalescence of all the elements required for great achievement was not at hand.

When a Scientist Challenges the Insolvable

Harvey's book on the *Generation of Animals* was almost five times as long as *de Motu Cordis*. Yet its place in history will never be the scientific landmark achieved by *de Motu Cordis*, for it failed in its goal. Its historical importance is as a lasting monument to the mind of any great scientist who challenges an unknown that is insolvable. Yet, one cannot conceive of a more noble quest than to explain the origin of life. It was this same quest that had also dominated much of Aristotle's thoughtful energy; and hardly any progress had come from the efforts of a myriad of other scientists on the same topic during the 2000 years between the lives of Aristotle and of Harvey.

Harvey's approach was to let his mind roam endlessly and obsessively through any and all knowledge even remotely related to animal reproduction, knowledge that was firm and unchallengeable from scientific history or from colloquial understanding of the processes involved. And his own scientific nature drove him to clear and precise experimental observations, beginning with detailed and intricate characterization of the development of the chick from the fertilized egg, followed by painstaking serial dissections and description of each stage of gestation in the doe, and finally by pathological studies in the human female.

Harvey considered incessantly the act of procreation between the cock and hen, and the buck and doe, and the male and female of the human species. And he mulled over the role of sexual desire as, or as not, a necessary accompaniment to successful fertilization. Indeed, he seemed to have much more information on this subject than would have been expected of a circumspect scientist, stating: "Even during the season of jocund masking in Venus's domains, male animals in general are depressed by intercourse, and become submissive and pusillanimous, as if reminded that in imparting life to others, they were contributing to their own destruction." And observing about the human female, "although some of warmer temperament shed a fluid in the sexual embrace, still that this is fruitful semen, or is a necessary requisite to conception, I do not believe."

Yet, there always remained a gaping, unexplained hiatus between the act of copulation and the first, slightest physical evidence of a newly developed being—a period of five days from the beginning of incubation of the egg until the slightest speck of an embryo could be seen even with a magnifying glass; and a minimum period of six to eight weeks after fertilization of the doe before even a trace of a conceptus could be found in the uterus.

Nor could Harvey find any evidence that the female testes (the ovaries) played any role in reproduction, observing that "the female testicles, as they are called, whether they be examined before or after intercourse, neither swell nor vary from their usual condition; they show no trace of being of the slightest use either in the business of intercourse or in that of generation."

Nor could he find a material role for semen in fertilization, stating: "And repeated examination led me to the conclusion that none of the semen whatsoever reached this seat [the seat of fertilization in the cavity of the uterus]." Also: "I therefore regard it as demonstrated that after fertile intercourse among viviparous as well as oviparous animals, there are no remains in the uterus either of the male or female emitted in the act, nothing produced by any mixture of these two fluids..."

Therefore, whence came the embryo? Harvey could only hypothesize that "the woman, after contact with the spermatic fluid in coitu, seems to receive influence, and to become fecundated without the co-operation of any sensible corporal agent, in the same way as iron touched by the magnet is endowed with its powers and can attract other iron to itself. When this virtue is once received the woman exercises a plastic power of generation..."

Thus, Harvey imagined that there resided in woman a "vital principle," always there but set to the motion of generating a new being only in response to the act of the male. This vital principle was passed from mother to daughter, for, as Harvey philosophized, "The eternity of things is connected with the reciprocal interchange of generation and decay; and as the sun, now in the east and then in the west, completes the measure of time by ceaseless revolutions, so are the fleeting things of mortal existence made eternal through incessant change, and kinds and species are perpetuated though individuals die."

Yet, since the embryo begins only in a prescribed point in the woman's body and always begins as an isolated speck, then it follows that the woman's vital principle first gives rise to "a particular genital particle, in virtue of which, as from a beginning all the other parts proceed... which is the author and original of sense and motion, and every manifestation of life."

But what was this primary vital principle, the thread of life? Harvey believed, "that the privilege of priority belongs to the blood alone; the blood being that which is first seen of the newly engendered being—I have indeed ascertained by numerous experiments—that the blood is the element of the body in which, so long as the vital heat has not entirely departed, the power of returning to life is continued."

Harvey was wrong, but he was also partly right. There *is* a thread of life passed successively from generation to generation, but through the primordial genital epithelium, not the blood. There *is* a primordial particle, the fertilized ovum, from which all other parts of the generated being are engendered as night follows day. And there *is* that magic influence of the male semen to set into motion the female vital principle to generate the baby.

But so much of this occurs below the visual minimum of the naked eye that Harvey's speculative role of blood to replace the germinal epithelium is to be excused. After all, Harvey had proved to virtually everyone of reason that the blood circulates through the body even though he had never seen the capillaries!

Harvey's Place in History

There is no doubt that the greatest discovery ever in the science of circulatory physiology was the discovery that blood is pumped in a circuitous manner through the body.

Would this discovery have come about in a few years without Harvey? The answer is: undoubtedly it would have. In fact, only 33 years after publication of Harvey's book Marcello Malpighi was able to see with his crude microscope the actual flow of blood in capillaries of the lungs. Also, almost three-quarters of a century before the publication of Harvey's book, Servetus, Columbus, and Caesalpinus had all put forth strong logical evidence for blood flow through the lungs from the right heart to the left heart.

Yet, it was Harvey alone who synthesized these many new tides of thinking into a total picture of circulatory function, not dwelling on a single segment of the circulation but discussing it in the whole, both giving evidence that the heart does indeed pump blood, and adding quantification to the amounts of blood pumped, amounts far greater than could fit with any of the previous theories—also giving evidence for equally large amounts of blood flow through the porosities of the tissues, which Harvey called *porositates carnis*, and which were the yet unseen tissue capillaries that by force of Harvey's logic had to exist.

Thus, in this beginning period of new ideas about the function of the circulation, the totality of Harvey's efforts stood out conspicuously above those of all others. This is what was required to break through the entrenched thought of antiquity that began in Aristotelian times almost 400 years before the birth of Christ and extended for 2000 years, first through the age of Galen, then through the entire period of the Middle Ages, and even surviving the first 100 years of the Renaissance until the time of Harvey.

The date 1628, when Harvey's book on the circulation of blood appeared, truly marks the Renaissance for circulatory science, leading during the next generation to thorough devastation of the Galenic scheme that blood ebbs forth and backward in the arteries and veins, substituting forever thereafter the continuous circulation of the blood around the body.

If we add a few other basic essentials to Harvey's concept of circulatory function, we have today's physiology of the circulation. For instance, it was up to Ludwig, Starling, and Landis to explain and quantify the principles of capillary exchange, which told us how it was possible for blood to remain in the circulatory system without leaking into the tissues. With Cannon, Dale, and Heymans came nervous and endocrine control of the heart and circulation. And more recently, a horde of quantitative physiologists, representing a coalescence of physiology, engineering, physics, and chemistry, have led to at least speculative understanding of the systems aspects of overall circulatory regulation—regulation of local tissue blood flow, regulation of cardiac output, regulation of arterial pressure, and regulation of the body fluid volumes.

All the newer knowledge of the circulation simply adds to Harvey's own fundamental concept that the circulation system is to serve the body—that every small structure and every slightest function of the circulation has a purpose. For Harvey frequently alluded to the essentiality of nature's purpose by stating at multiple points in his text, "for nature, doing nothing in vain," "nature, ever perfect and divine, doing nothing in vain," "as perfect nature does nothing in vain."

NOTE

*This account of Harvey's work and times is a condensation from several detailed books and articles written by medical historians who have spent years studying Harvey and his work. Because of the large number of separate facts presented in this condensation, and because most of the facts have come from several different ones of the sources, it has not been practical to reference each separately. Instead, at the end of this introductory chapter is a concise *Additional Reading List* of books and articles that cover thoroughly the life of Harvey, his achievements, and his place in medical history.

ADDITIONAL READING LIST

Leake, Chauncey D. Translation of William Harvey's *Anatomical Studies on the Motion of the Heart and Blood*, with extensive annotation and prefatorial comments. Fourth edition, 150 pp. Springfield, Ill.: Charles C. Thomas, 1958.

O'Malley, C. D., Poynter, F. N. L., and Russel, K. F. *William Harvey—Lectures on the Whole of Anatomy*, a translation with extensive annotation. 239 pp. Berkeley: University of California Press, 1961.

Whitteridge, Gweneth. *The Anatomical Lectures of William Harvey*, a translation with extensive annotation and introductory material. 504 pp. London: E. & S. Livingstone Ltd.

Keynes, Geoffrey. *The Life of William Harvey*. 483 pp. Oxford: Oxford University Press, 1966.

Pagel, Walter. *William Harvey's Biological Ideas, Selected Aspects and Historical Background*. 394 pp. Basel/New York: S. Karger AG, 1967.

Whitteridge, Gweneth. *William Harvey and the Circulation of the Blood*. 269 pp. New York: American Elsevier Inc., 1971.

Whitteridge, Gweneth. "William Harvey—The Man and His Work." Pp. 317–34 in C. J. Dickinson and J. Marks, eds., *Developments in Cardiovascular Medicine*, to celebrate the 400th anniversary of the birth of William Harvey Lancaster.: MTP Press Limited, 1978.

THE

SYDENHAM SOCIETY

INSTITUTED

MDCCCXLIII

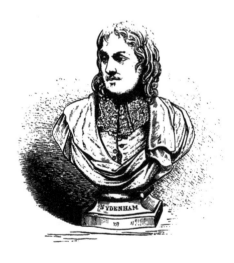

LONDON

MDCCCXLVII.

THE WORKS

OF

WILLIAM HARVEY, M.D.

PHYSICIAN TO THE KING, PROFESSOR OF ANATOMY AND SURGERY
TO THE COLLEGE OF PHYSICIANS

TRANSLATED FROM THE LATIN

WITH

A LIFE OF THE AUTHOR

BY

ROBERT WILLIS, M.D.

MEMBER OF THE ROYAL COLLEGES OF PHYSICIANS AND SURGEONS OF ENGLAND,
CORRESPONDING MEMBER OF THE ROYAL ACADEMY OF SCIENCES OF
GÖTTINGEN, OF THE IMPERIAL SOCIETY OF PHYSICIANS
AND SURGEONS OF VIENNA, AND OF THE
NATIONAL INSTITUTE OF AMERICA,
ETC. ETC.

LONDON

PRINTED FOR THE SYDENHAM SOCIETY

MDCCCXLVII.

JOHNSON REPRINT CORPORATION

New York and London

1965

First reprinting, 1965, Johnson Reprint Corporation

PREFACE.

When, at the instance of the governing body of the Sydenham Society, I undertook to edit the Works of the immortal Discoverer of the Circulation of the Blood, in English, I believed that the chief of these Works were already extant in our language, in such a shape as would make little more from an editor necessary than a careful revision of the text. I had unwarily adopted the idea, very gratuitously originated by Aubrey, that Harvey was what is called an indifferent scholar, and that the English versions of his writings were the proper originals, the Latin versions the translations. Having access to the handsome edition of Harvey's Works in Latin, revised by Drs. Lawrence and Mark Akenside, and published by the College of Physicians in 1766, I had always referred to that when the course of my studies led me to consult Harvey. Of the English versions, or any other edition, I knew little or nothing. On proceeding to my new duty of English editor, however, I immediately saw that the masterwork of Harvey on the MOTIONS of the HEART and BLOOD, far from having the character of an originally English writing, must have been rendered into English by one but little conversant with the subject, that it was both extremely rebutting in point of style and full of egregious errors, and that nothing short of an entirely new translation could do justice to this admirable treatise, or secure for it, at the present day, the attention it deserved. Full of zeal, and making of my task a labour of love, I had soon completed a new translation of the Exercises on the Heart and Blood, with equal pleasure and profit to myself.

The work on GENERATION came next under review. ✱The English version of this I had heard it positively asserted was the original, was Harvey's own; here therefore my business of editor would properly begin. But I had not gone through a couple of pages of the text, before difficulties like those already experienced met me again. That the statement above referred to was erroneous, speedily became apparent; and a little inquiry enabled me to discover that the English version of the Exercises on Generation was the work of a physician named Llewellen. Though not incorrect generally, there was, nevertheless, a great deal that I wished had been otherwise rendered; and then the scientific and professional language of two centuries back looked strangely when examined by the eye, and had an unusual sound when tried upon the ear. Only anxious to present to my brethren in the most appropriate and attractive form possible, the writings of him who had still met me in his Works and with his contemplative look in his Portrait as a kind of divinity in medicine, I even girded myself up for the long and laborious enterprise of translating anew into our mother tongue the work on Generation, and at length achieved my task, not without difficulty.

The short paper on the ANATOMY of THOMAS PARR appears in the Philosophical Transactions in English; but it stands there as a translation; and having now translated so much myself, I even thought it would be well to translate that also, and so it was achieved.

The LETTERS, though frequently quoted, have never appeared in English before. They will be found both highly interesting and important. To render them was a light and pleasant task. — In a word, the English reader is now presented with an entirely new translation of the writings of William Harvey; everything of our illustrious countryman worthy of publication that has come down to us, being here included.[1]

The reader will perceive that I have abstained from annotation and commentary in the course of my labour. The purpose of the Council of the Sydenham Society, as I understood it, was to give the Works of William Harvey in English now, as he himself gave them in Latin two centuries ago. Entirely approving of this intention, I felt that anything like corrections of statements and opinions, which could so readily have been made under the lights of modern physiology, would have been impertinencies, and I therefore abstained from them. To have carried out and completed the history of Harvey's two grand subjects, would also have been easy; but

---

[1] A certain MS. of Harvey's, frequently referred to as bearing the date of 1616, and containing the heads of his first course of Lectures at the College of Physicians on the Heart and Blood, is not now in existence, or at all events is not now to be found. At the present time there are only two MSS. at the British Museum which bear Harvey's name. Of these, one contains notes on the Muscles, Vessels, and Nerves, and on the Locomotion of Animals ; the other may be characterized as a book of Receipts or Prescriptions, and though partly the work of a contemporary, contains notes of cases that occurred after Harvey's death. The former MS. is as certainly in Harvey's handwriting as the latter is not. In Dr. Lawrence's* time there must have been a third MS. entitled 'De Anatomia Universa,' and it was here, in the index viz. which referred to the principal facts in the anatomy of the heart and of the circulation of the blood, that the dates April 16, 17, 18, an. 1616, were encountered. Mr. Pettigrew (Portrait Gallery, vol. iv, Harvey, p. 8), with the assistance of Sir Fred. Madden, made search for this MS. a few years ago, but failed to meet with it. A renewed search for this important document has been attended with no better success.

---

* Vide his Life of Harvey, prefixed to the edition by the College of Physicians p. xxxi.

this would have been almost as obviously out of place as commentary, and the inclination towards such an agreeable undertaking was also resisted.

It appeared, nevertheless, that the Works of our great physiological discoverer might be advantageously prefaced by some account of his Life and Writings. One great motive with me, indeed, for undertaking the office of Editor of the Works of Harvey was, that I might thus find a fitting opportunity for writing his life, a task which, in other circumstances than those that now surround me, it had still been a cherished purpose with me to perform. The Life of Harvey, by one who had maintained a familiarity with anatomy and physiology, had always seemed to me a desideratum in our medical literature.

This portion of my work I have only achieved with an effort, and at something like disadvantage. Incessantly engaged by night and by day in the laborious and responsible duties of a country practice, enjoying nothing of learned leisure, but snatching from the hours that should rightfully be given to rest, the time that was necessary to composition, remote too from means of information which I must nevertheless send for and consult—for I could not draw entirely upon memory and old recollections of Harvey, I have been much longer about this work than its length might indicate. In spite of many disadvantages, however, I trust it will be found that I have included everything of moment in my narrative of the life of Harvey; that I have set his claims to the whole and sole merit of the discovery of the Circulation in a new and clearer light than they have yet been seen; and that I have done more than any preceding biographer in exhibiting his moral nature; for truly he was as noble in nature as he was intellectually great.

The Wills of great men have always been looked on as calculated to throw light on the character of their authors; and I have, therefore, great pleasure in presenting to the medical world, for the first time, the Will of William Harvey.

It only remains for me, in conclusion, to explain and to apologise for the long delay that has taken place in the appearance of this volume. The work was, in fact, nearly three-fourths done more than a year ago; but with the change made in my sphere of action about that time, all aptitude for literary labour seemed to forsake me,—the bow, to use a common metaphor, became unbent, and for a while resisted every effort to string it anew; and, then, when restrung at length, how constantly was I hindered in my purpose to use it! With this brief explanation, which will be so well appreciated by the great majority of my fellow members of the Sydenham Society, I confidently throw myself on their kind consideration, and pray them to pardon the delay that has occurred.

R. WILLIS.

BARNES, SURREY;
Feb. 15*th*, 1847.

TABLE OF CONTENTS.

AN ANATOMICAL DISQUISITION ON THE MOTION OF THE HEART AND BLOOD IN ANIMALS.

ANATOMICAL EXERCISES ON THE GENERATION OF ANIMALS; TO
WHICH ARE ADDED, ESSAYS ON PARTURITION; ON THE MEM-
BRANES, AND FLUIDS OF THE UTERUS; AND ON CONCEPTION.

ON ANIMAL GENERATION.

	PAGE
Wherefore we begin with the history of the hen's egg	169
Of the seat of generation	171
Of the upper part of the hen's uterus, or the ovary	172
Of the infundibulum	179
Of the external portion of the uterus of the common fowl	180
Of the uterus of the fowl	190
Of the abdomen of the common fowl and of other birds	195
Of the situation and structure of the remaining parts of the fowl's uterus	198
Of the extrusion of the egg, or parturition of the fowl, in general	201
Of the increase and nutrition of the egg	202
Of the covering or shell of the egg	204
Of the remaining parts of the egg	211
Of the diversities of eggs	216
Of the production of the chick from the egg of the hen	225
The first examination of the egg; or of the effect of the first day's incu-	
bation upon the egg	228
Second inspection of the egg	232
The third inspection of the egg	234
The fourth inspection of the egg	243
The fifth inspection of the egg	252
The sixth inspection	256
The inspection after the tenth day	257
The inspection after the fourteenth day	259
Of the exclusion of the chick, or the birth from the egg	264

LETTERS.

THE LIFE OF WILLIAM HARVEY, M.D.

WILLIAM HARVEY, the immortal discoverer of the Circulation of the Blood, was the eldest son of Thomas Harvey and
Joan Halke, of Folkstone, in Kent, where he was born on the
1st of April, 1578.[1] Of the parents of Harvey, little is
known. His father, in our printed accounts, is generally designated Gentleman,[2] and must have been in easy circumstances ; inasmuch as he had a numerous family, consisting
of seven sons and two daughters, all the males of which he felt
himself competent to launch upon life in courses that imply
the possession of money wealth. William, the first-born,
adopted the profession of physic. Five of his brothers,—
Thomas, Daniel, Eliab, Michael, and Matthew—were merchants, and not merchants in a small and niggardly way—
non tenues et sordidi, as Dr. Lawrence has it in his Life of
Harvey,[3] but of weight and substance — magni et copiosi,
trading especially with Turkey or the Levant, then the main
channel through which the wealth of the East flowed into
Europe. The Harveys were undoubtedly men of consideration in the city of London, and several of them, in the end,

---

[1] The birthday in some of the lives is stated to be the 2d of April, for no better
reason apparently than that All-fools' Day should not lose its character by giving
birth to a great man. William Harvey, I believe, was born on the 1st of April.

[2] In the register of William Harvey's matriculation at Cambridge his father is
styled Yeoman Cantianus—Kentish yeoman.

[3] Prefixed to the Latin edition of Harvey's Works published by the Royal
College of Physicians, in two vols. 4to, 1766.

became possessed of the most ample independent fortunes.[1] The son, whose name does not appear in the list given above, was John, the immediate junior to William. He, too, was a man of note in his day, having been one of the King's receivers for Lincolnshire, having sat as member of parliament for Hythe, and for some time held the office of King's footman. Of the two sisters—Sarah died young; of the fate of Anne, or Amy, nothing is known.

Great men seem, in almost all authenticated instances, to have had noble-minded women for their mothers. We have not a word of his age or generation to assist us in forming an estimate of Harvey's male progenitor; but the inscription on his mother's monumental tablet, in Folkstone church, assures us that she, at least, was a woman of such mark and likelihood, that it was held due to her memory to leave her moral portrait to posterity in these beautiful words, penned, it may be, by her illustrious eldest son:

"A. D. 1605, Nov. 8th, dyed in yᵉ 50th yeere of her age,
JOAN, Wife of THO: HARVEY. Mother of 7 Sones & 2 Daughters.
A Godly harmles Woman: A chaste loveing Wife:
A charitable quiet Neighbour: A cõfortable frendly Matron:
A pͬovident diligent Huswyfe: A careful teͬder-harted Mother.
Deere to her Husband; Reverensed of her Children:
Beloved of her Neighbours: Elected of God.
Whose Soule Rest in Heaven: her Body in this Grave:
To Her a Happy Advantage: to Hers an Unhappy Loss."

[1] To show the esteem in which the Brothers Harvey were held, I may mention among other things that Ludovic Roberts dedicates his excellent and comprehensive work entitled 'The Merchant's Mapp of Commerce' (Folio, London, 1638) to "The thrice worthy and worshipful William Harvey, Dr. of Physic, John Harvey, Esq., Daniel Harvey, Mercht., Michael Harvey, Mercht., Mathew Harvey, Mercht., Brethren, and John Harvey, Mercht., onely sonne to Mr. Thomas Harvey, Mercht., deceased." The dedication is quaint, in the spirit of the times, but full of right-mindedness, respectfulness, and love for his former masters and present friends, in which relations the Harveys stood to Roberts. Thomas Harvey died in 1622, as appears by his monumental tablet in St. Peter-le-Poore's church, in the city of London. Eliab and Daniel lived rich and respected, the former near Chigwell, co. Essex, the latter at Combe, near Croydon, co. Surrey. Michael Harvey retired to Longford, co. Essex. Matthew Harvey died in London.

Epitaphs may not always be authorities implicitly to be relied on; but we unhesitatingly accept of everything to the credit of William Harvey's mother as a portion of our faith.

At ten years of age, Harvey was put to the grammar school of Canterbury, having, doubtless, already imbibed the rudiments of his English education at home under the eye of his excellent mother. In the grammar school of Canterbury he was, of course, initiated into a knowledge of the Latin and Greek languages—the routine practice then as now; and there he seems to have remained until he was about fifteen years of age. At sixteen he was removed to Caius-Gonvil College, Cambridge,[1] where he spent from three to four years in the study of classics, dialectics, and physics, such discipline being held peculiarly calculated to fit the mind of the future physician for entering on the study of the difficult science of medicine. At nineteen (1597) he took his degree of B.A. aud quitted the University. Cambridge, in Harvey's time, was a school of logic and divinity rather than of physic. Then, even as at the present day, the student of physic obtained the principal part of his medical education from another than his alma mater. In the 16th and 17th centuries, France and Italy boasted medical schools of higher repute than any in Europe; and to one or other of these must the young Englishman who dedicated himself to physic repair, in order to furnish himself with the lore that was indispensable in his profession. Harvey chose Italy; and Padua, about the year 1598, numbering such men as Fabricius of Aquapendente, Julius Casserius, aud Jo. Thomas Minadous among its professors, Harvey's preference of that school was well founded. There, then, it was, under these aud other able masters, that our Harvey

---

[1] "Gul. Harvey, Filius Thomæ Harvey, Yeoman Cantianus, ex Oppido Folkston, educatus in Ludo Literario Cantuar.; natus annos 16, admissus pensionarius minor in commeatum scholarium ultimo die Mai, 1593." (Regist. Coll. Caii Cantab. 1593.)

drank in the elementary knowledge which served him as a
foundation for that induction which has made his name immortal; for without detracting from the glory of Harvey, but
merely in recognizing the means to an end, we may admit that,
but for the lessons of his master, Fabricius, Harvey might
have passed through life, not unnoticed, indeed,—for such as
Harvey was in himself, he must still have been remarkable,—
but his name unconnected with one of the most admirable
and useful inferences ever given to the world.

Having passed five years at Padua, Harvey, then in the
twenty-fourth year of his age (1602), finally obtained his di-
ploma as doctor of physic, with licence to practise and to teach
arts and medicine in every land and seat of learning. Having
returned to England in the course of the same year, and submitted to the requisite forms, he also received his doctor's degree
from his original University of Cambridge; and then coming
to London, and taking to himself a wife in his six and twentieth
year, he entered on the practice of his profession.

History is all but silent in regard to the woman of our
great anatomist's choice. We only know that she was the
daughter of a physician of the day, Dr. Lancelot Browne, and
that Harvey's union with her proved childless. He himself
mentions his wife incidentally as having a remarkable pet
parrot, which must also, if we may infer so much from the
pains he takes in specifying its various habits and accomplishments, have been a particular favorite of his own.[1]

In 1604, Harvey joined the College of Physicians, his name
appearing on the roll of candidates for the fellowship in that
year; and three years afterwards, 1607, the term of his pro-

---

[1] Vide On Generation, p. 186. That Harvey outlived his wife is certain from his
Will, in which she is affectionately mentioned as his "deare deceased loving wife."
She must have been alive in 1645, the year in which Harvey's brother John died,
and left her £50.

bation having passed, he was duly admitted to the distinction
to which he aspired.

We do not now lose sight of Harvey for any length of time :
for a number of years, in the beginning of his career, he was
probably occupied, like young physicians of the present day,
among the poor in circumstance and afflicted in body, taking vast
pains without prospect of pecuniary reward, but actuated by the
ennobling sense of lightening the sum of human misery, and
carried away, uncaring personal respects, by that ardent love of
his profession which distinguishes every true votary of the art
medical.   Harvey, however, had not only zeal, talents, and
accomplishments ; he had, what was no less needful to success :
powerful friends, united brothers, with the will and the ability
to help him forward in the career he had chosen.

In the beginning of 1609, he made suit for the reversion
of the office of physician to St. Bartholomew's Hospital, then
held by Dr. Wilkinson, and backing his suit by such powerful
missives as the king's letters recommendatory to the governors
of the house, and farther, producing testimonials of compe-
tency from Dr. Adkinson, President of the College of Physicians, and others, his petition was granted, and he was
regularly chosen physician in futuro of St. Bartholomew's
Hospital.   Dr. Wilkinson having died in the course of the
year, Harvey was first appointed to discharge the physician's
duties ad interim, and by and by he was formally elected to
the vacant office, 14th October, 1609.

In his new position Harvey must have found ample scope
for acquiring tact and readiness in the practical details of his
profession; though St. Bartholomew's Hospital in his day
appears to have borne a nearer resemblance to the dispensary
of these times than to the hospital as we now understand the
term.   Harvey was now in his thirty-second year, and, brought
before the public at so suitable an age, in an office of such
responsibility, he must soon have risen into eminence as a

physician and come into practice. Harvey, indeed, appears subsequently to have been physician to many of the most distinguished men of his age, among others to the Lord Chancellor Bacon, to Thomas Howard, Earl of Arundel, &c.

In the year 1615, Harvey, then in the thirty-seventh year of his age, was happily chosen to deliver the lectures on anatomy and surgery at the College of Physicians, founded by Dr. Richard Caldwal, and it is generally allowed that in the very first course he gave, which commenced in the month of April of the following year, he presented a detailed exposition of the views concerning the circulation of the blood, which have made his name immortal. Long years had indeed been labouring at the birth which then first saw the light; civilized Europe, ancient and modern, had been slowly contributing and accumulating materials for its production; Harvey at length appeared, and the idea took fashion in his mind and emerged complete, like Pallas, perfect from the brain of Jove.

The circulation, it would seem, continued to form one of the subjects in the lectures on anatomy, which Harvey went on delivering for many years afterwards at the College of Physicians; but it was not till 1628 that he gave his views to the world at large in his celebrated treatise on the 'Motion of the Heart and Blood,'[1] having already, as he tells us in his preface, for nine years and more, gone on demonstrating the subject before his learned auditory, illustrating it by new and additional arguments, and freeing it from the objections raised by the skilful among anatomists.

Some few years after his appointment as their lecturer by the College of Physicians, Harvey must have been chosen one of the physicians extraordinary to the reigning sovereign, James I. The fame of Harvey's new views of the motions

---

[1] Exercitatio Anatomica de Motu Cordis et Sanguinis, 4to, Francof. ad Mœn., 1628.

of the heart and blood could not but speedily have reached
the wide-open ears of King James, and this of itself, to lay no
stress on the powerful city interest of the illustrious anatomist,
might suffice to ensure him such a mark of distinction as that
just named.   Of the precise date of his appointment as
physician extraordinary to the king we are not informed; but
in the letter of James bearing date the 3d of February, 1623,
it is spoken of as a thing foregone—that had taken place
some time ago; for in this letter Doctor Harvey is charged in
common with the physicians in ordinary, with the care of the
king's health; and he is further guaranteed the reversion of the
office of ordinary physician whenever, by death or otherwise,
a vacancy should occur.   To the promised dignity, however,
Harvey did not attain for several years, not till after the
demise of James, and when Charles had already occupied the
throne of his father for some five or six years.

Harvey may now be said to have become rather closely
connected with the court; but whether this connexion proved
truly advantageous to him as a philosopher and physiologist
may fairly be questioned.   The time and service which the
court physician must necessarily give to royalty and greatness
interfere materially with the leisure and privacy that are
indispensable to study and meditation.   But Harvey, who
appears to have been a man of singular self-possession, not to
be diverted from his purpose by trifling or merely ceremonial
considerations, always speaks of his master Charles in terms
of unfeigned love and respect; and everything induces us to
believe that Charles in turn loved and honoured his physician.
The sovereign seems even to have taken a remarkable interest
in the inquiries of the physiologist ; to have had several exhi-
bitions prepared of the punctum saliens in the embryo chick
and deer, and to have witnessed the dissections of many of the
does which he so liberally placed at Harvey's disposal whilst
the anatomist was prosecuting his inquiries into the subject of

generation. Whatever the defects in Charles's public and political character, he must always be admitted to have been a man of elegant tastes, and of amiable temper and refined manners in private. It was certainly worthy of the Prince who appreciated, whilst he commanded, the talents of a Vandyke and a Rubens, that he also prized and encouraged the less brilliant, but not less useful genius of a Harvey.

Harvey, as a physician, must now have been at the zenith of his reputation; he was physician in ordinary to the king, and we have seen him in the same position towards some of the foremost men of the age. His general practice, too, must have been extensive, and, if we look at the sum he is stated to have left behind him in money, his emoluments large. But he had not any lengthened harvest for all his early pains; his connexion with the court by and by came in the way of his continuing to improve his position; and then, grievous to relate, the appearance of the admirable Exercises on the Heart and Blood gave a decided and severe check to his professional prosperity. John Aubrey tells us he had "heard him (Harvey) say, that after his book on the 'Circulation of the Blood' came out, he fell mightily in his practice; 'twas believed by the vulgar that he was crack-brained, and all the physitians were against him." [1] Writing many years afterwards, when the cause particularly indicated above had conspired to make Harvey's practice less, Aubrey informs us further, that "though all his profession would allow him to be an excellent anatomist, I never heard any that admired his therapeutique way. I knew several practitioners in this town that would not have given threepence for one of his bills (prescriptions), and [who said] that a man could hardly tell by his bills what he did aim at." [2] So has it mostly been with those who have added to the sum of human knowledge!

[1] Aubrey, Lives of Eminent Persons, 8vo, London, 1813.
[2] Ib., vol. ii, p. 383.

The empiric under the title of the practical man, in his unsuspecting ignorance, sets himself up and is admitted as arbiter wherever there is difficulty : blind himself, he leads the blinded multitude the way he lists.   He who laid the foundation of modern medical science lost his practice for his pains, and the routineer, with an appropriate salve for every sore, a pill and potion for each particular ache and ail, would not give threepence for one of his prescriptions ! did not admire his therapeutique way ! ! and could not tell what he did aim at ! ! !   Ignorance and presumption have never hesitated to rend the veil that science and modesty, all in supplying the means, have still owned their inability to raise.   If Harvey faltered, who of his contemporaries could rightfully presume to walk secure ?   And yet did each and all of them, unconscious of the darkness, tread their twilight paths assuredly ; whilst he, the divinity among them, with his eyes unsealed, felt little certain of his way.   So has it still been with medicine ; and the world must make many a lusty onward stride in knowledge before it can be otherwise.

The first interruption to his ordinary professional pursuits and avocations which Harvey seems to have suffered through his connexion with the court, occurred in the beginning of 1630, when he was engaged "to accompany the young Duke of Lenox in his travels beyond seas."   In anticipation of a removal from London, apparently, Harvey had already, in December 1629, resigned his office of treasurer to the College of Physicians, which he seems to have filled for several years.

Of the course of Harvey's travels with the Duke of Lennox we have not been able to gain any information.   Their way probably led them to the Continent, and it may have been on this occasion and in this company that he visited Venice, as we know from himself that he did in the course of one of his journeys.   Harvey must have been in England again in 1632 and 1633 ; for in the former year he was formally chosen physician to Charles, and in the latter we find his absence, "by reason of his attendance on the king's majesty," from St. Bartholomew's Hospital complained of by the surgeons of that institution, and Dr. Andrews appointed by the governors as his substitute, but "without prejudice to him in his yearly fee or in any other respect."[1] Such considerate treatment satisfies us of the esteem in which Harvey was held.

In the early part of 1633 Charles determined to visit his ancient kingdom of Scotland, for the ostensible purpose of being crowned King of Scots. Upon this occasion Harvey accompanied him, as matter of course, we may presume. But the absence of the court from London was not of long duration; and in the early autumn of the same year we are pleased to find Harvey again at his post in St. Bartholomew's Hospital, engaged in his own province and propounding divers rules and regulations for the better government of the house and its officers,[2] which of themselves give us an excellent insight into the state of the hospital, as well as of the relative positions of the several departments of the healing art two centuries ago. The doctor's treatment of the poor chirurgeons in these rules is sufficiently despotic it must be admitted; but the chirurgeons in their acquiescence showed that they merited no better handling. The only point on which they proved restive, indeed, was the revealment of their SECRETS to the physician; a great outrage in days when every man had his secrets, and felt fully justified in keeping them to himself. But surgery in the year 1633 had not shown any good title to an independent existence. The surgeon of those days was

---

[1] Vide Records of Harvey from the Journals of St. Bartholomew's Hospital, pub. by James Paget, 8vo, London, 1846. Harvey, on his appointment to attend the Duke of Lennox, applied to have Dr. Smith chosen his substitute; but the governors proved recusant: "It was thought fit that they should have further knowledge and satisfaction of the sufficiency of the said Mr. Smith;" and they very shortly afterwards gave Dr. Andrews, first, the reversion of Harvey's office, and by and by they formally appointed him Harvey's deputy or substitute.

[2] Vide Mr. Paget's publication already quoted, p. 13.

but the hand or instrument of the physician; the dignitary mostly applied to his famulus when he required a wen removed, or a limb lopped, or a broken head plastered; though Harvey it seems did not feel himself degraded by taking up the knife or practising midwifery.[1] Nevertheless, in these latter days Royal Colleges of Physicians have been seen arrogating superiority over Royal Colleges of Surgeons, and Royal Colleges both of Physicians and Surgeons combining to keep the practitioner of obstetrics under.

From the year 1633 Harvey appears to have devoted much of his time to attendance upon the king and retainers of the court, so that we have little or no particular information of his movements for several years. We know, however, from Aubrey, that he accompanied Thomas Howard, Earl of Arundel, whose physician he was, in his extraordinary embassy to the emperor, in the year 1636.[2] In the course of this journey, Harvey had an opportunity of visiting several of the principal cities of Germany, and of making the acquaintance of many of the leading medical men of the time. The place of date of one of Harvey's letters, that namely to Caspar Hofmann, from Nuremberg, in the month of May, 1636, has not been noticed; but his presence with the Earl of Arundel at once accounts for it; and we therefore see that Harvey's offer to demonstrate to the distinguished professor of Nuremberg, the anatomical particulars which made the circulation of the blood a necessary conclusion was no vain boast, made at a distance,

---

[1] Vide his procedure for the removal of a sarcocele, 'On Generation,' p. 254. "My Lady Howard had a cancer in her breast, which he did cut off and seared." (Aubrey, Lives, p. 386.) He speaks of having been called to a young woman in labour in a state of coma (On Generation, p. 534); and in another place (Ib. p. 437) he says, in connexion with the subject of labour, 'Haud inexpertus loquuor,'— I speak not without experience. Vide also p. 545, where he passes his fingers into the uterus and brings away "a mole of the size of a goose's egg;" and p. 546, where he dilates the uterine orifice with an iron instrument, and uses a speculum, &c.

[2] The embassy left England the 7th of April, and returned about Christmas of the same year. Vide Crowne's 'True Relation,' &c., 4to, London, 1637.

bùt a substantial proposition in presence of his opponent, and
which there is tradition at least to assure us he was called
upon to fulfil.—Harvey is reported to have made a public demonstration of his anatomical views at Nuremberg, satisfactory
to all present save Caspar Hofmann himself; to whom, as he
still continued to urge objections, the futile nature of which
we in these days can readily understand, Harvey is further related to have deigned no other answer than by laying down
the scalpel and retiring, conduct which we find in entire conformity with our estimate of the character of the man.[1]

On his return to England, in the winter of 1636, Harvey must
have resumed his place near the person of the sovereign, and
by and by, as in duty bound, accompanied him on his first
hostile expedition into Scotland in 1639, when matters
were happily accommodated between the King and his Scottish
subjects, whom he had driven to take up arms so righteously
in defence of their religious liberties. Harvey, as physician to
the person, may be further presumed to have been with Charles
when he marched towards the Border the following year, so
memorable in the annals of English history, when the war
with the Scots was renewed, when the king's authority received
the first check at the battle of Newbury, and when Charles,
returning to his capital after his defeat, encountered the still
more formidable opposition of the English Parliament.

Harvey may now be said to have become fairly involved with
the Court. From the total absence of his name in the transactions of the times, it is nevertheless interesting to observe
how completely he kept himself aloof from all the intrigues

---

[1] Slegel (P. M.) De Sanguinis Motu Comment., 4to, Hamb. 1650, informs us in his
Preface, that, whilst living with Hofmann in 1638, he had sedulously tried to bring
him to admit the circulation; Slegel goes on to say, however, that it was in vain,
and indeed that Harvey himself had failed to convince him : " Neque tantum valuit
Harveus, *vel coram* (i. e. in his presence) cum salutaret Hofmannum in itinere
Germanico, vel literis," &c. The old man, nevertheless, seems not to have been
altogether deaf to reason ; Slegel had hopes of him at last had he but lived : " Nec
dubito quin concessisset tandem in nostra castra."

and dealings of the party with which he was connected. He must have held himself exclusively to the discharge of his professional duties. In the course of these he doubtless attended Charles in his third visit to Scotland in the summer of 1641, when he essayed the arts of diplomacy with little better effect than he had already attempted the weight of prerogative in the first, and the force of arms in the second visit.

On returning to London in the autumn of the same year, Charles soon brought matters to a crisis between himself and his English subjects, in the persons of their representatives, and nothing soon remained for him but to unfurl his standard and proclaim himself at war with his people. This was accordingly done in the course of the ensuing summer. But the Parliament did not yet abandon a seeming care of the royal person, and Harvey informs us himself, that he now attended the king, not only with the consent, but by the desire, of the parliament. The battle of Edge-hill, which followed, and in which the sun of fortune shone with a partial and fitful gleam upon the royal arms, is especially interesting to us from our Harvey having been present, though he still took no part in the affair, and seems indeed to have felt very little solicitude either about its progress or its issue, if the account of Aubrey may be credited. "When King Charles," says Aubrey, "by reason of the tumults, left London, he (Harvey) attended him, and was at the fight of Edge-hill with him ; and during the fight the Prince and Duke of York were committed to his care. He told me that he withdrew with them under a hedge, and tooke out of his pockett a booke and read. But he had not read very long before a bullet of a great gun grazed on the ground neare him, which made him remove his station."[1] The act of reading a book pending an important battle, the result of which was greatly to influence his master's fortunes, certainly shows a wonderful degree of coolness and a remarkable indifference

[1] Lives, &c., vol. ii, p. 379.

to everything like military matters. Harvey's own candid
character, and the confidence so obviously reposed in him
when he was intrusted with the care of the Prince and the
Duke of York, forbid us to interpret the behaviour into any
lukewarmness or indifference as to the issue; but Harvey,
throughout his whole career, was a most peaceful man : he never
had the least taste for literary controversy, and can scarcely
be said to have replied to any of those who opposed his views;
and in his indifference about the fight of Edge-hill he only
further shows us that he was not

> " Of those who build their faith upon
> The holy text of pike and gun,
> And prove their doctrine orthodox
> By apostolic blows and knocks."

With his fine understanding and freedom from party and
sectarian views of every kind, he probably saw that an appeal
to arms was not the way for political right to be elicited, or
for a sovereign to settle matters with his subjects. Harvey
had certainly no turn for politics,[1] and when we refer to
Aubrey we find that the fight of Edge-hill was hardly ended
before our anatomist had crept back into his shell, and become
absorbed in the subjects that formed the proper business of his
life. " I first saw him (Harvey) at Oxford, 1642, after Edge-
hill fight," says our authority, " but was then too young to be
acquainted with so great a doctor. I remember he came several times to our college (Trin.) to George Bathurst, B.D., who
had a hen to hatch eggs in his chamber, which they opened
dayly to see the progress and way of generation." The
zealous political partisan would have found no leisure for researches like these in such stirring times as marked the out-

---

[1] The author of the life of Harvey in the 'General Dictionary, Historical and
Critical' (folio, Lond. 1738), the original of all our other lives of Harvey, is certainly in error when he recognizes Harvey as the type of the Physician who takes
part in the Dialogue of Hy. Neville's Plato Redivivus, and assumes that he " relieved
his abstruser studies by conversations in politics." In a third edition of Neville's
work I find it stated that the physician who did so was Dr. Lower.

break of the civil war in England; the politician had then other than pullets' eggs to hatch.

The king's physician, not to speak of the author of a new doctrine of the motions of the heart and blood, was sure to find favour in the eyes of the high church dignitaries of Oxford; and we accordingly find that, besides being everywhere handsomely received and entertained, Harvey had the honorary degree of Doctor of Physic conferred on him. Oxford, indeed, when the king and court were driven from the metropolis, which was now wholly in the hands of the popular party, became the head-quarters of the royal army and principal residence of the king for several years. And here Harvey seems to have quietly settled himself down and again turned his attention to his favorite subjects. Nor was the honorary distinction of doctor of physic from the university, which has been mentioned, the only mark of favour he received. Sir Nathaniel Brent, Warden of Merton College, yielding to his natural bias, forsook Oxford when it was garrisoned by the king, and began to take a somewhat active part in the proceedings of the popular party; he came forward in especial as a witness against Archbishop Laud, on the trial of that dignitary. Merton College being thus left without a head, upon the suggestion, as it is said, of the learned antiquary and mathematician, John Greaves, and in virtue of a letter of the king, Harvey was elected warden some time in the course of 1645. This appointment was doubtless merited by Harvey for his constant and faithful service to Charles; but it may also have been bestowed in some measure as a retort upon the Parliament, which, the year before, had entertained a motion for the supercession of Harvey in his office of physician to St. Bartholomew's Hospital.[1]

---

[1] Feb. 12, an. 164⅘. "A motion this day made for Dr. Mieklethwayte to be recommended to the warden and masters of St. Bartholomew's Hospital, to be physician, in the place of Dr. Harvey, who hath withdrawn himself from his charge, and is retired to the party in arms against the Parliament." (Journals of the House of Commons, iii, 397.)

Harvey, however, did not long enjoy his new office or its
emoluments ; for Oxford having surrendered to the Parliamentary forces under Fairfax the following year, Harvey, of
course, resigned his charge, and immediately afterwards betook
himself to London. Sir Nathaniel Brent, on the contrary,
returned to Oxford; and the star of the Parliamentarians
being now in the ascendant, Merton College was not slow to
reinstate its old Presbyterian warden in the room of its late
royalist head.[1]

From the date of the surrender of Oxford (July, 1646),
Harvey followed the fortunes of Charles no longer. Of his reasons for quitting the service of his old master we know nothing.
He probably felt anxious for repose ; at sixty-eight, which was
Harvey's age, a man begins to find that an easy chair is a fitter
resting-place than the bare ground, a ceiled roof more suitable
covering than the open sky—prospects which a continuance of
the strife held out. Harvey, besides, as we have seen, had no
stomach for contention in any shape or form, not even in the

---

[1] I find a kind of obloquy commonly thrown on the memory of Nathaniel Brent
for what is styled his desertion of Charles ; but he never deserted Charles ; he never
belonged to him. Brent, forsooth, had received knighthood at the royal hands in
former years ; but knighthoods were sometimes forced upon men in those days for
the sake of the fees, and often as means of attaching men of mark and likelihood.
The truth is that Brent, who was a profound lawyer and scholar, as well as a
traveller, was greatly attached to Archbishop Abbott, who had patronized and advanced him through the whole course of his life. In the differences that took place
between Abbott, in common with all moderate men, and Archbishop Laud, Brent
naturally sided with his friend, led to do so, however, not by blind attachment only,
but by natural constitution of mind, which appears to have abhorred the notion of a
theocracy in the civil government of England, and to have been unfitted to comprehend the divinity that some conceive to inhere in despotism. Brent was, in fact,
a man of such note, that Charles had tried to win him to his party many years before
by various attentions and the free gift of knighthood; but this was in times when
men were not required to take a side, when they stood naturally neutral. When the
time came that it behoved him to show under what flag he meant to fight, Brent
was not wanting to his natural bias and to independence. He therefore left Oxford
when it was taken possession of by the royal forces, among other adherents of the
popular cause, and was simply true to his principles, in nothing false to a patron
or benefactor.

literary arena; and he now probably resolved himself to follow the advice he had once given to his young friend Charles Scarborough, " to leave off gunning,"[1] and dedicate himself wholly to more congenial pursuits.   And then Charles had long made it apparent, even to the most ardent of his adherents, that no faith was to be put in his promise, no trust to be reposed in his royal word.   The wise old man, verging on the age of threescore years and ten, doubtless saw that it was better for him to retire from a responsible office, now become most irksome and thankless, and seek privacy and leisure for the remainder of his days.   These Harvey found awaiting him in the houses of his affectionate brothers—now in the house of Eliab, in the City, or at Roehampton, and then in the house of Daniel, in the 'suburban' village of Lambeth, or at Combe near Croydon in Surrey, in each of which Harvey had his own apartments.   The Harveys appear to have been united from first to last in the closest bonds of brotherly love,[2] and to have had a common interest in many of their undertakings; and Eliab, as we shall see, employed the small capital,

---

[1] " Prithee leave off thy gunning and stay here ; I will bring thee into practice." (Aubrey, Op. cit. p. 381.)

[2] On the monumental tablet of Thomas, the first of the brothers who died, in the church of St. Peter's-le-Poore, the mottos, doubtless supplied by a surviving member of the family, show this feeling.   The inscription is as follows :

As in a Sheafe of Arrows.
Vis unita fortior.
The band of Love
The Unitor of Brethren.
Here Lyeth the body of Thomas Harvey,
Of London, Merchant,
Who departed this life
The 2nd of Feby. An. Dom.
1622.
(Stow's London, third edit., fol. Lond. 1633.)

John Harvey, Esq., who died in 1645, left his brother William's wife £50.   Eliab Harvey attended particularly to his brother William's interests ; and William at his death returned Eliab's kindness by leaving him his residuary legatee.

which his brother William must have accumulated before the civil wars broke out, to such purpose, that the doctor actually died a rich man. With his brothers, then, retreating now to the "leads" of the house in the heart of the metropolis, now to the "caves" of the one at Combe, did Harvey continue to pass his days—but not in idleness; for the work on Generation, with the subject of which we saw him busied at Oxford several years before, must have found him in ample occupation. Nor was the love of ease so great in William Harvey, even at the advanced age of seventy-one, if we may credit some of the accounts, as to hinder him from again visiting the Continent, and making his way as far as Italy, a journey in which it is said he was attended by his friend the accomplished scholar and gentleman, Dr. Ent.[1]

In the beginning of 1651 appeared the second of Harvey's great works, that, namely, On Animal Generation.[2] In this publication we have abundant proof of our author's unabated industry and devotion to physiological science; and in the long and admirable letter to P. M. Slegel, of Hamburg, written shortly after the appearance of the work, we have pleasing evidence of the integrity of Harvey's faculties at the advanced age of seventy-three.

The year after the publication of the work on Generation, i. e. 1652, when Harvey was looked up to by common consent as the most distinguished anatomist and physician of his age, the College of Physicians came to the resolution of placing his statue in their hall then occupying a site at Amen-corner; and measures being immediately taken in conformity with this purpose, it was carried into effect by the end of the year,

[1] This rather arduous undertaking in those days was accomplished, according to Aubrey, about the year 1649. But I have found so much to excite doubt in Aubrey's Notes, that I greatly suspect the accuracy of his statement about the journey to Italy.

[2] De Generatione Animalium, 4to, London, 1651.

when the statue, with the following complimentary inscription on the pedestal, was displayed :

GULIELMO HARVEIO
Viro monumentis suis immortali
Hoc insuper Collegium Medicorum Londinense
posuit.
Qui enim Sanguini motum
ut et
Animalibus ortum dedit,
Meruit esse
Stator Perpetuus.[1]

Harvey, in acknowledgment, it may have been, of the distinguished honour done him by his friends and colleagues, appears about this time to have commenced the erection at his own cost of a handsome addition to the College of Physicians.   It was, as Aubrey informs us, "a noble building of Roman architecture (of rustic work, with Corinthian pilasters), comprising a great parlour, a kind of convocation house for the fellows to meet in below, and a library above. On the outside, on the frieze, in letters three inches long, was this inscription : Suasu et cura Fran. Prujeani, Præsidis, et Edmundi Smith, elect. inchoata et perfecta est hæc fabrica, An. MDCLIII."[2]   Nor was Harvey content merely to erect this building ; he, further, furnished the library with books, and the museum with numerous objects of curiosity and a variety of surgical instruments.   On the ceremony of this handsome addition to the College of Physicians being opened, which took place on the 2d of February, 1653, a sumptuous entertainment was provided at Harvey's expense, at which he received the pre-

---

[1] This statue perished with the building, in the great fire of London in 1666, and seems never to have been replaced.   The hall of the present College of Physicians is not graced as was the old one in Harvey's time.   The only sculptures of Harvey that I know of are busts, in the theatre of the College of Physicians and on his monument in Hempstead church, but of dates posterior to their subject, that at the College of Physicians being apparently after the portrait by Jansen in the library, and, as I am informed, by a sculptor of the name of Seemacher.

[2] Aubrey, l. c. p. 378.

sident and fellows, and made over to them, on the spot, his whole interest in the structure.

Dr. Prujean, the president of the college, going out of office, as usual, at Michaelmas the next year (1654), Harvey was unanimously chosen to fill the vacant chair. Having been absent when the election took place, a deputation proceeded to his apartments to apprize him of the honour his colleagues had done themselves and him, and to say that they awaited his answer on the following day. Every act of Harvey's public life that has come down to us is marked not merely by propriety but by grace. He attended the comitia or assembly of the college next day; thanked his colleagues for the distinguished honour of which they had thought him worthy—the honour, as he said, of filling the foremost place among the physicians of England; but the concerns of the college, he proceeded, were too weighty to be intrusted to one like him, laden with years and infirm in health; and if he might be acquitted of arrogance in presuming to give advice in such circumstances, he would say that the college could not do better than rein-state in the authority which he had but just laid down, their late president, Dr. Prujean, under whose prudent management and fostering care the affairs of the college had greatly prospered. This noble counsel had fitting response: Harvey's advice being adopted by general consent, Dr. Prujean was forthwith re-elected president.

The College of Physicians were justly proud of their great associate, and Harvey, in his turn, was undoubtedly attached to the college. Here, indeed, as their lecturer on anatomy and surgery, he had first propounded the views which had won him such distinguished credit in his life, and which have left his name as a deathless word on the lips of men; here he consorted with his nearest and dearest friends, receiving from all those remarks of respectful consideration that were so justly his due; and here, in fine, the first place among the first men of his profession had been tendered to him, and gracefully declined. To a mind like Harvey's, and with the opportunity afforded him of making so graceful a concession, the foremost place was certainly a higher distinction unaccepted, than it had been enjoyed.—The excuse for declining the office of president was not merely personal: it was not alone that he was an old man, infirm in health, and incompetent for so great a trust; but, the affairs of the college had greatly thriven under the prudent management and constant care of the late president, and it was no more than right that he who had but just laid down should be re-established in authority.

Harvey, we have said, was childless; his wife, though we have not the date of her death, he had certainly lost by this time. His only surviving brother Eliab was rich; his nephews were prosperous merchants and on the road to the independence and titles which several of them afterwards achieved: he, therefore, determined to make the College of Physicians not only heirs to his paternal estate, worth, at that time, 56*l.* per annum, but to bestow it on them in free gift during his life. This purpose he carried into effect by means of a formal instrument, which he delivered to the college in the month of July, 1656; the special provisions in the deed settling one sum, by way of salary for the librarian, and another sum, for the delivery of a solemn oration annually, in commemoration of those who had approved themselves bene-factors to the college, and, by extension, who had added aught to the sum of medical science in the course of the bygone year.[1]

[1] There is much information on the life of Harvey in the inscription upon the copper-plate which was attached to his portrait in the old College of Physicians. I give it entire, anxious to set before the reader every authentic word of his times that was uttered of Harvey. This inscription, but, unless I mistake, abbreviated, may be found in printed letters under the bust of Harvey in the theatre of the Royal College of Physicians:

GULIELMUS HARVÆUS,

Anglus natus, Galliæ, Italiæ, Germaniæ hospes,

Ubique Amor et Desiderium,

Quem omnis terra expetisset Civem,

Having thus accompanied Harvey over so much of the way in his mortal career, let us, before proceeding further, briefly advert to his WRITINGS, to the influence they had in the republic of letters during his life-time, to the fruits they have since produced, and to the impression still made on the mind that holds communion through their means with the mind that dictated them so many years ago.—The intellectual endowment of a man necessarily appears in his writings; it is not always from them that so true a conception of his moral character can be formed. Harvey, however, though in his long life he accomplished but a small fraction of all his literary designs, has still left us sufficient from which to form an estimate of him as a philosopher, as a physiologist, and it

Medicinæ Doctor, Coll. Med. Lond. Socius et Consiliarius,
Anatomes, Chirurgiæque Professor,
Regis Jacobi Familiæ, Caroloque Regi Medicus,
Gestis clarus, omissisque honoribus,
Quorum alios tulit, oblatos renuit alios,
Omnes meruit.
Laudatis priscorum ingeniis par;
Quos honoravit maxime imitando,
Docuitque posteros exemplo.
Nullius lacessivit famam,
Veritatis studens magis quam gloriæ,
Hanc tamen adeptus
Industria, sagacitate, successu nobilis
Perpetuos sanguinis æstus
Circulari gyro fugientis, seque sequentis,
Primus promulgavit mundo.
Nec passus ultrà mortales sua ignorare primordia,
Aureum edidit de ovo atque pullo librum,
Albæ gallinæ filium.
Sic novis inventis Apollineam ampliavit artem,
Atque nostrum Apollinis sacrarium augustius esse
Tandem voluit;
Suasu enim et cura D. D. Dni. Francisci Prujeani Præsidis
Et Edmundi Smith Electoris
An. MDCLIII,
Senaculum, et de nomine suo Musæum horto superstruxit,
Quorum alterum plurimis libris et Instrumentis Chirurgicis,
Alterum omnigena supellectile ornavit et instruxit,
Medicinæ Patronus simul et Alumnus.

may also be said as a man. Let us take a brief survey of his writings, then, and wind up our account of his life with such personal notices as we can gather from contemporaries, or as we can infer from his own conduct and written word.

ON THE HEART AND BLOOD.

Harvey's great work, though by no means the largest in bulk, is the one on the Motions of the Heart and Blood. It has been said, happily, by a recent critical writer, that "men were already practising what Bacon came to inculcate," viz. induction upon data carefully collected and considered ; and it would not be easy to adduce a more striking example of

Non hic anhela substitit Herois Virtus, impatiens vinci
Accessit porro Munificentiæ decus :
Suasu enim et consilio D^{ui.} D^{ris.} Edv. Alstoni Præsidis,
Anno MDCLVI
Rem nostram angustam prius, annuo LVI. l. reditu auxit,
Paterni Fundi ex asse hæredem collegium dicens ;
Quo nihil Illi charius Nobisve honestius.
Unde ædificium sartum tectum perennare,
Unde Bibliothecario honorarium suum, suumque Oratori
Quotannis pendi ;
Unde omnibus sociis annuum suum convivium,
Et suum denique (quot menses) conviviolum censoribus parari,
Jussit.
Ipse etiam pleno theatro gestiens se hæreditate exuere,
In manus Præsidis syngrapham tradidit.
Interfuitque Orationi veterum Benefactorum novorumque Illicio,
Et Philotesio Epulo ;
Illius auspicium et pars maxima ;
Hujus conviva simul et convivator.
Sic postquam satis sibi, satis nobis, satis gloriæ,
Amicis solum non satis, nec satis patriæ, vixerat,
Cœlicolûm atria subiit
Jun. iii, MDCLVII.
Quem pigebat superis reddere, sed pudebat negare :
Ne mireris igitur Lector,
Si quem marmoreum illic stare vides,
Hic totam implevit tabulam.
Abi et merere alteram.

the way in which ultimate rational truth is arrived at by a succession of inferences than is contained in Harvey's Essay on the Heart and Blood. Had Bacon written his Novum Organum from Harvey's work as a text, he would scarcely have expressed himself otherwise than as he has done, or given different rules for philosophizing than those which he has laid down in his celebrated treatise.[1]

In his introduction, and by way of clearing the ground, Harvey exposes the views of preceding physiologists, ancient and modern, in regard to the motions of the heart, lungs, and blood, to the state of the arteries, &c.—in short, he gives the accredited physiology of the thoracic viscera, with comments, which prove it a mass of unintelligible and irreconcilable confusion. There is room, therefore, for another interpretation, consonant with reason and with anatomical fact, and susceptible of demonstration by the senses. When he first essayed himself to comprehend the motions of the heart, and to make out the uses of the organ from the dissection of living animals, he found the subject so beset with difficulties that he was almost inclined at one time to say with Fracastorius, that these motions and their purpose could be comprehended by God alone. By degrees, however, by repeating his observations, using greater care, and giving more concentrated attention, he at last discovers a way out of the labyrinth, and a means of explaining simply all that had previously appeared so obscure. Hence the occasion of his writing. Such is the burthen of the proem and first chapter. With Harvey's admirable work now put in an accessible shape into his hands, we should (did we proceed with an analysis) but anticipate the intelligent reader in the great pleasure he will have in following the author through the different steps of his argument

---

[1] The Novum Organum appeared in 1620. Though Harvey's work was not published till 1628, he had developed his subject in 1616, and there is every reason to believe, actually written the 'Exercit. de Motu Cordis et Sanguinis' before 1619.

until the conclusion is reached, and the inference presents itself as inevitable, namely, that the blood must circle round and round in one determinate course, in the body as in the lungs, incessantly. For Harvey, it must be here observed, left the doctrine of the circulation as an inference or induction only, not as a sensible demonstration. He adduced certain circumstances, and quoted various anatomical facts which made a continuous transit of the blood from the arteries into the veins, from the veins into the arteries, a necessary consequence; but he never saw this transit; his idea of the way in which it was accomplished was even defective; he had no notion of the one order of sanguiferous vessels ending by uninterrupted continuity, or by an intermediate vascular network, in the other order. This was the demonstration of a later day, and of one who first saw the light in the course of the very year when Harvey's work on the Heart was published.[1]

The appearance of Harvey's book on the Motion of the Heart and Blood seems almost immediately to have attracted the attention of all the better intellects among the medical men of Europe. The subject was not one, indeed, greatly calculated to interest the mass of mere practitioners; had it been a book of receipts it would have had a better chance with them; but the anatomists and physiologists and scientific physicians would seem at once to have taken it up and canvassed its merits. The conclusions come to in the work, there can be no question, took the medical world by surprise; it was not prepared for such a proposition as a ceaseless circular movement of the blood, with the heart for the propelling organ; for the latter point, be it understood, was even as great a novelty as the former.

Coming unexpectedly, and differing so widely from the ancient and accepted notions, we cannot wonder that Harvey's views were at first rejected almost universally. The older

---

[1] Malpighi, born at Crevalcuore, Bologna, the 10th of March, 1628.

intellects, in possession of the seats and places of authority, regarded them as idle dreams; and upon the faith of this conclusion, their author was set down and treated by the vulgar as a crackbrained innovator. Two years, however, elapsed before aught in contravention of the new doctrines saw the light, and this came at length not from any of the more mature anatomists of Europe—their minds were made up, the thing was absurd—but from a young physician, of the name of Primerose, of Scottish descènt, but French by birth. Primerose had been a pupil of Joannes Riolanus, professor of anatomy in the University of Paris; he had doubtless listened to his master's demonstration of the absurdity of the Harveian doctrine of the circulation, and by and by he set himself down, by way apparently of exercising his ingenuity, to try the question, not by fact and experiment, but by the precepts he had imbibed from his teacher and the texts of the ancients The essay of Primerose[1] may be regarded as a defence of the physiological ideas of Galen against the innovations of Harvey It is remarkable for any characteristic rather than that of a candid spirit in pursuit of truth; it abounds in obstinate denials, and sometimes in what may be termed dishonest perversions of simple matters of fact, and in its whole course appeals not once to experiment as a means of investigation.—Harvey, having already, and in the very outset of his work, demonstrated the notions untenable which it was Primerose's purpose to reassert and defend, of course deigned him no reply; he could never dream of going over the barren ground he had already trodden, in the hope of convincing such an antagonist.

Æmylius Parisanus, a physician of Venice, was the next to assail the Harveian doctrine of the circulation,[2] and still with

---

[1] Entitled 'Exercitationes et Animadversiones in Librum Harvei de Motu Cordis et Sanguinis,' 4to, London, 1630.

[2] In his work entitled 'Lapis Lydius de Motu Cordis et Sanguinis,' folio, Venet. 1635.

the old instruments,—the authority of Galen and the ancients generally. Parisanus perceived Harvey's views as directly contravening an hypothesis to which he had formerly committed himself, namely, that the spleen was the organ of sanguification and the furnisher of nutriment to the heart; on this ground may Parisanus have been led to enter the lists against the new opinions. But he proved a most flimsy antagonist. Ignorant of some of the commonest points of anatomy, and frequently misinterpreting the writer he combats, writing himself in a style the most elaborately involved, and consequently obscure, it is frequently difficult even to guess at his meaning. Like his countryman of the poet, Signor Gratiano, he

" Speaks an infinite deal of nothing; more than any man in all Venice : his reasons are two grains of wheat hid in two bushels of chaff; you shall seek all day ere you find them ; and when you have them they are not worth the search."

Had not Dr. Ent, in his Apology for the Circulation, given the name a place on his title-page, Parisanus's opposition would scarcely have merited mention here.

Nearly at the same time with Parisanus, Caspar Hofmann, the learned and laborious professor of Nuremberg, attracted particular attention, both in his teaching and his writings, as the opponent of the Harveian doctrine. The opposition here is the more remarkable from Hofmann's having shaken himself wholly free from the authority of Galen, and, as Slegel says, even admitted the lesser circulation of the blood through the lungs; but this must have been at a later period of his life, for in his works, up to Harvey's time, the idea he had of the motion of the blood may be gathered from his likening it to a lake or sea agitated by the wind, the veins being the conduits of the nutrient blood, the arteries of the vital spirits. Hofmann was an adversary whom Harvey held worthy of notice; and accordingly we have seen that our immortal countryman took advantage of the opportunity, whilst attending the Earl of Arundel and his party, to visit Hofmann at Nuremberg, and make a demonstration of the new views before him. Unhappily this was done in vain, for Hofmann continued unconvinced, though, towards the end of his very long life, he did show some signs of yielding.[1]

Joannes Veslingius, professor in the University of Padua, and one of the best anatomists of the age, about this time, addressed two letters to Harvey, in which he politely but candidly states his objections to the new doctrine. One great difficulty with Veslingius was the remarkable difference between the colour of the arterial and the venous blood. It did not seem possible to him that the fluid, which was of a bright scarlet in the arteries, could be the same as the dark-coloured fluid which is found in the veins. In the course of his letter, Veslingius takes occasion to animadvert on the uncivil tone and indifferent style of the productions of Primerose and Parisanus.[2]

But the theory of the double circulation was not now to meet with opposition only; the comprehensive intellect that had seized and worked that theorem to a rational demonstration was no longer to be left alone against the world in its defence. Roger Drake, a young Englishman, had the honour of appearing in his inaugural dissertation, proposed under the auspices of Joannes Walæus, the distinguished professor of Leyden, in 1639, as the enlightened advocate of the Harveian views; and in the course of the same year, H. Regius (Leroy) also came forward at Utrecht with certain Theses favorable to the doctrine of the circulation. Ten years had not lessened Primerose's enmity to Harvey and his views; for, on the appearance of these academical essays, he speedily showed himself again in the field as their opponent, publishing distinct animadver-

---

[1] Vide Slegel, De Sang. Motu in Præf.

[2] Veslingius's letters may be found in his Observationes Anatomicæ et Epist. Med. ex schedis pothumis, 12mo, Hafn. 1664. It is much to be regretted that the replies which Harvey doubtless wrote to these epistles have not been preserved.

sions upon each of the inaugural dissertations in the course of the year.[1] Regius (Leroy), a man of much less mind and information than Drake, if we may decide from their works, was, in turn, not slow to encounter Primerose;[2] and the spirit in which he did so, as well as the temper and taste of the reply which Primerose, true to his controversial nature, very soon produced,[3] may, to a certain extent, be imagined from the titles of their several productions, which are given below.

Still more illustrious advocates of the Harveian circulation presented themselves in Werner Rolfink,[4] professor of anatomy at Jena, and the celebrated Renatus Descartes. Rolfink, from his position and his popularity as a teacher, had immense influence in disseminating the new doctrine over Europe; and Descartes, under the ægis of his powerful name, was no less effective by means of his writings.[5] Opposed in his advocacy of the Harveian views by Vopiscus Fortunatus Plempius, professor of Louvain, Descartes made himself still more thoroughly master of the subject, and when he next appears as its advocate, which he does by and by, he even appeals to the experiments he had made on living animals in support of his convictions and conclusions.

The controversy on the circulation had been carried on up to this time abroad rather than at home; Harvey seems to have won over to his side all the men of his own country who, by their education and acquirements, might have been fitted to array themselves against him : his lectures at the College of Physicians had apparently satisfied all his contemporaries. But now one of Harvey's own countrymen made his appear-

[1] Animadversiones in J. Walæi (Drake) Disputationem quam pro Circulatione Sanguinis proposuit, 4to, Amst. 1639. Animad. in Theses quas pro Circulat. Sang. Hen. Regius proposuit, 4to, Leidæ, 1640.

[2] Spongia qua eluuntur sordes Animad. quas Jac. Primirosius advers. Theses, &c., edidit. 4to, Leidæ, 1640.

[3] Antidotum adversus Spongiam Venenatam Hen. Regii, 4to, Leidæ, 1640.

[4] Epist. duæ ad Th. Bartholinum de Motu Chyli et Sanguinis, 8vo, Leid. 1641.

[5] Epist. Cartesii, 4to, Amst. 1668.

ance as the vindicator of the circulation from the misrepresen-
tations and misapprehensions of its adversaries. This was Dr.
afterwards Sir George Ent, a good scholar, a respectable anatomist, conversant with physical science generally, a gentleman
by his position and profession, acquainted with all the leading
men of letters and science of his time, and in particular,
enjoying the friendship of William Harvey. Ent's work is
entitled 'An Apology for the Circulation of the Blood, with a
Reply to Æmylius Parisanus.'[1] In his letter to Harvey, which
stands in front of the work, Ent lets it appear that he was anxious
to come before the world as the advocate of the circulation ;
he first thought of making Primerose the particular object of his
animadversions, but as this opponent had already been very
effectually handled by Henry Leroy, he preferred taking Parisanus to task, the rather as in dealing with him he could also
controvert Primerose where it was necessary.—Ent's Apology
is, undoubtedly, a learned, though perhaps a somewhat pompous
and pedantic book ; still the writer occasionally shows both
wit and fancy in handling his antagonist, and always learning
enough in dealing with his subject. "Nothing, indeed," to quote
Dr. Lawrence,[2] " can be more unlike than Parisanus and Ent ;
and it is not wonderful, therefore, that one utterly ignorant
of physical science confronted by one thoroughly conversant
therein—that one, without power of utterance, opposed by one
gifted with eloquence—that one, sluggish and inert, in the
hands of one active and full of energy, should be effectually vanquished and overcome." We may imagine, nay, we may be
certain, that Harvey was not unacquainted with Ent's purpose
to appear as the advocate of his discovery, nor with the Apology
before it saw the light.

Having observed the appearance of certain academical dis-

---

[1] Apologia pro Circuitione Sanguinis, qua respondetur Æmylio Parisano, 8vo,
Lond. 1641.

[2] Harvei vita, ad cap. Operum, London, 1766.

sertations in defence of the circulation, we perceive the apostles of all new truths, namely, the youthful, at work. Were there not successive generations of men, the world would stand still; the death of the individual was not merely a necessary condition to the enjoyment of life by successive generations, but essential also to the onward progress of mankind. No man who had attained to the age of 40 years, it is said, was found to adopt the doctrine of the circulation; it had to win its way under the safeguard of the Drakes and Leroys especially, that is to say, of the youthful and unprejudiced spirits of the age.

Twenty years after the publication of the ʻ Exercitatio de Motu Cordis et Sanguinis,ʼ Joannes Riolanus, the younger, was delivered of his ʻ Encheiridium Anatomicumʼ (8vo. Lugd. Batav. 1648), in which he makes a vain attempt to supplant the Harveian doctrine by a new and most extraordinary one of his own, so incongruous and unlikely, that in these days we are irresistibly led to form no very high estimate of the intellect that could have engendered it. It looks to us, indeed, at this time, like condescension on the part of the great English anatomist, that he noticed the abortion of such a tyro in animal physics as the French professor here approves himself. Harvey's genius could surely have felt no real respect for the illogical intellect of Riolan. But Harvey, when he noticed Riolan's publication, was in want of a good occasion for a farther development of his own views; and so he seized on the Parisian professor, respectable from his position in the university, and as physician to the queen mother of France, and made him his vehicle—his placard bearer. Harvey, besides, was personally acquainted with Riolan, who had accompanied Mary de Medicis to England on a visit to her daughter the Queen of Charles the First; on which occasion Harvey and Riolan had even held conversations on the subject of the circulation, to which it is said that Riolan when face to face with the propounder, made no objection.

Riolan is by no means totally opposed to a circulation of the blood; he would only limit it to certain arbitrary regions, into which he divides the body : whilst it goes forward in one, it has no existence in another. The nature of his ideas can be gathered from Harvey's comments on them in his First Disquisition, addressed to the Coryphæus of Anatomists, as he politely designates the Parisian professor.

Having disposed of the original notions of the author of the 'Encheiridium Anatomicum,' in this first disquisition, Harvey, in his second, returns to his own views, which he proceeds still further to illustrate and confirm by additional arguments, observations, and experiments. In this admirable essay, we obtain innumerable glimpses of the clearness of Harvey's judgment, of his admirable powers of observation, and the diligent and excellent use he made of them; we at the same time become aware of the great loss we have sustained through the destruction of his Medical Observations. Riolan, in his Encheiridium, proposed to point out in the structure of the healthy body the seats of the various diseases, and to discuss their nature in conformity with the opinions that had been entertained of them. This was obviously at once a barren and an impracticable route : the matters he had in hand could never have been other than abstractions, and his own observations criticisms on opinions, never on facts. How much more natural and judicious the course which Harvey proposes to himself, when he informs us that in his ' Medical Anatomy' he meant, "from the many dissections he had made of the bodies of persons worn out by serious and strange affections, to relate how and in what way the internal organs were changed in their situation, size, structure, figure, consistency, and other sensible qualities, from their natural forms and appearances, such as they are usually described by anatomists; and in what various and remarkable ways they were affected. For even as the dissection of healthy and well-constituted bodies contributes essentially to the advancement of philosophy and sound physiology, so does the inspection of diseased and cachectic subjects powerfully assist philosophical pathology." This was precisely what Morgagni lived, in some considerable measure, to achieve, and it is that which it has been the business of modern pathology, through the illustrious line of the Baillies, Laennecs, Andrals, Louis, Cruveilhiers, Carswells, Richard Brights, and many others, to render more and more complete.

Riolan never replied to Harvey ; but neither did the Parisian Professor attempt to vindicate his views, nor did he exhibit such candour as to own himself otherwise convinced or converted. His doctrine had no abettors, and never bore fruit ; it stood a barren ear amidst the lusty, green, and copious harvest, that had already sprung up and overspread the lands.

Harvey must now, indeed, have seen his views assured of general reception at no distant date. The same year in which he himself answered Riolan, Dr. James de Back, of Amsterdam, published his work on the Heart,[1] which is written entirely in harmony with the Harveian doctrines, and the celebrated Lazarus Riverius, Professor of Medicine in the University of Montpellier, publicly defended and taught the circulation of the blood.[2] The following year, Paul Marquard Slegel, of Hamburg, produced his commentary on the Motion of the Blood,[3] in which he addresses himself particularly to a refutation of Riolanus, whose scholar he had been, and at the same time shows himself so thoroughly at home in the general ques-

---

[1] De Corde, Amst. 1649 ; in English, 12mo, Lond. 1653.

[2] A candour for which he was by and by summoned by an adherent of the old school to resign his chair.

[3] De Sanguinis Motu Commentarius, 4to, Hamb. 1650.

d

tion, that he is able to throw additional light on it by new and ingenious considerations and experiments.

Harvey appears to have been pleased with Slegel's production; for by and by he sends the Hamburger his new work on Generation, accompanied by an admirable letter, which has happily been preserved.[1] No one in reading that remarkable epistle could suppose that the pen which set it down was in the hand of a man in the 75th year of his age.

The young men of 1628 and 1630, who had been educated in unbelief of the circulation, were now coming into possession of professorial chairs and places of distinction; and having long escaped from leading-strings and made inquiry for themselves, were beginning in many of the European universities to proclaim the better faith through further knowledge that had sprung up within them. Harvey had himself received the seeds of his discovery in Italy; but the fructifying mother was slow to recognize him whom she had so powerfully concurred to form. It was not till 1651 that Harvey's views were in any way admitted beyond the Alps, when Trullius, a Roman professor, expounded and taught them. About the same time, John Pecquet,[2] of Dieppe, and Thomas Bartholin, the Dane,[3] men of original mind in the one case, of extensive learning and great research in the other, gave in their adhesion to the new doctrine, and spread it far and near by their writings. The victory for the circulation may finally be said to have been won, when Plempius, of Louvain, the old antagonist of Descartes on the subject, retracted all he had formerly written against it, convinced of its truth, as he so candidly informs us, by the very pains he took to satisfy himself of its erroneousness, and publicly proclaimed his conversion: "Primum mihi hoc inventum non

---

[1] Vide p. 596.

[2] Experimenta nova Anatomica. Acced. de Motu Sanguinis Diss., 8vo, Paris, 1651.

[3] Anatomia ex Casp. Bartholini Parent. Institut. ad Sanguinis Circulationem, tertium Reformata, 8vo, Leid. 1651.

placuit," says the worthy Plempius—" This discovery did not please me at all at first, as I publicly testified both by word of mouth and in my writings; but by and by, when I gave myself up with firmer purpose to refute and expose it, lo ! I refute and expose myself, so convincing, not to say merely persuasive, are the arguments of the author : I examine the whole thing anew and with greater care, and having at length made the dissection of a few live dogs, I find that all his statements are most true."[1]

From the first promulgation of the doctrine of the circulation, its progress towards ultimate general acknowledgment can scarcely be said for a moment to have been interrupted. The hostility of the Primeroses and Parisanuses and Riolans never interfered with it in fact ; the more candid spirits were rather led to inquire, by the virulence of these weak and inconsistent opponents, who thus hastened the catastrophe of their own discomfiture, and the triumph of the truth. If men's minds were once in danger of being led astray, it was only for an instant, and not so much through the opposition of enemies, as by an erroneous generalization, which a short interval of time sufficed to correct. Cæcilius Folius, a Venetian physician, having met with one of those anomalous instances of pervious foramen ovale in an adult, immediately and without looking farther, jumped to the conclusion that this structure or arrangement was normal, and that the blood passed in all cases by the route he had discovered, from the right to the left side of the heart. Many Italians received with favour the account which Folius immediately published of his discovery ;[2] and the natural philosopher, Gassendi, having about the same period had another instance of the kind which Folius encountered, shown to him, concurred with this writer in his views, and by a variety of arguments and objections, strove to damage, and did temporarily damage,

---

[1] Plempius, Fundamenta Medicinæ, fol. Lovan. 1652, p. 128.

[2] Sanguinis a dextro in sinistrum Cordis Ventriculum defluentis facilis reperta via, fol. Venet. 1639.

the Harveian doctrine.[1]   But this was only for a brief season ;
for Domenic de Marchettis[2] soon after showed that Folius had
mistaken an extremely rare occurrence for a general fact, and
that if the open foramen ovale might afford a passage from
the right to the left side of the heart in one case, closed it
would suffer no such transit in hundreds of other instances.
Gassendi, moreover, by getting still more out of his depth,
soon afterwards showed that familiarity with general physics
did not imply a particular knowledge of anatomy, nor give the
power of reasoning sagely on subjects of special physiology ;
so that in his eagerness to assail Harvey he did injury in the end
only to his own reputation.   In short, Harvey in his lifetime
had the high satisfaction of witnessing his discovery generally
received, and inculcated as a canon in most of the medical schools
of Europe ; he is, therefore, one of the few—his friend Thomas
Hobbes says, he was the only one within his knowledge—"Solus
quod sciam,"[3] who lived to see the new doctrine which he had
promulgated victorious over opposition, and established in
public opinion.   Harvey's views, then, were admitted ; the
circulation of the blood, through the action of the heart, was
received as an established fact ; but envy and detraction now
began their miserable work.   The fact was so; but it was none of
Harvey's discovering ; the fact was so, but it was of no great
moment in itself, and the merit of arriving at it was small ;
the way had been amply prepared for such a conclusion.

Let us look as impartially as we may at each of these statements.

They who deny the originality of Harvey's induction, very
commonly confound the idea of a Motion of the blood, with
the idea of a Continuous Motion in a Circle.   It would seem

---

[1] Gassendi, 'De Septo Cordis pervio,' published in a collection by Severinus Pinæus, 12mo, Leid. 1640.

[2] D. de Marchettis, Anatomia, 8vo, Padova, 1652.

[3] Elementa Philosophiæ in Præfat.

that even from remote antiquity, and by common consent, mankind had recognized the blood to be in motion. We have this fact declared to us by all antiquity, and it is even particularly referred to in various passages of the grand observer of his age, the depositary of the popular science of all preceding ages—Shakespeare. Brutus speaks thus to Portia:

> " You are my true and honourable wife;
> As dear to me as are the ruddy drops
> That visit my sad heart ;"

language not more touching and beautiful than physiologically correct. And again, with more of involution and ellipsis, yet with a meaning that is unmistakable, Warwick, by the bedside of the murdered Gloster, proceeds,—

> " See how the blood is settled in his face !
> —Oft have I seen a timely-parted ghost,
> Of ashy semblance, meagre, pale and bloodless,
> —Being all descended to the labouring heart,
> Who in the conflict that he holds with death,
> Attracts the same for aidance gainst the enemy ;
> Which with the heart there cools, and ne'er returneth
> To blush and beautify the cheek again—
> —But see, his face is black and full of blood," &c.

These passages have actually been cited, to prove that Shakespeare was not unacquainted with the circulation; and there have not been wanting some[1] who have even argued that Shakespeare had his knowledge direct from the fountain-head— from Harvey himself, with whom, for several years at least, he was contemporaneous.[2]

The passages quoted above are referred to all the more willingly, from their having preceded the teaching of Harvey by a few years only ; but Shakespeare probably referred to

---

[1] Thomas Nimmo, Esq., of New Amsterdam, Berbice: " On a passage in Shakespeare's Julius Cæsar." The Shakespeare Society's Papers, vol. ii, p. 109.

[2] Shakespeare died in 1616, the year when Harvey began to lecture at the College of Physicians. Harvey and Shakespeare may very well have been acquainted, —let us hope that they were,—but there is no authority for saying that they were friends.

nothing more than the accredited opinion that the blood was in motion within the vessels, particularly the veins of the body. In ancient times, indeed, the veins were regarded, as they are esteemed by the vulgar at the present hour, as the principal vessels of the body; they only were once believed to contain true blood; the arteries were held to contain at best but a little blood, different from that of the veins, and mixed accidentally in some sort with the vital spirits, of which they were the proper conduits.

In former times, farther,—times anterior to Harvey whether more remotely or more nearly,—the liver, as the organ of the hæmapoësis, was regarded as the source of all the veins, i. e. of all the proper blood-vessels; the heart, as the generator of heat and the vital spirits, was viewed as the mere cistern of the blood, whence it was propelled by the act of inspiration, and whither it reverted during the act of expiration, its flow to this part of the body or to that, being mainly determined by certain excitations there inherent or specially set up. By and by, however, the liver was given up as the origin of the venous system generally; but such anatomists as Jacobus Sylvius, Realdus Columbus, Bartholomæus Eustachius, and Gabriel Fallopius, may be found opposing Vesalius in regard to the origin of the vena cava, and asserting that it takes its rise from the liver, not from the heart, as the great reformer in modern anatomy had maintained.

In the progress of anatomical investigation, the valves in the interior of the heart, at the roots of the two great cardiac arterial trunks, and in the course of the veins at large, were perceived and their probable uses and actions canvassed. The general and prevalent notion was that they served to break or moderate the force of the current in the interior of the vessels or parts where they were encountered; though Berengarius of Carpi,[1] in describing the cardiac valves, had already said that the effect of the tricuspid valves, between the right auricle and ventricle, must be to prevent the blood in the former cavity

---

[1] Comment. super Anatomiam Mundini, 4to, Bonon. 1521.

from escaping into the latter; whilst the office of the semi-lunar valves, at the origins of the pulmonic artery and aorta, he declared, from their position, must be to prevent the entrance of the blood of the great arterial trunks into the heart. Fabricius, the master of Harvey, may be said to have perfected anatomical knowledge in regard to the valves of the veins—for he by no means first directed attention to their existence, or discovered them, as is generally asserted. Fabricius believed that their function was to act as obstacles to congestions of blood, as strengtheners of the veins and preventives to their becoming over-distended.

Another long and much agitated point in the anatomy of the sanguiferous system, was the state of the septum ventriculorum of the heart, in respect of permeability or impermeability. The reason of the vast importance attached to this point was connected with the ancient, and, in Harvey's time, generally accredited hypothesis of the Three Spirits—the natural, the vital, and the animal. The hypothesis to be brought into play, was presumed to require the intermixture in the heart of the two kinds of blood that were held appropriate to the two ventricles and to the arteries and veins respectively, and that were farther believed to meet in the cavities of the cranium, thorax, and abdomen, from which they returned to the heart by the way they came, for a fresh supply of the spirits (now exhausted or enfeebled), under the agency of which all the important operations of the body were believed to be accomplished.

Now, Galen, the author of this hypothesis, in order to obtain an admixture of the two kinds of blood, feigned and described the partition between the two ventricles, either as perforated like a sieve, or as filled with depressions of depth sufficient to entitle them to be viewed as constituting a kind of third ventricle—the last assumption doubtless to accommodate each order of spirits with its own particular officine or workshop.

With the revival of anatomical knowledge in modern Europe, however, the partition of the ventricles was soon perceived not to be porous or cribriform, but, as was first said, to be so nearly solid that any filtration of blood through it was well nigh impossible (Berengarius, 1521), and next, to be so completely solid that all permeation of blood was impossible (Vesalius, 1555), and another means must therefore be found for securing the necessary admixture of the two kinds of blood in order to effect the engenderment of the natural, animal, and vital spirits.

Such was the state of anatomical science and physiological belief on this particular point when Michael Servetus came upon the stage, and suggested the transit of the blood through the lungs from the right side of the heart to the left, with a view of meeting the difficulty which the undeniable solidity of the septum ventriculorum opposed to the presumed necessary admixture of the two kinds of blood. Servetus's idea, conse‐ quently—if at the distance of three hundred years we may presume to follow the mental process that led to the penning of the remarkable and often-quoted passage which occurs in his works—appears to be nothing more than a suggestion or proposition as a means of meeting a difficulty; it is very much as though he had said : If you cannot go straight through, you must even go round about. To so much and to no more, do Servetus's claims to be considered a discoverer, in the sense we would attach to that word, amount. The passage from the ‘Restitutio Christianismi’ of Servetus, 1553, if viewed from the point proposed, will not fail to set his title to be regarded as the discoverer of the lesser circulation in its true light—in a light under which it has not yet been seen. We translate so much of the passage as bears on the question under review. “ The vital spirit has its origin in the left ventricle, the lungs assisting especially in its generation. It is a subtile spirit * * * It is engendered from the mixture that takes place in the lungs of the inspired air with the elaborated subtile blood which the right ventricle of the heart communicates to the left. But this communication takes place, not by the middle septum of the heart, as is commonly believed, but by a remarkable artifice ; the subtile blood of the right side of the heart is agitated in a lengthened course through the lungs, whereby it is elaborated, from which it is thrown of a crimson colour, and from the vena arteriosa (pulmonary artery) is transfused into the arteria venosa (pulmonary veins) ; it is then mixed in the arteria venosa itself with the inspired air, and by the act of expiration is purified from fuliginous vapours, when, having become the fit recipient of the vital spirit, it is at length attracted by the diastole. Now, that the communication and preparation take place as stated through the lungs, is proclaimed by the various conjunctions and communications of the arterial vein with the venous artery. The remarkable size of the arterial vein (pulmonary artery) confirms this, a vessel which could neither have its actual constitution nor dimensions, nor transmit such a quantity of the purest blood direct from the heart itself, for the mere nourishment of the lungs. Neither would the heart supply the lungs in such proportion, (especially when we see the lungs in the embryo nourished from another source) by reason of those membranes or valves which remain unopened until the hour of birth, as Galen teaches. The blood, consequently, from the moment of birth, is sent, and in such quantity is sent, for another purpose from the heart into the lungs ; from the lungs also it is not simple air that is sent to the heart, but air mixed with blood is transmitted through the arteria venosa (pulmonary vein). In the lungs consequently does the mixture take place. The crimson colour is imparted to the spirituous blood by the lungs, not by the heart. There is not room enough in the left ventricle of the heart for so important and so great an admixture ; neither is there space there for the elaboration into the crimson colour. Finally, the septum medium, seeing that it is without vessels and properties, is not adapted to accomplish that communication and elaboration, although something may transude through it."

The discussion in this passage from Servetus obviously concerns the generation of the vital spirit, not the pulmonic circulation properly so called—that is altogether secondary and subordinate. His mention of "numerous communications between the vena arteriosa and the arteria venosa," is plainly conjectural; neither he, nor any one else for a century after him, saw such communications. The course through the lungs, then, as suggested by Servetus, was a mere hypothetical proposal for getting over the difficulty of the solid, or nearly solid, septum ventriculorum. As to the means by which such a transfusion as he suggests, is effected, Servetus, as he was profoundly ignorant himself, so does he leave his readers entirely in the dark. The transmission of the blood from the right to the left side of the heart, which Servetus proposed, is in fact, no great improvement on the old efflux and reflux, like the tides of Euripus, betwixt Attica and Euboea. He had no conception of a circle of the blood beginning and ending in the heart. On the contrary, he regarded the liver as the fountain-head of the blood; and if he has any reference to a moving power in connexion with the heart, it is nothing more than the diastole or dilatation of the organ that is named—a passive state therefore considered as an active and efficient cause, which is absurd.

The first modern anatomist of high repute, who treats particularly of the motion of the blood, may be said to be Realdus Columbus;[1] for Servetus, though educated to the medical profession, had long forsaken it for divinity, and only uses his old anatomical knowledge as a means of illustrating a theological dogma. Columbus, in treating of the heart and lungs, has certainly much that is remarkable, and much that is true;

---

[1] De Re Anatomica, fol. Venet. 1559.

and had he said nothing more than we find in single detached
sentences or paragraphs of his book, he must have been regarded as having gone a great length in the right direction.
The blood, he says, once it has entered the right ventricle
from the vena cava, can in no way again get back; for the
tricuspid valves are so placed that whilst they give a ready passage to the stream inwards, they effectually oppose its return.
The blood continuing to advance from the right ventricle into
the vena arteriosa or pulmonary artery, once there cannot flow
back upon the ventricle, for it is opposed by the sigmoid valves
situate at the root of the vessel. The blood, therefore, agitated
and mixed with the air in the lungs, and having thus
in some sort acquired the nature of spirit, is carried by the
arteria venosa or pulmonary vein into the left ventricle, from
whence, being received into the aorta, it is, by the ramifications of this vessel, transmitted to all parts of the body.

This much taken by itself looks very like an exposition of
the circulation of the blood as understood at the present time,
though we still see that the blood must be made to participate
in the nature of spirit before it enters the arteries, and is not
the blood which is contained in the veins, and which nourishes
the body; but when we go farther and turn to other parts of his
writings, we see that Columbus could never have conceived any
proper idea of the circulation. For example, he continues, with
Galen, to regard the liver as the origin of all the veins. The
vena portæ, he says, arising by innumerable roots from the concavity of the liver, proceeds to carry blood from this organ by
different branches to the stomach, spleen, and intestines, to the
end that it may convey nourishment in the first case, black bile
in the second, and in the third serve a double function—viz.
supply nourishment to the intestines at once, and by a kind
of imbibition, obtain nutritive matter, which is forthwith sent
back to the liver for elaboration into blood. The vena cava
again, he describes as arising from the convex aspect of the

liver, whence, by its ramifications, it carries the blood that is
requisite to nourish and maintain every part of the body.

This of itself is enough. But when, in addition, we find
that Columbus denies the muscular nature of the heart, we are
fully qualified to form a true estimate of the conception which
he could have had of the motion of the blood, and of his right
to be regarded as the discoverer of its ceaseless circular movement.

The next who is brought upon the scene with the imputed
honour of having had a knowledge, not only of the lesser, but
of the greater or systemic circulation also, is Andreas
Cæsalpinus,[1] of Arezzo. The account which this celebrated
peripatetic philosopher gives of the passage of the blood from
the right to the left side of the heart is essentially the same as
that given by Columbus. From the right ventricle the blood
passes into the pulmonic artery, and from this, by numerous
anastomoses, into the pulmonic veins, which transmit it to the
left ventricle. Cæsalpinus says well that it is absurd to call the
pulmonary artery by the name of vena arteriosa, on the mere
ground of its taking its departure, like the vena cava, from
the right ventricle; it is a true artery, and is, in all respects,
analogous to the aorta. The title of arteria venosa, again,
given to the pulmonic vein is not less ridiculous; inasmuch
as this vessel, though it end in the left ventricle, has all the
properties of the veins at large.

So far it looks as if Cæsalpinus had an exact idea of the
pulmonary circulation; indeed, he uses the word Circulation
in reference to the transit of the blood through the lungs;
but when we discover him still speaking of the permeation
of the septum ventriculorum by the blood, our faith in the
extent and accuracy of his knowledge begins to waver.

With reference to the greater or systemic circulation, again,

---

[1] Quæstiones Peripateticæ, fol. Florent. 1569; Quæst. Medicinales, fol. Venet.
1593; De Plantis, Florent. 1583.

Cæsalpinus speaks of the swelling of the veins between the circle of pressure and the extremities of the vessels, when a ligature is thrown round a limb ; and he even goes so far as to state that the common opinion which admitted a progressive motion—i. e. a motion from trunks to branches—of the blood in the veins was erroneous. Did we go no farther we should be led to conclude, as in Columbus's case, that Cæsalpinus believed in the continuous movement of the blood in the veins in one direction only ; and, as he has already spoken of the exit of the blood from the left ventricle, and of its reception by the aorta for general distribution, it might forthwith be inferred that, possessed of the essential elements of the greater circulation, he must, as matter of course, have been familiar with this as an ultimate result. And such an inference has indeed been drawn for him by high authority ; but Cæsalpinus came not himself to any such conclusion ; it was arrived at by others in his behalf, and after the lapse of almost a century from the date of his first publication. When we find Cæsalpinus, in other and closely connected passages of his writings, singing the old cuckoo note about a flux and reflux of the blood in the veins, and even using the accredited word—Euripus —to express his idea of its tide-like nature ; when we further perceive that he was ignorant of the existence of the valves of the veins, and finally arrive at his explanation of the cause of the swelling which takes place in the veins of an extremity beyond a ligature,—the cause with him consisting in an effort of the blood to get back to the focus or centre, lest, through the compression of the veins, it should be cut off and suffocated, —we not only feel that we were warranted in entertaining a wholesome scepticism of the conclusion come to by the admirers of Cæsalpinus in regard to his knowledge of a circulation of the blood ; but waxing in our infidelity as we become farther acquainted with his thoughts on the constitution of the blood, we find everything opposed to the likelihood of his having arrived at the same result as Harvey; and, at length, we discover that he neither had nor could have had any true knowledge of the circulation. Starting from the Aristotelian doctrines of growth and nutrition (of which so much will be found in Harvey's work on Generation), Cæsalpinus held that there were two kinds of blood, one for the growth, another for the nourishment of the body. The blood which went to augment the body, and which he designated alimentum auctivum, or aliment of increase, flowed from the liver into the vena cava, which he seems to have thought was connected with the heart only, ut inde virtus omnis a corde descendat— that a sufficiency of virtue might be thereby communicated to it. The auctive blood, he farther thought, was attracted into the ventricles of the heart by the inherent heat of the organ. The dilatation of the heart and arteries he imagined to be due to " an effervescence of the spirit ;" and the cause of their " collapse"—not systole, be it observed, in the active sense— was the appropriation by the parts of the body of the nutritive and augmentative matter. Again, though Cæsalpinus speaks of the intercommunication of the minute arteries and veins, he still thought that it was only during sleep that the blood mixed with the spirits passed from the former into the latter class of vessels; for it is during sleep, he says, that the veins become distended, whilst the pulsations of the arteries are then moderated. He plainly sees no connexion between a delivery by the artery and a filling by the vein. It is along with all this, and as if to settle the question of the kind of knowledge Cæsalpinus had of the movement of the blood, that he uses the old word Euripus, to express his idea of its alternating or tide-like motion.

Cæsalpinus, let us add, had no conception of the heart as the efficient cause of any motion which the blood might have.

In the often-quoted passage from the work ' De Plantis,'[1] it is still the spirit inherent in, or associated with, the blood, that is the cause of its motion.

Cæsalpinus, consequently, tried by a very moderately searching criticism, presents himself to us as but very little farther advanced than the ancients in his ideas on the motion of the blood.—The interpretation which successive generations of men give to a passage in a writer, some century or two old, is very apt to be in consonance with the state of knowledge at the time, in harmony with the prevailing ideas of the day, and, doubtless, often differs signally from the meaning that was in the mind of the man who composed it.   The world saw nothing of the circulation of the blood in Servetus, Columbus, Cæsalpinus, or—Shakespeare, until after William Harvey had taught and written.

The truth is, that some of the foremost grounds of Harvey's claims to rank as a discoverer are very commonly overlooked.   We always associate his name and fame with the development of the ultimate fact of the circulation of the blood. But Harvey, as a step to this conclusion, first demonstrated the heart as the means by which the circulation was effected; and he farther showed that there was but *one* kind of blood, common to both the arteries and the veins.   Up to his time the heart was regarded as the passive cistern of the blood; and the elaboratory of the vital spirits; it was not known as the moving instrument in any efflux or reflux of the blood, or even of any lesser circulation that had been previously asserted or conjectured.   The moving power was still the respiratory act. Harvey may be said to have first broached, as he also essentially completed the physiology of the heart's actions.   The circular motion of the blood followed as a necessary corollary from these.   The "motion of the heart" has even precedence in the title of his immortal work; the chapter in which

---

[1] Qua autem ratione fiat alimenti attractio, &c.   De Plantis, lib. i, cap. 2, p. 3, 4to, Florent. 1583.

he first enters properly on his subject (Chap. 2), is devoted
to its consideration. And then, no physiologist up to Harvey's
time had questioned the existence of two kinds of blood, one
appropriate to each order of vessels, and answering different
ends in the economy.

The only name still wanting in this historical sketch, till
we come to Harvey, is that of Fabricius of Aquapendente, his
teacher in anatomy. Fabricius had given particular attention,
among other subjects, to the anatomy of the valves of the
veins, which he entitled ostila venarum. Fabricius, indeed,
possessed so thorough a knowledge of the valvular elements of
the vascular system, that it is really astonishing, as an able
writer[1] has remarked, that he should not have had clearer ideas
on the functions, among other things, of the pulmonary veins,
and should have continued a rigid adherent to the prejudices
which prevailed before his time. Fabricius could observe, and
he could describe; but he wanted the combining intellect that
infers, the imagination that leads to new ideas—to discovery.
Though he did little himself, however, to advance the sum of
human knowledge, he proved a tooth in the wheel that has
since put in motion the whole machinery of modern medical
science.   He it was who sowed the seed, little dreaming of its
kind, which, finding one spot of congenial soil, sprung up a
harvest that has continued to nurture the world of physiological
science to the present hour.[2]

[1] Sprengel, Geschichte der Arzneikunde, ii Abschnitt, 4 Kapitel.

[2] I pass by unnoticed in my text several names that have been very gratuitously
associated with the discovery of the circulation, such as that of Father Paul the
Venetian, Walter Warner and Mr. Prothero, Honoratus Faber, &c. The claims of
Father Paul have been satisfactorily explained by Dr. Ent in his 'Apology,' who has
shown that instead of Harvey borrowing from the Monk, the Monk, through the
Venetian ambassador to London, who was Harvey's friend, had borrowed from
Harvey.   The others do not require serious mention.   Dr. Freind has given
an excellent summary of the entire doctrine of the circulation in his Harveian
Oration, to which it is with much pleasure that I refer the reader for other information. I also pass by the still-recurring denials by obtuse and ill-informed individuals
of the truth, or of the sufficiency of the evidence of the truth, of the Harveian cir-

Having now disposed of the claims that have been set up in behalf of one or another as the discoverer of the circulation, and shown, we trust satisfactorily, that these are all alike untenable, we should now proceed to discuss the question of the cui bono?—but this meets us in so forbidding an aspect, brimful as is our mind with a sense of the all-importance of the knowledge we had from Harvey, and seems so little to belong to our subject, that we gladly pass it by unnoticed; though it be only to find ourselves encountered by that other topic, but little more congenial to our mood of mind and intimate persuasion : The merit of Harvey as a discoverer. Few, very few have been found to question this ; but as one man of undeniable learning and eminence in his profession,[1] has very strangely, as it seems to us, been led to do so, it will not be impertinent if we cast away a few words on this matter.

Discovery is of several, particularly of two kinds: one sensible or perceptive ; another rational or inductive ; the former an act of simple consciousness through an impression made on one or more of the senses ; the latter a conclusion come to by the higher powers of the understanding dealing with data previously acquired by the senses and perceptive faculties.—We look through a telescope, for example, and we perceive a star which no one else had seen before ; we note the fact, and so become discoverers of a new star. The merit here is not, surely, very great, though the added fact may be highly important. Again, one of the planets is subject to such perturbations in its course that to compose exact tables of its orbit is held impossible. These perturbations are referable to none of the known perturbing causes. A great astronomer suggests the influence of an exterior and unknown planet as their cause. A

culation. Those who *can* not see, must, contrary to the popular adage, be admitted to be still blinder than those who *will* not see.

[1] Dr. William Hunter. Introductory Lectures, p. 59, (4to. Lond. 1784,) to which the reader is referred for a singularly inconsistent and extraordinary string of passages.

consummate mathematician and physical astronomer makes trial of this suggestion : he assumes the ascertained perturbations as elements, he combines these under the guidance of knowledge and reason, and at length he says, if the cause suggested be well founded, there or thereabouts must it exist ; and lo ! on turning the far-seeing tube to the point in space which he had indicated, there in verity gleams a new world, then first seen, though launched by God from Eternity to circle on the verge of our creation ; and he who bade us look becomes the discoverer of a new planet. Who will dispute the merit here ? Truly, man does show the God within him when he uses his faculties —God-like in themselves—in such God-like fashion. But Harvey's merit, according to our idea, was of the selfsame description in another sphere. The facts he used were familiarly known, most of them to his predecessors for nearly a century, all of them to his teachers and immediate contemporaries; yet did no one, mastering these facts in their connexion and sequence, rising superior to prejudice, groundless hypothesis, and erroneous reasoning, draw the inference that now meets the world as irresistible, until the combining mind of Harvey gave it shape and utterance. To our apprehension Harvey was as far above his fellows as the eye of poetic intelligence, that exultingly absorbs the beauties of the starry sky and the green earth, is above the mere physical sense that distinguishes light from dark. The late Dr. Barclay, a fervent admirer of Harvey, whose name he never uttered without the epithet immortal, has put the question of Harvey's merit both happily and eloquently, and it affords us pleasure to quote the passage from the writings of our old and honoured teacher in anatomy. " The late Dr. Hunter," says Dr. Barclay,[1] " has rather invidiously introduced Harvey along with Copernicus and Columbus, to show that his merit as a discoverer was comparatively low. But what did Copernicus, and what did

[1] On the Arteries, Introduction, p. ix.

Columbus? Not in possession of more numerous facts than their contemporaries, but endowed with nobler and more vigorous intellects, the one developed the intricate system of the heavenly bodies and the other discovered an unheard-of continent. Was it not in the same way, by the exertion of superior intellect, that Harvey made his immortal discovery? I know not what has happened in the world unseen; but if I may judge from the records of history and the annals of fame, the spirit of Bacon, the spirits of Columbus, Copernicus and Newton have not been ashamed to welcome and associate with the congenial spirit of Harvey." To this fine passage there is little to be added: Harvey's discovery was of the rational and inductive and therefore higher class, according to our estimate; it was made in virtue of the intellectual powers which peculiarly distinguish man, possessed in a state of the highest perfection.

THE WORK ON GENERATION.

In our account of Harvey's public career we found him busy with the subject of Generation at Oxford in 1642; but he had certainly turned his attention that way at a much earlier period, for one of the chief causes of his regret, as expressed to Dr. Ent, for the destruction of his papers during the civil war, is the loss of his Observations on the Generation of Insects, which could only have been made and reduced to form many years previously, probably before his engagement to accompany the Duke of Lennox on his travels. And then we see that all his notes on the gestation of the hind or doe were made in the palmy days of the first Charles, before the differences between him and the people of these countries had come to the arbitrement of arms. Harvey probably occupied a good deal of his leisure in arranging and writing the work on Generation, after quitting the service of Charles in 1646; his practice at this period was not extensive, and he seems to have passed much of his time in the country. Harvey appears to have been little inclined to the publication of this work, and only to have ventured it out of his hands with reluctance. Without the solicitations of Ent, indeed, it would certainly have been left unpublished during his lifetime. Ent, however, succeeded in carrying off the prize which his illustrious friend had showed him, and lost no time in getting it into types, taking on himself the task of correcting the press, and sending it forth according to his own ideas in fitting form, with a frontispiece, and a highflown dedication to the President and Fellows of the College of Physicians. Ent's account of his interview with Harvey on the occasion of obtaining his consent to the publication, though highly theatrical, is still extremely interesting. Saluting the great anatomist, and asking if all were well with him, Harvey answers, somewhat impatiently as it seems : " How can it, whilst the Commonwealth is full of distractions, and I myself am still in the open sea? And truly," he continues, " did I not find solace in my studies, and a balm for my spirit in the memory of my observations of former years, I should feel little desire for longer life." (p. 145.) Let the reader turn to the page from which the above quotation is taken, and to the one which follows it, for thoughts and views that clearly bespeak the greatness of intellect, the nobleness of sentiment that distinguished William Harvey. When Ent proceeds to say that the learned world, aware of his indefatigable industry, were eagerly looking for other works at his hands, the fervid genius of the poet or discoverer still appears in his reply : " And would you be the man," said Harvey, smiling, " who should recommend me to quit the peaceful haven, where I now pass my life, and launch again upon the faithless sea? You know full well what a storm my former lucubrations raised. Much better is it oftentimes to grow wise at home and in private, than by pub-

lishing what you have amassed with infinite labour, to stir up
tempests that may rob you of peace and quiet for the rest of
your days." (p. 147.)   By and by, however, he produces his
Exercises on the Generation of Animals, and though he makes
many difficulties at first, urging, among other things, that the
work must be held incomplete, as containing nothing on the
generation of insects, Ent, nevertheless, prevails in the end,
and receives the papers with full authority, either speedily to
commit them to the press, or to delay their publication to
a future time.   Ent set about his office of midwife, as he has
it, forthwith, and the following year (1651) saw the birth of
the work on Generation.

Physiological science generally was not sufficiently advanced
in Harvey's time to admit of a truly great and enduring work
being produced on a subject so abstruse, and involving so
many particulars as that of Generation.   On the doctrine
of the circulation the dawn had long been visible; Harvey
came and the sun arose.   On the subject of animal reproduction, all was night and darkness two centuries ago; and though
the light has still been waxing in strength since Harvey wrote,
it is only in these times that we have seen it brightening into
something like the day.   In Harvey's time the very means and
instruments that were indispensable to the investigation were
not yet known, or were used of powers inadequate to bring
the prime facts within the cognizance of the senses.   Harvey
doubtless did as much as any man living could have accomplished when he wrote.   He announced the general truth : Omne
animal ex ovo ; he showed the cicatricula of the egg as the
point where the reproductive process begins ; he corrected
numerous errors into which his master Fabricius had fallen ;
he further pointed out the path of observation and experiment
as the only one that could lead to satisfactory results in the
investigation of a subject which gradually displayed itself as
one of natural history ; and, it may be added, by his wan-

derings in the labyrinth of the metaphysics of physiological
science, he did enough to deter any one from attempting to
tread such barren ground again.   In his work on the Heart
and Blood, Harvey had all the essential facts of the subject
clearly before him, and he used them at once in such masterly-
wise, that he left little or nothing for addition either by himself
or others.   Secure of his footing here, he could well dispense
with " vital spirits," " innate heat," and other inscrutable agen-
cies, he could leave " adequate and efficient causes," and other
metaphysical phantoms on one side—it was physics that he
was dealing with, and the physician was at home.   With the
information we now possess, we see clearly how indifferently
weaponed was the physiologist of the year 1647 for encountering
such a subject as Animal Generation ; a Leeuwenhoek and a
De Graaf, a Spallanzani and a Haighton, a Wolff, a Purkinje,
a Von Baer, a Valentin, a Rudolph Wagner, a Bischoff, and
many more, had successively to appear, before the facts of the
subject could be ascertained, and a Schleiden and a Schwann
were further necessary as ultimate interpreters of the things
observed before they could be either rightly or wholly understood.   No wonder then that The Physiologist of the 17th century, meets us in the guise of one rather puzzled with the burthen he has made up his mind to bear, and, contrary to his former
wont, eking out the lack of positive knowledge by reiterated
disquisitions on topics where certainty is unattainable.

   It is rather curious, moreover, to find Harvey, in his work
on Generation, not entirely escaping the pitfall of which he
was so well aware, and which he shunned so successfully in
his earlier production.   In the work on the Heart, he sets out
with the certainty that the whole of the notions of the
ancients on the heart and blood are untenable; and then,
taking Nature for his guide, his fine intellect never once suffers
him to stray from the right path.   In the book on Generation,
on the other hand, he begins by putting himself in some sort

into the harness of Aristotle, and taking the bit of Fabricius between his teeth; and then, either assuming the ideas of the former as premises, or those of the latter as topics of discussion or dissent, he labours on endeavouring to find Nature in harmony with the Stagyrite, or at variance with the professor of Padua—for, in spite of many expressions of respect and deference for his old master, Harvey evidently delights to find Fabricius in the wrong. Finally, so possessed is he by scholastic ideas, that he winds up some of his opinions upon animal reproduction by presenting them in the shape of logical syllogisms.

The age of Harvey, then, was not competent to produce a work on generation,—it was still an impossible undertaking. Yet has Harvey written a remarkable book; one that teems with interesting observation, and that presents the author to us in the character of the elegant writer, the scholar, and the poet as well as the discoverer—if, indeed, poet and discoverer, though variously applied, be not identical terms. Besides the points already referred to, as immediately connected with his subject, we here find Harvey anticipating modern surgery, by applying a ligature to the main artery of a tumour which he wished to extirpate, and so making its subsequent removal much more easy. Here, too, we find him, a century and a half before his contemporaries, in the most rapidly progressive period in the history of human knowledge, throwing out the first hint of the true use of the lungs. Hitherto the lungs had been regarded as surrounding the heart for the purpose of ventilating the blood and tempering or moderating its heat, the heart being viewed as the focus or hearth of the innate heat; and Harvey himself generally uses language in harmony with these ideas; but in one instance, the lightning of genius giving him a glimpse of the truth, he says, " Air is given neither for the cooling nor the nutrition of animals * * * it is as if heat were rather enkindled within the fœtus [at birth] than repressed by the influence of the air."[1]

Had William Harvey possessed this idea in his earlier years, and pursued it as he did that of the blood never moving in the veins but in one recurrent course, he would at least have prepared the way for another grand discovery in physiology : demonstrating the erroneousness of the current physiological notions on the use of the lungs, he would have led the van in the investigation of their proper office ; and, had everything else permitted, he might even have anticipated Joseph Black in explaining the source of animal heat.   But this was an impossibility at the time : chemistry, in Harvey's day, mostly in the hands of adepts and charlatans, transmuters of the base metals, and searchers after the philosopher's stone and the elixir of life, could have no attractions for the clear intellect of the demonstrator of the circulation of the blood.   No wonder, therefore, that Harvey "did not care for chymistrey," or that "he was wont to speak against the chymists" (Aubrey, l. c. p. 385) ; this anecdote is but another proof of Harvey's sagacity.   Harvey then could only show himself in advance of his age by questioning its opinions on the office of the lungs as he does; the state of chemical science in the middle of the 17th century did not admit of his doing more.   Harvey, however, well knew the vivifying force of heat : he saw it the immediate indispensable agent in the reproduction of a living sentient being, as it is probably employed by the Creator as mainspring in the elaborate mechanism of the automatic animal body.

The short piece on the ANATOMY of THOMAS PARR, is interesting in itself; and in giving us a glimpse of Harvey's style of pathological reasoning, confirms us in our faith in the

[1] On Generation, p. 530.

great physiologist as a practitioner of medicine. If knowledge will not help, how should the want of it avail?

The LETTERS of Great men generally serve to make us more intimately acquainted with them than without such aid we could have become. This is more especially the case as respects the letters that are written in the ease and confidence of private friendship. It is greatly to be regretted that so few of the letters of this description that flowed from the pen of Harvey should have come down to us. Those addressed to Giovanni Nardi, however, show us what an affectionate and elegant mind our Harvey possessed; how mindful he always appears of former kindnesses to himself and to those that were near to him; how anxious that he should be cherished in the memory of his friends, even as he cherishes them in his own !

The other letters we possess are mostly upon professional —physiological topics; though the one addressed from Nuremberg to Caspar Hofmann may, perhaps, be held an exception; for in this letter the manly and candid character of Harvey displays itself conspicuously. In his own city he challenges the Nuremberg professor to the proof. " If you would see with your own eyes the things I assert of the circulation, I promise to show them to you with the opportunity afforded me." We have seen that Harvey accompanied the Earl of Arundel in his extraordinary embassy to the Emperor, in 1636, and may probably have been one of the party of which three members were barbarously murdered on their way, from Nuremberg to Ratisbon, as Crowne[1] informs us. Hence the solicitude which Hollar, the artist, who also accompanied the ambassador, informed Aubrey the Earl of Arundel expressed for his physician's safety: "For he would still be making of excursions into the woods, making observations of strange trees, plants, earths, &c., and sometimes like to be lost; so that my

---

[1] A True Relation, &c., p. 46.

lord ambassador would be really angry with him, for there was not only danger of wild beasts but of thieves."[1]

The burthen of the long and able letter to Slegel, of Hamburg, is still the Circulation. The one addressed to Morison, and the two to Horst, treat of the discovery of the receptaculum chyli and thoracic duct by Pecquet. Harvey has been held wanting to his greatness in having refused his assent to the facts of the distinct existence and special office of the lymphatic system. But, non omnia possumus omnes; Harvey had his own work laid out for him, and the lymphatic system was not a part of it. Aselli's book on the 'Lacteal Viens,'[2] was even published before Harvey's own Exercises on the Heart and Blood had appeared, and must have been familiar to our physiologist; but that he failed to perceive the import of that discovery, and never inquired particularly into it, cannot surely be rightly laid to him as a charge; and then, when the newly-discovered system of vessels acquired extension from the researches of Pecquet, Rudbeck, and Bartholin, Harvey felt that he was both too old and too infirm to enter on the examination of so extensive and delicate an anatomical question. In entire consistency with his noble nature, however, and in striking contrast with his own opponents, he nowhere formally denies the existence of the new lymphatic vessels; nor does he once oppose the authority of his name to the investigation of the truth. On the contrary, he states his objections, "not as being obstinately wedded to his own opinion, but that he may show what can readily be urged in opposition to the advocates of the new ideas. Nor do I doubt," he proceeds, "but that many things now hidden in the well of Democritus, will by and by be drawn up into day by the ceaseless industry of a coming age."[3]

[1] Aubrey, Op. cit. p. 384. In the printed work the phrase runs thus: "Not only danger of thieves, but of wild beasts." Crowne's anecdote suggests the proper reading.

[2] De Venis Lacteis. 4to, Milan, 1622.

[3] First Letter to J. D. Horst.

The letter to Vlackveld was written the very year, within a few weeks indeed, of his death.   It is even touching—it is in vain, he says, to his correspondent, that he would apply the spur; he has already felt his right to demand his release from duty; yet would he still be honorably considered by his contemporaries, and he begs his friend Vlackveld to love him to the last.

We have taken occasion from time to time in the course of our narrative, to glance at the mental and moral constitution, and also at the personal character, of Harvey, principally by way of inference from his conduct on particular occasions, and from what appears in his writings.   Happily we have in addition a few particulars from the pen of a contemporary, John Aubrey,[1] which, though perchance they do not harmonize in every respect with the facts in his public life and the portrait he gives us of himself in his works, are nevertheless extremely interesting, and cannot be left unnoticed in a Life of Harvey.

" In person," Aubrey informs us, " Harvey was not tall, but of the lowest stature ; round faced ; olivaster (like wainscot) complexion ; little eye, round, very black, full of spirit ; his hair black as a raven, but quite white 20 years before he died."   The portrait we have of Harvey by Cornelius Jansen, in the library of the Royal College of Physicians, as well as of one, we presume by Bemmel, now in the possession of Dr. Richard Bright, corresponds with this account : the temperament is nervous-bilious ; the forehead is compact and square, and of greater width than usual between the temples ; the expression is highly intellectual, contemplative, and manly.

" In temper," Aubrey says, " he was like the rest of his brothers, very choleric, and, in his younger days, he wore a dagger, as the fashion then was, which he would be apt to draw

---

[1] Letters and Lives of Eminent Persons, 2 vols. 8vo, London, 1813.

out upon every occasion." We cannot suppose that this was offensively, but merely in the way of gesticulation, and to lend force to his words; for in his public and literary life, Harvey showed everything but a choleric nature : he seems, indeed, at all times to have had his temper under entire control. The way in which Harvey himself speaks of the robbery of his apartments and the destruction of his papers, has nothing of bitterness or acrimony in it. With the opportunity presenting itself to him— as when he sends Nardi the books on the Troubles in England —he is not tempted to utter even a splenetic word against the party which had been all along opposed to his friends, and by which he had suffered so severely. Harvey was, probably, a marked man by Cromwell and his adherents; but had he been so disposed he could have indulged in a little vitupera-tion without risk of molestation. The government of England in the Protector's time was still no tyranny.

Harvey appears not to have esteemed the fair sex very highly. He would say, that " we Europeans knew not how to order or govern our women, and that the Turks were the only people who used them wisely." But, indeed, if Aubrey may be trusted, he did not think very much of mankind in general : he was wont to say, that " man was but a great mischievous baboon." Harvey, however, wived young, and in his age he seems still to have thought that the old man was best tended by the gentle hand of a woman not too far stricken in years.[1]

Harvey, in his own family circle, must have been affec-tionate and kind,—characteristics of all his brothers—who appear as we have said to have lived together through their lives in perfect amity and peace. But our Harvey's sympa-thies were not limited to his immediate relatives : attachment, friendship was an essential ingredient in his nature. His will from first to last is a piece of beautiful humanity, and more than one widow and helpless woman is there provided for.

[1] Vide Aubrey, Op. cit. p. 381.

He seems to have been very anxious to live in the memory of his sisters-in-law and of his nephews and nieces, whose legacies are mostly given to the end that they may buy something to keep in remembrance of him. To Dr. Ent he was much attached, and, besides his bookcases, there are ' five pounds to buy a ring.' Dr. Scarborough, who also stood high in Harvey's favour, has his ' silver instruments of surgery and his best velvet gown.'

We cannot fancy that Harvey was at any time very eager in the pursuit of wealth. Aubrey tells us that, " For twenty years before he died, he took no care of his worldly concerns; but his brother Eliab, who was a very wise and prudent manager, ordered all, not only faithfully, but better than he could have done for himself." The effect of this good management was that Harvey lived, towards the end of his life, in very easy circumstances. Having no costly establishment to maintain, for he always lived with one or other of his brothers in his latter days, and no family to provide for, he could afford to be munificent, as we have seen him, to the College of Physicians, and at his death he is reported to have left as much as 20,000*l.* to his faithful steward and kind brother Eliab, who always meets us as the guardian angel of our anatomist, in a worldly and material point of view. Honoured be the name and the memory of Eliab Harvey for his good offices to one so worthy !

Though of competent estate, in the enjoyment of the highest reputation, and trusted by two sovereign Princes in succession, Harvey never suffered his name to be coupled with any of those lower-grade titles that were so freely conferred in the time of both the First and Second Charles. When we associate Harvey's name with a title at all, it is with the one he fairly won from his masters of Padua : by his contemporaries he is always spoken of as Dr. Harvey ; we in the present day rightly class him with our Shakespeares, and our Miltons, and speak of him as Harvey. Harvey, indeed, had no love of ostentation or display. The very buildings he erected, were built "at the suggestion and under the auspices" of others.

Harvey's mind was largely imbued with the imaginative faculty : how finely he brings in the classical allusion to "the Sicilian sea, dashing among the rocks around Charybdis, hissing and foaming and tossed hither and thither," in illustration of those who reason against the evidence of their senses. (p. 130.) And then what unbounded confidence he has in Nature (p. 153), and how keenly alive he is to her beauties in every sphere : Nature has not been sedulous to deck out animals only with ornaments ; she has further thrown an infinite variety of beautiful dyes over the lowly and insensate herbs and flowers. (p. 426.)

In Harvey the religious sentiments appear to have been active ; the exordium to his will is unusually solemn and grand. He also evinces true and elevated piety throughout the whole course of his work on Generation, and seizes every opportunity of giving utterance to his sense of the immediate agency and omnipotence of Deity. He appears, with the ancient philosophers, to have regarded the universe and its parts as actuated by a Supreme and all-pervading Intelligence. He was a great admirer of Virgil, whose works were frequently in his hands, and whose religious philosophy he seems also, in a great measure, to have adopted. The following beautiful and often-quoted passage of his favorite author may be said to embody his ideas on this subject, as they appear repeatedly in the course of the work on Generation :—

" Principio cœlum ac terras camposque liquentes,
Lucentemque globum lunæ, Titaniaque astra,
Spiritus intus alit, totamque infusa per artus
Mens agitat molem, et magno se corpore miscet."

—The heavens and earth, and ocean's liquid plains,
The moon's bright orb, and the Titanian stars,
Are fed by intrinsic spirit : deep infused
Through all, mind mingles with and actuates the mass.

Upon the purely Deistic notions of antiquity, however, Harvey unquestionably ingrafted the special faith in Christianity. In connexion with the subject of the "term utero-gestation," he adduces the highest recorded examples as the rule, and speaks of "Christ, our Saviour, of men the most perfect;"[1] in the will he farther "most humbly renders his soul to Him that gave it, and to his blessed Lord and Saviour Christ Jesus."

Harvey was very inquisitive into natural things and natural phenomena. When he accompanied the Earl of Arundel, we have seen that he would still be wandering in the woods, making observations on the strange trees and herbs, and minerals he encountered. His industry in collecting facts was unwearied, and the accuracy with which he himself observed appears in every page of his writings; though we sometimes meet him amiably credulous in regard to the observations of others,—as in that instance where he suffers himself to be imposed upon by the traveller's tale of the "Genus humanum caudatum"—the race of the human kind with tails.[2] Harvey was the first English comparative anatomist; in other words, he was the first physiologist England produced whom superiority of natural endowment led to perceive the relations between the meanest and the highest of created things, and who made the simplicity of structure and of function in the one, a means of explaining the complexity of structure and of function in the other. "Had anatomists," he says, "only been as conversant with the dissection of the lower animals as they are with that of the human body, many matters that have hitherto kept them in a perplexity of doubt would, in my opinion, have met them freed from every kind of difficulty." (On the Heart, p. 35.) Harvey makes frequent and most effectual use of his knowledge of comparative anatomy in his earlier work; and if the reader will turn to the one on

[1] On Generation, p. 529.   [2] Ib. p. 182.

Generation (p. 423), and peruse what is said on the subject of 'parts not essential to the being of the individual,' and will then visit the Hunterian Museum in Lincoln's Inn Fields, he will find that the great comparative anatomist and physiologist of the 19th century had a herald in the great comparative anatomist and physiologist of the 17th century. Aubrey mentions particularly Harvey's having "often said that of all the losses he sustained, no grief was so crucifying to him as the loss of his papers (containing notes of his dissections of the frog, toad, and other animals,) which, together with his goods in his lodgings at Whitehall, were plundered at the beginning of the rebellion." Harvey's store of individual knowledge must have been great; and he seems never to have flagged in his anxiety to learn more. He made himself master of Oughtred's 'Clavis Mathematica' in his old age, according to Aubrey, who found him "perusing it, and working problems not long before he dyed."

Aubrey says "he understood Greek and Latin pretty well, but was no critique, and he wrote very bad Latin. The Circuitus Sanguinis was, as I take it, done into Latin by Sir George Ent, as also his booke de Generatione Animalium; but a little booke, in 12mo, against Riolan (I thinke) wherein he makes out his doctrine clearer, was writ by himself, and that, as I take it, at Oxford."[1] Aubrey, in his gossiping, is doing injustice both to the scholarship and to the candour of Harvey. He heard or knew that Harvey wrote an indifferent hand, and this forsooth he turns into writing indifferent Latin. Every-thing points to the year 1619 as the period when the book De Motu Cordis et Sanguinis (Aubrey does not even know the title!) was written; Ent, born in 1603, was then a lad of sixteen, and in all likelihood had never heard of Harvey's name; in 1628, when the work came forth at Frankfort, he was but twenty-five, and scarcely emancipated from the leading

[1] Aubrey, l. c. p. 383.

strings of his instructors. The Exercises to Riolan, which Aubrey cites as a specimen of Harvey's own latinity, are at least as well written as the Exercises on the Heart. And then our authority evidently speaks at random in regard to the time and place when these Exercises were composed. Harvey never resided at Oxford after 1646, and Riolan's Encheiridium Anatomicum, to which Harvey's Two Exercises were an answer, did not appear till 1648! Harvey's reply could not have been written by anticipation. It came out at Cambridge the year after Riolan's work—in 1649.

With regard to the work on Generation, again, had Ent received it in English and turned it into Latin, this fact would certainly have been stated; whereas, there is only the information that he played the midwife's part, and over-looked the press. More than this, from what Ent says, it is evident that the printer worked from Harvey's own MS. "As our author writes a bad hand," says Ent, "which no one without practice can easily read, I have taken some pains to prevent the printer committing any very grave blunders through this,—a point which, I observe, has not been suffi-ciently attended to in a small work of his (The Exercitatio ad Riolanum) which lately appeared."[1] Harvey was a man of the most liberal education, and lived in an age when every man of liberal education wrote and conversed in Latin with ease at least, if not always with elegance. Harvey's Latin is generally easy, often elegant, and not unfrequently copious and imaginative; he never seems to feel in the least fettered by the language he is using.

Harvey, if eager in the acquirement of knowledge, was also ready at all times to communicate what he knew, " and," as Aubrey has it, " to instruct any that were modest and respectful to him. In order to my journey (I was at that time bound for

---

[1] Epistle Dedicatory to the work on Generation.

f

Italy) he dictated to me what to see, what company to keep, what bookes to read, how to manage my studies—in short, he bid me go to the fountain head and read Aristotle, Cicero, Avicenna, and did call the Neoteriques s—t-breeches."[1]

Harvey was not content merely to gather knowledge; he digested and arranged it under the guidance of the faculties which compare and reason. "He was always very contemplative," pursues Aubrey, "and was wont to frequent the leads of Cockaine-house, which his brother Eliab had bought, having there his several stations in regard to the sun and the wind, for the indulgence of his fancy. At the house at Combe, in Surrey," which, by the way, appears to have been purchased of Mr. Cockaine, as well as the mansion in the city, "he had caves made in the ground, in which he delighted in the summer time to meditate. He also loved darkness," telling Aubrey, "'that he could then best contemplate.' His thoughts working, would many times keep him from sleeping, in which case his way was to rise from his bed and walk about his chamber in his shirt, till he was pretty cool, and then return to his bed and sleep very comfortably." He treated the principal bodily ailment with which he was afflicted (gout) somewhat in the same manner. The fever of the mind being subdued by the application of cold air to the body at large, the fever in the blood, induced by gout, was abated by the use of cold water to the affected member: "He would then sitt with his legges bare, though it were frost, on the leads of Cockaine-house, putt them into a payle of water till he was almost dead with cold, and betake himself to his stove, and so 'twas gone."[2]

Harvey, besides being physician to the king and household, held the same responsible situation in the families of many of the most distinguished among the nobles and men of eminence

---

[1] Aubrey, p. 383.   [2] Ibid., p. 384.

of his time—among others to the Lord Chancellor Bacon, whom, Aubrey informs us, " he esteemed much for his witt and style, but would not allow to be a great philosopher. Said he to me, ' He writes philosophy like a Lord Chancellor' —speaking in derision." Harvey's penetration never failed him : the philosopher of fact cared not for the philosopher of prescription ; he who was dealing with the Things, and, through his own inherent powers, exhibiting the Rule, thought little of him who was at work upon abstractions, and who only inculcated the Rule from the use which he saw others making of it. Bacon has many admirers, but there are not wanting some in these present times who hold, with his illustrious contemporary, that " he wrote philosophy like a Lord Chancellor."

Harvey was also acquainted with all the men of letters and science of his age—with Hobbes, Dryden, Cowley, Boyle, and the rest.   Dryden, in his metrical epistle to Dr. Charleton, has these lines, of no great merit or significance :—

> " The circling streams once thought but pools of blood,
> (Whether life's fuel or the body's food,)
> From dark oblivion Harvey's name shall save."

Cowley is more happy in his ode on Dr. Harvey :—

> " Thus Harvey sought for truth in Truth's own book
> —Creation—which by God himself was writ ;
> And wisely thought 'twas fit
> Not to read comments only upon it,
>   But on th' original itself to look.
> Methinks in Art's great circle others stand
> Lock'd up together hand in hand :
>   Every one leads as he is led,
>   The same bare path they tread,
> A dance like that of Fairies, a fantastic round,
> With neither change of motion nor of ground.
>   Had Harvey to this road confined his wit,
>   His noble circle of the blood had been untrodden yet."

Cowley and Harvey must often have encountered ; both

had the confidence of the king, but in very different ways: Cowley lent himself to the privacies and intrigues of the royal family and its adherents, for whom he even consented to play the base part of spy upon their opponents. He was also the cypher-letter writer, and the decypherer of the royal correspondence, and thus mixed up with all the littlenesses of the court party, by whom he must have been, as matter of course, despised, as he was subsequently neglected. Harvey was a man of another stamp, composed of a different clay; and it gives us a high sense of his independence and true nobility of nature that in the midst of faction and intrigue, he is never found associated with aught that is unworthy of the name of man in his best estate. The war of party and the work of destruction might be going on around; Harvey, under a hedge, and within reach of shot, was cooly engaged with his book, or in the chamber of his friend Dr. Bathurst, wrapt in contemplation of the mysteries of Generation.

Harvey appears to have possessed, in a remarkable degree, the power of persuading and conciliating those with whom he came in contact. In the whole course of his long life we hear nothing either of personal enemies or personal enmities; "Man" he says "comes into the world naked and unarmed, as if nature had destined him for a social creature and ordained that he should live under equitable laws and in peace; as if she had desired that he should be guided by reason rather than be driven by force."[1] The whole of the opposition to his new views on the circulation was got up at a distance; all within his own sphere were of his way of thinking. His brethren of the College of Physicians appear to have revered him. The congregated fellows must have risen to their feet by common consent as he came among them on the memorable occasion after they had elected him their president.

---

[1] On Generation, p. 425.

Among other tastes or habits which Harvey had, Aubrey informs us that " he was wont to drink coffee, which he and his brother Eliab did before coffee-houses were in fashion in London."[1]   This was probably a cherished taste with Harvey. In his will he makes a special reservation of his " coffey-pot;" —his niece Mary West and her daughter have all his plate except this precious utensil, which, with the residue, he evidently desired should descend to his brother Eliab as a memorial doubtless of the pleasure they had often enjoyed together over its contents—the brewage from the ' sober berry.'

In visiting his patients, Harvey " rode on horseback with a foot-cloath, his men following on foot, as the fashion then was, which was very decent, now quite discontinued.   The judges rode also with their foot-cloathes to Westminster Hall, which ended at the death of Sir Robert Hyde, Lord Chief Justice; Anthony Earl of Shaftesbury would have revived it, but several of the judges being old and ill horsemen would not agree to it."[2]

Harvey appears to have preserved his faculties unimpaired to the very last.   Aubrey, as we have seen, found the anatomist perusing Oughtred's ' Clavis Mathematica,' and working the problems not long before he died ; and the registers of the College of Physicians further assure us that Harvey, when very far stricken in years, still lost little or nothing of his old activity of mind.   He continued to deliver his lectures till within a year or two of his death, when he was succeeded by his friend Sir Charles Scarborough, and he never failed at the comitia of the college when anything of moment was under consideration.

Accumulating years, however, and repeated attacks of gout, to which Harvey had long been a martyr, at length asserted their mastery over the declining body, and William Harvey, the great in intellect, the noble in nature, finally ceased to be,

---

[1] Op. cit. p. 384.   [2] Aubrey, ib. p. 386.

lxxxvi THE LIFE OF HARVEY.

on the 3d of June, 1657, in the eightieth year of his age.
About ten o'clock in the morning, as Aubrey tells us, on
attempting to speak, he found that he had lost the power of
utterance, that, in the language of the vulgar, he had the
dead palsy in his tongue. He did not lose his other faculties,
however; but knowing that his end was approaching, he sent
for his nephews, to each of whom he gave some token of remembrance,—his watch to one, his signet ring to another,
and so on. He farther made signs to Sambroke, his apothe-
cary, to let him blood in the tongue; but this did little or no
good, and by and by, in the evening of the day on which he
was stricken, he died; "the palsy," as Aubrey has it, "giving
him an easy passport."[1]

The funeral took place a few days afterwards, the body
being attended far beyond the walls of the city by a long train
of his friends of the College of Physicians, and the remains
were finally deposited "in a vault at Hempstead, in Essex,
which his brother Eliab had built; he was lapt in lead, and on
his breast, in great letters, his name—DR. WILLIAM HARVEY.
* * * I was at his funeral," continues Aubrey, "and
helpt to carry him into the vault." And there, at this hour, he
lies, the lead that laps him little changed, and showing indis-

---

[1] Aubrey gives a positive denial to "the scandall that ran strongly against him
(Harvey), viz. that he made himself away, to put himself out of his paine, by
opium." Aubrey proceeds: "The scandall aforesaid is from Sir Charles Scarborough's saying that he (Harvey) had, towards his latter end, a preparation of
opium and I know not what, which he kept in his study to take if occasion should
serve, to put him out of his paine, and which Sir Charles promised to give him.
This I believe to be true; but do not at all believe thát he really did give it him.
The palsey did give him an easie passeport." (l. c. p. 385.)

Harvey, if he meditated anything of the kind above alluded to, would not be the
only instance on record of even a strong-minded man shrinking from a struggle
which he knows must prove hopeless, from which there is no issue but one. Nature,
as the physician knows, does often kill the body by a very lingering and painful process. In his practice he is constantly required to smooth the way for the unhappy
sufferer. In his own case he may sometimes wish to shorten it. Such requests as
Harvey may be presumed to have made to Scarborough, are frequently enough preferred to medical men: it is needless to say that they are never granted.

tinctly the outline of the form within; for he lies not in an ordinary coffin, but the cerements that surround the body immediately invested in their turn by the lead.

So lived, so died one of the great men whom God, in virtue of his eternal laws, bids to appear on earth from time to time to enlighten, and to ennoble mankind.[1]

---

[1] On the Tablet placed in Hempstead church to Harvey's memory are inscribed these words:

GULIELMUS HARVEIUS,
Cui tam colendo Nomini assurgunt omnes Academiæ;
Qui diuturnum sanguinis motum
Post tot annorum Millia,
Primus invenit;
Orbi salutem, sibi immortalitatem
Consequutus.
Qui ortum et generationem Animalium solus omnium
A Pseudo-philosophiâ liberavit.
Cui debet
Quod sibi innotuit humanum Genus, seipsam Medicina.
Screniss. Majestat. Jacobi et Carolo Britanniarum
Monarchis Archiatrus et charissimus.
Collegii Med. Lond. Anatomes et Chirurgiæ Professor
Assiduus et felicissimus:
Quibus illustrem construxit Bibliothecam,
Suoque dotavit et ditavit Patrimonio.
Tandem
Post triumphales
Contemplando, sanando, inveniendo
Sudores,
Varias domi forisque statuas,
Quum totum circuit Microcosmum,
Medicinæ Doctor et Medicorum,
Improles obdormivit,
III Junii anno salutis cIↃIↃcLVII, Ætat. LXXX.
Annorum et Famæ satur.

THE LAST WILL AND TESTAMENT OF
WILLIAM HARVEY. M.D.

*Extracted from the Registry of the Prerogative Court
of Canterbury.*

IN the name of the Almighty and Eternal God Amen I
WILLIAM HARVEY of London Doctor of Physicke doe by
these presents make and ordaine this my last Will and testament in manner and forme following Revoking hereby all
former and other wills and testaments whatsoever   Imprimis
I doe most humbly render my soule to Him that gave it
and to my blessed Lord and Saviour Christ Jesus and my
bodie to the Earth to be buried at the discretion of my
executor herein after named   The personall estate which
at the time of my decease I shalbe in any way possessed of
either in Law or equitie be it in goods householdstuffe readie
moneys debts duties arrearages of rents or any other wayes
whatsoever and whereof I shall not by this present will or by
some Codicill to be hereunto annexed make a particular gift
and disposition I doe after my debts Funeralls and Legacies
paid and discharged give and bequeath the same vnto my
loving brother Mr. Eliab Harvey merchant of London whome
I make Executor of this my last will and testament   And
whereas I have lately purchased certaine lands in North-
amptonshire or thereabouts commonly knowne by the name
of Oxon grounds and formally belonging vnto to the Earl of
Manchester and certaine other grounds in Leicestershire commonly called or knowne by the name of Baron Parke and
sometime heretofore belonging vnto Sir Henry Hastings

Knight both which purchases were made in the name of several persons nominated and trusted by me and by two severall deeds of declaracon vnder the hands and seales of all persons any waye parties or privies to the said trusts are declared to be first vpon trust and to the intent that I should be permitted to enioye all the rents and profits and the benefit of the collaterall securitie during my life and from and after my decease   Then upon trust and for the benefit of such person and persons and of and for such estate and estates and Interests   And for raysing and payment of such summe and summes of Money Rents Charges Annuities and yearly payments to and for such purposes as from time to time by any writing or writings to be by me signed and sealed in the presence of Two or more credible witnesses or by my last will and testament in writing should declare limit direct or appoint   And further in trust that the said Mannors and lands and everie part thereof together with the Collaterall securitie should be assigned conveyed and assured vnto such persons and for suche Estates as the same should by me be limited and directed charged and chargeable neverthelec with all Annuities rents and summes of money by me limited and appointed if any such shalbe   And in default of such appointment then to Eliab Harvey his heires executors and Assignes or to such as he or they shall nominate as by the said two deeds of declaracon both of them bearing date the tenth day of July in the year of our Lord God one Thousand six hundred Fiftie and one more at large it doth appeare I doe now hereby declare limit direct and appoint that with all convenient speed after my decease there shalbe raised satisfied and paid these severall summes of money Rents Charges and Annuities herein after expressed and likewise all such other summes of Money Rents Charges or Annuities which at any time hereafter in any Codicill to be hereunto annexed shall happen to be limited or expressed

And first I appoint so much money to be raised and laid out vpon that building which I have already begun to erect within the Colledge of Physicians in London as will serve to finish the same according to the designe already made   Item I give and bequeath vnto my lo sister in Law Mrs Eliab Harvey one hundred pounds to buy something to keepe in remembrance of me   Item   I give to my Niece Mary Pratt all that Linnen householdstuffe and furniture which I have at Coome neere Croydon for the vse of Will Foulkes and to whom his keeping shalbe assigned after her death or before me at any time   Item   I give vnto my Niece Mary West and her daughter Amy West halfe the Linnen I shall leave at London in 'my chests and Chambers together with all my plate excepting my Coffey pot   Item   I give to my lo sister Eliab all the other halfe of my Linnen which I shall leave behind me   Item   I give to my lo sister Daniell at Lambeth and to everie one of her children severally the summe of fiftie pounds   Item   I give to my lo Coosin Mr Hencage Finch for his paines counsell and advice about the contriving of this my will one hundred pounds   Item   I give to all my little Godchildren Nieces and Nephews severally to everie one Fiftie pounds   Item   I give and bequeath to the towne of Foulkestone where I was borne two hundred pounds to be bestowed by the advice of the Mayor thereof and my Executor for the best vse of the poore   Item   I give to the poore of Christ hospitall in Smithfield thirtie pounds Item   I give to Will Harvey my godsonne the sonne of my brother Mich Harvey deceased one hundred pounds and to his brother Michaell Fiftie pounds   Item   I give to my Nephew Tho Cullen and his children one hundred pounds and to his brother my godsonne Will Cullen one hundred pounds   Item I give to my Nephew Jhon Harvey the sonne of my lo brother Tho Harvey deceased two hundred pounds   Item   I give to my Servant John Raby for his diligence in my ser-

vice and sicknesse twentie pounds   And to Alice Garth my
Servant Tenne pounds over and above what I am already
owing unto her by my bill which was her mistresses legacie
Item   I give among the poor children of Amy Rigdon
daughter of my lo vncle Mr Tho Halke twentie pounds Item
among other my poorest kindred one hundred pounds to be
distributed at the appointment of my Executor   Item   I give
among the servants of my sister Dan at my Funeralls Five
pounds   And likewise among the servants of my Nephew
Dan Harvey at Coome as much   Item   I give to my Cousin
Mary Tomes Fifty pounds   Item   I give to my lo Friend
Mr Prestwood one hundred pounds   Item   I give to everíe
one of my lo brother Eliab his sonnes and daughters severally
Fiftie pounds apiece   All which legacies and gifts aforesaid
are chiefly to buy something to keepe in remembrance of me
Item   I give among the servants of my brother Eliab which
shalbe dwelling with him at the time of my decease tenne
pounds Furthermore I give and bequeath vnto my Sister
Eliabs Sister Mrs Coventrey a widowe during her natural life
the yearly rent or summe of twentie pounds   Item   I give to
my Niece Mary West during her naturall life the yearly rent
or summe of Fortie pounds   Item   I give for the ɯse and
behoofe and better ordering of Will Foulkes for and during
the term of his life vnto my Niece Mary Pratt the yearly
rent of tenne pounds which summe if it happen my said
Niece shall dye before him I desire may be paid to them to
whome his keeping shalbe appointed   Item   I will that the
twentie pounds which I yearly allowe him my brother Galen
Browne may be continued as a legacie from his sister during
his naturall life   Item   I will that the payments to Mr
Samuel Fentons children out of the profits of Buckholt
Lease be orderly performed as my deere deceased lo wife gave
order so long as that lease shall stand good   Item   I give
vnto Alice Garth during her naturall life the yearly rent or

summe of twentie pounds   Item   To John Raby during his naturall life sixteene pounds yearly rent   All which yearly rents or summes to be paid halfe yearly at the two most vsuall feasts in the yeare viz Michaelmas and our Lady day without any deduction for or by reason of any manner of taxes to be any way hereafter imposed   The first payment of all the said rents or Annuities respectively to beginne at such of those feasts which shall first happen next after my decease Thus I give the remainder of my lands vnto my lo brother Eliab and his heires   All my legacies and gifts &c. being performed and discharged   Touching my bookes and householdstuffe Pictures and apparell of which I have not already disposed I give to the Colledge of Physicians all my bookes and papers and my best Persia long Carpet and my blue sattin imbroyedyed Cushion one paire of brasse Andirons with fireshovell and tongues of brasse for the ornament of the meeting roome I have erected for that purpose   Item   I give my velvet gowne to my lo friend Mr Doctor Scarbrough desiring him and my lo friend Mr Doctor Ent to looke over those scattered remnant of my poore Librarie and what bookes papers or rare collections they shall thinke fit to present to the Colledge and the rest to be Sold and with the money buy better   And for their paines I give to Mr Doctor Ent all the presses and shelves he please to make use of and five pounds to buy him a ring to keepe or weare in remembrance of me   And to Doctor Scarbrough All my little silver instruments of surgerie   Item I give all my Chamber furniture tables bed bedding hangings which I have at Lambeth to my Sister Dan and her daughter Sarah   And all that at London to my lo Sister Eliab and her daughter or my godsonne Eliab as she shall appoint Lastly   I desire my executor to assigne over the custode of Will Fowkes after the death of my Niece Mary Pratt if she happen to dye before him vnto the Sister of the said William my Niece Mary West   Thus I have finished my last

Will in three pages two of them written with own hand and my name subscribed to everie one with my hand and seal to the last

WILL HARVEY

Signed sealed and published as the last will and testament of me William Harvey In the presence of us Edward Dering   Henneage Finch   Richard Flud   Francis Finche Item   I have since written a Codicill with my owne hand in a sheet of paper to be added hereto with my name thereto subscribed and my seale.

ITEM I will that the sumes and charges here specified be added and annexed vnto my last will and testament published heretofore in the presence of Sir Edward Dering and Mr Henneage Finch and others and as a Codicill by my Executor in like manner to be performed whereby I will and bequeath to John Denn sonne of Vincent Denne the summe of thirtie pounds.   Item to my good friend Mr Tho Hobbs to buy something to keepe in remembrance of me tenne pounds and to Mr Kennersley in like manner twentie pounds   Item what moneys shalbe due to me from Mr Hen Thompson his fees being discharged I give to my friend Mr Prestwood   Item what money is of mine viz one hundred pounds in the hands of my Cosin Rigdon I give halfe thereof to him towards the marriage of his niece and the other halfe to be given to Mrs Coventrey for her sonne Walter when he shall come of yeares and for vse my Cosin Rigdon giving securitie I would he should pay none   Item what money shalbe due to me and Alice Garth my servant on a pawne now in the hands of Mr Prestwood I will after my decease shall all be given my said servant for her diligence about me in my siknesse and service both interest and principall   Item if in case it so fall out that my good friend Mrs Coventrey during her widowhood shall not dyet on freecost with my brother or Sister Eliab

Harvey Then I will and bequeath to her one hundred marke yearly during her widowhood   Item   I will and bequeath to my loving Cosin Mr Henneage Finch (more than heretofore) to be for my godsonne Will Finche one hundred pounds Item I will and bequeath yearly during her life a rent of thirtie pounds vnto Mrs Jane Nevison Widdowe in case she shall not preferre her selfe in marriage to be paid quarterly by even porcons the first to beginn at Christmas Michaelmas or Lady day or Midsummer which first happens after my decease   Item I give to my Goddaughter Mrs Eliz Glover daughter of my Cosin Toomes the yearly rent of tenne pounds from my decease vnto the end of five years   Item to her brother Mr Rich Toomes thirty pounds as a legacie   Item I give to John Cullen sonne of Tho Cullen deceased all what I have formerly given his father and more one hundred pounds Item I will that what I have bequeathed to my Niece Mary West be given to her husband my Cosin Rob West for his daughter Amy West   Item what should have bene to my Sister Dan deceased I will be given my lo Niece her daughter in Law   Item   I give my Cosin Mrs Mary Ranton fortie pounds to buy something to keep in remembrance of me Item to my nephews Michaell and Will the sonnes of my brother Mich one hundred pounds to either of them   Item all the furniture of my chamber and all the hangings I give to my godsonne Mr Eliab Harvey at his marriage and all my red damaske furniture and plate to my Cosin Mary Harvey Item I give my best velvet gowne to Doctor Scarbrowe.

WILL HARVEY.

Memorandum that upon Sunday the twentie eighth day of December in the yeare of our Lord one thousand sixe hundred fiftie sixe I did againe peruse my last will which formerly conteined three pages and hath now this fourth page added to it   And I doe now this present Sunday

December 28 1656 publish and declare these foure pages whereof the three last are written with my owne hand to be my last will In the presence of Henneage Finch John Raby.

THIS WILL with the Codicill annexed was proved at London on the second day of May In the yeare of our Lord God one Thousand six hundred fiftie nine before the Judge for probate of wills and granting Adcons lawfully authorized By the oath of Eliab Harvey the Brother and sole executor therein named To whom Administracon of all and singular the goods Chattells and debts of the said deceased was granted and committed He being first sworne truely to administer.[1]

CHAS. DYNELEY ⎫
JOHN IGGULDEN ⎬ *Deputy*
W. F. GOSTLING ⎭ *Registers.*

---

[1] The will of Harvey is without date. But was almost certainly made some time in the course of 1652. He speaks of certain deeds of declaration bearing date the 10th of July, 1651; and he provides money for the completion of the buildings which he has "already begun to erect within the College of Physicians." Now these structures were finished in the early part of 1653. The will was, therefore, written between July 1651, and Febraruy 1653. The codicil is also undated: but we may presume that it was added shortly before Sunday the 28th of December 1656, the day on which Harvey reads over the whole document and formally declares and publishes it as his last will and testament in the presence of his friend Henneage Finch, and his faithful servant John Raby.

AN ANATOMICAL DISQUISITION

ON THE

MOTION OF THE HEART AND BLOOD IN ANIMALS.

TO

THE MOST ILLUSTRIOUS AND INDOMITABLE PRINCE,

CHARLES,

KING OF GREAT BRITAIN, FRANCE, AND IRELAND,

DEFENDER OF THE FAITH.

MOST ILLUSTRIOUS PRINCE!

The heart of animals is the foundation of their life, the sovereign of everything within them, the sun of their microcosm, that upon which all growth depends, from which all power proceeds. The King, in like manner, is the foundation of his kingdom, the sun of the world around him, the heart of the republic, the fountain whence all power, all grace doth flow. What I have here written of the motions of the heart I am the more emboldened to present to your Majesty, according to the custom of the present age, because almost all things human are done after human examples, and many things in a King are after the pattern of the heart. The knowledge of his heart, therefore, will not be useless to a Prince, as embracing a kind of Divine example of his functions,—and it has still been usual with men to compare small things with great.   Here, at all events, best of Princes, placed as you are on the pinnacle of human affairs, you may at once contemplate the prime mover in the body of man, and the emblem of your own sovereign power. Accept therefore, with your wonted clemency, I most humbly beseech you, illustrious Prince, this, my new Treatise on the Heart; you, who are yourself the new light of this age, and indeed its very heart; a Prince abounding in virtue and in grace, and to whom we gladly refer all the blessings which England enjoys, all the pleasure we have in our lives.

Your Majesty's most devoted servant,

WILLIAM HARVEY.

[LONDON . . . .
1628.]

To his very dear Friend, DOCTOR ARGENT, the excellent
and accomplished President of the Royal College of
Physicians, and to other learned Physicians, his most
esteemed Colleagues.

I have already and repeatedly presented you, my learned
friends, with my new views of the motion and function of the
heart, in my anatomical lectures; but having now for nine
years and more confirmed these views by multiplied demonstrations in your presence, illustrated them by arguments, and
freed them from the objections of the most learned and skilful
anatomists, I at length yield to the requests, I might say entreaties, of many, and here present them for general consideration in this treatise.

Were not the work indeed presented through you, my learned
friends, I should scarce hope that it could come out scatheless
and complete; for you have in general been the faithful witnesses of almost all the instances from which I have either
collected the truth or confuted error; you have seen my dissections, and at my demonstrations of all that I maintain to
be objects of sense, you have been accustomed to stand by
and bear me out with your testimony.   And as this book alone
declares the blood to course and revolve by a new route, very
different from the ancient and beaten pathway trodden for so
many ages, and illustrated by such a host of learned and distinguished men, I was greatly afraid lest I might be charged
with presumption did I lay my work before the public at home,

or send it beyond seas for impression, unless I had first proposed its subject to you, had confirmed its conclusions by ocular demonstrations in your presence, had replied to your doubts and objections, and secured the assent and support of our distinguished President.   For I was most intimately persuaded, that if I could make good my proposition before you and our College, illustrious by its numerous body of learned individuals, I had less to fear from others; I even ventured to hope that I should have the comfort of finding all that you had granted me in your sheer love of truth, conceded by others who were philosophers like yourselves.   For true philosophers, who are only eager for truth and knowledge, never regard themselves as already so thoroughly informed, but that they welcome further information from whomsoever and from whencesoever it may come; nor are they so narrow-minded as to imagine any of the arts or sciences transmitted to us by the ancients, in such a state of forwardness or completeness, that nothing is left for the ingenuity and industry of others; very many, on the contrary, maintain that all we know is still infinitely less than all that still remains unknown; nor do philosophers pin their faith to others' precepts in such wise that they lose their liberty, and cease to give credence to the conclusions of their proper senses.   Neither do they swear such fealty to their mistress Antiquity, that they openly, and in sight of all, deny and desert their friend Truth.   But even as they see that the credulous and vain are disposed at the first blush to accept and to believe everything that is proposed to them, so do they observe that the dull and unintellectual are indisposed to see what lies before their eyes, and even to deny the light of the noonday sun.   They teach us in our course of philosophy as sedulously to avoid the fables of the poets and the fancies of the vulgar, as the false conclusions of the sceptics.   And then the studious, and good, and true, never suffer their minds to be warped by the passions of hatred and envy, which unfit men duly to weigh the arguments that are advanced in behalf of truth, or to appreciate the proposition that is even fairly demonstrated ; neither do they think it unworthy of them to change their opinion if truth and undoubted demonstration require them so to do; nor do they esteem it discreditable to desert error, though sanctioned by the highest antiquity ; for they know full well that to err, to be deceived, is human; that many things are discovered by accident, and that many may be learned indifferently from any quarter, by an old man from a youth, by a person of understanding from one of inferior capacity.

My dear colleagues, I had no purpose to swell this treatise into a large volume by quoting the names and writings of anatomists, or to make a parade of the strength of my memory, the extent of my reading, and the amount of my pains; because I profess both to learn and to teach anatomy, not from books but from dissections; not from the positions of philosophers but from the fabric of nature ; and then because I do not think it right or proper to strive to take from the ancients any honour that is their due, nor yet to dispute with the moderns, and enter into controversy with those who have excelled in anatomy and been my teachers. I would not charge with wilful falsehood any one who was sincerely anxious for truth, nor lay it to any one's door as a crime that he had fallen into error. I avow myself the partisan of truth alone ; and I can indeed say that I have used all my endeavours, bestowed all my pains on an attempt to produce something that should be agreeable to the good, profitable to the learned, and useful to letters.

Farewell, most worthy Doctors,
And think kindly of your Anatomist,
WILLIAM HARVEY.

1 §

AN ANATOMICAL DISQUISITION

ON THE

MOTION OF THE HEART AND BLOOD IN ANIMALS.

INTRODUCTION.

As we are about to discuss the motion, action, and use of the heart and arteries, it is imperative on us first to state what has been thought of these things by others in their writings, and what has been held by the vulgar and by tradition, in order that what is true may be confirmed, and what is false set right by dissection, multiplied experience, and accurate observation.

Almost all anatomists, physicians, and philosophers, up to the present time, have supposed, with Galen, that the object of the pulse was the same as that of respiration, and only differed in one particular, this being conceived to depend on the animal, the respiration on the vital faculty; the two, in all other respects, whether with reference to purpose or to motion, comporting themselves alike. Whence it is affirmed, as by Hieronymus Fabricius of Aquapendente, in his book on ' Respiration,' which has lately appeared, that as the pulsation of the heart and arteries does not suffice for the ventilation and refrigeration of the blood, therefore were the lungs fashioned to surround the heart. From this it appears, that whatever has hitherto been said upon the systole and diastole, on the motion of the heart and arteries, has been said with especial reference to the lungs.

But as the structure and movements of the heart differ from those of the lungs, and the motions of the arteries from those of the chest, so seems it likely that other ends and offices will thence arise, and that the pulsations and uses of the heart, likewise of the arteries, will differ in many respects from the heavings and uses of the chest and lungs. For did the arterial pulse and the respiration serve the same ends; did the arteries

in their diastole take air into their cavities, as commonly stated,
and in their systole emit fuliginous vapours by the same pores
of the flesh and skin ; and further, did they, in the time intermediate between the diastole and the systole, contain air, and at
all times either air, or spirits, or fuliginous vapours, what should
then be said to Galen, who wrote a book on purpose to show
that by nature the arteries contained blood, and nothing but
blood ; neither spirits nor air, consequently, as may be readily
gathered from the experiments and reasonings contained in the
same book ?   Now if the arteries are filled in the diastole with
air then taken into them (a larger quantity of air penetrating
when the pulse is large and full), it must come to pass, that if
you plunge into a bath of water or of oil when the pulse is
strong and full, it ought forthwith to become either smaller or
much slower, since the circumambient bath will render it either
difficult or impossible for the air to penetrate.   In like manner,
as all the arteries, those that are deep-seated as well as those
that are superficial, are dilated at the same instant, and with
the same rapidity, how were it possible that air should penetrate to the deeper parts as freely and quickly through the
skin, flesh, and other structures, as through the mere cuticle ?
And how should the arteries of the fœtus draw air into their
cavities through the abdomen of the mother and the body of
the womb ?   And how should seals, whales, dolphins and other
cetaceans, and fishes of every description, living in the depths
of the sea, take in and emit air by the diastole and systole of
their arteries through the infinite mass of waters ?   For to say
that they absorb the air that is infixed in the water, and emit their
fumes into this medium, were to utter something very like a mere
figment.   And if the arteries in their systole expel fuliginous
vapours from their cavities through the pores of the flesh and
skin, why not the spirits, which are said to be contained in these
vessels, at the same time, since spirits are much more subtile
than fuliginous vapours or smoke ? And further, if the arteries
take in and cast out air in the systole and diastole, like the
lungs in the process of respiration, wherefore do they not do the
same thing when a wound is made in one of them, as is done
in the operation of arteriotomy ?   When the windpipe is divided, it is sufficiently obvious that the air enters and returns
through the wound by two opposite movements ; but when an

artery is divided, it is equally manifest that blood escapes in one continuous stream, and that no air either enters or issues. If the pulsations of the arteries fan and refrigerate the several parts of the body as the lungs do the heart, how comes it, as is commonly said, that the arteries carry the vital blood into the different parts, abundantly charged with vital spirits, which cherish the heat of these parts, sustain them when asleep, and recruit them when exhausted? and how should it happen that, if you tie the arteries, immediately the parts not only become torpid, and frigid, and look pale, but at length cease even to be nourished? This, according to Galen, is because they are deprived of the heat which flowed through all parts from the heart, as its source; whence it would appear that the arteries rather carry warmth to the parts than serve for any fanning or refrigeration. Besides, how can the diastole [of the arteries] draw spirits from the heart to warm the body and its parts, and, from without, means of cooling or tempering them? Still further, although some affirm that the lungs, arteries, and heart have all the same offices, they yet maintain that the heart is the workshop of the spirits, and that the arteries contain and transmit them; denying, however, in opposition to the opinion of Columbus, that the lungs can either make or contain spirits; and then they assert, with Galen, against Erasistratus, that it is blood, not spirits, which is contained in the arteries.

These various opinions are seen to be so incongruous and mutually subversive, that every one of them is not unjustly brought under suspicion. That it is blood and blood alone which is contained in the arteries is made manifest by the experiment of Galen, by arteriotomy, and by wounds; for from a single artery divided, as Galen himself affirms in more than one place, the whole of the blood may be withdrawn in the course of half an hour, or less. The experiment of Galen alluded to is this: " If you include a portion of an artery between two ligatures, and slit it open lengthways, you will find nothing but blood;" and thus he proves that the arteries contain blood only. And we too may be permitted to proceed by a like train of reasoning: if we find the same blood in the arteries that we find in the veins, which we have tied in the same way, as I have myself repeatedly ascertained, both in the dead body and in living animals, we may fairly conclude that the arteries con-

tain the same blood as the veins, and nothing but the same
blood.   Some, whilst they attempt to lessen the difficulty here,
affirming that the blood is spirituous and arterious, virtually
concede that the office of the arteries is to carry blood from the
heart into the whole of the body, and that they are therefore
filled with blood; for spirituous blood is not the less blood on
that account.   And then no one denies that the blood as such,
even the portion of it which flows in the veins, is imbued with
spirits.   But if that portion which is contained in the arteries
be richer in spirits, it is still to be believed that these spirits are
inseparable from the blood, like those in the veins; that the blood
and spirits constitute one body (like whey and butter in milk, or
heat [and water] in hot water), with which the arteries are charged,
and for the distribution of which from the heart they are provided, and that this body is nothing else than blood.   But if this
blood be said to be drawn from the heart into the arteries by
the diastole of these vessels, it is then assumed that the arteries
by their distension are filled with blood, and not with the ambient air, as heretofore; for if they be said also to become
filled with air from the ambient atmosphere, how and when, I
ask, can they receive blood from the heart?   If it be answered:
during the systole; I say, that seems impossible; the arteries
would then have to fill whilst they contracted; in other words,
to fill, and yet not become distended.   But if it be said: during
the diastole, they would then, and for two opposite purposes, be
receiving both blood and air, and heat and cold; which is improbable.   Further, when it is affirmed that the diastole of the
heart and arteries is simultaneous, and the systole of the two is
also concurrent, there is another incongruity.   For how can
two bodies mutually connected, which are simultaneously distended, attract or draw anything from one another; or, being
simultaneously contracted, receive anything from each other?
And then, it seems impossible that one body can thus attract another body into itself, so as to become distended,
seeing that to be distended is to be passive, unless, in the
manner of a sponge, previously compressed by an external
force, whilst it is returning to its natural state.   But it is
difficult to conceive that there can be anything of this kind in
the arteries.   The arteries dilate, because they are filled like
bladders or leathern bottles; they are not filled because they

expand like bellows. This I think easy of demonstration; and indeed conceive that I have already proved it. Nevertheless, in that book of Galen headed ' Quod Sanguis continetur in Arteriis,' he quotes an experiment to prove the contrary: An artery having been exposed, is opened longitudinally, and a reed or other pervious tube, by which the blood is prevented from being lost, and the wound is closed, is inserted into the vessel through the opening. " So long," he says, " as things are thus arranged, the whole artery will pulsate; but if you now throw a ligature about the vessel and tightly compress its tunics over the tube, you will no longer see the artery beating beyond the ligature." I have never performed this experiment of Galen's, nor do I think that it could very well be performed in the living body, on account of the profuse flow of blood that would take place from the vessel which was operated on; neither would the tube effectually close the wound in the vessel without a ligature; and I cannot doubt but that the blood would be found to flow out between the tube and the vessel. Still Galen appears by this experiment to prove both that the pulsative faculty extends from the heart by the walls of the arteries, and that the arteries, whilst they dilate, are filled by that pulsific force, because they expand like bellows, and do not dilate because they are filled like skins. But the contrary is obvious in arteriotomy and in wounds; for the blood spurting from the arteries escapes with force, now farther, now not so far, alternately, or in jets; and the jet always takes place with the diastole of the artery, never with the systole. By which it clearly appears that the artery is dilated by the impulse of the blood; for of itself it would not throw the blood to such a distance, and whilst it was dilating; it ought rather to draw air into its cavity through the wound, were those things true that are commonly stated concerning the uses of the arteries. Nor let the thickness of the arterial tunics impose upon us, and lead us to conclude that the pulsative property proceeds along them from the heart. For in several animals the arteries do not apparently differ from the veins; and in extreme parts of the body, where the arteries are minutely subdivided, as in the brain, the hand, &c., no one could distinguish the arteries from the veins by the dissimilar characters of their coats; the tunics of both are identical. And then, in an aneurism proceeding from a wounded or eroded artery, the pulsation is precisely the same as in the other arteries, and yet it has no proper arterial tunic. This the learned Riolanus testifies to, along with me, in his Seventh Book.

Nor let any one imagine that the uses of the pulse and the respiration are the same, because under the influence of the same causes, such as running, anger, the warm bath, or any other heating thing, as Galen says, they become more frequent and forcible together. For, not only is experience in opposition to this idea, though Galen endeavours to explain it away, when we see that with excessive repletion the pulse beats more forcibly, whilst the respiration is diminished in amount; but in young persons the pulse is quick, whilst respiration is slow. So is it also in alarm, and amidst care, and under anxiety of mind; sometimes, too, in fevers, the pulse is rapid, but the respiration is slower than usual.

These and other objections of the same kind may be urged against the opinions mentioned. Nor are the views that are entertained of the offices and pulse of the heart, perhaps, less bound up with great and most inextricable difficulties. The heart, it is vulgarly said, is the fountain and workshop of the vital spirits, the centre from whence life is dispensed to the several parts of the body; and yet it is denied that the right ventricle makes spirits; it is rather held to supply nourishment to the lungs; whence it is maintained that fishes are without any right ventricle (and indeed every animal wants a right ventricle which is unfurnished with lungs), and that the right ventricle is present solely for the sake of the lungs.

1. Why, I ask, when we see that the structure of both ventricles is almost identical, there being the same apparatus of fibres, and braces, and valves, and vessels, and auricles, and in both the same infarction of blood, in the subjects of our dissections, of the like black colour, and coagulated—why, I say, should their uses be imagined to be different, when the action, motion, and pulse of both are the same? If the three tricuspid valves placed at the entrance into the right ventricle prove obstacles to the reflux of the blood into the vena cava, and if the three semilunar valves which are situated at the commencement of the pulmonary artery be there, that they may prevent the return of the blood into the ventricle; wherefore, when we find similar structures in connexion with the left ventricle, should we deny that they are

there for the same end, of preventing here the egress, there the regurgitation of the blood?

2. And again, when we see that these structures, in point of size, form, and situation, are almost in every respect the same in the left as in the right ventricle, wherefore should it be maintained that things are here arranged in connexion with the egress and regress of spirits, there, i. e. in the right, of blood. The same arrangement cannot be held fitted to favour or impede the motion of blood and of spirits indifferently.

3. And when we observe that the passages and vessels are severally in relation to one another in point of size, viz., the pulmonary artery to the pulmonary veins; wherefore should the one be imagined destined to a private or particular purpose, that to wit, of nourishing the lungs, the other to a public and general function?

4. And, as Realdus Columbus says, how can it be conceived that such a quantity of blood should be required for the nutrition of the lungs; the vessel that leads to them, the vena arteriosa or pulmonary artery being of greater capacity than both the iliac veins?

5. And I ask further; as the lungs are so close at hand, and in continual motion, and the vessel that supplies them is of such dimensions, what is the use or meaning of the pulse of the right ventricle? and why was nature reduced to the necessity of adding another ventricle for the sole purpose of nourishing the lungs?

When it is said that the left ventricle obtains materials for the formation of spirits, air to wit, and blood, from the lungs and right sinuses of the heart, and in like manner sends spirituous blood into the aorta, drawing fuliginous vapours from thence, and sending them by the arteria venosa into the lungs, whence spirits are at the same time obtained for transmission into the aorta, I ask how, and by what means, is the separation effected? and how comes it that spirits and fuliginous vapours can pass hither and thither without admixture or confusion? If the mitral cuspidate valves do not prevent the egress of fuliginous vapours to the lungs, how should they oppose the escape of air? and how should the semilunars hinder the regress of spirits from the aorta upon each supervening diastole of the heart? and, above all, how can they say that the spirituous blood is sent from the arteria venalis (pulmonary veins) by the left ventricle into the lungs without any obstacle to its passage from the mitral valves, when they have previously asserted that the air entered by the same vessel from the lungs into the left ventricle, and have brought forward these same mitral valves as obstacles to its retrogression? Good God! how should the mitral valves prevent regurgitation of air and not of blood?

Further, when they dedicate the vena arteriosa (or pulmonary artery), a vessel of great size, and having the tunics of an artery, to none but a kind of private and single purpose, that, namely, of nourishing the lungs, why should the arteria venalis (or pulmonary vein), which is scarcely of similar size, which has the coats of a vein, and is soft and lax, be presumed to be made for many—three or four, different uses? For they will have it that air passes through this vessel from the lungs into the left ventricle; that fuliginous vapours escape by it from the heart into the lungs; and that a portion of the spirituous or spiritualized blood is distributed by it to the lungs for their refreshment.

If they will have it that fumes and air—fumes flowing from, air proceeding towards the heart—are transmitted by the same conduit, I reply, that nature is not wont to institute but one vessel, to contrive but one way for such contrary motions and purposes, nor is anything of the kind seen elsewhere.

If fumes or fuliginous vapours and air permeate this vessel, as they do the pulmonary bronchia, wherefore do we find neither air nor fuliginous vapours when we divide the arteria venosa? why do we always find this vessel full of sluggish blood, never of air? whilst in the lungs we find abundance of air remaining.

If any one will perform Galen's experiment of dividing the trachea of a living dog, forcibly distending the lungs with a pair of bellows, and then tying the trachea securely, he will find, when he has laid open the thorax, abundance of air in the lungs, even to their extreme investing tunic, but none in either the pulmonary veins, or left ventricle of the heart. But did the heart either attract air from the lungs, or did the lungs transmit any air to the heart, in the living dog, by so much the more ought this to be the case in the experiment just referred to. Who, indeed, doubts that, did he inflate the lungs of a subject in the dissecting-room, he would instantly see the air making its way by this route, were there actually any such passage for it? But this office of the pulmonary veins, namely, the transference of air from the lungs to the heart, is held of such importance, that

Hieronymus Fabricius, of Aquapendente, maintains the lungs were made for the sake of this vessel, and that it constitutes the principal element in their structure.

But I should like to be informed wherefore, if the pulmonary vein were destined for the conveyance of air, it has the structure of a blood-vessel here. Nature had rather need of annular tubes, such as those of the bronchia, in order that they might always remain open, not have been liable to collapse ; and that they might continue entirely free from blood, lest the liquid should interfere with the passage of the air, as it so obviously does when the lungs labour from being either greatly oppressed or loaded in a less degree with phlegm, as they are when the breathing is performed with a sibilous or rattling noise.

Still less is that opinion to be tolerated which (as a two-fold matter, one aëreal, one sanguineous, is required for the composition of vital spirits,) supposes the blood to ooze through the septum of the heart from the right to the left ventricle by certain secret pores, and the air to be attracted from the lungs through the great vessel, the pulmonary vein; and which will have it, consequently, that there are numerous pores in the septum cordis adapted for the transmission of the blood. But, in faith, no such pores can be demonstrated, neither in fact do any such exist. For the septum of the heart is of a denser and more compact structure than any portion of the body, except the bones and sinews. But even supposing that there were foramina or pores in this situation, how could one of the ventricles extract anything from the other—the left, e. g. obtain blood from the right, when we see that both ventricles contract and dilate simultaneously? Wherefore should we not rather believe that the right took spirits from the left, than that the left obtained blood from the right ventricle, through these foramina? But it is certainly mysterious and incongruous that blood should be supposed to be most commodiously drawn through a set of obscure or invisible pores, and air through perfectly open passages, at one and the same moment. And why, I ask, is recourse had to secret and invisible porosities, to uncertain and obscure channels, to explain the passage of the blood into the left ventricle, when there is so open a way through the pulmonary veins? I own it has always appeared extraordinary to me that they should have chosen to make, or rather to imagine, a way through

2

the thick, hard, and extremely compact substance of the septum cordis, rather than to take that by the open vas venosum or pulmonary vein, or even through the lax, soft and spongy substance of the lungs at large. Besides, if the blood could permeate the substance of the septum, or could be imbibed from the ventricles, what use were there for the coronary artery and vein, branches of which proceed to the septum itself, to supply it with nourishment? And what is especially worthy of notice is this: if in the fœtus, where everything is more lax and soft, nature saw herself reduced to the necessity of bringing the blood from the right into the left side of the heart by the foramen ovale, from the vena cava through the arteria venosa, how should it be likely that in the adult she should pass it so commodiously, and without an effort, through the septum ventriculorum, which has now become denser by age?

Andreas Laurentius,[1] resting on the authority of Galen[2] and the experience of Hollerius, asserts and proves that the serum and pus in empyema, absorbed from the cavities of the chest into the pulmonary vein, may be expelled and got rid of with the urine and fæces through the left ventricle of the heart and arteries. He quotes the case of a certain person affected with melancholia, and who suffered from repeated fainting fits, who was relieved from the paroxysms on passing a quantity of turbid, fetid, and acrid urine; but he died at last, worn out by the disease; and when the body came to be opened after death, no fluid like that he had micturated was discovered either in the bladder or in the kidneys; but in the left ventricle of the heart and cavity of the thorax plenty of it was met with; and then Laurentius boasts that he had predicted the cause of the symptoms. For my own part, however, I cannot but wonder, since he had divined and predicted that heterogeneous matter could be discharged by the course he indicates, why he could not or would not perceive, and inform us that, in the natural state of things, the blood might be commodiously transferred from the lungs to the left ventricle of the heart by the very same route.

Since, therefore, from the foregoing considerations and many others to the same effect, it is plain that what has heretofore been said concerning the motion and function of the heart and

---

[1] Lib. ix, cap. xi, quest. 12.

[2] De Locis Affectis., lib. vi, cap. 7.

arteries must appear obscure, or inconsistent or even impossible to him who carefully considers the entire subject; it will be proper to look more narrowly into the matter; to contemplate the motion of the heart and arteries, not only in man, but in all animals that have hearts; and further, by frequent appeals to vivisection, and constant ocular inspection, to investigate and endeavour to find the truth.

CHAPTER I.

THE AUTHOR'S MOTIVES FOR WRITING.

WHEN I first gave my mind to vivisections, as a means of discovering the motions and uses of the heart, and sought to discover these from actual inspection, and not from the writings of others, I found the task so truly arduous, so full of difficulties, that I was almost tempted to think, with Fracastorius, that the motion of the heart was only to be comprehended by God. For I could neither rightly perceive at first when the systole and when the diastole took place, nor when and where dilatation and contraction occurred, by reason of the rapidity of the motion, which in many animals is accomplished in the twinkling of an eye, coming and going like a flash of lightning; so that the systole presented itself to me now from this point, now from that; the diastole the same; and then everything was reversed, the motions occurring, as it seemed, variously and confusedly together. My mind was therefore greatly unsettled, nor did I know what I should myself conclude, nor what believe from others; I was not surprised that Andreas Laurentius should have said that the motion of the heart was as perplexing as the flux and reflux of Euripus had appeared to Aristotle.

At length, and by using greater and daily diligence, having frequent recourse to vivisections, employing a variety of animals for the purpose, and collating numerous observations, I thought that I had attained to the truth, that I should extricate myself and escape from this labyrinth, and that I had discovered what I so much desired, both the motion and the use of the heart and arteries; since which time I have not hesitated to expose my views upon these subjects, not only in private to my friends, but also in public, in my anatomical lectures, after the manner of the Academy of old.

These views, as usual, pleased some more, others less; some chid and calumniated me, and laid it to me as a crime that I had dared to depart from the precepts and opinion of all anatomists; others desired further explanations of the novelties, which they said were both worthy of consideration, and might perchance be found of signal use. At length, yielding to the requests of my friends, that all might be made participators in my labours, and partly moved by the envy of others, who, receiving my views with uncandid minds and understanding them indifferently, have essayed to traduce me publicly, I have been moved to commit these things to the press, in order that all may be enabled to form an opinion both of me and my labours. This step I take all the more willingly, seeing that Hieronymus Fabricius of Aquapendente, although he has accurately and learnedly delineated almost every one of the several parts of animals in a special work, has left the heart alone untouched. Finally, if any use or benefit to this department of the republic of letters should accrue from my labours, it will, perhaps, be allowed that I have not lived idly, and, as the old man in the comedy says :

> For never yet hath any one attained
> To such perfection, but that time, and place,
> And use, have brought addition to his knowledge;
> Or made correction, or admonished him,
> That he was ignorant of much which he
> Had thought he knew; or led him to reject
> What he had once esteemed of highest price.

So will it, perchance, be found with reference to the heart at this time; or others, at least, starting from hence, the way pointed out to them, advancing under the guidance of a happier genius, may make occasion to proceed more fortunately, and to inquire more accurately.

CHAPTER II.

OF THE MOTIONS OF THE HEART, AS SEEN IN THE DISSECTION OF LIVING ANIMALS.

IN the first place, then, when the chest of a living animal is laid open and the capsule that immediately surrounds the heart is slit up or removed, the organ is seen now to move, now to be at rest;—there is a time when it moves, and a time when it is motionless.

These things are more obvious in the colder animals, such as toads, frogs, serpents, small fishes, crabs, shrimps, snails and shell-fish. They also become more distinct in warm-blooded animals, such as the dog and hog, if they be attentively noted when the heart begins to flag, to move more slowly, and, as it were, to die: the movements then become slower and rarer, the pauses longer, by which it is made much more easy to perceive and unravel what the motions really are, and how they are performed. In the pause, as in death, the heart is soft, flaccid, exhausted, lying, as it were, at rest.

In the motion, and interval in which this is accomplished, three principal circumstances are to be noted:

1. That the heart is erected, and rises upwards to a point, so that at this time it strikes against the breast and the pulse is felt externally.

2. That it is everywhere contracted, but more especially towards the sides, so that it looks narrower, relatively longer, more drawn together. The heart of an eel taken out of the body of the animal and placed upon the table or the hand, shows these particulars; but the same things are manifest in the heart of small fishes and of those colder animals where the organ is more conical or elongated.

3. The heart being grasped in the hand, is felt to become harder during its action. Now this hardness proceeds from tension, precisely as when the forearm is grasped, its tendons are perceived to become tense and resilient when the fingers are moved.

4. It may further be observed in fishes, and the colder blooded animals, such as frogs, serpents, &c., that the heart,

when it moves, becomes of a paler colour, when quiescent of a deeper blood-red colour.

From these particulars it appeared evident to me that the motion of the heart consists in a certain universal tension—both contraction in the line of its fibres, and constriction in every sense. It becomes erect, hard, and of diminished size during its action; the motion is plainly of the same nature as that of the muscles when they contract in the line of their sinews and fibres; for the muscles, when in action, acquire vigour and tenseness, and from soft become hard, prominent and thickened: in the same manner the heart.

We are therefore authorized to conclude that the heart, at the moment of its action, is at once constricted on all sides, rendered thicker in its parietes and smaller in its ventricles, and so made apt to project or expel its charge of blood. This, indeed, is made sufficiently manifest by the fourth observation preceding, in which we have seen that the heart, by squeezing out the blood it contains becomes paler, and then when it sinks into repose and the ventricle is filled anew with blood, that the deeper crimson colour returns. But no one need remain in doubt of the fact, for if the ventricle be pierced the blood will be seen to be forcibly projected outwards upon each motion or pulsation when the heart is tense.

These things, therefore, happen together or at the same instant: the tension of the heart, the pulse of its apex, which is felt externally by its striking against the chest, the thickening of its parietes, and the forcible expulsion of the blood it contains by the constriction of its ventricles.

Hence the very opposite of the opinions commonly received, appears to be true; inasmuch as it is generally believed that when the heart strikes the breast and the pulse is felt without, the heart is dilated in its ventricles and is filled with blood; but the contrary of this is the fact, and the heart, when it contracts [and the shock is given], is emptied. Whence the motion which is generally regarded as the diastole of the heart, is in truth its systole. And in like manner the intrinsic motion of the heart is not the diastole but the systole; neither is it in the diastole that the heart grows firm and tense, but in the systole, for then only, when tense, is it moved and made vigorous.

Neither is it by any means to be allowed that the heart only moves in the line of its straight fibres, although the great Vesalius, giving this notion countenance, quotes a bundle of osiers bound into a pyramidal heap in illustration; meaning, that as the apex is approached to the base, so are the sides made to bulge out in the fashion of arches, the cavities to dilate, the ventricles to acquire the form of a cupping-glass and so to suck in the blood. But the true effect of every one of its fibres is to constringe the heart at the same time that they render it tense; and this rather with the effect of thickening and amplifying the walls and substance of the organ than enlarging its ventricles. And, again, as the fibres run from the apex to the base, and draw the apex towards the base, they do not tend to make the walls of the heart bulge out in circles, but rather the contrary; inasmuch as every fibre that is circularly disposed, tends to become straight when it contracts; and is distended laterally and thickened, as in the case of muscular fibres in general, when they contract, that is, when they are shortened longitudinally, as we see them in the bellies of the muscles of the body at large. To all this let it be added, that not only are the ventricles contracted in virtue of the direction and condensation of their walls, but farther, that those fibres, or bands, styled nerves by Aristotle, which are so conspicuous in the ventricles of the larger animals, and contain all the straight fibres, (the parietes of the heart containing only circular ones,) when they contract simultaneously, by an admirable adjustment all the internal surfaces are drawn together, as if with cords, and so is the charge of blood expelled with force.

Neither is it true, as vulgarly believed, that the heart by any dilatation or motion of its own, has the power of drawing the blood into the ventricles; for when it acts and becomes tense, the blood is expelled; when it relaxes and sinks together it receives the blood in the manner and wise which will by and by be explained.

CHAPTER III.

OF THE MOTIONS OF ARTERIES, AS SEEN IN THE DISSECTION
OF LIVING ANIMALS.

In connexion with the motions of the heart these things are further to be observed having reference to the motions and pulses of the arteries :

1. At the moment the heart contracts, and when the breast is struck, when in short the organ is in its state of systole, the arteries are dilated, yield a pulse, and are in the state of diastole. In like manner, when the right ventricle contracts and propels its charge of blood, the arterial vein [the pulmonary artery] is distended at the same time with the other arteries of the body.

2. When the left ventricle ceases to act, to contract, to pulsate, the pulse in the arteries also ceases; further, when this ventricle contracts languidly, the pulse in the arteries is scarcely perceptible. In like manner, the pulse in the right ventricle failing, the pulse in the vena arteriosa [pulmonary artery] ceases also.

3. Further, when an artery is divided or punctured, the blood is seen to be forcibly propelled from the wound at the moment the left ventricle contracts; and, again, when the pulmonary artery is wounded, the blood will be seen spouting forth with violence at the instant when the right ventricle contracts.

So also in fishes, if the vessel which leads from the heart to the gills be divided, at the moment when the heart becomes tense and contracted, at the same moment does the blood flow with force from the divided vessel.

In the same way, finally, when we see the blood in arteriotomy projected now to a greater, now to a less distance, and that the greater jet corresponds to the diastole of the artery and to the time when the heart contracts and strikes the ribs, and is in its state of systole, we understand that the blood is expelled by the same movement.

From these facts it is manifest, in opposition to commonly received opinions, that the diastole of the arteries corresponds with the time of the heart's systole; and that the arteries are

filled and distended by the blood forced into them by the contraction of the ventricles; the arteries, therefore, are distended,
because they are filled like sacs or bladders, and are not filled
because they expand like bellows. It is in virtue of one and
the same cause, therefore, that all the arteries of the body
pulsate, viz. the contraction of the left ventricle; in the same
way as the pulmonary artery pulsates by the contraction of the
right ventricle.

Finally, that the pulses of the arteries are due to the impulses
of the blood from the left ventricle, may be illustrated by blowing into a glove, when the whole of the fingers will be found
to become distended at one and the same time, and in their
tension to bear some resemblance to the pulse. For in the
ratio of the tension is the pulse of the heart, fuller, stronger,
more frequent as that acts more vigorously, still preserving the
rhythm and volume, and order of the heart's contractions. Nor
is it to be expected that because of the motion of the blood, the
time at which the contraction of the heart takes place, and that
at which the pulse in an artery (especially a distant one,) is
felt, shall be otherwise than simultaneous: it is here the same
as in blowing up a glove or bladder; for in a plenum, (as in a
drum, a long piece of timber, &c.) the stroke and the motion
occur at both extremities at the same time. Aristotle,[1] too,
has said, "the blood of all animals palpitates within their veins,
(meaning the arteries,) and by the pulse is sent everywhere
simultaneously." And further,[2] "thus do all the veins pulsate
together and by successive strokes, because they all depend upon
the heart; and, as it is always in motion, so are they likewise
always moving together, but by successive movements." It is
well to observe with Galen, in this place, that the old philosophers called the arteries veins.

I happened upon one occasion to have a particular case under
my care, which plainly satisfied me of this truth: A certain
person was affected with a large pulsating tumour on the right
side of the neck, called an aneurism, just at that part where
the artery descends into the axilla, produced by an erosion of
the artery itself, and daily increasing in size; this tumour was
visibly distended as it received the charge of blood brought to

[1] De Animal. iii, cap. 9.   [2] De Respirat. cap. 20.

it by the artery, with each stroke of the heart: the connexion of parts was obvious when the body of the patient came to be opened after his death. The pulse in the corresponding arm was small, in consequence of the greater portion of the blood being diverted into the tumour and so intercepted.

Whence it appears that wherever the motion of the blood through the arteries is impeded, whether it be by compression or infarction, or interception, there do the remote divisions of the arteries beat less forcibly, seeing that the pulse of the arteries is nothing more than the impulse or shock of the blood in these vessels.

CHAPTER IV.

OF THE MOTION OF THE HEART AND ITS AURICLES, AS SEEN IN THE BODIES OF LIVING ANIMALS.

BESIDES the motions already spoken of, we have still to consider those that appertain to the auricles.

Caspar Bauhin and John Riolan,[1] most learned men and skilful anatomists, inform us from their observations, that if we carefully watch the movements of the heart in the vivisection of an animal, we shall perceive four motions distinct in time and in place, two of which are proper to the auricles, two to the ventricles. With all deference to such authority I say, that there are four motions distinct in point of place, but not of time; for the two auricles move together, and so also do the two ventricles, in such wise that though the places be four, the times are only two. And this occurs in the following manner:

There are, as it were, two motions going on together; one of the auricles, another of the ventricles; these by no means taking place simultaneously, but the motion of the auricles preceding, that of the heart itself following; the motion appearing to begin from the auricles and to extend to the ventricles. When all things are becoming languid, and the heart is dying, as also in fishes and the colder blooded animals, there is a short pause between these two motions, so that the heart aroused, as it were, appears to respond to the motion, now more quickly,

---

[1] Bauhin, lib. ii, cap. 21. Riolan, lib. viii, cap. 1.

now more tardily; and at length, and when near to death, it ceases to respond by its proper motion, but seems, as it were, to nod the head, and is so obscurely moved that it appears rather to give signs of motion to the pulsating auricle, than actually to move. The heart, therefore, ceases to pulsate sooner than the auricles, so that the auricles have been said to outlive it, the left ventricle ceasing to pulsate first of all; then its auricle, next the right ventricle; and, finally, all the other parts being at rest and dead, as Galen long since observed, the right auricle still continues to beat; life, therefore, appears to linger longest in the right auricle. Whilst the heart is gradually dying, it is sometimes seen to reply, after two or three contractions of the auricles, roused as it were to action, and making a single pulsation, slowly, unwillingly, and with an effort.

But this especially is to be noted, that after the heart has ceased to beat, the auricles however still contracting, a finger placed upon the ventricles perceives the several pulsations of the auricles, precisely in the same way and for the same reason, as we have said, that the pulses of the ventricles are felt in the arteries, to wit, the distension produced by the jet of blood. And if at this time, the auricles alone pulsating, the point of the heart be cut off with a pair of scissors, you will perceive the blood flowing out upon each contraction of the auricles. Whence it is manifest how the blood enters the ventricles, not by any attraction or dilatation of the heart, but thrown into them by the pulses of the auricles.

And here I would observe, that whenever I speak of pulsations as occurring in the auricles or ventricles, I mean contractions: first the auricles *contract*, and then and subsequently the heart itself *contracts*. When the auricles contract they are seen to become whiter, especially where they contain but little blood; but they are filled as magazines or reservoirs of the blood, which is tending spontaneously and, by the motion of the veins, under pressure towards the centre; the whiteness indicated is most conspicuous towards the extremities or edges of the auricles at the time of their contractions.

In fishes and frogs, and other animals which have hearts with but a single ventricle, and for an auricle have a kind of bladder much distended with blood, at the base of the organ, you may very plainly perceive this bladder contracting first, and the contraction of the heart or ventricle following afterwards.

But I think it right to describe what I have observed of an opposite character: the heart of an eel, of several fishes, and even of some [of the higher] animals taken out of the body, beats without auricles; nay, if it be cut in pieces the several parts may still be seen contracting and relaxing; so that in these creatures the body of the heart may be seen pulsating, palpitating, after the cessation of all motion in the auricle. But is not this perchance peculiar to animals more tenacious of life, whose radical moisture is more glutinous, or fat and sluggish, and less readily soluble? The same faculty indeed appears in the flesh of eels, generally, which even when skinned and embowelled, and cut into pieces, are still seen to move.

Experimenting with a pigeon upon one occasion, after the heart had wholly ceased to pulsate, and the auricles too had become motionless, I kept my finger wetted with saliva and warm for a short time upon the heart, and observed, that under the influence of this fomentation it recovered new strength and life, so that both ventricles and auricles pulsated, contracting and relaxing alternately, recalled as it were from death to life.

Besides this, however, I have occasionally observed, after the heart and even its right auricle had ceased pulsating,—when it was in articulo mortis in short, that an obscure motion, an undulation or palpitation, remained in the blood itself, which was contained in the right auricle, this being apparent so long as it was imbued with heat and spirit. And indeed a circumstance of the same kind is extremely manifest in the course of the generation of animals, as may be seen in the course of the first seven days of the incubation of the chick: A drop of blood makes its appearance which palpitates, as Aristotle had already observed; from this, when the growth is further advanced and the chick is fashioned, the auricles of the heart are formed, which pulsating henceforth give constant signs of life. When at length, and after the lapse of a few days, the outline of the body begins to be distinguished, then is the ventricular part of the heart also produced; but it continues for a time white and apparently bloodless, like the rest of the animal; neither does it pulsate or give signs of motion. I have seen a similar condition of the heart in the human fœtus about the beginning of the third month, the heart being then whitish and bloodless, although its auricles contained a considerable quantity of purple blood. In the same way in the egg, when the chick was formed and had increased in size, the heart too increased and acquired ventricles, which then began to receive and to transmit blood.

And this leads me to remark, that he who inquires very particularly into this matter will not conclude that the heart, as a whole, is the primum vivens, ultimum moriens—the first part to live, the last to die, but rather its auricles, or the part which corresponds to the auricles in serpents, fishes, &c., which both lives before the heart[1] and dies after it.

Nay, has not the blood itself or spirit an obscure palpitation inherent in it, which it has even appeared to me to retain after death? and it seems very questionable whether or not we are to say that life begins with the palpitation or beating of the heart. The seminal fluid of all animals—the prolific spirit, as Aristotle observed, leaves their body with a bound and like a living thing; and nature in death, as Aristotle[2] further remarks, retracing her steps, reverts to whence she had set out, returns at the end of her course to the goal whence she had started; and as animal generation proceeds from that which is not animal, entity from non-entity, so, by a retrograde course, entity, by corruption, is resolved into non-entity; whence that in animals, which was last created, fails first; and that which was first, fails last.

I have also observed, that almost all animals have truly a heart, not the larger creatures only, and those that have red blood, but the smaller, and [seemingly] bloodless ones also, such as slugs, snails, scallops, shrimps, crabs, crayfish, and many others; nay, even in wasps, hornets and flies, I have, with the aid of a magnifying glass, and at the upper part of what is called the tail, both seen the heart pulsating myself, and shown it to many others.

But in the exsanguine tribes the heart pulsates sluggishly and deliberately, contracting slowly as in animals that are moribund, a fact that may readily be seen in the snail, whose

---

[1] [The reader will observe that Harvey, when he speaks of the *heart*, always means the ventricles or ventricular portion of the organ.—ED.]

[2] De Motu Animal. cap. 8.

heart will be found at the bottom of that orifice in the right side of the body which is seen to be opened and shut in the course of respiration, and whence saliva is discharged, the incision being made in the upper aspect of the body, near the part which corresponds to the liver.

This, however, is to be observed: that in winter and the colder season, exsanguine animals, such as the snail, show no pulsations; they seem rather to live after the manner of vegetables, or of those other productions which are therefore designated plant-animals.

It is also to be noted that all animals which have a heart, have also auricles, or something analogous to auricles; and further, that wherever the heart has a double ventricle there are always two auricles present, but not otherwise. If you turn to the production of the chick in ovo, however, you will find at first no more than a vesicle or auricle, or pulsating drop of blood; it is only by and by, when the development has made some progress, that the heart is fashioned: even so in certain animals not destined to attain to the highest perfection in their organization, such as bees, wasps, snails, shrimps, crayfish, &c., we only find a certain pulsating vesicle, like a sort of red or white palpitating point, as the beginning or principle of their life.[1]

We have a small shrimp in these countries, which is taken in the Thames and in the sea, the whole of whose body is transparent; this creature, placed in a little water, has frequently afforded myself and particular friends an opportunity of observing the motions of the heart with the greatest distinctness, the external parts of the body presenting no obstacle to our view, but the heart being perceived as though it had been seen through a window.

I have also observed the first rudiments of the chick in the course of the fourth or fifth day of the incubation, in the guise of a little cloud, the shell having been removed and the egg immersed in clear tepid water. In the midst of the cloudlet in question there was a bloody point so small that it disappeared during the contraction and escaped the sight, but in the re-

---

[1] [The Editor begs here to be allowed to remark on Harvey's obvious perception of the correspondence between that permanent condition of an organ in the lower, and its transitory condition in the higher animals.—ED.]

laxation it reappeared again, red and like the point of a pin;
so that betwixt the visible and invisible, betwixt being and not
being, as it were, it gave by its pulses a kind of representation
of the commencement of life.[1]

CHAPTER V.

OF THE MOTION, ACTION, AND OFFICE OF THE HEART.

FROM these and other observations of the like kind, I am
persuaded it will be found that the motion of the heart is as
follows :

First of all, the auricle contracts, and in the course of its
contraction throws the blood, (which it contains in ample quantity as the head of the veins, the store-house and cistern of the
blood,) into the ventricle, which being filled, the heart raises
itself straightway, makes all its fibres tense, contracts the ventricles, and performs a beat, by which beat it immediately sends
the blood supplied to it by the auricle into the arteries; the
right ventricle sending its charge into the lungs by the vessel
which is called vena arteriosa, but which, in structure and function, and all things else, is an artery; the left ventricle sending its charge into the aorta, and through this by the arteries
to the body at large.

These two motions, one of the ventricles, another of the auricles, take place consecutively, but in such a manner that there
is a kind of harmony or rhythm preserved between them, the
two concurring in such wise that but one motion is apparent,
especially in the warmer blooded animals, in which the movements in question are rapid.   Nor is this for any other reason
than it is in a piece of machinery, in which, though one wheel gives
motion to another, yet all the wheels seem to move simultaneously; or in that mechanical contrivance which is adapted to
firearms, where the trigger being touched, down comes the flint,
strikes against the steel, elicits a spark, which falling among the

---

[1] [At the period Harvey indicates, a rudimentary auricle and ventricle exist, but
are so transparent that unless with certain precautions their parietes cannot be seen.
The filling and emptying of them, therefore, give the appearance of a speck of blood
alternately appearing and disappearing.—ED.]

powder, it is ignited, upon which the flame extends, enters the barrel, causes the explosion, propels the ball, and the mark is attained—all of which incidents, by reason of the celerity with which they happen, seem to take place in the twinkling of an eye. So also in deglutition : by the elevation of the root of the tongue, and the compression of the mouth, the food or drink is pushed into the fauces, the larynx is closed by its own muscles, and the epiglottis, whilst the pharynx, raised and opened by its muscles no otherwise than is a sac that is to be filled, is lifted up, and its mouth dilated ; upon which, the mouthful being received, it is forced downwards by the transverse muscles, and then carried farther by the longitudinal ones. Yet are all these motions, though executed by different and distinct organs, performed harmoniously, and in such order, that they seem to constitute but a single motion and act, which we call deglutition.

Even so does it come to pass with the motions and action of the heart, which constitute a kind of deglutition, a transfusion of the blood from the veins to the arteries. And if any one, bearing these things in mind, will carefully watch the motions of the heart in the body of a living animal, he will perceive not only all the particulars I have mentioned, viz., the heart becoming erect, and making one continuous motion with its auricles; but farther, a certain obscure undulation and lateral inclination in the direction of the axis of the right ventricle, [the organ] twisting itself slightly in performing its work. And indeed every one may see, when a horse drinks, that the water is drawn in and transmitted to the stomach at each movement of the throat, the motion being accompanied with a sound, and yielding a pulse both to the ear and the touch ; in the same way it is with each motion of the heart, when there is the delivery of a quantity of blood from the veins to the arteries, that a pulse takes place, and can be heard within the chest.

The motion of the heart, then, is entirely of this description, and the one action of the heart is the transmission of the blood and its distribution, by means of the arteries, to the very extremities of the body ; so that the pulse which we feel in the arteries is nothing more than the impulse of the blood derived from the heart.

Whether or not the heart, besides propelling the blood, giving it motion locally, and distributing it to the body, adds anything else to it,—heat, spirit, perfection,—must be inquired into by and by, and decided upon other grounds. So much may suffice at this time, when it is shown that by the action of the heart the blood is transfused through the ventricles from the veins to the arteries, and distributed by them to all parts of the body.

So much, indeed, is admitted by all [physiologists], both from the structure of the heart and the arrangement and action of its valves. But still they are like persons purblind or groping about in the dark; and then they give utterance to diverse, contradictory, and incoherent sentiments, delivering many things upon conjecture, as we have already had occasion to remark.

The grand cause of hesitation and error in this subject appears to me to have been the intimate connexion between the heart and the lungs. When men saw both the vena arteriosa [or pulmonary artery] and the arteriæ venosæ [or pulmonary veins] losing themselves in the lungs, of course it became a puzzle to them to know how or by what means the right ventricle should distribute the blood to the body, or the left draw it from the venæ cavæ. This fact is borne witness to by Galen, whose words, when writing against Erasistratus in regard to the origin and use of the veins and the coction of the blood, are the following:[1] "You will reply," he says, "that the effect is so; that the blood is prepared in the liver, and is thence transferred to the heart to receive its proper form and last perfection; a statement which does not appear devoid of reason; for no great and perfect work is ever accomplished at a single effort, or receives its final polish from one instrument. But if this be actually so, then show us another vessel which draws the absolutely perfect blood from the heart, and distributes it as the arteries do the spirits over the whole body." Here then is a reasonable opinion not allowed, because, forsooth, besides not seeing the true means of transit, he could not discover the vessel which should transmit the blood from the heart to the body at large!

But had any one been there in behalf of Erasistratus, and of that opinion which we now espouse, and which Galen himself acknowledges in other respects consonant with reason, to have pointed to the aorta as the vessel which distributes the blood from

---

[1] De Placitis Hippocratis et Platonis, vi.

the heart to the rest of the body, I wonder what would have been the answer of that most ingenious and learned man? Had he said that the artery transmits spirits and not blood, he would indeed sufficiently have answered Erasistratus, who imagined that the arteries contained nothing but spirits; but then he would have contradicted himself, and given a foul denial to that for which he had keenly contended in his writings against this very Erasistratus, to wit, that blood in substance is contained in the arteries, and not spirits; a fact which he demonstrated not only by many powerful arguments, but by experiments.

But if the divine Galen will here allow, as in other places he does, "that all the arteries of the body arise from the great artery, and that this takes its origin from the heart; that all these vessels naturally contain and carry blood; that the three semilunar valves situated at the orifice of the aorta prevent the return of the blood into the heart, and that nature never connected them with this, the most noble viscus of the body, unless for some most important end;" if, I say, this father of physic admits all these things,—and I quote his own words,—I do not see how he can deny that the great artery is the very vessel to carry the blood, when it has attained its highest term of perfection, from the heart for distribution to all parts of the body. Or would he perchance still hesitate, like all who have come after him, even to the present hour, because he did not perceive the route by which the blood was transferred from the veins to the arteries, in consequence, as I have already said, of the intimate connexion between the heart and the lungs? And that this difficulty puzzled anatomists not a little, when in their dissections they found the pulmonary artery and left ventricle full of thick, black, and clotted blood, plainly appears, when they felt themselves compelled to affirm that the blood made its way from the right to the left ventricle by sweating through the septum of the heart. But this fancy I have already refuted. A new pathway for the blood must therefore be prepared and thrown open, and being once exposed, no further difficulty will, I believe, be experienced by any one in admitting what I have already proposed in regard to the pulse of the heart and arteries, viz. the passage of the blood from the veins to the arteries, and its distribution to the whole of the body by means of these vessels.

CHAPTER VI.

OF THE COURSE BY WHICH THE BLOOD IS CARRIED FROM THE
VENA CAVA INTO THE ARTERIES, OR FROM THE RIGHT INTO
THE LEFT VENTRICLE OF THE HEART.

SINCE the intimate connexion of the heart with the lungs,
which is apparent in the human subject, has been the probable
cause of the errors that have been committed on this point,
they plainly do amiss who, pretending to speak of the parts of
animals generally, as anatomists for the most part do, confine
their researches to the human body alone, and that when it is
dead. They obviously act no otherwise than he who, having
studied the forms of a single commonwealth, should set about
the composition of a general system of polity; or who, having
taken cognizance of the nature of a single field, should imagine
that he had mastered the science of agriculture; or who, upon
the ground of one particular proposition, should proceed to draw
general conclusions.

Had anatomists only been as conversant with the dissection of
the lower animals as they are with that of the human body, the
matters that have hitherto kept them in a perplexity of doubt
would, in my opinion, have met them freed from every kind of
difficulty.

And, first, in fishes, in which the heart consists of but a
single ventricle, they having no lungs, the thing is sufficiently
manifest. Here the sac, which is situated at the base of the heart,
and is the part analogous to the auricle in man, plainly throws
the blood into the heart, and the heart, in its turn, conspicuously transmits it by a pipe or artery, or vessel analogous to an
artery; these are facts which are confirmed by simple ocular
inspection, as well as by a division of the vessel, when the blood
is seen to be projected by each pulsation of the heart.

The same thing is also not difficult of demonstration in those animals that have either no more, or, as it were, no more than a single
ventricle to the heart, such as toads, frogs, serpents, and lizards,
which, although they have lungs in a certain sense, as they have
a voice, (and I have many observations by me on the admirable
structure of the lungs of these animals, and matters appertain-

ing, which, however, I cannot introduce in this place,) still their anatomy plainly shows that the blood is transferred in them from the veins to the arteries in the same manner as in higher animals, viz., by the action of the heart; the way, in fact, is patent, open, manifest; there is no difficulty, no room for hesitating about it; for in them the matter stands precisely as it would in man, were the septum of his heart perforated or removed, or one ventricle made out of two; and this being the case, I imagine that no one will doubt as to the way by which the blood may pass from the veins into the arteries.

But as there are actually more animals which have no lungs than there are which be furnished with them, and in like manner a greater number which have only one ventricle than there are which have two, it is open to us to conclude, judging from the mass or multitude of living creatures, that for the major part, and generally, there is an open way by which the blood is transmitted from the veins through the sinuses or cavities of the heart into the arteries.

I have, however, cogitating with myself, seen further, that the same thing obtained most obviously in the embryos of those animals that have lungs; for in the fœtus the four vessels belonging to the heart, viz., the vena cava, the vena arteriosa or pulmonary artery, the arteria venalis or pulmonary vein, and the arteria magna or aorta, are all connected otherwise than in the adult; a fact sufficiently known to every anatomist. The first contact and union of the vena cava with the arteria venosa or pulmonary veins, which occurs before the cava opens properly into the right ventricle of the heart, or gives off the coronary vein, a little above its escape from the liver, is by a lateral anastomosis; this is an ample foramen, of an oval form, communicating between the cava and the arteria venosa, or pulmonary vein, so that the blood is free to flow in the greatest abundance by that foramen from the vena cava into the arteria venosa or pulmonary vein, and left auricle, and from thence into the left ventricle; and farther, in this foramen ovale, from that part which regards the arteria venosa, or pulmonary vein, there is a thin tough membrane, larger than the opening, extended like an operculum or cover; this membrane in the adult blocking up the foramen, and adhering on all sides, finally closes it up, and almost obliterates every trace of it. This membrane, however, is so contrived in the fœtus, that falling loosely upon itself, it permits a ready access to the lungs and heart, yielding a passage to the blood which is streaming from the cava, and hindering the tide at the same time from flowing back into that vein.   All things, in short, permit us to believe that in the embryo the blood must constantly pass by this foramen from the vena cava into the arteria venosa, or pulmonary vein, and from thence into the left auricle of the heart; and having once entered there, it can never regurgitate.

Another union is that by the vena arteriosa, or pulmonary artery, and is effected when that vessel divides into two branches after its escape from the right ventricle of the heart. It is as if to the two trunks already mentioned a third were superadded, a kind of arterial canal, carried obliquely from the vena arteriosa, or pulmonary artery, to perforate and terminate in the arteria magna or aorta. In the embryo, consequently, there are, as it were, two aortas, or two roots of the arteria magna, springing from the heart. This canalis arteriosus shrinks gradually after birth, and is at length and finally almost entirely withered, and removed, like the umbilical vessels.

The canalis arteriosus contains no membrane or valve to direct or impede the flow of the blood in this or in that direction: for at the root of the vena arteriosa, or pulmonary artery, of which the canalis arteriosus is the continuation in the fœtus, there are three sigmoid or semilunar valves, which open from within outwards, and oppose no obstacle to the blood flowing in this direction or from the right ventricle into the pulmonary artery and aorta; but they prevent all regurgitation from the aorta or pulmonic vessels back upon the right ventricle; closing with perfect accuracy, they oppose an effectual obstacle to everything of the kind in the embryo. So that there is also reason to believe that when the heart contracts, the blood is regularly propelled by the canal or passage indicated from the right ventricle into the aorta.

What is commonly said in regard to these two great communications, to wit, that they exist for the nutrition of the lungs, is both improbable and inconsistent; seeing that in the adult they are closed up, abolished, and consolidated, although the lungs, by reason of their heat and motion, must then be presumed to require a larger supply of nourishment. The same may be said in regard to the assertion that the heart in the embryo does not pulsate, that it neither acts nor moves, so that nature was forced to make these communications for the nutrition of the lungs. This is plainly false; for simple inspection of the incubated egg, and of embryos just taken out of the uterus, shows that the heart moves precisely in them as in adults, and that nature feels no such necessity. I have myself repeatedly seen these motions, and Aristotle is likewise witness of their reality. " The pulse," he observes, " inheres in the very constitution of the heart, and appears from the beginning, as is learned both from the dissection of living animals, and the formation of the chick in the egg."[1] But we further observe, that the passages in question are not only pervious up to the period of birth in man, as well as in other animals, as anatomists in general have described them, but for several months subsequently, in some indeed for several years, not to say for the whole course of life; as, for example, in the goose, snipe, and various birds, and many of the smaller animals. And this circumstance it was, perhaps, that imposed upon Botallus, who thought he had discovered a new passage for the blood from the vena cava into the left ventricle of the heart; and I own that when I met with the same arrangement in one of the larger members of the mouse family, in the adult state, I was myself at first led to something of a like conclusion.

From this it will be understood that in the human embryo, and in the embryos of animals in which the communications are not closed, the same thing happens, namely, that the heart by its motion propels the blood by obvious and open passages from the vena cava into the aorta through the cavities of both the ventricles; the right one receiving the blood from the auricle, and propelling it by the vena arteriosa, or pulmonary artery, and its continuation, named the ductus arteriosus, into the aorta; the left, in like manner, charged by the contraction of its auricle, which has received its supply through the foramen ovale from the vena cava, contracting, and projecting the blood through the root of the aorta into the trunk of that vessel.

In embryos, consequently, whilst the lungs are yet in a state of inaction, performing no function, subject to no motion any

---

[1] Lib. de Spiritu, cap. v.

more than if they had not been present, nature uses the two ventricles of the heart as if they formed but one, for the transmission of the blood. The condition of the embryos of those animals which have lungs, whilst these organs are yet in abeyance and not employed, is the same as that of those animals which have no lungs.

So clearly, therefore, does it appear in the case of the fœtus, viz., that the heart by its action transfers the blood from the vena cava into the aorta, and that by a route as obvious and open, as if in the adult the two ventricles were made to communicate by the removal of their septum. Since, then, we find that in the greater number of animals, in all, indeed, at a certain period of their existence, the channels for the transmission of the blood through the heart are so conspicuous, we have still to inquire wherefore in some creatures—those, namely, that have warm blood, and that have attained to the adult age, man among the number—we should not conclude that the same thing is accomplished through the substance of the lungs, which in the embryo, and at a time when the function of these organs is in abeyance, nature effects by the direct passages described, and which, indeed, she seems compelled to adopt through want of a passage by the lungs; or wherefore it should be better (for nature always does that which is best) that she should close up the various open routes which she had formerly made use of in the embryo and fœtus, and still uses in all other animals; not only opening up no new apparent channels for the passage of the blood, therefore, but even entirely shutting up those which formerly existed.

And now the discussion is brought to this point, that they who inquire into the ways by which the blood reaches the left ventricle of the heart and pulmonary veins from the vena cava, will pursue the wisest course if they seek by dissection to discover the causes why in the larger and more perfect animals of mature age, nature has rather chosen to make the blood percolate the parenchyma of the lungs, than as in other instances chosen a direct and obvious course—for I assume that no other path or mode of transit can be entertained. It must be either because the larger and more perfect animals are warmer, and when adult their heat greater—ignited, as I might say, and requiring to be damped or mitigated; therefore it may be that the blood is sent through the lungs, that it may be tempered by the air that is inspired, and prevented from boiling up, and so becoming extinguished, or something else of the sort. But to determine these matters, and explain them satisfactorily, were to enter on a speculation in regard to the office of the lungs and the ends for which they exist; and upon such a subject, as well as upon what pertains to eventilation, to the necessity and use of the air, &c., as also to the variety and diversity of organs that exist in the bodies of animals in connexion with these matters, although I have made a vast number of observations, still, lest I should be held as wandering too wide of my present purpose, which is the use and motion of the heart, and be charged with speaking of things beside the question, and rather complicating and quitting than illustrating it, I shall leave such topics till I can more conveniently set them forth in a treatise apart. And now, returning to my immediate subject, I go on with what yet remains for demonstration, viz., that in the more perfect and warmer adult animals, and man, the blood passes from the right ventricle of the heart by the vena arteriosa, or pulmonary artery, into the lungs, and thence by the arteriæ venosæ, or pulmonary veins, into the left auricle, and thence into the left ventricle of the heart. And, first, I shall show that this may be so, and then I shall prove that it is so in fact.

CHAPTER VII.

THE BLOOD PERCOLATES THE SUBSTANCE OF THE LUNGS FROM THE RIGHT VENTRICLE OF THE HEART INTO THE PULMONARY VEINS AND LEFT VENTRICLE.

THAT this is possible, and that there is nothing to prevent it from being so, appears when we reflect on the way in which water percolating the earth produces springs and rivulets, or when we speculate on the means by which the sweat passes through the skin, or the urine through the parenchyma of the kidneys. It is well known that persons who use the Spa waters, or those of La Madonna, in the territories of Padua, or others of an acidulous or vitriolated nature, or who simply swallow drinks by the gallon, pass all off again within an hour or two by urine. Such a quantity of liquid must take some short time in the concoction: it must pass through the liver; (it is allowed by all that the juices of the food we consume pass twice through this organ in the course of the day;) it must flow through the veins, through the parenchyma of the kidneys, and through the ureters into the bladder.

To those, therefore, whom I hear denying that the blood, aye the whole mass of the blood may pass through the substance of the lungs, even as the nutritive juices percolate the liver, asserting such a proposition to be impossible, and by no means to be entertained as credible, I reply, with the poet, that they are of that race of men who, when they will, assent full readily, and when they will not, by no manner of means; who, when their assent is wanted, fear, and when it is not, fear not to give it.

The parenchyma of the liver is extremely dense, so is that of the kidney; the lungs, again, are of a much looser texture, and if compared with the kidneys are absolutely spongy. In the liver there is no forcing, no impelling power; in the lungs the blood is forced on by the pulse of the right ventricle, the necessary effect of whose impulse is the distension of the vessels and pores of the lungs. And then the lungs, in respiration, are perpetually rising and falling; motions, the effect of which must needs be to open and shut the pores and vessels, precisely as in the case of a sponge, and of parts having a spongy structure, when they are alternately compressed and again are suffered to expand. The liver, on the contrary, remains at rest, and is never seen to be dilated and constricted. Lastly, if no one denies the possibility of the whole of the ingested juices passing through the liver, in man, oxen, and the larger animals generally, in order to reach the vena cava, and for this reason, that if nourishment is to go on, these juices must needs get into the veins, and there is no other way but the one indicated, why should not the same arguments be held of avail for the passage of the blood in adults through the lungs? Why not, with Columbus, that skilful and learned anatomist, maintain and believe the like, from the capacity and structure of the pulmonary vessels; from the fact of the pulmonary veins and ventricle corresponding with them, being always found to contain blood, which must needs have come from the veins, and by no other passage save through the lungs? Columbus, and we also, from what precedes, from dissections, and other arguments, conceive the thing to be clear. But as there are some who admit nothing unless upon authority, let them learn that the truth I am contending for can be confirmed from Galen's own words, namely, that not only may the blood be transmitted from the pulmonary artery into the pulmonary veins, then into the left ventricle of the heart, and from thence into the arteries of the body, but that this is effected by the ceaseless pulsation of the heart and the motion of the lungs in breathing.

There are, as every one knows, three sigmoid or semilunar valves situated at the orifice of the pulmonary artery, which effectually prevent the blood sent into the vessel from returning into the cavity of the heart. Now Galen, explaining the uses of these valves, and the necessity for them, employs the following language :[1] " There is everywhere a mutual anastomosis and inosculation of the arteries with the veins, and they severally transmit both blood and spirit, by certain invisible and undoubtedly very narrow passages. Now if the mouth of the vena arteriosa, or pulmonary artery, had stood in like manner continually open, and nature had found no contrivance for closing it when requisite, and opening it again, it would have been impossible that the blood could ever have passed by the invisible and delicate mouths, during the contractions of the thorax, into the arteries ; for all things are not alike readily attracted or repelled ; but that which is light is more readily drawn in, the instrument being dilated, and forced out again when it is contracted, than that which is heavy ; and in like manner is anything drawn more rapidly along an ample conduit, and again driven forth, than it is through a narrow tube. But when the thorax is contracted, the pulmonary veins, which are in the lungs, being driven inwardly, and powerfully compressed on every side, immediately force out some of the spirit they contain, and at the same time assume a certain portion of blood by those subtile mouths ; a thing that could never come to pass were the blood at liberty to flow back into the heart through the great orifice of the pulmonary artery. But its return through this great opening being prevented, when it is compressed on every side, a certain portion of it distils into the pulmonary veins

---

[1] De Usu partium, lib. vi, cap. 10.

by the minute orifices mentioned." And shortly afterwards, in the very next chapter, he says : " The more the thorax contracts, the more it strives to force out the blood, the more exactly do these membranes (viz., the sigmoid valves) close up the mouth of the vessel, and suffer nothing to regurgitate." The same fact he has also alluded to in a preceding part of the tenth chapter : " Were there no valves, a three-fold inconvenience would result, so that the blood would then perform this lengthened course in vain ; it would flow inwards during the diastoles of the lungs, and fill all their arteries ; but in the systoles, in the manner of the tide, it would ever and anon, like the Euripus, flow backwards and forwards by the same way, with a reciprocating motion, which would nowise suit the blood. This, however, may seem a matter of little moment ; but if it meantime appear that the function of respiration suffer, then I think it would be looked upon as no trifle, &c." And again, and shortly afterwards : " And then a third inconvenience, by no means to be thought lightly of, would follow, were the blood moved backwards during the expirations, had not our Maker instituted those supplementary membranes [the sigmoid valves]." Whence, in the eleventh chapter, he concludes : " That they have all a common use, (to wit, the valves,) and that it is to prevent regurgitation or backward motion; each, however, having a proper function, the one set drawing matters from the heart, and preventing their return, the other drawing matters into the heart, and preventing their escape from it. For nature never intended to distress the heart with needless labour, neither to bring aught into the organ which it had been better to have kept away, nor to take from it again aught which it was requisite should be brought. Since, then, there are four orifices in all, two in either ventricle, one of these induces, the other educes." And again he says : " Farther, since there is one vessel, consisting of a simple tunic, implanted in the heart, and another, having a double tunic, extending from it, (Galen is here speaking of the right side of the heart, but I extend his observations to the left side also,) a kind of reservoir had to be provided, to which both belonging, the blood should be drawn in by the one, and sent out by the other."

This argument Galen adduces for the transit of the blood by the right ventricle from the vena cava into the lungs ; but we can use it with still greater propriety, merely changing the terms, for the passage of the blood from the veins through the heart into the arteries. From Galen, however, that great man, that father of physicians, it clearly appears that the blood passes through the lungs from the pulmonary artery into the minute branches of the pulmonary veins, urged to this both by the pulses of the heart and by the motions of the lungs and thorax ; that the heart, moreover, is incessantly receiving and expelling the blood by and from its ventricles, as from a magazine or cistern, and for this end is furnished with four sets of valves, two serving for the induction and two for the eduction of the blood, lest, like the Euripus, it should be incommodiously sent hither and thither, or flow back into the cavity which it should have quitted, or quit the part where its presence was required, and so the heart be oppressed with labour in vain, and the office of the lungs be interfered with.[1] Finally, our position that the blood is continually passing from the right to the left ventricle, from the vena cava into the aorta, through the porous structure of the lungs, plainly appears from this, that since the blood is incessantly sent from the right ventricle into the lungs by the pulmonary artery, and in like manner is incessantly drawn from the lungs into the left ventricle, as appears from what precedes and the position of the valves, it cannot do otherwise than pass through continuously. And then, as the blood is incessantly flowing into the right ventricle of the heart, and is continually passed out from the left, as appears in like manner, and as is obvious both to sense and reason, it is impossible that the blood can do otherwise than pass continually from the vena cava into the aorta.

Dissection consequently shows distinctly what takes place [in regard to the transit of the blood] in the greater number of animals, and indeed in all, up to the period of their [fœtal] maturity ; and that the same thing occurs in adults is equally certain, both from Galen's words, and what has already been said on the subject, only that in the former the transit is effected by open and obvious passages, in the latter by the obscure porosities of the lungs and the minute inoscula-

---

[1] See the Commentary of the learned Hofmann upon the Sixth Book of Galen, 'De Usu partium,' a work which I first saw after I had written what precedes.

tions of vessels. Whence it appears that, although one ventricle of the heart, the left to wit, would suffice for the distribution of the blood over the body, and its eduction from the vena cava, as indeed is done in those creatures that have no lungs, nature, nevertheless, when she ordained that the same blood should also percolate the lungs, saw herself obliged to add another ventricle, the right, the pulse of which should force the blood from the vena cava through the lungs into the cavity of the left ventricle. In this way, therefore, it may be said that the right ventricle is made for the sake of the lungs, and for the transmission of the blood through them, not for their nutrition; seeing it were unreasonable to suppose that the lungs required any so much more copious a supply of nutriment, and that of so much purer and more spirituous a kind, as coming immediately from the ventricle of the heart, than either the brain with its peculiarly pure substance, or the eyes with their lustrous and truly admirable structure, or the flesh of the heart itself, which is more commodiously nourished by the coronary artery.

CHAPTER VIII.

OF THE QUANTITY OF BLOOD PASSING THROUGH THE HEART FROM THE VEINS TO THE ARTERIES; AND OF THE CIRCULAR MOTION OF THE BLOOD.

THUS far I have spoken of the passage of the blood from the veins into the arteries, and of the manner in which it is transmitted and distributed by the action of the heart; points to which some, moved either by the authority of Galen or Columbus, or the reasonings of others, will give in their adhesion. But what remains to be said upon the quantity and source of the blood which thus passes, is of so novel and unheard-of character, that I not only fear injury to myself from the envy of a few, but I tremble lest I have mankind at large for my enemies, so much doth wont and custom, that become as another nature, and doctrine once sown and that hath struck deep root, and respect for antiquity influence all men : Still the die is cast, and my trust is in my love of truth, and the candour that inheres in cultivated minds. And sooth to say, when I surveyed my mass of evidence, whether derived from vivisections, and my various reflections on them, or from the ventricles of the heart and the vessels that enter into and issue from them, the symmetry and size of these conduits,—for nature doing nothing in vain, would never have given them so large a relative size without a purpose,—or from the arrangement and intimate structure of the valves in particular, and of the other parts of the heart in general, with many things besides, I frequently and seriously bethought me, and long revolved in my mind, what might be the quantity of blood which was transmitted, in how short a time its passage might be effected, and the like; and not finding it possible that this could be supplied by the juices of the ingested aliment without the veins on the one hand becoming drained, and the arteries on the other getting ruptured through the excessive charge of blood, unless the blood should somehow find its way from the arteries into the veins, and so return to the right side of the heart; I began to think whether there might not be A MO-TION, AS IT WERE, IN A CIRCLE. Now this I afterwards found to be true; and I finally saw that the blood, forced by the action of the left ventricle into the arteries, was distributed to the body at large, and its several parts, in the same manner as it is sent through the lungs, impelled by the right ventricle into the pulmonary artery, and that it then passed through the veins and along the vena cava, and so round to the left ventricle in the manner already indicated. Which motion we may be allowed to call circular, in the same way as Aristotle says that the air and the rain emulate the circular motion of the superior bodies; for the moist earth, warmed by the sun, evaporates; the vapours drawn upwards are condensed, and descending in the form of rain, moisten the earth again; and by this arrangement are generations of living things produced; and in like manner too are tempests and meteors engendered by the circular motion, and by the approach and recession of the sun.

And so, in all likelihood, does it come to pass in the body, through the motion of the blood; the various parts are nourished, cherished, quickened by the warmer, more perfect, vaporous, spirituous, and, as I may say, alimentive blood; which, on the contrary, in contact with these parts becomes cooled, coagulated, and, so to speak, effete; whence it returns to its sovereign the heart, as if to its source, or to the inmost home of the body, there to recover its state of excellence or perfection. Here it resumes its due fluidity and receives an infusion of natural heat—powerful, fervid, a kind of treasury of life, and is impregnated with spirits, and it might be said with balsam; and thence it is again dispersed; and all this depends on the motion and action of the heart.

The heart, consequently, is the beginning of life; the sun of the microcosm, even as the sun in his turn might well be designated the heart of the world; for it is the heart by whose virtue and pulse the blood is moved, perfected, made apt to nourish, and is preserved from corruption and coagulation; it is the household divinity which, discharging its function, nourishes, cherishes, quickens the whole body, and is indeed the foundation of life, the source of all action. But of these things we shall speak more opportunely when we come to speculate upon the final cause of this motion of the heart.

Hence, since the veins are the conduits and vessels that transport the blood, they are of two kinds, the cava and the aorta; and this not by reason of there being two sides of the body, as Aristotle has it, but because of the difference of office; nor yet, as is commonly said, in consequence of any diversity of structure, for in many animals, as I have said, the vein does not differ from the artery in the thickness of its tunics, but solely in virtue of their several destinies and uses. A vein and an artery, both styled vein by the ancients, and that not undeservedly, as Galen has remarked, because the one, the artery to wit, is the vessel which carries the blood from the heart to the body at large, the other or vein of the present day bringing it back from the general system to the heart; the former is the conduit from, the latter the channel to, the heart; the latter contains the cruder, effete blood, rendered unfit for nutrition; the former transmits the digested, perfect, peculiarly nutritive fluid.

CHAPTER IX.

THAT THERE IS A CIRCULATION OF THE BLOOD IS CONFIRMED
FROM THE FIRST PROPOSITION.

But lest any one should say that we give them words only, and make mere specious assertions without any foundation, and desire to innovate without sufficient cause, three points present themselves for confirmation, which being stated, I conceive that the truth I contend for will follow necessarily, and appear as a thing obvious to all. First,—the blood is incessantly transmitted by the action of the heart from the vena cava to the arteries in such quantity, that it cannot be supplied from the ingesta, and in such wise that the whole mass must very quickly pass through the organ; Second,—the blood under the influence of the arterial pulse enters and is impelled in a continuous, equable, and incessant stream through every part and member of the body, in much larger quantity than were sufficient for nutrition, or than the whole mass of fluids could supply; Third,—the veins in like manner return this blood incessantly to the heart from all parts and members of the body. These points proved, I conceive it will be manifest that the blood circulates, revolves, propelled and then returning, from the heart to the extremities, from the extremities to the heart, and thus that it performs a kind of circular motion.

Let us assume either arbitrarily or from experiment, the quantity of blood which the left ventricle of the heart will contain when distended to be, say two ounces, three ounces, one ounce and a half—in the dead body I have found it to hold upwards of two ounces. Let us assume further, how much less the heart will hold in the contracted than in the dilated state; and how much blood it will project into the aorta upon each contraction; —and all the world allows that with the systole something is always projected, a necessary consequence demonstrated in the third chapter, and obvious from the structure of the valves; and let us suppose as approaching the truth that the fourth, or fifth, or sixth, or even but the eighth part of its charge is thrown into the artery at each contraction; this would give either half an ounce, or three drachms, or one drachm of blood as propelled by the heart at each pulse into the aorta; which quantity, by reason of the valves at the root of the vessel, can by no means return into the ventricle. Now in the course of half an hour, the heart will have made more than one thousand beats, in some as many as two, three, and even four thousand. Multiplying the number of drachms propelled by the number of pulses, we shall have either one thousand half ounces, or one thousand times three drachms, or a like proportional quantity of blood, according to the amount which we assume as propelled with each stroke of the heart, sent from this organ into the artery; a larger quantity in every case than is contained in the whole body! In the same way, in the sheep or dog, say that but a single scruple of blood passes with each stroke of the heart, in one half hour we should have one thousand scruples, or about three pounds and a half of blood injected into the aorta; but the body of neither animal contains above four pounds of blood, a fact which I have myself ascertained in the case of the sheep.

Upon this supposition, therefore, assumed merely as a ground for reasoning, we see the whole mass of blood passing through the heart, from the veins to the arteries, and in like manner through the lungs.

But let it be said that this does not take place in half an hour, but in an hour, or even in a day; any way it is still manifest that more blood passes through the heart in consequence of its action, than can either be supplied by the whole of the ingesta, or than can be contained in the veins at the same moment.

Nor can it be allowed that the heart in contracting sometimes propels and sometimes does not propel, or at most propels but very little, a mere nothing, or an imaginary something: all this, indeed, has already been refuted; and is, besides, contrary both to sense and reason. For if it be a necessary effect of the dilatation of the heart that its ventricles become filled with blood, it is equally so that, contracting, these cavities should expel their contents; and this not in any trifling measure, seeing that neither are the conduits small, nor the contractions few in number, but frequent, and always in some certain proportion, whether it be a third or a sixth, or an eighth, to the total capacity of the ventricles, so that a like proportion

4

of blood must be expelled, and a like proportion received with
each stroke of the heart, the capacity of the ventricle contracted always bearing a certain relation to the capacity of the
ventricle when dilated.   And since in dilating, the ventricles
cannot be supposed to get filled with nothing, or with an imaginary something; so in contracting they never expel nothing
or aught imaginary, but always a certain something, viz. blood,
in proportion to the amount of the contraction.   Whence it
is to be inferred, that if at one stroke the heart in man, the
ox or the sheep, ejects but a single drachm of blood, and there
are one thousand strokes in half an hour, in this interval there
will have been ten pounds five ounces expelled: were there with
each stroke two drachms expelled, the quantity would of course
amount to twenty pounds and ten ounces; were there half an
ounce, the quantity would come to forty-one pounds and eight
ounces; and were there one ounce it would be as much as
eighty-three pounds and four ounces; the whole of which, in
the course of one half hour, would have been transfused from
the veins to the arteries.   The actual quantity of blood expelled
at each stroke of the heart, and the circumstances under which
it is either greater or less than ordinary, I leave for particular
determination afterwards, from numerous observations which
I have made on the subject.

Meantime this much I know, and would here proclaim to
all that the blood is transfused at one time in larger, at another in smaller quantity; and that the circuit of the blood is
accomplished now more rapidly, now more slowly, according to
the temperament, age, &c. of the individual, to external and
internal circumstances, to naturals and non-naturals,—sleep,
rest, food, exercise, affections of the mind, and the like.   But
indeed, supposing even the smallest quantity of blood to be
passed through the heart and the lungs with each pulsation, a
vastly greater amount would still be thrown into the arteries
and whole body, than could by any possibility be supplied by
the food consumed; in short it could be furnished in no other
way than by making a circuit and returning.

This truth, indeed, presents itself obviously before us when
we consider what happens in the dissection of living animals;
the great artery need not be divided, but a very small branch
only, (as Galen even proves in regard to man,) to have the whole

of the blood in the body, as well that of the veins as of the arteries, drained away in the course of no long time—some half hour or less. Butchers are well aware of the fact and can bear witness to it; for, cutting the throat of an ox and so dividing the vessels of the neck, in less than a quarter of an hour they have all the vessels bloodless—the whole mass of blood has escaped. The same thing also occasionally occurs with great rapidity in performing amputations and removing tumours in the human subject.

Nor would this argument lose any of its force, did any one say that in killing animals in the shambles, and performing amputations, the blood escaped in equal, if not perchance in larger quantity by the veins than by the arteries. The contrary of this statement, indeed, is certainly the truth; the veins, in fact, collapsing, and being without any propelling power, and further, because of the impediment of the valves, as I shall show immediately, pour out but very little blood; whilst the arteries spout it forth with force abundantly, impetuously, and as if it were propelled by a syringe. And then the experiment is easily tried of leaving the vein untouched, and only dividing the artery in the neck of a sheep or dog, when it will be seen with what force, in what abundance, and how quickly, the whole blood in the body, of the veins as well as of the arteries, is emptied. But the arteries receive blood from the veins in no other way than by transmission through the heart, as we have already seen; so that if the aorta be tied at the base of the heart, and the carotid or any other artery be opened, no one will now be surprised to find it empty, and the veins only replete with blood.

And now the cause is manifest, wherefore in our dissections we usually find so large a quantity of blood in the veins, so little in the arteries; wherefore there is much in the right ventricle, little in the left; circumstances which probably led the ancients to believe that the arteries (as their name implies) contained nothing but spirits during the life of an animal. The true cause of the difference is this perhaps : that as there is no passage to the arteries, save through the lungs and heart, when an animal has ceased to breathe and the lungs to move, the blood in the pulmonary artery is prevented from passing into the pulmonary veins, and from thence into the left ventricle of the heart; just as we have already seen the same transit prevented in the embryo, by the want of movement in the lungs and the alternate opening and shutting of their minute orifices and invisible pores. But the heart not ceasing to act at the same precise moment as the lungs, but surviving them and continuing to pulsate for a time, the left ventricle and arteries go on distributing their blood to the body at large and sending it into the veins; receiving none from the lungs, however, they are soon exhausted, and left, as it were, empty. But even this fact confirms our views, in no trifling manner, seeing that it can be ascribed to no other than the cause we have just assumed.

Moreover it appears from this that the more frequently or forcibly the arteries pulsate, the more speedily will the body be exhausted in an hemorrhagy. Hence, also, it happens, that in fainting fits and in states of alarm, when the heart beats more languidly and with less force, hemorrhages are diminished or arrested.

Still further, it is from this that after death, when the heart has ceased to beat, it is impossible by dividing either the jugular or femoral veins and arteries, by any effort to force out more than one half of the whole mass of the blood. Neither could the butcher, did he neglect to cut the throat of the ox which he has knocked on the head and stunned, until the heart had ceased beating, ever bleed the carcass effectually.

Finally, we are now in a condition to suspect wherefore it is that no one has yet said anything to the purpose upon the anastomosis of the veins and arteries, either as to where or how it is effected, or for what purpose. I now enter upon the investigation of the subject.

CHAPTER X.

THE FIRST POSITION: OF THE QUANTITY OF BLOOD PASSING FROM THE VEINS TO THE ARTERIES. AND THAT THERE IS A CIRCUIT OF THE BLOOD, FREED FROM OBJECTIONS, AND FARTHER CONFIRMED BY EXPERIMENT.

So far our first position is confirmed, whether the thing be referred to calculation or to experiment and dissection, viz., that the blood is incessantly infused into the arteries in larger quantities than it can be supplied by the food; so that the whole passing over in a short space of time, it is matter of necessity that the blood perform a circuit, that it return to whence it set out.

But if any one shall here object that a large quantity may pass through and yet no necessity be found for a circulation, that all may come from the meat and drink consumed, and quote as an illustration the abundant supply of milk in the mammæ—for a cow will give three, four, and even seven gallons and more in a day, and a woman two or three pints whilst nursing a child or twins, which must manifestly be derived from the food consumed; it may be answered, that the heart by computation does as much and more in the course of an hour or two.

And if not yet convinced, he shall still insist, that when an artery is divided a preternatural route is, as it were, opened, and that so the blood escapes in torrents, but that the same thing does not happen in the healthy and uninjured body when no outlet is made; and that in arteries filled, or in their natural state, so large a quantity of blood cannot pass in so short a space of time as to make any return necessary;—to all this it may be answered, that from the calculation already made, and the reasons assigned, it appears, that by so much as the heart in its dilated state contains in addition to its contents in the state of constriction, so much in a general way must it emit upon each pulsation, and in such quantity must the blood pass, the body being healthy and naturally constituted.

But in serpents, and several fishes, by tying the veins some way below the heart, you will perceive a space between the ligature and the heart speedily to become empty; so that, unless you would deny the evidence of your senses, you must needs admit the return of the blood to the heart. The same thing will also plainly appear when we come to discuss our second position.

Let us here conclude with a single example, confirming all that has been said, and from which every one may obtain conviction through the testimony of his own eyes.

If a live snake be laid open, the heart will be seen pulsating quietly, distinctly, for more than an hour, moving like a worm, contracting in its longitudinal dimensions, (for it is of an oblong shape,) and propelling its contents; becoming of a paler colour in the systole, of a deeper tint in the diastole; and almost all things else by which I have already said that the truth I contend for is established, only that here everything takes place more slowly, and is more distinct. This point in particular may be observed more clearly than the noon-day sun : the vena cava enters the heart at its lower part, the artery quits it at the superior part; the vein being now seized either with forceps or between the finger and thumb, and the course of the blood for some space below the heart interrupted, you will perceive the part that intervenes between the fingers and the heart almost immediately to become empty, the blood being exhausted by the action of the heart; at the same time the heart will become of a much paler colour, even in its state of dilatation, than it was before; it is also smaller than at first, from wanting blood; and then it begins to beat more slowly, so that it seems at length as if it were about to die. But the impediment to the flow of blood being removed, instantly the colour and the size of the heart are restored.

If, on the contrary, the artery instead of the vein be compressed or tied, you will observe the part between the obstacle and the heart, and the heart itself, to become inordinately distended, to assume a deep purple or even livid colour, and at length to be so much oppressed with blood that you will believe it about to be choked; but the obstacle removed, all things immediately return to their pristine state—the heart to its colour, size, stroke, &c.

Here then we have evidence of two kinds of death: extinction from deficiency, and suffocation from excess. Examples of both have now been set before you, and you have had opportunity of viewing the truth contended for with your own eyes in the heart.

CHAPTER XI.

THE SECOND POSITION IS DEMONSTRATED.

THAT this may the more clearly appear to every one, I have here to cite certain experiments, from which it seems obvious that the blood enters a limb by the arteries, and returns from it by the veins; that the arteries are the vessels carrying the blood from the heart, and the veins the returning channels of the blood to the heart; that in the limbs and extreme parts of the body the blood passes either immediately by anastomosis from the arteries into the veins, or mediately by the pores of

the flesh, or in both ways, as has already been said in speaking
of the passage of the blood through the lungs; whence it appears manifest that in the circuit the blood moves from thence
hither, and from hence thither; from the centre to the extremities, to wit; and from the extreme parts back again to the centre.
Finally, upon grounds of calculation, with the same elements as
before, it will be obvious that the quantity can neither be accounted for by the ingesta, nor yet be held necessary to nutrition.

The same thing will also appear in regard to ligatures, and
wherefore they are said to *draw*; though this is neither from
the heat, nor the pain, nor the vacuum they occasion, nor indeed from any other cause yet thought of; it will also explain
the uses and advantages to be derived from ligatures in medicine, the principle upon which they either suppress or occasion
hemorrhage; how they induce sloughing and more extensive
mortification in extremities; and how they act in the castration
of animals and the removal of warts and fleshy tumours. But
it has come to pass, from no one having duly weighed and understood the causes and rationale of these various effects, that
though almost all, upon the faith of the old writers, recommend
ligatures in the treatment of disease, yet very few comprehend
their proper employment, or derive any real assistance from
them in effecting cures.

Ligatures are either very tight or of middling tightness. A
ligature I designate as tight or perfect when it is drawn so close
about an extremity that no vessel can be felt pulsating beyond
it. Such a ligature we use in amputations to control the flow
of blood; and such also are employed in the castration of animals and the removal of tumours. In the latter instances, all
afflux of nutriment and heat being prevented by the ligature,
we see the testes and large fleshy tumours dwindle, and die, and
finally fall off.

Ligatures of middling tightness I regard as those which compress a limb firmly all around, but short of pain, and in such
a way as still suffers a certain degree of pulsation to be felt in
the artery beyond them. Such a ligature is in use in bloodletting, an operation in which the fillet applied above the elbow
is not drawn so tight but that the arteries at the wrist may still
be felt beating under the finger.

Now let any one make an experiment upon the arm of a man,

either using such a fillet as is employed in bloodletting, or grasping the limb lightly with his hand, the best subject for it being one who is lean, and who has large veins, and the best time after exercise, when the body is warm, the pulse is full, and the blood carried in larger quantity to the extremities, for all then is more conspicuous; under such circumstances let a ligature be thrown about the extremity, and drawn as tightly as can be borne, it will first be perceived that beyond the ligature, neither in the wrist nor anywhere else, do the arteries pulsate, at the same time that immediately above the ligature the artery begins to rise higher at each diastole, to throb more violently, and to swell in its vicinity with a kind of tide, as if it strove to break through and overcome the obstacle to its current; the artery here, in short, appears as if it were preternaturally full. The hand under such circumstances retains its natural colour and appearance; in the course of time it begins to fall somewhat in temperature, indeed, but nothing is *drawn* into it.

After the bandage has been kept on for some short time in this way, let it be slackened a little, brought to that state or term of middling tightness which is used in bleeding, and it will be seen that the whole hand and arm will instantly become deeply suffused and distended, and the veins show themselves tumid and knotted; after ten or fifteen pulses of the artery, the hand will be perceived excessively distended, injected, gorged with blood, *drawn*, as it is said, by this middling ligature, without pain, or heat, or any horror of a vacuum, or any other cause yet indicated.

If the finger be applied over the artery as it is pulsating by the edge of the fillet, at the moment of slackening it, the blood will be felt to glide through, as it were, underneath the finger; and he, too, upon whose arm the experiment is made, when the ligature is slackened, is distinctly conscious of a sensation of warmth, and of something, viz., a stream of blood suddenly making its way along the course of the vessels and diffusing itself through the hand, which at the same time begins to feel hot, and becomes distended.

As we had noted, in connexion with the tight ligature, that the artery above the bandage was distended and pulsated, not below it, so, in the case of the moderately tight bandage, on the contrary, do we find that the veins below, never above, the fillet, swell, and become dilated, whilst the arteries shrink; and such is the degree of distension of the veins here, that it is only very strong pressure that will force the blood beyond the fillet, and cause any of the veins in the upper part of the arm to rise.

From these facts it is easy for every careful observer to learn that the blood enters an extremity by the arteries; for when they are effectually compressed nothing is *drawn* to the member; the hand preserves its colour; nothing flows into it, neither is it distended; but when the pressure is diminished, as it is with the bleeding fillet, it is manifest that the blood is instantly thrown in with force, for then the hand begins to swell; which is as much as to say, that when the arteries pulsate the blood is flowing through them, as it is when the moderately tight ligature is applied; but where they do not pulsate, as, when a tight ligature is used, they cease from transmitting anything; they are only distended above the part where the ligature is applied. The veins again being compressed, nothing can flow through them; the certain indication of which is, that below the ligature they are much more tumid than above it, and than they usually appear when there is no bandage upon the arm.

It therefore plainly appears that the ligature prevents the return of the blood through the veins to the parts above it, and maintains those beneath it in a state of permanent distension. But the arteries, in spite of its pressure, and under the force and impulse of the heart, send on the blood from the internal parts of the body to the parts beyond the bandage. And herein consists the difference between the tight and the medium bandage, that the former not only prevents the passage of the blood in the veins, but in the arteries also; the latter, however, whilst it does not prevent the pulsific force from extending beyond it, and so propelling the blood to the extremities of the body, compresses the veins, and greatly or altogether impedes the return of the blood through them.

Seeing, therefore, that the moderately tight ligature renders the veins turgid, and the whole hand full of blood, I ask, whence is this? Does the blood accumulate below the ligature coming through the veins, or through the arteries, or passing by certain secret pores? Through the veins it cannot come; still less can it come by any system of invisible pores; it must needs arrive by the arteries, then, in conformity with all that has been already said. That it cannot flow in by the veins appears plainly enough from the fact that the blood cannot be forced towards the heart unless the ligature be removed; when on a sudden all the veins collapse, and disgorge themselves of their contents into the superior parts, the hand at the same time resuming its natural pale colour,—the tumefaction and the stagnating blood have disappeared.

Moreover, he whose arm or wrist has thus been bound for some little time with the medium bandage, so that it has not only got swollen and livid but cold, when the fillet is undone is aware of something cold making its way upwards along with the returning blood, and reaching the elbow or the axilla. And I have myself been inclined to think that this cold blood rising upwards to the heart was the cause of the fainting that often occurs after bloodletting : fainting frequently supervenes even in robust subjects, and mostly at the moment of undoing the fillet, as the vulgar say, from the turning of the blood.

Farther, when we see the veins below the ligature instantly swell up and become gorged, when from extreme tightness it is somewhat relaxed, the arteries meantime continuing unaffected, this is an obvious indication that the blood passes from the arteries into the veins, and not from the veins into the arteries, and that there is either an anastomosis of the two orders of vessels, or pores in the flesh and solid parts generally that are permeable to the blood. It is farther an indication that the veins have frequent communications with one another, because they all become turgid together, whilst under the medium ligature applied above the elbow; and if any single small vein be pricked with a lancet, they all speedily shrink, and disburthening themselves into this they subside almost simultaneously.

These considerations will enable any one to understand the nature of the attraction that is exerted by ligatures, and perchance of fluxes generally; how, for example, the veins when compressed by a bandage of medium tightness applied above the elbow, the blood cannot escape, whilst it still continues to be driven in, to wit, by the forcing power of the heart, by which the parts are of necessity filled, gorged with blood. And how should it be otherwise? Heat and pain and the *vis vacui* draw, indeed; but in such wise only that parts are filled, not preternaturally distended or gorged, not so suddenly and violently overwhelmed with the charge of blood forced in upon them, that the flesh is lacerated and the vessels ruptured. Nothing of the kind as an effect of heat, or pain, or the vacuum force, is either credible or demonstrable.

Besides, the ligature is competent to occasion the afflux in question without either pain, or heat, or *vis vacui*. Were pain in any way the cause, how should it happen that, with the arm bound above the elbow, the hand and fingers should swell below the bandage, and their veins become distended? The pressure of the bandage certainly prevents the blood from getting there by the veins. And then, wherefore is there neither swelling nor repletion of the veins, nor any sign or symptom of attraction or afflux, above the ligature? But this is the obvious cause of the preternatural attraction and swelling below the bandage, and in the hand and fingers, that the blood is entering abundantly, and with force, but cannot pass out again.

Now is not this the cause of all tumefaction, as indeed Avicenna has it, and of all oppressive redundancy in parts, that the access to them is open, but the egress from them is closed? Whence it comes that they are gorged and tumefied. And may not the same thing happen in local inflammations, where, so long as the swelling is on the increase, and has not reached its extreme term, a full pulse is felt in the part, especially when the disease is of the more acute kind, and the swelling usually takes place most rapidly. But these are matters for after discussion. Or does this, which occurred in my own case, happen from the same cause. Thrown from a carriage upon one occasion, I struck my forehead a blow upon the place where a twig of the artery advances from the temple, and immediately, within the time in which twenty beats could have been made, I felt a tumour the size of an egg developed, without either heat or any great pain: the near vicinity of the artery had caused the blood to be effused into the bruised part with unusual force and quickness.

And now, too, we understand wherefore in phlebotomy we apply our fillet above the part that is punctured, not below it; did the flow come from above, not from below, the bandage in this case would not only be of no service, but would prove a positive hinderance; it would have to be applied below the orifice, in order to have the flow more free, did the blood descend by the veins from superior to inferior parts; but as it is elsewhere forced through the extreme arteries into the extreme veins, and the return in these last is opposed by the ligature, so do they fill and swell, and being thus filled and distended, they are made capable of projecting their charge with force, and to a distance, when any one of them is suddenly punctured; but the fillet being slackened, and the returning channels thus left open, the blood forthwith no longer escapes, save by drops; and, as all the world knows, if in performing phlebotomy the bandage be either slackened too much or the limb be bound too tightly, the blood escapes without force, because in the one case the returning channels are not adequately obstructed; in the other the channels of influx, the arteries, are impeded.

CHAPTER XII.

THAT THERE IS A CIRCULATION OF THE BLOOD IS SHOWN FROM THE SECOND POSITION DEMONSTRATED.

IF these things be so, another point which I have already referred to, viz., the continual passage of the blood through the heart will also be confirmed. We have seen, that the blood passes from the arteries into the veins, not from the veins into the arteries; we have seen, farther, that almost the whole of the blood may be withdrawn from a puncture made in one of the cutaneous veins of the arm if a bandage properly applied be used; we have seen, still farther, that the blood flows so freely and rapidly that not only is the whole quantity which was contained in the arm beyond the ligature, and before the puncture was made, discharged, but the whole which is contained in the body, both that of the arteries and that of the veins.

Whence we must admit, first, that the blood is sent along with an impulse, and that it is urged with force below the fillet; for it escapes with force, which force it receives from the pulse and power of the heart; for the force and motion of the blood are derived from the heart alone. Second, that the afflux proceeds from the heart, and through the heart by a course from the great veins [into the aorta]; for it gets into the parts below the ligature through the arteries, not through the veins; and the arteries nowhere receive blood from the veins, nowhere receive blood save and except from the left ventricle of the heart. Nor could so large a quantity of blood be drawn from one vein (a ligature having been duly applied), nor with such impetuosity, such readiness, such celerity, unless through the medium of the impelling power of the heart.

But if all things be as they are now represented, we shall feel ourselves at liberty to calculate the quantity of the blood, and to reason on its circular motion. Should any one, for instance, in performing phlebotomy, suffer the blood to flow in the manner it usually does, with force and freely, for some half hour or so, no question but that the greatest part of the blood being abstracted, faintings and syncopes would ensue, and that not only would the arteries but the great veins also be nearly emptied of their contents. It is only consonant with reason to conclude that in the course of the half hour hinted at, so much as has escaped has also passed from the great veins through the heart into the aorta. And further, if we calculate how many ounces flow through one arm, or how many pass in twenty or thirty pulsations under the medium ligature, we shall have some grounds for estimating how much passes through the other arm in the same space of time; how much through both lower extremities, how much through the neck on either side, and through all the other arteries and veins of the body, all of which have been supplied with fresh blood, and as this blood must have passed through the lungs and ventricles of the heart, and must have come from the great veins,—we shall perceive that a circulation is absolutely necessary, seeing that the quantities hinted at cannot be supplied immediately from the ingesta, and are vastly more than can be requisite for the mere nutrition of the parts.

It is still further to be observed, that the truths contended for are sometimes confirmed in another way; for having tied up the arm properly, and made the puncture duly, still, if from alarm or any other causes, a state of faintness supervenes, in which the heart always pulsates more languidly, the blood does not flow freely, but distils by drops only. The reason is, that with the somewhat greater than usual resistance offered to the transit of the blood by the bandage, coupled with the weaker action of the heart, and its diminished impelling power, the stream cannot make its way under the fillet; and farther, owing to the weak and languishing state of the heart, the blood is not transferred in such quantity as wont from the veins to the arteries through the sinuses of that organ. So also, and for the same reasons, are the menstrual fluxes of women, and indeed hemorrhagies of every kind, controlled. And now, a contrary state of things occurring, the patient getting rid of his fear and recovering his courage, the pulsific power is increased, the arteries begin again to beat with greater force, and to drive the blood even into the part that is bound; so that the blood now springs from the puncture in the vein, and flows in a continuous stream.

CHAPTER XIII.

THE THIRD POSITION IS CONFIRMED: AND THE CIRCULATION OF THE BLOOD IS DEMONSTRATED FROM IT.

THUS far have we spoken of the quantity of blood passing through the heart and the lungs in the centre of the body, and in like manner from the arteries into the veins in the peripheral parts and the body at large. We have yet to explain, however, in what manner the blood finds its way back to the heart from the extremities by the veins, and how and in what way these are the only vessels that convey the blood from the external to the central parts; which done, I conceive that the three fundamental propositions laid down for the circulation of the blood will be so plain, so well established, so obviously true, that they may claim general credence. Now the remaining position will be made sufficiently clear from the valves which are found in the cavities of the veins themselves, from the uses of these, and from experiments cognizable by the senses.

The celebrated Hieronymus Fabricius of Aquapendente, a most skilful anatomist, and venerable old man, or, as the learned Riolan will have it, Jacobus Silvius, first gave representations of the valves in the veins, which consist of raised or loose portions of the inner membranes of these vessels, of extreme delicacy, and a sigmoid or semilunar shape. They are situ-

ated at different distances from one another, and diversely in
different individuals ; they are connate at the sides of the veins ;
they are directed upwards or towards the trunks of the veins ;
the two—for there are for the most part two together—regard
each other, mutually touch, and are so ready to come into contact by their edges, that if anything attempt to pass from the
trunks into the branches of the veins, or from the greater vessels
into the less, they completely prevent it ; they are farther so arranged, that the horns of those that succeed are opposite the middle of the convexity of those that precede, and so on alternately.

The discoverer of these valves did not rightly understand their
use, nor have succeeding anatomists added anything to our
knowledge : for their office is by no means explained when we
are told that it is to hinder the blood, by its weight, from all
flowing into inferior parts ; for the edges of the valves in the
jugular veins hang downwards, and are so contrived that they
prevent the blood from rising upwards ; the valves, in a word,
do not invariably look upwards, but always towards the trunks
of the veins, invariably towards the seat of the heart.   I, and
indeed others, have sometimes found valves in the emulgent
veins, and in those of the mesentery, the edges of which were
directed towards the vena cava and vena portæ.   Let it be added
that there are no valves in the arteries [save at their roots],
and that dogs, oxen, &c., have invariably valves at the divisions
of their crural veins, in the veins that meet towards the top of
the os sacrum, and in those branches which come from the
haunches, in which no such effect of gravity from the erect
position was to be apprehended.   Neither are there valves in the
jugular veins for the purpose of guarding against apoplexy, as
some have said ; because in sleep the head is more apt to be
influenced by the contents of the carotid arteries.   Neither are
the valves present, in order that the blood may be retained in
the divarications or smaller trunks and minuter branches, and
not be suffered to flow entirely into the more open and capacious channels ; for they occur where there are no divarications ; although it must be owned that they are most frequent
at the points where branches join.   Neither do they exist for
the purpose of rendering the current of blood more slow from
the centre of the body; for it seems likely that the blood would
be disposed to flow with sufficient slowness of its own accord,

as it would have to pass from larger into continually smaller vessels, being separated from the mass and fountain head, and attaining from warmer into colder places.

But the valves are solely made and instituted lest the blood should pass from the greater into the lesser veins, and either rupture them or cause them to become varicose; lest, instead of advancing from the extreme to the central parts of the body, the blood should rather proceed along the veins from the centre to the extremities; but the delicate valves, while they readily open in the right direction, entirely prevent all such contrary motion, being so situated and arranged, that if anything escapes, or is less perfectly obstructed by the cornua of the one above, the fluid passing, as it were, by the chinks between the cornua, it is immediately received on the convexity of the one beneath, which is placed transversely with reference to the former, and so is effectually hindered from getting any farther.

And this I have frequently experienced in my dissections of the veins : if I attempted to pass a probe from the trunk of the veins into one of the smaller branches, whatever care I took I found it impossible to introduce it far any way, by reason of the valves; whilst, on the contrary, it was most easy to push it along in the opposite direction, from without inwards, or from the branches towards the trunks and roots.   In many places two valves are so placed and fitted, that when raised they come exactly together in the middle of the vein, and are there united by the contact of their margins; and so accurate is the adaptation, that neither by the eye nor by any other means of examination can the slightest chink along the line of contact be perceived. But if the probe be now introduced from the extreme towards the more central parts, the valves, like the floodgates of a river, give way, and are most readily pushed aside.   The effect of this arrangement plainly is to prevent all motion of the blood from the heart and vena cava, whether it be upwards towards the head, or downwards towards the feet, or to either side towards the arms, not a drop can pass; all motion of the blood, beginning in the larger and tending towards the smaller veins, is opposed and resisted by them; whilst the motion that proceeds from the lesser to end in the larger branches is favoured, or, at all events, a free and open passage is left for it.

But that this truth may be made the more apparent, let an arm be tied up above the elbow as if for phlebotomy (A, A, fig. 1).

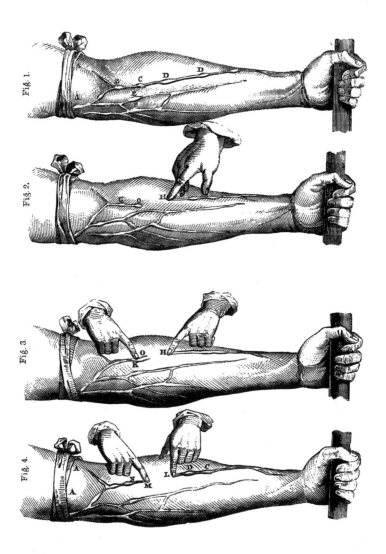

At intervals in the course of the veins, especially in labouring people and those whose veins are large, certain knots or ele-

5

vations (B, C, D, E, F,) will be perceived, and this not only at the places where a branch is received (E, F), but also where none enters (C, D): these knots or risings are all formed by valves, which thus show themselves externally. And now if you press the blood from the space above one of the valves, from H to O, (fig. 2,) and keep the point of a finger upon the vein inferiorly, you will see no influx of blood from above; the portion of the vein between the point of the finger and the valve O will be obliterated; yet will the vessel continue sufficiently distended above that valve (O, G). The blood being thus pressed out, and the vein emptied, if you now apply a finger of the other hand upon the distended part of the vein above the valve O, (fig. 3,) and press downwards, you will find that you cannot force the blood through or beyond the valve; but the greater effort you use, you will only see the portion of vein that is between the finger and the valve become more distended, that portion of the vein which is below the valve remaining all the while empty (H, O, fig. 3).

It would therefore appear that the function of the valves in the veins is the same as that of the three sigmoid valves which we find at the commencement of the aorta and pulmonary artery, viz., to prevent all reflux of the blood that is passing over them.

Farther, the arm being bound as before, and the veins looking full and distended, if you press at one part in the course of a vein with the point of a finger (L, fig. 4), and then with another finger streak the blood upwards beyond the next valve (N), you will perceive that this portion of the vein continues empty (L N), and that the blood cannot retrograde, precisely as we have already seen the case to be in fig. 2; but the finger first applied (H, fig. 2, L, fig. 4), being removed, immediately the vein is filled from below, and the arm becomes as it appears at D C, fig. 1. That the blood in the veins therefore proceeds from inferior or more remote to superior parts, and towards the heart, moving in these vessels in this and not in the contrary direction, appears most obviously. And although in some places the valves, by not acting with such perfect accuracy, or where there is but a single valve, do not seem totally to prevent the passage of the blood from the centre, still the greater number of them plainly do so; and then, where things appear contrived more negligently, this is compensated either by the more frequent occurrence or more perfect action of the succeeding valves or in some other way : the veins, in short, as they are the free and open conduits of the blood returning *to* the heart, so are they effectually prevented from serving as its channels of distribution *from* the heart.

But this other circumstance has to be noted : The arm being bound, and the veins made turgid, and the valves prominent, as before, apply the thumb or finger over a vein in the situation of one of the valves in such a way as to compress it, and prevent any blood from passing upwards from the hand; then, with a finger of the other hand, streak the blood in the vein upwards till it has passed the next valve above, (N, fig. 4,) the vessel now remains empty; but the finger at L being removed for an instant, the vein is immediately filled from below; apply the finger again, and having in the same manner streaked the blood upwards, again remove the finger below, and again the vessel becomes distended as before ; and this repeat, say a thousand times, in a short space of time.   And now compute the quantity of blood which you have thus pressed up beyond the valve, and then multiplying the assumed quantity by one thousand, you will find that so much blood has passed through a certain portion of the vessel ; and I do now believe that you will find yourself convinced of the circulation of the blood, and of its rapid motion.   But if in this experiment you say that a violence is done to nature, I do not doubt but that, if you proceed in the same way, only taking as great a length of vein as possible, and merely remark with what rapidity the blood flows upwards, and fills the vessel from below, you will come to the same conclusion.

CHAPTER XIV.

CONCLUSION OF THE DEMONSTRATION OF THE CIRCULATION.

AND now I may be allowed to give in brief my view of the circulation of the blood, and to propose it for general adoption.

Since all things, both argument and ocular demonstration, show that the blood passes through the lungs and heart by the action of the [auricles and] ventricles, and is sent for distribution to all parts of the body, where it makes its way into the veins and pores of the flesh, and then flows by the veins from the circumference on every side to the centre, from the lesser to the greater veins, and is by them finally discharged into the vena cava and right auricle of the heart, and this in such a quantity or in such a flux and reflux thither by the arteries, hither by the veins, as cannot possibly be supplied by the ingesta, and is much greater than can be required for mere purposes of nutrition; it is absolutely necessary to conclude that the blood in the animal body is impelled in a circle, and is in a state of ceaseless motion; that this is the act or function which the heart performs by means of its pulse; and that it is the sole and only end of the motion and contraction of the heart.

CHAPTER XV.

THE CIRCULATION OF THE BLOOD IS FURTHER CONFIRMED BY PROBABLE REASONS.

IT will not be foreign to the subject if I here show further, from certain familiar reasonings, that the circulation is matter both of convenience and necessity. In the first place, since death is a corruption which takes place through deficiency of heat,[1] and since all living things are warm, all dying things cold, there must be a particular seat and fountain, a kind of home and hearth, where the cherisher of nature, the original of the native fire, is stored and preserved; whence heat and life are dispensed to all parts as from a fountain head;

---

[1] Aristoteles De Respiratione, lib. ii et iii: De Part. Animal. et alibi.

whence sustenance may be derived; and upon which concoction and nutrition, and all vegetative energy may depend. Now, that the heart is this place, that the heart is the principle of life, and that all passes in the manner just mentioned, I trust no one will deny.

The blood, therefore, required to have motion, and indeed such a motion that it should return again to the heart; for sent to the external parts of the body far from its fountain, as Aristotle says, and without motion, it would become congealed. For we see motion generating and keeping up heat and spirits under all circumstances, and rest allowing them to escape and be dissipated. The blood, therefore, become thick or congealed by the cold of the extreme and outward parts, and robbed of its spirits, just as it is in the dead, it was imperative that from its fount and origin, it should again receive heat and spirits, and all else requisite to its preservation—that, by returning, it should be renovated and restored.

We frequently see how the extremities are chilled by the external cold, how the nose and cheeks and hands look blue, and how the blood, stagnating in them as in the pendent or lower parts of a corpse, becomes of a dusky hue; the limbs at the same time getting torpid, so that they can scarcely be moved, and seem almost to have lost their vitality. Now they can by no means be so effectually, and especially so speedily restored to heat and colour and life, as by a new afflux and appulsion of heat from its source. But how can parts attract in which the heat and life are almost extinct? Or how should they whose passages are filled with condensed and frigid blood, admit fresh aliment—renovated blood—unless they had first got rid of their old contents? Unless the heart were truly that fountain where life and heat are restored to the refrigerated fluid, and whence new blood, warm, imbued with spirits, being sent out by the arteries, that which has become cooled and effete is forced on, and all the particles recover their heat which was failing, and their vital stimulus well-nigh exhausted.

Hence it is that if the heart be unaffected, life and health may be restored to almost all the other parts of the body; but the heart being chilled, or smitten with any serious disease, it seems matter of necessity that the whole animal fabric should suffer and fall into decay. When the source is corrupted,

there is nothing, as Aristotle says,[1] which can be of service
either to it or aught that depends on it.   And hence, by the
way, it may perchance be wherefore grief, and love, and envy,
and anxiety, and all affections of the mind of a similar kind
are accompanied with emaciation and decay, or with cacochemy
and crudity, which engender all manner of diseases and consume the body of man.   For every affection of the mind that
is attended with either pain or pleasure, hope or fear, is the cause
of an agitation whose influence extends to the heart, and there induces change from the natural constitution, in the temperature,
the pulse and the rest, which impairing all nutrition in its
source and abating the powers at large, it is no wonder that
various forms of incurable disease in the extremities and in the
trunk are the consequence, inasmuch as in such circumstances
the whole body labours under the effects of vitiated nutrition
and a want of native heat.

Moreover, when we see that all animals live through food concocted in their interior, it is imperative that the digestion and
distribution be perfect; and, as a consequence, that there be a
place and receptacle where the aliment is perfected and whence
it is distributed to the several members.   Now this place is the
heart, for it is the only organ in the body which contains blood
for the general use; all the others receive it merely for their
peculiar or private advantage, just as the heart also has a supply
for its own especial behoof in its coronary veins and arteries; but
it is of the store which the heart contains in its auricles and
ventricles that I nere speak; and then the heart is the only
organ which is so situated and constituted that it can distribute
the blood in due proportion to the several parts of the body,
the quantity sent to each being according to the dimensions of
the artery which supplies it, the heart serving as a magazine or
fountain ready to meet its demands.

Further, a certain impulse or force, as well as an impeller or
forcer, such as the heart, was required to effect this distribution
and motion of the blood; both because the blood is disposed
from slight causes, such as cold, alarm, horror, and the like, to
collect in its source, to concentrate like parts to a whole, or
the drops of water spilt upon a table to the mass of liquid;

_____
[1] De Part. Animal. iii.

and then because it is forced from the capillary veins into the smaller ramifications, and from these into the larger trunks by the motion of the extremities and the compression of the muscles generally. The blood is thus more disposed to move from the circumference to the centre than in the opposite direction, were there even no valves to oppose its motion; whence that it may leave its source and enter more confined and colder channels, and flow against the direction to which it spontaneously inclines, the blood requires both force and an impelling power. Now such is the heart and the heart alone, and that in the way and manner already explained.

CHAPTER XVI.

THE CIRCULATION OF THE BLOOD IS FURTHER PROVED FROM CERTAIN CONSEQUENCES.

THERE are still certain phenomena, which, taken as consequences of this truth assumed as proven, are not without their use in exciting belief, as it were, *a posteriore;* and which, although they may seem to be involved in much doubt and obscurity, nevertheless readily admit of having reasons and causes assigned for them. The phenomena alluded to are those that present themselves in connexion with contagions, poisoned wounds, the bites of serpents and rabid animals, lues venerea and the like. We sometimes see the whole system contaminated, though the part first infected remains sound; the lues venerea has occasionally made its attack with pains in the shoulders and head, and other symptoms, the genital organs being all the while unaffected; and then we know that the wound made by a rabid dog having healed, fever and a train of disastrous symptoms nevertheless supervene. Whence it appears that the contagion impressed upon or deposited in a particular part, is by and by carried by the returning current of blood to the heart, and by that organ is sent to contaminate the whole body.

In tertian fever, the morbific cause seeking the heart in the first instance, and hanging about the heart and lungs, renders the patient short-winded, disposed to sighing, indisposed to exertion; because the vital principle is oppressed and the blood forced into the lungs and rendered thick, does not pass through their substance, (as I have myself seen in opening the bodies of those who had died in the beginning of the attack,) when the pulse is always frequent, small, and occasionally irregular; but the heat increasing, the matter becoming attenuated, the passages forced, and the transit made, the whole body begins to rise in temperature, and the pulse becomes fuller, stronger —the febrile paroxysm is fully formed, whilst the preternatural heat kindled in the heart, is thence diffused by the arteries through the whole body along with the morbific matter, which is in this way overcome and dissolved by nature.

When we perceive, further, that medicines applied externally exert their influence on the body just as if they had been taken internally, the truth we are contending for is confirmed. Colocynth and aloes [applied externally] move the belly, cantharides excites the urine, garlic applied to the soles of the feet assists expectoration, cordials strengthen, and an infinite number of examples of the same kind might be cited. It will not, therefore, be found unreasonable perchance, if we say that the veins, by means of their orifices, absorb some of the things that are applied externally and carry this inwards with the blood, not otherwise, it may be, than those of the mesentery imbibe the chyle from the intestines and carry it mixed with the blood to the liver. For the blood entering the mesentery by the coeliac artery, and the superior and inferior mesenterics, proceeds to the intestines, from which, along with the chyle that has been attracted into the veins, it returns by their numerous ramifications into the vena portæ of the liver, and from this into the vena cava, and this in such wise that the blood in these veins has the same colour and consistency as in other veins, in opposition to what many believe to be the fact. Nor indeed can we imagine two contrary motions in any capillary system—the chyle upwards, the blood downwards. This could scarcely take place, and must be held as altogether improbable. But is not the thing rather arranged as it is by the consummate providence of nature? For were the chyle mingled with the blood, the crude with the concocted, in equal proportions, the result would not be concoction, transmutation, and sanguification, but rather, and because they are severally active and passive, a mixture or

combination, or medium compound of the two, precisely as
happens when wine is mixed with water and syrup. But when
a very minute quantity of chyle is mingled with a very large
quantity of circulating blood, a quantity of chyle that bears no
kind of proportion to the mass of blood, the effect is the same,
as Aristotle says, as when a drop of water is added to a cask of
wine, or the contrary; the mass does not then present itself as
a mixture, but is still sensibly either wine or water. So in the
mesenteric veins of an animal we do not find either chyme or
chyle and blood, blended together or distinct, but only blood,
the same in colour, consistency, and other sensible properties,
as it appears in the veins generally. Still as there is a certain
though small and inappreciable proportion of chyle or unconcocted matter mingled with this blood, nature has interposed
the liver, in whose meandering channels it suffers delay and
undergoes additional change, lest arriving prematurely and crude
at the heart, it should oppress the vital principle. Hence in
the embryo, there is almost no use for the liver, but the
umbilical vein passes directly through, a foramen or anastomosis
existing from the vena portæ, so that the blood returns from the
intestines of the fœtus, not through the liver, but into the umbilical vein mentioned, and flows at once into the heart, mingled
with the natural blood which is returning from the placenta;
whence also it is that in the development of the fœtus the liver
is one of the organs that is last formed; I have observed all
the members perfectly marked out in the human fœtus, even
the genital organs, whilst there was yet scarcely any trace of
the liver. And indeed at the period when all the parts, like
the heart itself in the beginning, are still white, and save in the
veins there is no appearance of redness, you shall see nothing
in the seat of the liver but a shapeless collection, as it were, of
extravasated blood, which you might take for the effects of a
contusion or ruptured vein.

But in the incubated egg there are, as it were, two umbilical
vessels, one from the albumen passing entire through the liver,
and going straight to the heart; another from the yelk, ending
in the vena portæ; for it appears that the chick, in the first
instance, is entirely formed and nourished by the white; but
by the yelk after it has come to perfection and is excluded from
the shell; for this part may still be found in the abdomen of

the chick many days after its exclusion, and is a substitute for the milk to other animals.

But these matters will be better spoken of in my observations on the formation of the fœtus, where many propositions, the following among the number, will be discussed : Wherefore is this part formed or perfected first, that last ?—and of the several members : what part is the cause of another? And many points having special reference to the heart, such as : Wherefore does it first acquire consistency, and appear to possess life, motion, sense, before any other part of the body is perfected, as Aristotle says in his third book, De partibus Animalium? And so also of the blood : Wherefore does it precede all the rest ? And in what way does it possess the vital and animal principle ? And show a tendency to motion, and to be impelled hither and thither, the end for which the heart appears to be made ? In the same way, in considering the pulse : Wherefore one kind of pulse should indicate death, another recovery? And so of all the other kinds of pulse, what may be the cause and indication of each. So also in the consideration of crises and natural critical discharges; of nutrition, and especially the distribution of the nutriment; and of defluxions of every description. Finally, reflecting on every part of medicine, physiology, pathology, semeiotics, therapeutics, when I see how many questions can be answered, how many doubts resolved, how much obscurity illustrated, by the truth we have declared, the light we have made to shine, I see a field of such vast extent in which I might proceed so far, and expatiate so widely, that this my tractate would not only swell out into a volume, which was beyond my purpose, but my whole life, perchance, would not suffice for its completion.

In this place, therefore, and that indeed in a single chapter, I shall only endeavour to refer the various particulars that present themselves in the dissection of the heart and arteries to their several uses and causes; for so I shall meet with many things which receive light from the truth I have been contending for, and which, in their turn, render it more obvious. And indeed I would have it confirmed and illustrated by anatomical arguments above all others.

There is but a single point which indeed would be more correctly placed among our observations on the use of the spleen, but which it will not be altogether impertinent to notice in this place incidentally. From the splenic branch which passes into the pancreas, and from the upper part, arise the posterior coronary, gastric, and gastroepiploic veins, all of which are distributed upon the stomach in numerous branches and twigs, just as the mesenteric vessels are upon the intestines; in like manner, from the inferior part of the same splenic branch, and along the back of the colon and rectum proceed the hemorrhoidal veins. The blood returning by these veins, and bringing the cruder juices along with it, on the one hand from the stomach, where they are thin, watery, and not yet perfectly chylified; on the other thick and more earthy, as derived from the fæces, but all poured into this splenic branch, are duly tempered by the admixture of contraries; and nature mingling together these two kinds of juices, difficult of coction by reason of most opposite defects, and then diluting them with a large quantity of warm blood, (for we see that the quantity returned from the spleen must be very large when we contemplate the size of its arteries,) they are brought to the porta of the liver in a state of higher preparation; the defects of either extreme are supplied and compensated by this arrangement of the veins.

CHAPTER XVII.

THE MOTION AND CIRCULATION OF THE BLOOD ARE CONFIRMED FROM THE PARTICULARS APPARENT IN THE STRUCTURE OF THE HEART, AND FROM THOSE THINGS WHICH DISSECTION UNFOLDS.

I do not find the heart as a distinct and separate part in all animals; some, indeed, such as the zoophytes, have no heart; this is because these animals are coldest, of no great bulk, of soft texture or of a certain uniform sameness or simplicity of structure; among the number I may instance grubs and earthworms, and those that are engendered of putrefaction and do not preserve their species. These have no heart, as not requiring any impeller of nourishment into the extreme parts; for they have bodies which are connate and homogeneous, and without limbs; so that by the contraction and relaxation of the whole body they assume and expel, move and remove the aliment. Oysters, mussels, sponges, and the whole genus of zoophytes or plant-animals have no heart; for the whole body is used as a heart, or the whole animal is a heart.   In a great number of animals, almost the whole tribe of insects, we cannot see distinctly by reason of the smallness of the body; still in bees, flies, hornets, and the like, we can perceive something pulsating with the help of a magnifying glass; in pediculi, also, the same thing may be seen, and as the body is transparent, the passage of the food through the intestines, like a black spot or stain, may be perceived by the aid of the same magnifying glass.

In some of the bloodless[1] and colder animals, further, as in snails, whelks, shrimps, and shell-fish, there is a part which pulsates—a kind of vesicle or auricle without a heart—slowly indeed, and not to be perceived save in the warmer season of the year.   In these creatures this part is so contrived that it shall pulsate, as there is here a necessity for some impulse to distribute the nutritive fluid, by reason of the variety of organic parts, or of the density of the substance; but the pulsations occur unfrequently, and sometimes in consequence of the cold not at all, an arrangement the best adapted to them as being of a doubtful nature, so that sometimes they appear to live, sometimes to die; sometimes they show the vitality of an animal, sometimes of a vegetable.   This seems also to be the case with the insects which conceal themselves in winter, and lie, as it were, defunct, or merely manifesting a kind of vegetative exist-ence.   But whether the same thing happens in the case of certain animals that have red blood, such as frogs, tortoises, serpents, swallows, may be made a question without any kind of impropriety.

In all the larger and warmer, because [red-]blooded animals, there was need of an impeller of the nutritive fluid, and that perchance possessing a considerable amount of power.   In fishes, serpents, lizards, tortoises, frogs, and others of the same kind there is a heart present, furnished with both an auricle and a ventricle, whence it is perfectly true, as Aristotle has observed,[2] that no [red-]blooded animal is without a heart, by the im-pelling power of which the nutritive fluid is forced, both with greater vigour and rapidity to a greater distance; it is not

[¹ i. e. Not having red blood.—Ed.]   ² De Part. Animal. lib. iii.

merely agitated by an auricle as it is in lower forms. And then in regard to animals that are yet larger, warmer, and more perfect, as they abound in blood, which is ever hotter and more spirituous, and possess bodies of greater size and consistency, they require a larger, stronger, and more fleshy heart, in order that the nutritive fluid may be propelled with yet greater force and celerity. And further, inasmuch as the more perfect animals require a still more perfect nutrition, and a larger supply of native heat, in order that the aliment may be thoroughly concocted and acquire the last degree of perfection, they required both lungs and a second ventricle, which should force the nutritive fluid through them.

Every animal that has lungs has therefore two ventricles to its heart, one right, another left; and wherever there is a right, there also is there a left ventricle; but the contrary of this does not hold good: where there is a left there is not always a right ventricle. The left ventricle I call that which is distinct in office, not in place from the other, that one namely which distributes the blood to the body at large, not to the lungs only. Hence the left ventricle seems to form the principal part of the heart; situated in the middle, more strongly marked, and constructed with greater care, the heart seems formed for the sake of the left ventricle, and the right but to minister to it; for the right neither reaches to the apex of the heart, nor is it nearly of such strength, being three times thinner in its walls, and in some sort jointed on to the left, (as Aristotle says;) though indeed it is of greater capacity, inasmuch as it has not only to supply material to the left ventricle, but likewise to furnish aliment to the lungs.

It is to be observed, however, that all this is otherwise in the embryo, where there is not such a difference between the two ventricles; but as in a double nut, they are nearly equal in all respects, the apex of the right reaching to the apex of the left, so that the heart presents itself as a sort of double-pointed cone. And this is so, because in the fœtus, as already said, whilst the blood is not passing through the lungs from the right to the left cavities of the heart, but flowing by the foramen ovale and ductus arteriosus, directly from the vena cava into the aorta, whence it is distributed to the whole body, both ventricles have in fact the same office to perform, whence their equality of constitution. It is only when the lungs come to be used, and it is requisite that the passages indicated should be blocked up, that the difference in point of strength and other things between the two ventricles begin to be apparent: in the altered circumstances the right has only to throw the blood through the lungs, whilst the left has to impel it through the whole body.

There are further within the heart numerous braces, so to speak, fleshy columns and fibrous bands, which Aristotle, in his third book on Respiration, and the Parts of Animals, entitles nerves. These are variously extended, and are either distinct or contained in grooves in the walls and partition, where they occasion numerous pits or depressions. They constitute a kind of small muscles, which are superadded and supplementary to the heart, assisting it to execute a more powerful and perfect contraction, and so proving subservient to the complete expulsion of the blood. They are in some sort like the elaborate and artful arrangement of ropes in a ship, bracing the heart on every side as it contracts, and so enabling it more effectually and forcibly to expel the charge of blood from its ventricles. This much is plain, at all events, that some animals have them strongly marked, others have them less so; and, in all that have them, they are more numerous and stronger in the left than in the right ventricle ; and whilst some have them in the left, there are yet none present in the right ventricle. In the human subject, again, these fleshy columns and braces are more numerous in the left than in the right ventricle, and they are more abundant in the ventricles than in the auricles ; occasionally, indeed, in the auricles there appear to be none present whatsoever. In large, more muscular and hardier bodies, as of countrymen, they are numerous; in more slender frames and in females they are fewer.

In those animals in which the ventricles of the heart are smooth within, and entirely without fibres or muscular bands, or anything like foveæ, as in almost all the smaller birds, the partridge and the common fowl, serpents, frogs, tortoises, and also fishes, for the major part, there are no chordæ tendineæ, nor bundles of fibres, neither are there any tricuspid valves in the ventricles.

Some animals have the right ventricle smooth internally, but the left provided with fibrous bands, such as the goose, swan, and larger birds ; and the reason here is still the same as elsewhere : as the lungs are spongy, and loose, and soft, no great amount of force is required to force the blood through them ; hence the right ventricle is either without the bundles in question, or they are fewer and weaker, not so fleshy or like muscles ; those of the left ventricle, however, are both stronger and more numerous, more fleshy and muscular, because the left ventricle requires to be stronger, inasmuch as the blood which it propels has to be driven through the whole body. And this, too, is the reason why the left ventricle occupies the middle of the heart, and has parietes three times thicker and stronger than those of the right. Hence all animals—and among men it is not otherwise—that are endowed with particularly strong frames, and that have large and fleshy limbs at a great distance from the heart, have this central organ of greater thickness, strength, and muscularity. And this is both obvious and necessary. Those, on the contrary, that are of softer and more slender make have the heart more flaccid, softer, and internally either sparely or not at all fibrous. Consider farther the use of the several valves, which are all so arranged, that the blood once received into the ventricles of the heart shall never regurgitate, once forced into the pulmonary artery and aorta shall not flow back upon the ventricles. When the valves are raised and brought together they form a three cornered line, such as is left by the bite of a leech ; and the more they are forced, the more firmly do they oppose the passage of the blood. The tricuspid valves are placed, like gate-keepers, at the entrance into the ventricles from the venæ cavæ and pulmonary veins, lest the blood when most forcibly impelled should flow back ; and it is for this reason that they are not found in all animals ; neither do they appear to have been constructed with equal care in all the animals in which they are found ; in some they are more accurately fitted, in others more remissly or carelessly contrived, and always with a view to their being closed under a greater or a slighter force of the ventricle. In the left ventricle, therefore, and in order that the occlusion may be the more perfect against the greater impulse, there are only two valves, like a mitre, and produced into an elongated cone, so that they come together and touch to their middle ; a circumstance which perhaps led Aristotle into the error of supposing this ventricle to be double, the division taking place transversely. For the same reason, indeed, and that the blood may not regurgitate upon the pulmonary veins, and thus the force of the ventricle in propelling the blood through the system at large come to be neutralized, it is that these mitral valves excel those of the right ventricle in size and strength, and exactness of closing. Hence, too, it is essential that there can be no heart without a ventricle, since this must be the source and storehouse of the blood. The same law does not hold good in reference to the brain. For almost no genus of birds has a ventricle in the brain, as is obvious in the goose and swan, the brains of which nearly equal that of a rabbit in size; now rabbits have ventricles in the brain, whilst the goose has none. In like manner, wherever the heart has a single ventricle, there is an auricle appended, flaccid, membranous, hollow, filled with blood; and where there are two ventricles, there are likewise two auricles. On the other hand, however, some animals have an auricle without any ventricle; or at all events they have a sac analogous to an auricle; or the vein itself, dilated at a particular part, performs pulsations, as is seen in hornets, bees, and other insects, which certain experiments of my own enable me to demonstrate have not only a pulse, but a respiration in that part which is called the tail, whence it is that this part is elongated and contracted now more rarely, now more frequently, as the creature appears to be blown and to require a larger quantity of air. But of these things, more in our Treatise on Respiration.

It is in like manner evident that the auricles pulsate, contract, as I have said before, and throw the blood into the ventricles; so that wherever there is a ventricle an auricle is necessary, not merely that it may serve, according to the general belief, as a source and magazine for the blood: for what were the use of its pulsations had it nothing to do save to contain? No; the auricles are prime movers of the blood, especially the right auricle, which is "the first to live, the last to die;" as already said; whence they are subservient to sending the blood into the ventricle, which, contracting incontinently, more readily and forcibly expels the blood already in motion; just as the ball-player can strike the ball more forcibly and further if he takes it on the rebound than if he simply threw it. Moreover, and contrary to the general opinion, since neither the heart nor anything else can dilate or distend itself so as to draw aught into its cavity during the diastole, unless, like a sponge, it has been first compressed, and as it is returning to its primary condition; but in animals all local motion proceeds from, and has its original in the contraction of some part: it is consequently by the contraction of the auricles that the blood is thrown into the ventricles, as I have already shown, and from thence, by the contraction of the ventricles, it is propelled and distributed. Which truth concerning local motions, and how the immediate moving organ in every motion of an animal primarily endowed with a motive spirit (as Aristotle has it,[1]) is contractile; and in what way the word νεῦρον is derived from νεύω, nuto, contraho; and how Aristotle was acquainted with the muscles, and did not unadvisedly refer all motion in animals to the nerves, or to the contractile element, and therefore called those little bands in the heart nerves—all this, if I am permitted to proceed in my purpose of making a particular demonstration of the organs of motion in animals from observations in my possession, I trust I shall be able to make sufficiently plain.

But that we may go on with the subject we have in hand, viz., the use of the auricles in filling the ventricles: we should expect that the more dense and compact the heart, the thicker its parietes, the stronger and more muscular must be the auricle to force and fill it, and *vice versa*. Now this is actually so: in some the auricle presents itself as a sanguinolent vesicle, as a thin membrane containing blood, as in fishes, in which the sac that stands in lieu of the auricle, is of such delicacy and ample capacity, that it seems to be suspended or to float above the heart; in those fishes in which the sac is somewhat more fleshy, as in the carp, barbel, tench, and others, it bears a wonderful and strong resemblance to the lungs.

In some men of sturdier frame and stouter make, the right auricle is so strong, and so curiously constructed within of bands and variously interlacing fibres, that it seems to equal the ventricle of the heart in other subjects; and I must say that I am astonished to find such diversity in this particular in different individuals. It is to be observed, however, that in the fœtus the auricles are out of all proportion large,

---

[1] In the book, de Spiritu, and elsewhere.

which is because they are present before the heart [the ventricular portion] makes its appearance or suffices for its office even when it has appeared, and they therefore have, as it were, the duty of the whole heart committed to them, as has already been demonstrated. But what I have observed in the formation of the fœtus as before remarked (and Aristotle had already confirmed all in studying the incubated egg,) throws the greatest light and likelihood upon the point. Whilst the fœtus is yet in the guise of a soft worm, or, as is commonly said, in the milk, there is a mere bloody point or pulsating vesicle, a portion apparently of the umbilical vein, dilated at its commencement or base; by and by, when the outline of the fœtus is distinctly indicated, and it begins to have greater bodily consistence, the vesicle in question having become more fleshy and stronger, and changed its position, passes into the auricles, over or upon which the body of the heart begins to sprout, though as yet it apparently performs no duty; but when the fœtus is farther advanced, when the bones can be distinguished from the soft parts, and movements take place, then it has also a heart internately which pulsates, and, as I have said, throws blood by either ventricle from the vena cava into the arteries.

Thus nature, ever perfect and divine, doing nothing in vain, has neither given a heart where it was not required, nor produced it before its office had become necessary; but by the same stages in the development of every animal, passing through the constitutions of all, as I may say (ovum, worm, fœtus), it acquires perfection in each. These points will be found elsewhere confirmed by numerous observations on the formation of the fœtus.

Finally, it was not without good grounds that Hippocrates, in his book, ' De Corde,' intitles it a muscle; as its action is the same, so is its function, viz., to contract and move something else, in this case, the charge of blood.

Farther, as in muscles at large, so can we infer the action and use of the heart from the arrangement of its fibres and its general structure. All anatomists admit with Galen that the body of the heart is made up of various courses of fibres running straight, obliquely, and transversely, with reference to one another; but in a heart which has been boiled the arrangement of the fibres is seen to be different: all the fibres in the parietes and septum are circular, as in the sphincters;

those, again, which are in the columnæ extend lengthwise, and are oblique longitudinally; and so it comes to pass, that when all the fibres contract simultaneously, the apex of the cone is pulled towards its base by the columnæ, the walls are drawn circularly together into a globe, the whole heart in short is contracted, and the ventricles narrowed; it is therefore impossible not to perceive that, as the action of the organ is so plainly contraction, its function is to propel the blood into the arteries.

Nor are we the less to agree with Aristotle in regard to the sovereignty of the heart; nor are we to inquire whether it receives sense and motion from the brain? whether blood from the liver? whether it be the origin of the veins and of the blood? and more of the same description. They who affirm these propositions against Aristotle, overlook, or do not rightly understand the principal argument, to the effect that the heart is the first part which exists, and that it contains within itself blood, life, sensation, motion, before either the brain or the liver were in being, or had appeared distinctly, or, at all events, before they could perform any function. The heart, ready furnished with its proper organs of motion, like a kind of internal creature, is of a date anterior to the body: first formed, nature willed that it should afterwards fashion, nourish, preserve, complete the entire animal, as its work and dwelling place: the heart, like the prince in a kingdom, in whose hands lie the chief and highest authority, rules over all; it is the original and foundation from which all power is derived, on which all power depends in the animal body.

And many things having reference to the arteries farther illustrate and confirm this truth. Why does not the arteria venosa pulsate, seeing that it is numbered among the arteries? Or wherefore is there a pulse in the vena arteriosa? Because the pulse of the arteries is derived from the impulse of the blood. Why does an artery differ so much from a vein in the thickness and strength of its coats? Because it sustains the shock of the impelling heart and streaming blood. Hence, as perfect nature does nothing in vain, and suffices under all circumstances, we find that the nearer the arteries are to the heart, the more do they differ from the veins in structure; here they are both stronger and more ligamentous, whilst in extreme parts of the body, such as the feet and hands, the brain, the mesentery,

and the testicles, the two orders of vessels are so much alike
that it is impossible to distinguish between them with the eye.
Now this is for the following very sufficient reasons: for the
more remote vessels are from the heart, with so much the less
force are they impinged upon by the stroke of the heart, which
is broken by the great distance at which it is given. Add to
this, that the impulse of the heart exerted upon the mass of
blood, which must needs fill the trunks and branches of the
arteries, is diverted, divided, as it were, and diminished at
every subdivision; so that the ultimate capillary divisions of the
arteries look like veins, and this not merely in constitution but
in function; for they have either no perceptible pulse, or they
rarely exhibit one, and never save where the heart beats more
violently than wont, or at a part where the minute vessel is more
dilated or open than elsewhere. Hence it happens that at
times we are aware of a pulse in the teeth, in inflammatory
tumours, and in the fingers; at another time we feel nothing of
the sort. Hence, too, by this single symptom I have ascertained
for certain that young persons, whose pulses are naturally
rapid, were labouring under fever; in like manner, on compressing the fingers in youthful and delicate subjects during
a febrile paroxysm, I have readily perceived the pulse there.
On the other hand, when the heart pulsates more languidly,
it is often impossible to feel the pulse not merely in the fingers,
but at the wrist, and even at the temple; this is the case in
persons afflicted with lipothymiæ and asphyxia, and hysterical
symptoms, as also in persons of very weak constitution and in
the moribund.

And here surgeons are to be advised that, when the blood
escapes with force in the amputation of limbs, in the removal
of tumours, and in wounds, it constantly comes from an artery;
not always per saltum, however, because the smaller arteries
do not pulsate, especially if a tourniquet has been applied.

And then the reason is the same wherefore the pulmonary
artery has not only the structure of an artery, but wherefore it
does not differ so widely in the thickness of its tunics from the
veins as the aorta: the aorta sustains a more powerful shock from
the left ventricle than the pulmonary artery does from the right;
and the tunics of this last vessel are thinner and softer than
those of the aorta in the same proportion as the walls of the

right ventricle of the heart are weaker and thinner than those of the left ventricle; and in like manner, in the same degree in which the lungs are softer and laxer in structure than the flesh and other constituents of the body at large, do the tunics of the branches of the pulmonary artery differ from the tunics of the vessels derived from the aorta. And the same proportion in these several particulars is universally preserved. The more muscular and powerful men are, the firmer their flesh, the stronger, thicker, denser, and more fibrous their heart, in the same proportion are the auricles and arteries in all respects thicker, closer, and stronger. And again, and on the other hand, in those animals the ventricles of whose heart are smooth within, without villi or valves, and the walls of which are thinner, as in fishes, serpents, birds, and very many genera of animals, in all of them the arteries differ little or nothing in the thickness of their coats from the veins.

Farther, the reason why the lungs have such ample vessels, both arteries and veins, (for the capacity of the pulmonary veins exceeds that of both the crural and jugular vessels,) and why they contain so large a quantity of blood, as by experience and ocular inspection we know they do, admonished of the fact indeed by Aristotle, and not led into error by the appearances found in animals which have been bled to death,—is, because the blood has its fountain, and storehouse, and the workshop of its last perfection in the heart and lungs. Why, in the same way we find in the course of our anatomical dissections the arteria venosa and left ventricle so full of blood, of the same black colour and clotted character, too, as that with which the right ventricle and pulmonary artery are filled, inasmuch as the blood is incessantly passing from one side of the heart to the other through the lungs. Wherefore, in fine, the pulmonary artery or vena arteriosa has the constitution of an artery, and the pulmonary veins or arteriæ venosæ have the structure of veins; because, in sooth, in function and constitution, and everything else, the first is an artery, the others are veins, in opposition to what is commonly believed; and why the pulmonary artery has so large an orifice, because it transports much more blood than is requisite for the nutrition of the lungs.

All these appearances, and many others, to be noted in the course of dissection, if rightly weighed, seem clearly to illustrate and fully to confirm the truth contended for throughout these pages, and at the same time to stand in opposition to the vulgar opinion ; for it would be very difficult to explain in any other way to what purpose all is constructed and arranged as we have seen it to be.

AN ANATOMICAL DISQUISITION

ON THE

CIRCULATION OF THE BLOOD.

TO

JOHN RIOLAN, Jun., of Paris;

A MOST SKILFUL PHYSICIAN; THE CORYPHÆUS OF ANATOMISTS; REGIUS
PROFESSOR OF ANATOMY AND BOTANY IN THE UNIVERSITY OF PARIS;
DEAN OF THE SAME UNIVERSITY; AND FIRST PHYSICIAN TO
THE QUEEN, MOTHER OF LOUIS XIII.

BY WILLIAM HARVEY, AN ENGLISHMAN,

PROFESSOR OF ANATOMY AND SURGERY IN THE ROYAL COLLEGE OF
PHYSICIANS OF LONDON; AND PRINCIPAL PHYSICIAN TO
HIS MOST SERENE MAJESTY THE KING.

CAMBRIDGE, 1649.

THE FIRST ANATOMICAL DISQUISITION ON THE CIRCULA-
TION OF THE BLOOD, ADDRESSED TO JO. RIOLAN.

SOME few months ago there appeared a small anatomical and pathological work from the pen of the celebrated Riolanus, for which, as sent to me by the author himself, I return him my grateful thanks.[1] I also congratulate this author on the highly laudable undertaking in which he has engaged. To demonstrate the seats of all diseases is a task that can only be achieved under favour of the highest abilities; for surely he enters on a difficult province who proposes to bring under the cognizance of the eyes those diseases which almost escape the keenest understanding. But such efforts become the prince of anatomists; for there is no science which does not spring from preexisting knowledge, and no certain and definite idea which has not derived its origin from the senses. Induced therefore by the subject itself, and the example of so distinguished an individual, which makes me think lightly of the labour, I also intend putting to press my Medical Anatomy, or Anatomy in its Application to Medicine. Not with the purpose, like Riolanus, of indicating the seats of diseases from the bodies of healthy subjects, and discussing the several diseases that make their appearance there, according to the views which others have entertained of them; but that I may relate from the many dissections I have made of the bodies of persons diseased, worn out by serious and strange affections, how and in what way the internal organs were changed in their situation, size, structure, figure, consistency, and other sensible qualities, from their natural forms and appearances, such as they are usually described by anatomists; and in what various and remarkable ways they were affected. For even as the dissection

---

[1] Encheiridium Anatomicum et Pathologicum. 12mo, Parisiis, 1648.

of healthy and well-constituted bodies contributes essentially to the advancement of philosophy and sound physiology, so does the inspection of diseased and cachectic subjects powerfully assist philosophical pathology. And, indeed, the physiological consideration of the things which are according to nature is to be first undertaken by medical men; since that which is in conformity with nature is right, and serves as a rule both to itself and to that which is amiss; by the light it sheds, too, aberrations and affections against nature are defined; pathology then stands out more clearly; and from pathology the use and art of healing, as well as occasions for the discovery of many new remedies, are perceived. Nor could any one readily imagine how extensively internal organs are altered in diseases, especially chronic diseases, and what monstrosities among internal parts these diseases engender. So that I venture to say, that the examination of a single body of one who has died of tabes or some other disease of long standing, or poisonous nature, is of more service to medicine than the dissection of the bodies of ten men who have been hanged.

I would not have it supposed by this that I in any way disapprove of the purpose of Riolanus, that learned and skilful anatomist; on the contrary, I think it deserving of the highest praise, as likely to be extremely useful to medicine, inasmuch as it illustrates the physiological branch of this science; but I have thought that it would scarcely turn out less profitable to the art of healing, did I place before the eyes of my readers not only the places, but the affections of these places, illustrating them as I proceed with observations, and recording the results of my experience derived from my numerous dissections.

But it is imperative on me first to dispose of those observations contained in the work referred to, which bear upon the circulation of the blood as discovered by me, and which seem to require especial notice at my hands. For the judgment of such a man, who is indeed the prince and leader of all the anatomists of the present age, in such a matter, is not to be lightly esteemed, but is rather to be held of greater weight and authority, either for praise or blame, than the commendations or censure of all the world besides.

Riolanus, then, admits our motion of the blood in animals,[1]

---

[1] Enchiridion, lib. iii, cap. 8.

and falls in with our conclusions in regard to the circulation; yet not entirely and avowedly; for he says[1] that the blood contained in the vena portæ does not circulate like that in the vena cava; and again he states[2] that there is some blood which circulates, and that the circulatory vessels are the aorta and vena cava; but then he denies that the continuations of these trunks have any circulation, " because the blood is effused into all the parts of the second and third regions, where it remains for purposes of nutrition; nor does it return to any greater vessels, unless forcibly drawn back when there is a great lack of blood in the main channels, or driven by a fit of passion when it flows to the greater circulatory vessels;" and shortly afterwards : " thus, as the blood of the veins naturally ascends incessantly or returns to the heart, so the blood of the arteries descends or departs from the heart; still, if the smaller veins of the arms and legs be empty, the blood filling the empty channels in succession, may descend in the veins, as I have clearly shown," he says, " against Harvey and Walæus." And as the authority of Galen and daily experience confirm the anastomoses of the arteries and veins, and the necessity of the circulation of the blood, " you perceive," he continues, " how the circulation is effected, without any perturbation or confusion of fluids and the destruction of the ancient system of medicine."

These words explain the motives by which this illustrious anatomist was actuated when he was led partly to admit, partly to deny the circulation of the blood; and why he only ventures on an undecided and inconclusive opinion of the subject; his fear is lest it destroy the ancient medicine. Not yielding implicitly to the truth, which it appears he could not help seeing, but rather guided by caution, he fears speaking plainly out, lest he offend the ancient physic, or perhaps seem to retract the physiological doctrines he supports in his Anthropology. The circulation of the blood does not shake, but much rather confirms the ancient medicine; though it runs counter to the physiology of physicians, and their speculations upon natural subjects, and opposes the anatomical doctrine of the use and action of the heart and lungs, and rest of the viscera. That this is so shall readily be made to appear, both from his own words and avowal, and partly also from what I shall supply;

[1] Euchiridion, lib. ii, cap. 21. [2] Ib. lib. iii, cap. 8.

viz., that the whole of the blood, wherever it be in the living body, moves and changes its place, not merely that which is in the larger vessels and their continuations, but that also which is in their minute subdivisions, and which is contained in the pores or interstices of every part; that it flows from and back to the heart ceaselessly and without pause, and could not pause for ever so short a time without detriment, although I admit that occasionally, and in some places, its motion is quicker or slower.[1]

In the first place, then, our learned anatomist only denies that the contents of the branches in continuation of the vena portæ circulate; but he could neither oppose nor deny this, did he not conceal from himself the force of his own arguments; for he says in his Third Book, chap. viii, " If the heart at each pulsation admits a drop of blood which it throws into the aorta, and in the course of an hour makes two thousand beats, it is a necessary consequence that the quantity of blood transmitted must be great." He is farther forced to admit as much in reference to the mesentery, when he sees that far more than single drops of blood are sent into the cœliac and mesenteric arteries at each pulsation; so that there must either be some outlet for the fluid, of magnitude commensurate with its quantity, or the branches of the vena portæ must give way. Nor can the explanation that is had recourse to with a view of meeting the difficulty, viz., that the blood of the mesentery ebbs and flows by the same channels, after the manner of Euripus, be received as either probable or possible. Neither can the reflux from the mesentery be effected by those passages and that system of translation, by which he will have it to disgorge itself into the aorta; this were against the force of the existing current, and by a contrary motion; nor can anything like pause or alternation be admitted, where there is very certainly an incessant influx: the blood sent into the mesentery must as inevitably go elsewhere as that which is poured into the heart. And this is obvious; were it otherwise, indeed, everything like a circulation might be overturned upon the same showing and by the same subterfuge; it might just as well be said that the blood contained in the left ventricle of the heart is propelled into the aorta during the systole, and flows back to it during the diastole,

[1] Vide Chapter III.

the aorta disgorging itself into the ventricle, precisely as the ventricle has disgorged itself into the aorta. There would thus be circulation neither in the heart nor in the mesentery, but an alternate flux and reflux, — a useless labour, as it seems. If, therefore, and for the reason assigned and approved by him, a circulation through the heart be argued for as a thing necessary, the argument has precisely the same force when applied to the mesentery : if there be no circulation in the mesentery, neither is there any in the heart ; for both affirmations, this in reference to the heart, that in reference to the mesentery, merely changing the words, stand or fall together, by force of the very same arguments.

He says : " The sigmoid valves prevent regurgitation into the heart ; but there are no valves in the mesentery." To this I reply, that the thing is not so ; for there is a valve in the splenic vein, and sometimes also in other veins. And besides, valves are not met with universally in veins ; there are few or none in the deep-seated veins of the extremities, but many in the subcutaneous branches. For where the blood is flowing naturally from smaller into greater branches, into which it is disposed to enter, the pressure of the circumjacent muscles is enough, and more than enough to prevent all retrograde movement, and it is forced on where the way lies open ; in such circumstances, what use were there for valves ? But the quantity of blood that is forced into the mesentery by each stroke of the heart, may be estimated in the same way as you estimate the quantity impelled into the hand when you bind a ligature with medium tightness about the wrist : if in so many beats the vessels of the hand become distended, and the whole extremity swells, you will find, that much more than a single drop of blood has entered with each pulse, and which cannot return, but must remain to fill the hand and increase its size. But analogy permits us to say, that the same thing takes place in reference to the mesentery and its vessels, in an equal degree at least, if not in a greater degree, seeing that the vessels of the mesentery are considerably larger than those of the carpus. And if any one will but think on the difficulty that is experienced with all the aid supplied by compresses, bandages, and a multiplied apparatus, in restraining the flow of blood from the smallest artery when wounded, with what force

it overcomes all obstacles and soaks through the whole apparatus, he will scarcely, I imagine, think it likely that there can
be any retrograde motion against such an impulse and influx
of blood, any retrograde force to meet and overcome a direct
force of such power.   Turning over these things in his mind,
I say, no one will ever be brought to believe that the blood
from the branches of the vena portæ can possibly make its way
by the same channels against an influx by the artery of such
impetuosity and force, and so unload the mesentery.

Moreover, if the learned anatomist does not think that the
blood is moved and changed by a circular motion, but that the
same fluid always stagnates in the channels of the mesentery,
he appears to suppose that there are two descriptions of blood,
serving different uses and ends; that the blood of the vena
portæ, and that of the vena cava are dissimilar in constitution, seeing that the one requires a circulation for its preservation, the other requires nothing of the kind; which
neither appears on the face of the thing, nor is its truth
demonstrated by him.   Our author then refers to " A fourth
order of mesenteric vessels, the lacteal vessels, discovered
by Asellius;" and having mentioned these, he seems to infer
that they extract all the nutriment from the intestines, and
transfer this to the liver, the workshop of the blood, whence,
having been concocted and changed into blood, (so he says in his
third book, chapter the 8th), the blood is transferred from the
liver to the right ventricle of the heart.   " Which things premised," he continues,[2] " all the difficulties which were formerly
experienced in regard to the distribution of the chyle and blood
by the same channel come to an end ; for the lacteal veins carry
the chyle to the liver, and as these canals are distinct, so may
they be severally obstructed."   But truly I would here ask:
how this milky fluid can be poured into and pass through the
liver, and how from thence gain the vena cava and the ventricle of the heart? when our author denies that the blood
of the vena portæ passes through the liver, and that so a circulation is established.   I pause for a reply.   I would fain know
how such a thing can be shown to be probable ; especially
when the blood appears to be both more spirituous or subtile

and penetrating than the chyle or milk contained in these lacteal vessels, and is further impelled by the pulsations of the arteries that it may find a passage by other channels.

Our learned author mentions a certain tract of his on the Circulation of the Blood : I wish I could obtain a sight of it ; perhaps I might retract. But had the learned writer been so disposed, I do not see but that having admitted the circular motion of the blood,[1] all the difficulties which were formerly felt in connexion with the distribution of the chyle and the blood by the same channels are brought to an equally satisfactory solution ; so much so indeed that there would be no necessity for inquiring after or laying down any separate vessels for the chyle. Even as the umbilical veins absorb the nutritive juices from the fluids of the egg and transport them for the nutrition and growth of the chick, in its embryo state, so do the meseraic veins suck up the chyle from the intestines and transfer it to the liver ; and why should we not maintain that they perform the same office in the adult ? For all the mooted difficulties vanish when we cease to suppose two contrary motions in the same vessels, and admit but one and the same continuous motion in the mesenteric vessels from the intestines to the liver.

I shall elsewhere state my views of the lacteal veins when I treat of the milk found in different parts of new-born animals, especially of the human subject ; for it is met with in the mesentery and all its glands, in the thymus, in the axillæ, also in the breasts of infants. This milk the midwifes are in the habit of pressing out, for the health, as they believe, of the infants. But it has pleased the learned Riolanus, not only to take away circulation from the blood contained in the mesentery ; he affirms that neither do the vessels in continuation of the vena cava, nor the arteries, nor any of the parts of the second and third regions, admit of circulation, so that he entitles and enumerates as circulating vessels the vena cava and aorta only. For this he appears to me to give a very indifferent reason:[2] " The blood," he says, " effused into all the parts of the second and third regions, remains there for their nutrition ; nor does it

---

[1] Enchiridion, lib. iii, cap. 8 : " The blood incessantly and naturally ascends or flows back to the heart in the veins, as in the arteries it descends or departs from the heart."

[2] Enchirid. lib. iii, cap. 8.

return to the great vessels, unless forcibly drawn back by an extreme dearth of blood in the great vessels, nor, unless carried by an impulse, does it flow to the circulatory vessels."

That so much of the blood must remain as is appropriated to the nutrition of the tissues, is matter of necessity; for it cannot nourish unless it be assimilated and become coherent, and form substance in lieu of that which is lost; but that the whole of the blood which flows into a part should there remain, in order that so small a portion should undergo transformation, is nowise necessary; for no part uses so much blood for its nutrition as is contained in its arteries, veins, and interstices. Nor because the blood is continually coming and going is it necessary to suppose that it leaves nothing for nutriment behind it. Consequently it is by no means necessary that the whole remain in order that nutrition be effected. But our learned author, in the same book, where he affirms so much, appears almost everywhere else to assert the contrary. In that paragraph especially where he describes the circulation in the brain, he says: "And the brain by means of the circulation sends back blood to the heart, and thus refrigerates the organ." And in the same way are all the more remote parts said to refrigerate the heart; thus in fevers, when the præcordia are scorched and burn with febrile heat, patients baring their limbs and casting off the bedclothes, seek to cool their heart; and the blood generally, tempered and cooled down, as our learned author states it to be with reference to the brain in particular, returns by the veins and refrigerates the heart. Our author, therefore, appears to insinuate a certain necessity for a circulation from every part, as well as from the brain, in opposition to what he had before said in very precise terms. But then he cautiously and ambiguously asserts, that the blood does not return from the parts composing the second and third regions, unless, as he says, it is drawn by force, and through a signal deficiency of blood in the larger vessels, &c., which is most true if these words be rightly understood; for by the larger vessels, in which the deficiency is said to cause the reflux, I think he must be held to mean the veins not the arteries; for the arteries are never emptied, save into the veins or interstices of parts, but are incessantly filled by the strokes of the heart; but in the vena cava and other returning channels, in which the blood glides rapidly on, hastening to the heart, there would speedily be a great deficiency of blood did not every part incessantly restore the blood that is incessantly poured into it. Add to this, that by the impulse of the blood which is forced with each stroke into every part of the second and third regions, that which is contained in the pores or interstices is urged into the smaller veins, from which it passes into larger vessels, its motion assisted besides by the motion and pressure of circumjacent parts; for from every containing thing compressed and constringed, contained matters are forced out. And thus it is that by the motions of the muscles and extremities, the blood contained in the minor vessels is forced onwards and delivered into the larger trunks. But that the blood is incessantly driven from the arteries into every part of the body, there gives a pulse and never flows back in these channels, cannot be doubted, if it be admitted that with each pulse of the heart all the arteries are simultaneously distended by the blood sent into them; and as our learned author himself allows that the diastole of the arteries is occasioned by the systole of the heart, and that the blood once out of the heart can never get back into the ventricles by reason of the opposing valves; if I say, our learned author believes that these things are so, it will be as manifestly true with regard to the force and impulse by which the blood contained in the vessels is propelled into every part of every region of the body. For wheresoever the arteries pulsate, so far must the impulse and influx extend, and therefore is the impulse felt in every part of each several region; for there is a pulse everywhere, to the very points of the fingers and under the nails, nor is there any part of the body where the shooting pain that accompanies each pulse of the artery, and the effort made to effect a solution of the continuity is not experienced when it is the seat of a phlegmon or furuncle.

But, further, that the blood contained in the pores of the living tissues returns to the heart, is manifest from what we observe in the hands and feet. For we frequently see the hands and feet, in young persons especially, during severe weather, become so cold that to the touch they feel like ice, and they are so benumbed and stiffened that they seem scarcely to retain a trace of sensibility or to be capable of any motion; still are they all the while surcharged with blood, and look red or livid. Yet can the extremities be warmed in no way, save by circulation; the chilled blood, which has lost its spirit and heat, being driven out, and fresh, warm, and vivified blood flowing in by the arteries in its stead, which fresh blood cherishes and warms the parts, and restores to them sense and motion; nor could the extremities be restored by the warmth of a fire or other external heat, any more than those of a dead body could be so recovered: they are only brought to life again, as it were, by an influx of internal warmth.   And this indeed is the principal use and end of the circulation; it is that for which the blood is sent on its ceaseless course, and to exert its influence continually in its circuit, to wit, that all parts dependent on the primary innate heat may be retained alive, in their state of vital and vegetative being, and apt to perform their functions; whilst, to use the language of physiologists, they are sustained and actuated by the inflowing heat and vital spirits.   Thus, by the aid of two extremes, viz. cold and heat, is the temperature of the animal body retained at its mean.   For as the air inspired tempers the too great heat of the blood in the lungs and centre of the body, and effects the expulsion of suffocating fumes, so in its turn does the hot blood, thrown by the arteries into all parts of the body, cherish and nourish and keep them in life, defending them from extinction through the power of external cold.

It would, therefore, be in some sort unfair and extraordinary did not every particle composing the body enjoy the advantages of the circulation and transmutation of the blood; the ends for which the circulation was mainly established by nature would no longer be effected.   To conclude then: you see how circulation may be accomplished without confusion or admixture of humours, through the whole body, and each of its individual parts, in the smaller as well as in the larger vessels; and all as matter of necessity and for the general advantage; without circulation, indeed, there would be no restoration of chilled and exhausted parts, no continuance of these in life; since it is apparent enough that the whole influence of the preservative heat comes by the arteries, and is the work of the circulation.

It, therefore, appears to me that the learned Riolanus speaks rather expediently than truly, when in his Enchiridion he denies a circulation to certain parts; it would seem as though he had wished to please the mass, and oppose none; to have written with such a bias rather than rigidly and in behalf of the simple truth. This is also apparent when he would have the blood to make its way into the left ventricle through the septum of the heart, by certain invisible and unknown passages, rather than through those ample and abundantly pervious channels, the pulmonary vessels, furnished with valves, opposing all reflux or regurgitation. He informs us that he has elsewhere discussed the reasons of the impossibility or inconvenience of this : I much desire to see his disquisition. It would be extraordinary, indeed, were the aorta and pulmonary artery, with the same dimensions, properties, and structure, not to have the same functions. But it would be more wonderful still were the whole tide of the blood to reach the left ventricle by a set of inscrutable passages of the septum, a tide which, in quantity must correspond, first to the influx from the vena cava into the right side of the heart, and next to the efflux from the left, both of which require such ample conduits. But our author has adduced these matters inconsistently, for he has established the lungs as an emunctory or passage from the heart;[1] and he says: "The lung is affected by the blood which passes through it, the sordes flowing along with the blood." And, again : "The lungs receive injury from distempered and ill-conditioned viscera; these deliver an impure blood to the heart, which it cannot correct except by multiplied circulations." In the same place, he further proceeds, whilst speaking against Galen of bloodletting in peripneumonia and the communication of the veins : "Were it true that the blood naturally passed from the right ventricle of the heart to the lungs, that it might be carried into the left ventricle and from thence into the aorta; and were the circulation of the blood admitted, who does not see that in affections of the lungs the blood would flow to them in larger quantity and would oppress them, unless it were taken away, first, freely, and then in repeated smaller quantities in order to relieve them, which indeed was the advice of Hippocrates, who, in affections of the lungs takes away blood from every part—the head, nose, tongue, arms and feet, in order that its quantity may be diminished and a diversion effected from the lungs ; he takes away blood till the body is almost bloodless. Now admitting the circu-

---

[1] Lib. iii, cap. 6.

lation, the lungs are most readily depleted by opening a vein; but rejecting it, I do not see how any revulsion of the blood can be accomplished by this means; for did it flow back by the pulmonary artery upon the right ventricle, the sigmoid valves would oppose its entrance, and any escape from the right ventricle into the vena cava is prevented by the tricuspid valves. The blood, therefore, is soon exhausted when a vein is opened in the arm or foot, if we admit the circulation; and the opinion of Fernelius is at the same time upset by this admission, viz. that in affections of the lungs it is better to bleed from the right than the left arm; because the blood cannot flow backwards into the vena cava unless the two barriers situated in the heart be first broken down."

He adds yet further in the same place :[2] " If the circulation of the blood be admitted, and it be acknowledged that this fluid generally passes through the lungs, not through the middle partition of the heart, a double circulation becomes requisite; one effected through the lungs, in the course of which the blood quitting the right ventricle of the heart passes through the lungs in order that it may arrive at the left ventricle; leaving the heart on the one hand, therefore, the blood speedily returns to it again; another and longer circulation proceeding from the left ventricle of the heart performs the circuit of the whole body by the arteries, and by the veins returns to the right side of the heart."

The learned anatomist might here have added a third and extremely short circulation, viz.—from the left to the right ventricle of the heart, with that blood which courses through the coronary arteries and veins, and by their ramifications is distributed to the body, walls, and septum of the heart.

" He who admits one circulation," proceeds our author, "cannot repudiate the other;" and he might, as it appears, have added, " the third." For why should the coronary arteries of the heart pulsate, if it were not to force on the blood by their pulsations ? and why should there be coronary veins, the end and office of all veins being to receive the blood brought by the arteries, were it not to deliver and discharge the blood sent into the substance of the heart ? In this consideration let it

<hr>

[1] Lib. iii, cap. 6.

be remembered that a valve is very commonly found at the orifice of the coronary vein, as our learned author himself admits,[1] preventing all ingress, but offering no obstacle to the egress of the blood. It therefore seems that he cannot do otherwise than admit this third circulation, who acknowledges a general circulation through the body, and that the blood also passes through the lungs and the brain.[2] Nor, indeed, can he deny a similar circulation to every other part of every other region. The blood flowing in under the influence of the arterial pulse, and returning by the veins, every particle of the body has its circulation.

From the words of our learned writer quoted above, consequently, his opinion may be gathered both of the general circulation, and then of the circulation through the lungs and the several parts of the body; for he who admits the first, manifestly cannot refuse to acknowledge the others. How indeed could he who has repeatedly asserted a circulation through the general system and the greater vessels, deny a circulation in the branches continuous with these vessels, or in the several parts of the second and third regions? as if all the veins, and those he calls greater circulatory vessels, were not enumerated by every anatomist, and by himself, as being within the second region of the body. Is it possible that there can be a circulation which is universal, and which yet does not extend through every part? Where he denies it, then, he does so hesitatingly, and vaccillates between negations, giving us mere words. Where he asserts the circulation, on the contrary, he speaks out heartily, and gives sufficient reasons, as becomes a philosopher; and then, when he relies on this opinion in a particular instance, he delivers himself like an experienced physician and honest man, and, in opposition to Galen and his favorite Fernelius, advises bloodletting as the chief remedy in dangerous diseases of the lungs.

No learned man and Christian, having doubts in such a case, would have recommended his experience to posterity, to the imminent risk, and even loss of human life; neither would he without very sufficient reasons, have repudiated the authority of Galen and Fernelius, which has usually such weight with

---

[1] Lib. iii, cap. 9.   [2] Lib. iv. cap. 2.

him. Whatever he has denied in the circulation of the blood, therefore, whether with reference to the mesentery or any other part, and with an eye to the lacteal veins or the ancient system of physic, or any other consideration, must be ascribed to his courtesy and modesty, and is to be excused.

Thus far, I think, it appears plain enough, from the very words and arguments of our author, that there is a circulation everywhere; that the blood, wherever it is, changes its place, and by the veins returns to the heart; so that our learned author seems to be of the same opinion as myself. It would therefore be labour in vain, did I here quote at greater length the various reasons which I have consigned in my work on the Motion of the Blood, in confirmation of my opinions, and which are derived from the structure of the vessels, the position of the valves, and other matters of experience and observation; and this the more, as I have not yet seen the treatise on the Circulation of the Blood of the learned writer; nor, indeed, have I yet met with a single argument of his, or more than his simple negation, which would lead me to see wherefore he should reject a circulation which he admits as universal, in certain parts, regions, and vessels.

It is true that by way of subterfuge he has recourse to an anastomosis of the vessels on the authority of Galen, and the evidence of daily experience. But so distinguished a personage, an anatomist so expert, so inquisitive, and careful, should first have shown anastomoses between the larger arteries and larger veins, and these, both obvious and ample, having mouths in relation with such a torrent as is constituted by the whole mass of the blood, and larger than the capacity of the continuous branches, (from which he takes away all circulation,) before he had rejected those that are familiarly known, that are more likely and more open; he ought to have clearly shown us where these anastomoses are, and how they are fashioned, whether they be adapted only to permit the access of the blood into the veins, and not to allow of its regurgitation, in the same way as we see the ureters connected with the urinary bladder, or in what other manner things are contrived. But —and here I speak over boldly perhaps—neither our learned author himself, nor Galen, nor any experience, has ever succeeded in making such anastomoses as he imagines, sensible to the eye.

I have myself pursued this subject of the anastomosis with all the diligence I could command, and have given not a little both of time and labour to the inquiry; but I have never succeeded in tracing any connexion between arteries and veins by a direct anastomosis of their orifices. I would gladly learn of those who give so much to Galen, how they dare swear to what he says. Neither in the liver, spleen, lungs, kidneys, nor any other viscus, is such a thing as an anastomosis to be seen; and by boiling, I have rendered the whole parenchyma of these organs so friable that it could be shaken like dust from the fibres, or picked away with a needle, until I could trace the fibres of every subdivision, and see every capillary filament distinctly. I can therefore boldly affirm, that there is neither any anastomosis of the vena portæ with the cava, of the arteries with the veins, or of the capillary ramifications of the biliary ducts, which can be traced through the entire liver, with the veins. This alone may be observed in the recent liver: all the branches of the vena cava ramifying through the convexity of the liver, have their tunics pierced with an infinity of minute holes, as is a sieve, and are fashioned to receive the blood in its descent. The branches of the porta are not so constituted, but simply spread out in subdivisions; and the distribution of these two vessels is such, that whilst the one runs upon the convexity, the other proceeds along the concavity of the liver to its outer margin, and all the while without anastomosing.

In three places only do I find anything that can be held equivalent to an anastomosis. From the carotids, as they are creeping over the base of the brain, numerous interlaced fibres arise, which afterwards form the choroid plexus, and passing through the lateral ventricles, finally unite and terminate in the third sinus, which performs the office of a vein. In the spermatic vessels, commonly called vasa præparantia, certain minute arteries proceeding from the great artery adhere to the venæ præparantes, which they accompany, and are at length taken in and included within their coats, in such a way that they seem to have a common ending, so that where they terminate on the upper portion of the testis, on that cone-shaped

process called the corpus varicosum et pampiniforme, it is altogether uncertain whether we are to regard their terminations
as veins, or as arteries, or as both.   In the same way are the
ultimate ramifications of the arteries which run to the umbilical vein, lost in the tunics of this vessel.

What doubt can there be, if by such channels the great
arteries, distended by the stream of blood sent into them, are
relieved of so great and obvious a torrent, but that nature
would not have denied distinct and visible passages, vortices,
and estuaries, had she intended to divert the whole current of
the blood, and had wished in this way to deprive the lesser
branches and the solid parts of all the benefit of the influx of
that fluid?

Finally, I shall quote this single experiment, which appears
to me sufficient to clear up all doubts about the anastomoses,
and their uses, if any exist, and to set at rest the question of
a passage of the blood from the veins to the arteries, by any
special channels, or by regurgitation.

Having laid open the thorax of an animal, and tied the vena
cava near the heart, so that nothing shall pass from that vessel
into its cavities, and immediately afterwards, having divided
the carotid arteries on both sides, the jugular veins being left untouched; if the arteries be now perceived to become empty but
not the veins, I think it will be manifest that the blood does nowhere pass from the veins into the arteries except through the
ventricles of the heart.   Were it not so, as observed by Galen,
we should see the veins as well as the arteries emptied in a very
short time, by the efflux from their corresponding arteries.

For what further remains, oh Riolanus! I congratulate both
myself and you: myself, for the opinion with which you have
graced my circulation; and you, for your learned, polished, and
terse production, than which nothing more elegant can be
imagined.   For the favour you have done me in sending me
this work, I feel most grateful, and I would gladly, as in duty
bound, proclaim my sense of its merits, but I confess myself
unequal to the task; for I know that the Enchiridion bearing
the name of Riolanus inscribed upon it, has thereby more of
honour conferred upon it than it can derive from any praise of
mine, which nevertheless I would yield without reserve.   The

famous book will live for ever; and when marble shall have mouldered, will proclaim to posterity the glory that belongs to your name.   You have most happily conjoined anatomy with pathology, and have greatly enriched the subject with a new and most useful osteology.   Proceed in your worthy career, most illustrious Riolanus, and love him who wishes that you may enjoy both happiness and length of days, and that all your admirable works may conduce to your eternal fame.

WILLIAM HARVEY.

A

SECOND DISQUISITION TO JOHN RIOLAN, JUN.,

IN WHICH

MANY OBJECTIONS

TO THE

CIRCULATION OF THE BLOOD

ARE REFUTED.

A SECOND DISQUISITION TO JOHN RIOLAN.

Ir is now many years, most learned Riolanus, since, with the aid of the press, I published a portion of my work. But scarce a day, scarce an hour, has passed since the birth-day of the Circulation of the blood, that I have not heard something for good or for evil said of this my discovery. Some abuse it as a feeble infant, and yet unworthy to have seen the light; others, again, think the bantling deserves to be cherished and cared for; these oppose it with much ado, those patronize it with abundant commendation; one party holds that I have completely demonstrated the circulation of the blood by experiment, observation, and ocular inspection, against all force and array of argument; another thinks it scarcely yet sufficiently illustrated —not yet cleared of all objections. There are some, too, who say that I have shown a vainglorious love of vivisections, and who scoff at and deride the introduction of frogs and serpents, flies, and others of the lower animals upon the scene, as a piece of puerile levity, not even refraining from opprobrious epithets.

To return evil speaking with evil speaking, however, I hold to be unworthy in a philosopher and searcher after truth; I believe that I shall do better and more advisedly if I meet so many indications of ill breeding with the light of faithful and conclusive observation. It cannot be helped that dogs bark and vomit their foul stomachs, or that cynics should be numbered among philosophers; but care can be taken that they do not bite or inoculate their mad humours, or with their dogs' teeth gnaw the bones and foundations of truth.

Detractors, mummers, and writers defiled with abuse, as I resolved with myself never to read them, satisfied that nothing solid or excellent, nothing but foul terms, was to be expected from them, so have I held them still less worthy of an answer. Let them consume on their own ill nature; they will scarcely find many well-disposed readers, I imagine, nor does God give that which is most excellent and chiefly to be desired—wisdom, to the wicked; let them go on railing, I say, until they are weary, if not ashamed.

If for the sake of studying the meaner animals you should even enter the bakehouse with Heraclitus, as related in Aristotle, I bid you approach; for neither are the immortal Gods absent here, and the great and almighty Father is sometimes most visible in His lesser, and to the eye least considerable works.[1]

In my book on the Motion of the Heart and Blood in Animals, I have only adduced those facts from among many other observations, by which either errors were best refuted, or truth was most strongly supported; I have left many proofs, won by dissection and appreciable to sense, as redundant and unnecessary; some of these, however, I now supply in brief terms, for the sake of the studious, and those who have expressed their desire to have them.

The authority of Galen is of such weight with all, that I have seen several hesitate greatly with that experiment before them, in which the artery is tied upon a tube placed within its cavity; and by which it is proposed to prove that the arterial pulse is produced by a power communicated from the heart through the coats of the arteries, and not from the shock of the blood contained within them; and thence, that the arteries dilate as bellows, are not filled as sacs. This experiment is spoken of by Vesalius, the celebrated anatomist; but neither Vesalius nor Galen says that he had tried the experiment, which, however, I did. Vesalius only prescribes, and Galen advises it, to those anxious to discover the truth, and for their better assurance, not thinking of the difficulties that attend its performance, nor of its futility when done; for indeed, although executed with the greatest skill, it supplies nothing in support of the opinion which

---

[1] [To those who hesitated to visit him in his kiln or bakehouse ('ιπνω, which some have said should be 'ιππω, rendered a dunghill) Heraclitus addressed the words in the text. Aristotle, who quotes them, has been defending the study of the lower animals.—Ed.]

maintains that the coats of the vessel are the cause of the pulse ; it much rather proclaims that this is owing to the impulse of the blood. For the moment you have thrown your ligature around the artery upon the reed or tube, immediately, by the force of the blood thrown in from above, it is dilated beyond the circle of the tube, by which the flow is impeded, and the shock is broken ; so that the artery which is tied only pulsates obscurely, being now cut off from the full force of the blood that flows through it, the shock being reverberated, as it were, from that part of the vessel which is above the ligature ; but if the artery below the ligature be now divided, the contrary of what has been maintained will be apparent, from the spurting of the blood impelled through the tube ; just as happens in the cases of aneurism, referred to in my book on the Motion of the Blood, which arise from an erosion of the coats of the vessel, and when the blood is contained in a membranous sac, formed not by the coats of the vessel dilated, but preternaturally produced from the surrounding tissues and flesh. The arteries beyond an aneurism of this kind will be felt beating very feebly, whilst in those above it and in the swelling itself the pulse will be perceived of great strength and fulness. And here we cannot imagine that the pulsation and dilatation take place by the coats of the arteries, or any power communicated to the walls of the sac ; they are plainly due to the shock of the blood.

But that the error of Vesalius, and the inexperience of those who assert their belief that the part below the tube does not pulsate when the ligature is tied, may be made the more apparent, I can state, after having made the trial, that the inferior part will continue to pulsate if the experiment be properly performed ; and whilst they say that when you have undone the ligature the inferior arteries begin again to pulsate, I maintain that the part below beats less forcibly when the ligature is untied than it did when the thread was still tight. But the effusion of blood from the wound confuses everything, and renders the whole experiment unsatisfactory and nugatory, so that nothing certain can be shown, by reason, as I have said, of the hemorrhage. But if, as I know by experience, you lay bare an artery, and control the divided portion by the pressure of your fingers, you may try many things at pleasure by which the truth will be made to appear. In the first place, you will feel the blood coming down in the artery at each pulsation, and visibly dilating the vessel. You may also at will suffer the blood to escape, by relaxing the pressure, and leaving a small outlet; and you will see that it jets out with each stroke, with each contraction of the heart, and with each dilatation of the artery, as I have said in speaking of arteriotomy, and the experiment of perforating the heart. And if you suffer the efflux to go on uninterruptedly, either from the simple divided artery or from a tube inserted into it, you will be able to perceive by the sight, and if you apply your hand, by the touch likewise, every character of the stroke of the heart in the jet; the rhythm, order, intermission, force, &c., of its pulsations, all becoming sensible there, no otherwise than would the jets from a syringe, pushed in succession and with different degrees of force, received upon the palm of the hand, be obvious to sight and touch. I have occasionally observed the jet from a divided carotid artery to be so forcible, that, when received on the hand, the blood rebounded to the distance of four or five feet.

But that the question under discussion, viz.—that the pulsific power does not proceed from the heart by the coats of the vessels, may be set in yet a clearer light, I beg here to refer to a portion of the descending aorta, about a span in length, with its division into the two crural trunks, which I removed from the body of a nobleman, and which is converted into a bony tube; by this hollow tube, nevertheless, did the arterial blood reach the lower extremities of this nobleman during his life, and cause the arteries in these to beat; and yet the main trunk was precisely in the same condition as is the artery in the experiment of Galen, when it is tied upon a hollow tube; where it was converted into bone it could neither dilate nor contract like bellows, nor transmit the pulsific power from the heart to the inferior vessels; it could not convey a force which it was incapable of receiving through the solid matter of the bone. In spite of all, however, I well remember to have frequently noted the pulse in the legs and feet of this patient whilst he lived, for I was myself his most attentive physician, and he my very particular friend. The arteries in the inferior extremities of this nobleman must therefore and of necessity have been dilated by the impulse of the blood like flaccid sacs, and not have expanded in the manner of bellows through the action of their tunics. It is obvious, that whether an artery be tied over a hollow tube, or its tunics be converted into a bony and unyielding canal, the interruption to the pulsific power in the inferior part of the vessel must be the same.

I have known another instance in which a portion of the aorta near the heart was found converted into bone, in the body of a nobleman, a man of great muscular strength. The experiment of Galen, therefore, or, at all events, a state analogous to it, not effected on purpose but encountered by accident, makes it sufficiently to appear, that compression or ligature of the coats of an artery does not interfere with the pulsative properties of its derivative branches; and indeed, if the experiment which Galen recommends were properly performed by any one, its results would be found in opposition to the views which Vesalius believed they would support.

But we do not therefore deny everything like motion to the tunics of the arteries; on the contrary, we allow them the same motions which we concede to the heart, viz., a diastole, and a systole or return from the distended to the natural state; this much we believe to be effected by a power inherent in the coats themselves. But it is to be observed, that they are not both dilated and contracted by the same, but by different causes and means; as may be observed of the motions of all parts, and of the ventricle of the heart itself, which is distended by the auricle, contracted by its own inherent power; so, the arteries are dilated by the stroke of the heart, but they contract or collapse of themselves.[1]

You may also perform another experiment at the same time : if you fill one of two basins of the same size with blood issuing per saltum from an artery, the other with venous blood from a vein of the same animal, you will have an opportunity of perceiving by the eye, both immediately and by and by, when the blood in either vessel has become cold, what differences there are between them. You will find that it is not as they believe who fancy that there is one kind of blood in the arteries and another in the veins, that in the arteries being of a more florid colour, more frothy, and imbued with an abundance of I know not what spirits, effervescing and swelling, and occupying a

---

[1] Vide Chapter III, of the Disquisition on the Motion of the Heart and Blood.

greater space, like milk or honey set upon the fire. For were the blood which is thrown from the left ventricle of the heart into the arteries, fermented into any such frothy and flatulent fluid, so that a drop or two distended the whole cavity of the aorta; unquestionably, upon the subsidence of this fermentation, the blood would return to its original quantity of a few drops; (and this, indeed, is the reason that some assign for the usually empty state of the arteries in the dead body;) and so should it be with the arterial blood in the cup, for so it is with boiling milk and honey when they come to cool. But if in either basin you find blood nearly of the same colour, not of very different consistency in the coagulated state, forcing out serum in the same manner, and filling the cups to the same height when cold that it did when hot, this will be enough for any one to rest his faith upon, and afford argument enough, I think, for rejecting the dreams that have been promulgated on the subject. Sense and reason alike assure us that the blood contained in the left ventricle is not of a different nature from that in the right. And then, when we see that the mouth of the pulmonary artery is of the same size as the aorta, and in other respects equal to that vessel, it were imperative on us to affirm that the pulmonary artery was distended by a single drop of spumous blood, as well as the aorta, and so that the right as well as the left side of the heart was filled with a brisk or fermenting blood.

The particulars which especially dispose men's minds to admit diversity in the arterial and venous blood are three in number: one, because in arteriotomy the blood that flows is of a more florid hue than that which escapes from a vein; a second, because in the dissection of dead bodies the left ventricle of the heart, and the arteries in general, are mostly found empty; a third, because the arterial blood is believed to be more spirituous, and being replete with spirit is made to occupy a much larger space. The causes and reasons, however, wherefore all these things are so, present themselves to us when we ask after them.

1st. With reference to the colour it is to be observed, that wherever the blood issues by a very small orifice, it is in some measure strained, and the thinner and lighter part, which usually swims on the top and is the most penetrating, is emitted.

Thus, in phlebotomy, when the blood escapes forcibly and to a distance, in a full stream, and from a large orifice, it is thicker, has more body, and a darker colour; but, if it flows from a small orifice, and only drop by drop, as it usually does when the bleeding fillet is untied, it is of a brighter hue; for then it is strained as it were, and the thinner and more penetrating portion only escapes; in the same way, in the bleeding from the nose, in that which takes place from a leech-bite, or from scarifications, or in any other way by diapedesis or transudation, the blood is always seen to have a brighter cast, because the thickness and firmness of the coats of the arteries render the outlet or outlets smaller, and less disposed to yield a ready passage to the outpouring blood; it happens also that when fat persons, are let blood, the orifice of the vein is apt to be compressed by the subcutaneous fat, by which the blood is made to appear thinner, more florid, and in some sort arterious. On the other hand, the blood that flows into a basin from a large artery freely divided, will look venous. The blood in the lungs is of a much more florid colour than it is in the arteries, and we know how it is strained through the pulmonary tissue.

2d. The emptiness of the arteries in the dead body, which probably misled Erasistratus in supposing that they only contained aereal spirits, is caused by this, that when respiration ceases the lungs collapse, and then the passages through them are closed; the heart, however, continues for a time to contract upon the blood, whence we find the left auricle more contracted, and the corresponding ventricle, as well as the arteries at large, appearing empty, simply because there is no supply of blood flowing round to fill them. In cases, however, in which the heart has ceased to pulsate and the lungs to afford a passage to the blood simultaneously, as in those who have died from drowning or syncope, or who die suddenly, you will find the arteries, as well as the veins, full of blood.

3d. With reference to the third point, or that of the spirits, it may be said that, as it is still a question what they are, how extant in the body, of what consistency, whether separate and distinct from the blood and solids, or mingled with these,— upon each and all of these points there are so many and such conflicting opinions, that it is not wonderful that the spirits, whose nature is thus left so wholly ambiguous, should serve as the common subterfuge of ignorance. Persons of limited information, when they are at a loss to assign a cause for anything, very commonly reply that it is done by the spirits; and so they bring the spirits into play upon all occasions; even as indifferent poets are always thrusting the gods upon the stage as a means of unravelling the plot, and bringing about the catastrophe.

Fernelius, and many others, suppose that there are aereal spirits and invisible substances. Fernelius proves that there are animal spirits, by saying that the cells in the brain are apparently unoccupied, and as nature abhors a vacuum, he concludes that in the living body they are filled with spirits, just as Erasistratus had held that, because the arteries were empty of blood, therefore they must be filled with spirits. But Medical Schools admit three kinds of spirits: the natural spirits flowing through the veins, the vital spirits through the arteries, and the animal spirits through the nerves; whence physicians say, out of Galen, that sometimes the parts of the brain are oppressed by sympathy, because the faculty with the essence, i. e., the spirit, is overwhelmed; and sometimes this happens independently of the essence. Farther, besides the three orders of influxive spirits adverted to, a like number of implanted or stationary spirits seem to be acknowledged; but we have found none of all these spirits by dissection, neither in the veins, nerves, arteries, nor other parts of living animals. Some speak of corporeal, others of incorporeal spirits; and they who advocate the corporeal spirits will have the blood, or the thinner portion of the blood, to be the bond of union with the soul, the spirit being contained in the blood as the flame is in the smoke of a lamp or candle, and held admixed by the incessant motion of the fluid; others, again, distinguish between the spirits and the blood. They who advocate incorporeal spirits have no ground of experience to stand upon; their spirits indeed are synonymous with powers or faculties, such as a concoctive spirit, a chylopoietic spirit, a procreative spirit, &c.—they admit as many spirits, in short, as there are faculties or organs.

But then the schoolmen speak of a spirit of fortitude, prudence, patience, and the other virtues, and also of a most holy spirit of wisdom, and of every divine gift; and they besides suppose that there are good and evil spirits that roam about or possess the body, that assist or cast obstacles in the way. They hold some diseases to be owing to a Cacodæmon or evil spirit, as there are others that are due to a cacochemy or defective assimilation.

Although there is nothing more uncertain and questionable, then, than the doctrine of spirits that is proposed to us, nevertheless physicians seem for the major part to conclude, with Hippocrates, that our body is composed or made up of three elements, viz., containing parts, contained parts, and causes of action, spirits being understood by the latter term. But if spirits are to be taken as synonymous with causes of activity, whatever has power in the living body and a faculty of action must be included under the denomination. It would appear, therefore, that all spirits were neither aereal substances, nor powers, nor habits; and that all were not incorporeal.

But keeping in view the points that especially interest us, others, as leading to tediousness, being left unnoticed, it seems that the spirits which flow by the veins or the arteries are not distinct from the blood, any more than the flame of a lamp is distinct from the inflammable vapour that is on fire; in short, that the blood and these spirits signify one and the same thing, though different,—like generous wine and its spirit; for as wine, when it has lost all its spirit, is no longer wine, but a vapid liquor or vinegar; so blood without spirit is not blood, but something else—clot or cruor; even as a hand of stone, or of a dead body, is no hand in the most complete sense, neither is blood void of the vital principle proper blood; it is immediately to be held as corrupt when deprived of its spirit. The spirit therefore which inheres in the arteries, and especially in the blood which fills them, is to be regarded either as its act or agent, in the same way as the spirit of wine in wine, and the spirit of aqua vitæ in brandy, or as a flame kindled in alcohol, which lives and feeds on, or is nourished by itself. The blood consequently, though richly imbued with spirits, does not swell, nor ferment, nor rise to a head through them, so as to require and occupy a larger space,—a fact that may be ascertained beyond the possibility of question by the two cups of equal size; it is to be regarded as wine, possessed of a large amount of spirits, or, in the Hippocratic sense, of signal powers of acting and effecting.

It is therefore the same blood in the arteries that is found in the veins, although it may be admitted to be more spirituous, possessed of higher vital force in the former than in the latter; but it is not changed into anything more vaporous, or more aereal, as if there were no spirits but such as are aereal, and no cause of action or activity that is not of the nature of flatus or wind. But neither the animal, natural, nor vital spirits which inhere in the solids, such as the ligaments and nerves (especially if they be of so many different species), and are contained within the viewless interstices of the tissues, are to be regarded as so many different aereal forms, or kinds of vapour.

And here I would gladly be informed by those who admit corporeal spirits, but of a gaseous or vaporous consistency, in the bodies of animals, whether or not they have the power of passing hither and thither, like distinct bodies independently of the blood? Or whether the spirits follow the blood in its motions, either as integral parts of the fluid or as indissolubly connected with it, so that they can neither quit the tissues nor pass hither nor thither without the influx and reflux, and motion of the blood? For if the spirits exhaling from the blood, like the vapour of water attenuated by heat, exist in a state of constant flow and succession as the pabulum of the tissues, it necessarily follows that they are not distinct from this pabulum, but are incessantly disappearing; whereby it seems that they can neither have influx nor reflux, nor passage, nor yet remain at rest without the influx, the reflux, the passage [or stasis] of the blood, which is the fluid that serves as their vehicle or pabulum.

And next I desire to know of those who tell us that the spirits are formed in the heart, being compounded of the vapours or exhalations of the blood (excited either by the heat of the heart or the concussion) and the inspired air, whether such spirits are not to be accounted much colder than the blood, seeing that both the elements of their composition, namely, air and vapour, are much colder? For the vapour of boiling water is much more bearable than the water itself; the flame of a candle is less burning than the red-hot snuff, and burning charcoal than incandescent iron or brass. Whence it would appear that spirits of this nature rather receive their heat from the blood, than that the blood is warmed by these spirits; such spirits are rather to be regarded as fumes and excrementitious effluvia proceeding from the body in the manner of odours, than in any way as natural artificers of the tissues; a conclusion which we are the more disposed to admit, when we see that they so speedily lose any virtue they may possess, and which they had derived from the blood as their source,—they are at best of a very frail and evanescent nature. Whence also it becomes probable that the expiration of the lungs is a means by which these vapours being cast off, the blood is fanned and purified; whilst inspiration is a means by which the blood in its passage between the two ventricles of the heart is tempered by the cold of the ambient atmosphere, lest, getting heated, and blown up with a kind of fermentation, like milk or honey set over the fire, it should so distend the lungs that the animal got suffocated; somewhat in the same way, perchance, as one labouring under a severe asthma, which Galen himself seems to refer to its proper cause when he says it is owing to an obstruction of the smaller arteries, viz., the vasa venosa et arteriosa. And I have found by experience that patients affected with asthma might be brought out of states of very imminent danger by having cupping-glasses applied, and a plentiful and sudden affusion of cold water [upon the chest]. Thus much—and perhaps it is more than was necessary—have I said on the subject of spirits in this place, for I felt it proper to define them, and to say something of their nature in a physiological disquisition.

I shall only further add, that they who descant on the calidum innatum or innate heat, as an instrument of nature available for every purpose, and who speak of the necessity of heat as the cherisher and retainer in life of the several parts of the body, who at the same time admit that this heat cannot exist unless connected with something, and because they find no substance of anything like commensurate mobility, or which might keep pace with the rapid influx and reflux of this heat (in affections of the mind especially), take refuge in spirits as most subtile substances, possessed of the most penetrating qualities, and highest mobility—these persons see nothing less than the wonderful and almost divine character of the natural operations as proceeding from the instrumentality of this common agent, viz., the calidum innatum; they farther regard these spirits as of a sublime, lucid, ethereal, celestial, or divine nature, and the bond of the soul; even as the vulgar and unlettered, when they do not comprehend the causes of various effects, refer them to the immediate interposition of the Deity. Whence they declare that the heat perpetually flowing into the several parts is in virtue of the influx of spirits through the channels of the arteries; as if the blood could neither move so swiftly, nor penetrate so intimately, nor cherish so effectually. And such faith do they put in this opinion, such lengths are they carried by their belief, that they deny the contents of the arteries to be blood! And then they proceed with trivial reasonings to maintain that the arterial blood is of a peculiar kind, or that the arteries are filled with such aereal spirits, and not with blood; all the while, in opposition to everything which Galen has advanced against Erasistratus, both on grounds of experiment and of reason. But that arterial blood differs in nothing essential from venous blood has been already sufficiently demonstrated; and our senses likewise assure us that the blood and spirits do not flow in the arteries separately and disjoined, but as one body.

We have occasion to observe so often as our hands, feet, or ears have become stiff and cold, that as they recover again by the warmth that flows into them, they acquire their natural colour and heat simultaneously; that the veins which had become small and shrunk, swell visibly and enlarge, so that when they regain their heat suddenly they become painful; from which it appears, that that which by its influx brings heat is the same which causes repletion and colour; now this can be and is nothing but blood.

When an artery and a vein are divided, any one may clearly see that the part of the vein towards the heart pours out no blood, whilst that beyond the wound gives a torrent; the divided artery, on the contrary, (as in my experiment on the carotids,) pours out a flood of pure blood from the orifice next the heart, and in jets as if it were forced from a syringe, whilst from the further orifice of the divided artery little or no blood escapes. This experiment therefore plainly proves in what direction the current sets in either order of vessels—towards the heart in the veins, from the heart in the arteries; it also shows with what velocity the current moves, not gradually and by drops, but even with violence.   And lest any one, by way of subterfuge, should take shelter in the notion of invisible spirits, let the orifice of the divided vessel be plunged under water or oil, when, if there be any air contained in it, the fact will be proclaimed by a succession of visible bubbles.   Hornets, wasps, and other insects of the same description plunged in oil, and so suffocated, emit bubbles of air from their tail whilst they are dying ; whence it is not improbable that they thus respire when alive; for all animals submerged and drowned, when they finally sink to the bottom and die, emit bubbles of air from the mouth and lungs.   It is also demonstrated by the same experiment, that the valves of the veins act with such accuracy, that air blown into them does not penetrate ; much less then can blood make its way through them :—it is certain, I say, that neither sensibly nor insensibly, nor gradually and drop by drop, can any blood pass from the heart by the veins.

And that no one may seek shelter in asserting that these things are so when nature is disturbed and opposed, but not when she is left to herself and at liberty to act ; that the same things do not come to pass in morbid and unusual states as in the healthy and natural condition ; they are to be met by saying, that if it were so, if it happened that so much blood was lost from the farther orifice of a divided vein because nature was disturbed, still that the incision does not close the nearer orifice, from which nothing either escapes or can be expressed, whether nature be disturbed or not.   Others argue in the same way, maintaining that, although the blood immediately spurts out in such profusion with every beat, when an artery is divided near the heart, it does not therefore follow that the blood is propelled by the pulse when the heart and artery are entire.   It is most probable, however, that every stroke impels something ; and that there would be no pulse of the container, without an impulse being communicated to the thing contained, seems certain.   Yet some, that they may seize upon a farther means of defence, and escape the necessity of admitting the circulation, do not fear to affirm that the arteries in the living body and in the natural state are already so full of blood, that they are incapable of receiving another drop ; and so also of the ventricles of the heart. But it is indubitable that, whatever the degree of distension and the extent of contraction of the heart and arteries, they are still in a condition to receive an additional quantity of blood forced into them, and that this is far more than is usually reckoned in grains or drops, seems also certain. For if the ventricles become so excessively distended that they will admit no more blood, the heart ceases to beat, (and we have occasional opportunities of observing the fact in our vivisections,) and, continuing tense and resisting, death by asphyxia ensues.

In the work on the Motion of the Heart and Blood, I have already sufficiently discussed the question as to whether the blood in its motion was attracted, or impelled, or moved by its own inherent nature. I have there also spoken at length of the action and office, of the dilatation and contraction of the heart, and have shown what these truly are, and how the heart contracts during the diastole of the arteries; so that I must hold those who take points for dispute from among them as either not understanding the subject, or as unwilling to look at things for themselves, and to investigate them with their own senses.[1]

For my part, I believe that no other kind of attraction can be demonstrated in the living body save that of the nutriment, which gradually and incessantly passes on to supply the waste that takes place in the tissues; in the same way as the oil rises in the wick of a lamp to be consumed by the flame. Whence I conclude that the primary and common organ of all sensible attraction and impulsion is of the nature of sinew (nervus), or fibre, or muscle, and this to the end that it may be contractile, that contracting it may be shortened, and so either stretch out, draw towards, or propel. But these topics will be better discussed elsewhere, when we speak of the organs of motion in the animal body.

To those who repudiate the circulation because they neither see the efficient nor final cause of it, and who exclaim, cui bono? I have yet to reply, having hitherto taken no note of the ground of objection which they take up. And first I own I am of opinion that our first duty is to inquire whether the thing be or not, before asking wherefore it is? for from the facts and circumstances which meet us in the circulation admitted, established, the ends and objects of its institution are especially

---

[1] Vide Chapter XIV.

to be sought. Meantime I would only ask, how many things we admit in physiology, pathology, and therapeutics, the causes of which are unknown to us? That there are many, no one doubts—the causes of putrid fevers, of revulsions, of the purgation of excrementitious matters, among the number.

Whoever, therefore, sets himself in opposition to the circulation, because, if it be acknowledged, he cannot account for a variety of medical problems, nor in the treatment of diseases and the administration of medicines, give satisfactory reasons for the phenomena that appear; or who will not see that the precepts he has received from his teachers are false; or who thinks it unseemly to give up accredited opinions; or who regards it as in some sort criminal to call in question doctrines that have descended through a long succession of ages, and carry the authority of the ancients;—to all of these I reply: that the facts cognizable by the senses wait upon no opinions, and that the works of nature bow to no antiquity; for indeed there is nothing either more ancient or of higher authority than nature.

To those who object to the circulation as throwing obstacles in the way of their explanations of the phenomena that occur in medical cases (and there are persons who will not be content to take up with a new system, unless it explains everything, as in astronomy), and who oppose it with their own erroneous assumptions, such as that, if it be true, phlebotomy cannot cause revulsion, seeing that the blood will still continue to be forced into the affected part; that the passage of excrementitious matters and foul humours through the heart, that most noble and principal viscus, is to be apprehended; that an efflux and excretion, occasionally of foul and corrupt blood, takes place from the same body, from different parts, even from the same part and at the same time, which, were the blood agitated by a continuous current, would be shaken and effectually mixed in passing through the heart, and many points of the like kind admitted in our medical schools, which are seen to be repugnant to the doctrine of the circulation,— to them I shall not answer farther here, than that the circulation is not always the same in every place, and at every time, but is contingent upon many circumstances: the more rapid or slower motion of the blood, the strength or weakness of the heart as the propelling organ, the quantity and quality or constitution of the blood, the rigidity or laxity of the tissues, and the like. A thicker blood, of course, moves more slowly through narrower channels; it is more effectually strained in its passage through the substance of the liver than through that of the lungs. It has not the same velocity through flesh and the softer parenchymatous structures and through sinewy parts of greater compactness and consistency : for the thinner and purer and more spirituous part permeates more quickly, the thicker more earthy and indifferently concocted portion moves more slowly, or is refused admission. The nutritive portion, or ultimate aliment of the tissues, the dew or cambium, is of a more penetrating nature, inasmuch as it has to be added everywhere, and to everything that grows and is nourished in its length and thickness, even to the horns, nails, hair and feathers; and then the excrementitious matters have to be secreted in some places, where they accumulate, and either prove a burthen or are concocted. But I do not imagine that the excrementitious fluids or bad humours when once separated, nor the milk, the phlegm, and the spermatic fluid, nor the ultimate nutritive part, the dew or cambium, necessarily circulate with the blood : that which nourishes every part adheres and becomes agglutinated to it. Upon each of these topics and various others besides, to be discussed and demonstrated in their several places, viz., in the physiology and other parts of the art of medicine, as well as of the consequences, advantages or disadvantages of the circulation of the blood, I do not mean to touch here; it were fruitless indeed to do so until the circulation has been established and conceded as a fact. And here the example of astronomy is by no means to be followed, in which from mere appearances or phenomena that which is in fact, and the reason wherefore it is so, are investigated. But as he who inquires into the cause of an eclipse must be placed beyond the moon if he would ascertain it by sense, and not by reason, still, in reference to things sensible, things that come under the cognizance of the senses, no more certain demonstration or means of gaining faith can be adduced than examination by the senses, than ocular inspection.

There is one remarkable experiment which I would have every one try who is anxious for truth, and by which it is clearly shown that the arterial pulse is owing to the impulse of the blood. Let a portion of the dried intestine of a dog or wolf, or any other animal, such as we see hung up in the druggists' shops, be taken and filled with water, and then secured at both ends like a sausage: by tapping with the finger at one extremity, you will immediately feel a pulse and vibration in any other part to which you apply the fingers, as you do when you feel the pulse at the wrist. In this way, indeed, and also by means of a distended vein, you may accurately either in the dead or living body, imitate and show every variety of the pulse, whether as to force, frequency, volume, rhythm, &c. Just as in a long bladder full of fluid, or in an oblong drum, every stroke upon one end is immediately felt at the other; so also in a dropsy of the belly and in abscesses under the skin, we are accustomed to distinguish between collections of fluid and of air, between anasarca and tympanites in particular. If a slap or push given on one side is clearly felt by a hand placed on the other side, we judge the case to be tympanites [?]; not, as falsely asserted, because we hear a sound like that of a drum, and this produced by flatus, which never happens[?] ; but because, as in a drum, every the slightest tap passes through and produces a certain vibration on the opposite side; for it indicates that there is a serous and ichorous substance present, of such a consistency as urine, and not any sluggish or viscid matter as in anasarca, which when struck retains the impress of the blow or pressure, and does not transmit the impulse.

Having brought forward this experiment I may observe, that a most formidable objection to the circulation of the blood rises out of it, which, however, has neither been observed nor adduced by any one who has written against me. When we see by the experiment just described, that the systole and diastole of the pulse can be accurately imitated without any escape of fluid, it is obvious that the same thing may take place in the arteries from the stroke of the heart, without the necessity for a circulation, but like Euripus, with a mere motion of the blood alternately backwards and forwards. But we have already satisfactorily replied to this difficulty; and now we venture to say that the thing could not be so in the arteries of a living animal ; to be assured of this it is enough to see that the right auricle is incessantly injecting the right ventricle of the heart with blood, the return of which is effectually prevented by the

tricuspid valves; the left auricle in like manner filling the left
ventricle, the return of the blood there being opposed by the
mitral valves; and then the ventricles in their turn are propelling the blood into either great artery, the reflux in each being
prevented by the sigmoid valves in its orifice. Either, consequently, the blood must move on incessantly through the
lungs, and in like manner within the arteries of the body, or
stagnating and pent up, it must rupture the containing vessels,
or choke the heart by over distension, as I have shown it to
do in the vivisection of a snake, described in my book on the
Motion of the Blood.   To resolve this doubt I shall relate two
experiments among many others, the first of which, indeed, I
have already adduced, and which show with singular clearness
that the blood flows incessantly and with great force and in
ample abundance in the veins towards the heart.   The internal jugular vein of a live fallow deer having been exposed,
(many of the nobility and his most serene majesty the king, my
master, being present,) was divided; but a few drops of blood
were observed to escape from the lower orifice rising up from
under the clavicle ; whilst from the superior orifice of the vein
and coming down from the head, a round torrent of blood
gushed forth.   You may observe the same fact any day in
practising phlebotomy: if with a finger you compress the vein
a little below the orifice, the flow of blood is immediately
arrested; but the pressure being removed, forthwith the flow
returns as before.

From any long vein of the forearm get rid of the blood as
much as possible by holding the hand aloft and pressing the
blood towards the trunk, you will perceive the vein collapsed
and leaving, as it were, in a furrow of the skin ; but now compress
the vein with the point of a finger, and you will immediately
perceive all that part of it which is towards the hand, to enlarge
and to become distended with the blood that is coming from the
hand.   How comes it when the breath is held and the lungs
thereby compressed, a large quantity of air having been taken in,
that the vessels of the chest are at the same time obstructed, the
blood driven into the face, and the eyes rendered red and suffused? Why is it, as Aristotle asks in his problems, that all the
actions are more energetically performed when the breath is
held than when it is given?   In like manner, when the frontal

and lingual veins are incised, the blood is made to flow more freely by compressing the neck and holding the breath.   I have several times opened the breast and pericardium of a man within two hours after his execution by hanging, and before the colour had totally left the face, and in presence of many witnesses, have demonstrated the right auricle of the heart and the lungs distended with blood; the auricle in particular of the size of a large man's fist, and so full of blood that it looked as if it would burst.   This great distension, however, had disappeared next day, the body having stiffened and become cold, and the blood having made its escape through various channels. These and other similar facts, therefore, make it sufficiently certain that the blood flows through the whole of the veins of the body towards the base of the heart, and that unless there was a further passage afforded it, it would be pent up in these channels, or would oppress and overwhelm the heart; as on the other hand, did it not flow outwards by the arteries, but was found regurgitating, it would soon be seen how much it would oppress.

I add another observation. A noble knight, Sir Robert Darcy, an ancestor of that celebrated physician and most learned man, my very dear friend Dr. Argent, when he had reached to about the middle period of life, made frequent complaint of a certain distressing pain in the chest, especially in the night season; so that dreading at one time syncope, at another suffocation in his attacks he led an unquiet and anxious life.   He tried many remedies in vain, having had the advice of almost every medical man.   The disease going on from bad to worse, he by and by became cachectic and dropsical, and finally, grievously distressed, he died in one of his paroxysms.   In the body of this gentleman, at the inspection of which there were present Dr. Argent, then president of the College of Physicians, and Dr. Gorge, a distinguished theologian and preacher, who was pastor of the parish, we found the wall of the left ventricle of the heart ruptured, having a rent in it of size sufficient to admit any of my fingers, although the wall itself appeared sufficiently thick and strong; this laceration had apparently been caused by an impediment to the passage of the blood from the left ventricle into the arteries.

I was acquainted with another strong man, who having received an injury and affront from one more powerful than himself, and upon whom he could not have his revenge, was so overcome with hatred and spite and passion, which he yet communicated to no one, that at last he fell into a strange distemper, suffering from extreme oppression and pain of the heart and breast, and the prescriptions of none of the very best physicians proving of any avail, he fell in the course of a few years into a scorbutic and cachectic state, became tabid and died. This patient only received some little relief when the whole of his chest was pummelled or kneaded by a strong man, as a baker kneads dough.   His friends thought him poisoned by some maleficent influence, or possesséd with an evil spirit. His jugular arteries, enlarged to the size of the thumb, looked like the aorta itself, or they were as large as the descending aorta; they had pulsated violently, and appeared like two long aneurisms. These symptoms had led to trying the effects of arteriotomy in the temples, but with no relief.   In the dead body I found the heart and aorta so much gorged and distended with blood, that the cavities of the ventricles equalled those of a bullock's heart in size.   Such is the force of the blood pent up, and such are the effects of its impulse.

We may therefore conclude, that although there may be impulse without any exit, as illustrated in the experiment lately spoken of, still that this could not take place in the vessels of living creatures without most serious dangers and impediments. From this, however, it is manifest that the blood in its course does not everywhere pass with the same celerity, neither with the same force in all places and at all times, but that it varies greatly according to age, sex, temperament, habit of body, and other contingent circumstances, external as well as internal, natural or non-natural.   For it does not course through intricate and obstructed passages with the same. readiness that it does through straight, unimpeded, and pervious channels. Neither does it run through close, hard, and crowded parts, with the same velocity as through spongy, soft, and permeable tissues.   Neither does it flow and penetrate with such swiftness when the impulse [of the heart] is slow and weak, as when this is forcible and frequent, in which case the blood is driven onwards with vigour and in large quantity.   Nor is the same blood, when it has become more consistent or earthy, so penetrative as when it is more serous and attenuated or liquid. And then it seems only reasonable to think that the blood in its circuit passes more slowly through the kidneys than through the substance of the heart; more swiftly through the liver than through the kidneys; through the spleen more quickly than through the lungs, and through the lungs more speedily than through any of the other viscera or the muscles, in proportion always to the denseness or sponginess of the tissue of each.

We may be permitted to take the same view of the influence of age, sex, temperament, and habit of body, whether this be hard or soft; of that of the ambient cold which condenses bodies, and makes the veins in the extremities to shrink and almost to disappear, and deprives the surface both of colour and heat; and also of that of meat and drink which render the blood more watery, by supplying fresh nutritive matter. From the veins, therefore, the blood flows more freely in phlebotomy when the body is warm than when it is cold. We also observe the signal influence of the affections of the mind when a timid person is bled and happens to faint: immediately the flow of blood is arrested, a deadly pallor overspreads the surface, the limbs stiffen, the ears sing, the eyes are dazzled or blinded, and, as it were, convulsed. But here I come upon a field where I might roam freely and give myself up to speculation. And, indeed, such a flood of light and truth breaks in upon me here; occasion offers of explaining so many problems, of resolving so many doubts, of discovering the causes of so many slighter and more serious diseases, and of suggesting remedies for their cure, that the subject seems almost to demand a separate treatise. And it will be my business in my 'Medical Observations,' to lay before my reader matter upon all these topics which shall be worthy of the gravest consideration.

And what indeed is more deserving of attention than the fact that in almost every affection, appetite, hope, or fear, our body suffers, the countenance changes, and the blood appears to course hither and thither. In anger the eyes are fiery and the pupils contracted; in modesty the cheeks are suffused with blushes; in fear, and under a sense of infamy and of shame, the face is pale, but the ears burn as if for the evil they heard or were to hear; in lust how quickly is the member distended with blood and erected! But, above all, and this is of the highest interest to the medical practitioner,—how speedily is pain relieved or removed by the detraction of blood, the application of cupping-glasses, or the compression of the artery which leads to a part? It sometimes vanishes as if by magic. But these are topics that I must refer to my 'Medical Observations,' where they will be found exposed at length and explained.

Some weak and inexperienced persons vainly seek by dialectics and far-fetched arguments, either to upset or establish things that are only to be founded on anatomical demonstration, and believed on the evidence of the senses. He who truly desires to be informed of the question in hand, and whether the facts alleged be sensible, visible, or not, must be held bound either to look for himself, or to take on trust the conclusions to which they have come who have looked; and indeed there is no higher method of attaining to assurance and certainty. Who would pretend to persuade those who had never tasted wine that it was a drink much pleasanter to the palate than water? By what reasoning should we give the blind from birth to know that the sun was luminous, and far surpassed the stars in brightness? And so it is with the circulation of the blood, which the world has now had before it for so many years, illustrated by proofs cognizable by the senses, and confirmed by various experiments. No one has yet been found to dispute the sensible facts, the motion, efflux and afflux of the blood, by like observations based on the evidence of sense, or to oppose the experiments adduced, by other experiments of the same character; nay, no one has yet attempted an opposition on the ground of ocular testimony.

There have not been wanting many who, inexperienced and ignorant of anatomy, and making no appeal to the senses in their opposition, have, on the contrary, met it with empty assertions, and mere suppositions, with assertions derived from the lessons of teachers and captious cavillings; many, too, have vainly sought refuge in words, and these not always very nicely chosen, but reproachful and contumelious; which, however, have no farther effect than to expose their utterer's vanity and weakness, and ill breeding and lack of the arguments that are to be sought in the conclusions of the senses, and false sophistical reasonings that seem utterly opposed to sense. Even as the waves of the Sicilian sea, excited by the blast, dash against the rocks around

Charybdis, and then hiss and foam, and are tossed hither and thither; so do they who reason against the evidence of their senses.

Were nothing to be acknowledged by the senses without evidence derived from reason, or occasionally even contrary to the previously received conclusions of reason, there would now be no problem left for discussion. Had we not our most perfect assurances by the senses, and were not their perceptions confirmed by reasoning, in the same way as geometricians proceed with their figures, we should admit no science of any kind; for it is the business of geometry, from things sensible, to make rational demonstration of things that are not sensible; to render credible or certain things abstruse and beyond sense from things more manifest and better known. Aristotle counsels us better when, in treating of the generation of bees, he says:[1] "Faith is to be given to reason, if the matters demonstrated agree with those that are perceived by the senses; when the things have been thoroughly scrutinized, then are the senses to be trusted rather than the reason." Whence it is our duty to approve or disapprove, to receive or reject everything only after the most careful examination; but to examine, to test whether anything have been well or ill advanced, to ascertain whether some falsehood does not lurk under a proposition, it is imperative on us to bring it to the proof of sense, and to admit or reject it on the decision of sense. Whence Plato in his Critias, says, that the explanation of those things is not difficult of which we can have experience; whilst they are not of apt scientific apprehension who have no experience.

How difficult is it to teach those who have no experience, the things of which they have not any knowledge by their senses! And how useless and intractable, and unimpregnable to true science are such auditors! They show the judgment of the blind in regard to colours, of the deaf in reference to concords. Who ever pretended to teach the ebb and flow of the tide, or from a diagram to demonstrate the measurements of the angles and the proportions of the sides of a triangle to a blind man, or to one who had never seen the sea nor a diagram? He who is not conversant with anatomy, inasmuch as he forms no

---

[1] De Generat. Animal. lib. iii, cap. x.

conception of the subject from the evidence of his own eyes, is virtually blind to all that concerns anatomy, and unfit to appreciate what is founded thereon; he knows nothing of that which occupies the attention of the anatomist, nor of the principles inherent in the nature of the things which guide him in his reasonings; facts and inferences as well as their sources are alike unknown to such a one. But no kind of science can possibly flow, save from some pre-existing knowledge of more obvious things; and this is one main reason why our science in regard to the nature of celestial bodies, is so uncertain and conjectural. I would ask of those who profess a knowledge of the causes of all things, why the two eyes keep constantly moving together, up or down, to this side or to that, and not independently, one looking this way another that; why the two auricles of the heart contract simultaneously, and the like? Are fevers, pestilence, and the wonderful properties of various medicines to be denied because their causes are unknown? Who can tell us why the fœtus in utero, breathing no air up to the tenth month of its existence, is yet not suffocated? born in the course of the seventh or eighth month, and having once breathed, it is nevertheless speedily suffocated if its respiration be interrupted. Why can the fœtus still contained within the uterus, or enveloped in the membranes, live without respiration; whilst once exposed to the air, unless it breathes it inevitably dies?[1]

Observing that many hesitate to acknowledge the circulation, and others oppose it, because, as I conceive, they have not rightly understood me, I shall here recapitulate briefly what I have said in my work on the Motion of the Heart and Blood. The blood contained in the veins, in its magazine, and where it is collected in largest quantity, viz., in the vena cava, close to the base of the heart and right auricle, gradually increasing in temperature by its internal heat, and becoming attenuated, swells and rises like bodies in a state of fermentation, whereby the auricle being dilated, and then contracting, in virtue of its pulsative power, forthwith delivers its charge into the right ventricle; which being filled, and the systole ensuing, the charge, hindered from returning into the auricle by the

---

[1] Vide Chapter VI, of the Disq. on the Motion of the Heart and Blood.

tricuspid valves, is forced into the pulmonary artery, which stands open to receive it, and is immediately distended with it. Once in the pulmonary artery, the blood cannot return, by reason of the sigmoid valves; and then the lungs, alternately expanded and contracted during inspiration and expiration, afford it passage by the proper vessels into the pulmonary veins; from the pulmonary veins, the left auricle, acting equally and synchronously with the right auricle, delivers the blood into the left ventricle; which acting harmoniously with the right ventricle, and all regress being prevented by the mitral valves, the blood is projected into the aorta, and consequently impelled into all the arteries of the body. The arteries, filled by this sudden push, as they cannot discharge themselves so speedily, are distended; they receive a shock, or undergo their diastole. But as this process goes on incessantly, I infer that the arteries both of the lungs and of the body at large, under the influence of such a multitude of strokes of the heart and injections of blood, would finally become so over-gorged and distended, that either any further injection must cease, or the vessels would burst, or the whole blood in the body would accumulate within them, were there not an exit provided for it.

The same reasoning is applicable to the ventricles of the heart: distended by the ceaseless action of the auricles, did they not disburthen themselves by the channels of the arteries, they would by and by become over-gorged, and be fixed and made incapable of all motion. Now this, my conclusion, is true and necessary, if my premises be true; but that these are either true or false, our senses must inform us, not our reason—ocular inspection, not any process of the mind.

I maintain further, that the blood in the veins always and everywhere flows from less to greater branches, and from every part towards the heart; whence I gather that the whole charge which the arteries receive, and which is incessantly thrown into them, is delivered to the veins, and flows back by them to the source whence it came. In this way, indeed, is the circulation of the blood established: by an efflux and reflux from and to the heart; the fluid being forcibly projected into the arterial system, and then absorbed and imbibed from every part by the veins, it returns through these in a continuous stream. That all this is so, sense assures us; and necessary inference from the perceptions of sense takes away all occasion for doubt.   Lastly, this is what I have striven, by my observations and experiments, to illustrate and make known; I have not endeavoured from causes and probable principles to demonstrate my propositions, but, as of higher authority, to establish them by appeals to sense and experiment, after the manner of anatomists.

And here I would refer to the amount of force, even of violence, which sight and touch make us aware of in the heart and greater arteries; and to the systole and diastole constituting the pulse in the large warm-blooded animals, which I do not say is equal in all the vessels containing blood, nor in all animals that have blood; but which is of such a nature and amount in all, that a flow and rapid passage of the blood through the smaller arteries, the interstices of the tissues, and the branches of the veins, must of necessity take place; and therefore there is a circulation.

For neither do the most minute arteries, nor the veins, pulsate; but the larger arteries and those near the heart pulsate, because they do not transmit the blood so quickly as they receive it.[1]   Having exposed an artery, and divided it so that the blood shall flow out as fast and freely as it is received, you will scarcely perceive any pulse in that vessel; and for the simple reason, that an open passage being afforded, the blood escapes, merely passing through the vessel, not distending it. In fishes, serpents, and the colder animals, the heart beats so slowly and feebly, that a pulse can scarcely be perceived in the arteries; the blood in them is transmitted gradually. Whence in them, as also in the smaller branches of the arteries in man, there is no distinction between the coats of the arteries and veins, because the arteries have to sustain no shock from the impulse of the blood.

An artery denuded and divided in the way I have indicated, sustains no shock, and therefore does not pulsate; whence it clearly appears that the arteries have no inherent pulsative power, and that neither do they derive any from the heart; but that they undergo their diastole solely from the impulse of the blood; for in the full stream, flowing to a distance, you may see the systole and diastole, all the motions of the heart—their order,

---

[1] Vide Chapter III, on the Motion of the Heart and Blood.

force, rhythm, &c.,[1] as it were in a mirror, and even perceive them by the touch. Precisely as in the water that is forced aloft, through a leaden pipe, by working the piston of a forcing-pump, each stroke of which, though the jet be many feet distant, is nevertheless distinctly perceptible,—the beginning, increasing strength, and end of the impulse, as well as its amount, and the regularity or irregularity with which it is given, being indicated, the same precisely is the case from the orifice of a divided artery; whence, as in the instance of the forcing engine quoted, you will perceive that the efflux is uninterrupted, although the jet is alternately greater and less. In the arteries, therefore, besides the concussion or impulse of the blood, the pulse or beat of the artery, which is not equally exhibited in all, there is a perpetual flow and motion of the blood, which returns in an unbroken stream to the point from whence it commenced—the right auricle of the heart.

All these points you may satisfy yourself upon, by exposing one of the longer arteries, and having taken it between your finger and thumb, dividing it on the side remote from the heart. By the greater or less pressure of your fingers, you can have the vessel pulsating less or more, or losing the pulse entirely, and recovering it at will. And as these things proceed thus when the chest is uninjured, so also do they go on for a short time when the thorax is laid open, and the lungs having collapsed, all the respiratory motions have ceased; here, nevertheless, for a little while you may perceive the left auricle contracting and emptying itself, and becoming whiter; but by and by growing weaker and weaker, it begins to intermit, as does the left ventricle also, and then it ceases to beat altogether, and becomes quiescent. Along with this, and in the same measure, does the stream of blood from the divided artery grow less and less, the pulse of the vessel weaker and weaker, until at last, the supply of blood and the impulse of the left ventricle failing, nothing escapes from it. You may perform the same experiment, tying the pulmonary veins, and so taking away the pulse of the left auricle, or relaxing the ligature, and restoring it at pleasure. In this experiment, too, you will observe what happens in moribund animals, viz., that the left

[1] Vide Chapter III, on the Motion of the Heart and Blood.

ventricle first ceases from pulsation and motion, then the left auricle, next the right ventricle, finally the right auricle; so that where the vital force and pulse first begin, there do they also last fail.

All of these particulars having been recognized by the senses, it is manifest that the blood passes through the lungs, not through the septum [in its course from the right to the left side of the heart], and only through them when they are moved in the act of respiration, not when they are collapsed and quiescent; whence we see the probable reason wherefore nature has instituted the foramen ovale in the fœtus, instead of sending the blood by the way of the pulmonary artery into the left auricle and ventricle, which foramen she closes when the new-born creature begins to breathe freely. We can also now understand why, when the vessels of the lungs become congested and oppressed, and in those who are affected with serious diseases, it should be so dangerous and fatal a symptom when the respiratory organs become implicated.

We perceive further, why the blood is so florid in the lungs, which is, because it is thinner, as having there to undergo filtration.

Still further; from the summary which precedes, and by way of satisfying those who are importunate in regard to the causes of the circulation, and incline to regard the power of the heart as competent to everything—as that it is not only the seat and source of the pulse which propels the blood, but also, as Aristotle thinks, of the power which attracts and produces it; moreover, that the spirits are engendered by the heart, and the influxive vital heat, in virtue of the innate heat of the heart, as the immediate instrument of the soul, or common bond and prime organ in the performance of every act of vitality; in a word, that the motion, perfection, heat, and every property besides of the blood and spirits are derived from the heart, as their fountain or original, (a doctrine as old as Aristotle, who maintained all these qualities to inhere in the blood, as heat inheres in boiling water or pottage,) and that the heart is the primary cause of pulsation and life; to those persons, did I speak openly, I should say that I do not agree with the common opinion; there are numerous particulars to be noted in the production of the parts of the body which incline me this way, but which it does not seem expedient to enter upon here. Before long, perhaps, I shall have occasion to lay before the world things that are more wonderful than these, and that are calculated to throw still greater light upon natural philosophy.

Meantime I shall only say, and, without pretending to demonstrate it, propound—with the good leave of our learned men, and with all respect for antiquity—that the heart, with the veins and arteries and the blood they contain, is to be regarded as the beginning and author, the fountain and original of all things in the body, the primary cause of life; and this in the same acceptation as the brain with its nerves, organs of sense and spinal marrow inclusive, is spoken of as the one and general organ of sensation. But if by the word heart the mere body of the heart, made up of its auricles and ventricles, be understood, then I do not believe that the heart is the fashioner of the blood; neither do I imagine that the blood has powers, properties, motion, or heat, as the gift of the heart; lastly, neither do I admit that the cause of the systole and contraction is the same as that of the diastole or dilatation, whether in the arteries, auricles, or ventricles; for I hold that that part of the pulse which is designated the diastole depends on another cause different from the systole, and that it must always and everywhere precede any systole; I hold that the innate heat is the first cause of dilatation, and that the primary dilatation is in the blood itself, after the manner of bodies in a state of fermentation, gradually attenuated and swelling, and that in the blood is this finally extinguished; I assent to Aristotle's example of gruel or milk upon the fire, to this extent, that the rising and falling of the blood does not depend upon vapours or exhalations, or spirits, or anything rising in a vaporous or aëreal shape, nor upon any external agency, but upon an internal principle under the control of nature.

Nor is the heart, as some imagine, anything like a chauffer or fire, or heated kettle, and so the source of the heat of the blood; the blood, instead of receiving, rather gives heat to the heart, as it does to all the other parts of the body; for the blood is the hottest element in the body; and it is on this account that the heart is furnished with coronary arteries and veins; it is for the same reason that other parts have vessels, viz., to secure the access of warmth for their due conservation and stimulation; so that the warmer any part is, the greater is its supply of blood, or otherwise; where the blood is in largest quantity, there also is the heat highest. For this reason is the heart, remarkable through its cavities, to be viewed as the elaboratory, fountain, and perennial focus of heat, and as comparable to a hot kettle, not because of its proper substance, but because of its contained blood; for the same reason, because they have numerous veins or vessels containing blood, are the liver, spleen, lungs, &c., reputed hot parts. And in this way do I view the native or innate heat as the common instrument of every function, the prime cause of the pulse among the rest. This, however, I do not mean to state absolutely, but only propose it by way of thesis. Whatever may be objected to it by good and learned men, without abusive or contemptuous language, I shall be ready to listen to—I shall even be most grateful to any one who will take up and discuss the subject.

These then, are, as it were, the very elements and indications of the passage and circulation of the blood, viz., from the right auricle into the right ventricle; from the right ventricle by the way of the lungs into the left auricle; thence into the left ventricle and aorta; whence by the arteries at large through the pores or interstices of the tissues into the veins, and by the veins back again with great rapidity to the base of the heart.

There is an experiment on the veins by which any one that chooses may convince himself of this truth: Let the arm be bound with a moderately tight bandage, and then, by opening and shutting the hand, make all the veins to swell as much as possible, and the integuments below the fillet to become red; and now let the arm and hand be plunged into very cold water, or snow, until the blood pent up in the veins shall have become cooled down; then let the fillet be undone suddenly, and you will perceive, by the cold blood returning to the heart, with what celerity the current flows, and what an effect it produces when it has reached the heart; so that you will no longer be surprised that some should faint when the fillet is undone after venesection.[1] This experiment shows that the veins swell below the ligature not with attenuated blood, or with blood raised by spirits or vapours, for the

---

[1] Vide Chapter XI, of the Motion of the Heart, &c.

immersion in the cold water would repress their ebullition, but with blood only, and such as could never make its way back into the arteries, either by open-mouthed communications or by devious passages; it shows, moreover, how and in what way those who are travelling over snowy mountains are sometimes stricken suddenly with death, and other things of the same kind.

Lest it should seem difficult for the blood to make its way through the pores of the various structures of the body, I shall add one illustration: The same thing happens in the bodies of those that are hanged or strangled, as in the arm that is bound with a fillet: all the parts beyond the noose,—the face, lips, tongue, eyes, and every part of the head appear gorged with blood, swollen and of a deep red or livid colour; but if the noose be relaxed, in whatever position you have the body, before many hours have passed you will perceive the whole of the blood to have quitted the head and face, and gravitated through the pores of the skin, flesh, and other structures, from the superior parts towards those that are inferior and dependent, until they become tumid and of a dark colour. But if this happens in the dead body, with the blood dead and coagulated, the frame stiffened with the chill of death, the passages all compressed or blocked up, it is easy to perceive how much more apt it will be to occur in the living subject, when the blood is alive and replete with spirits, when the pores are all open, the fluid ready to penetrate, and the passage in every way made easy.

When the ingenious and acute Descartes, (whose honourable mention of my name demands my acknowledgments,) and others, having taken out the heart of a fish, and put it on a plate before them, see it continuing to pulsate (in contracting), and when it raises or erects itself and becomes firm to the touch, they think it enlarges, expands, and that its ventricles thence become more capacious. But, in my opinion, they do not observe correctly; for, at the time the heart gathers itself up, and becomes erect, it is certain that it is rather lessened in every one of its dimensions; that it is in its systole, in short, not in its diastole. Neither, on the contrary, when it collapses and sinks down, is it then properly in its state of diastole and distension, by which the ventricles become more capacious. But as we do not say that the heart is in the state of diastole in the dead body, as having sunk relaxed after the systole, but is then collapsed, and without all motion—in short is in a state of rest, and not distended. It is only truly distended, and in the proper state of diastole, when it is filled by the charge of blood projected into it by the contraction of the auricles; a fact which sufficiently appears in the course of vivisections. Descartes therefore does not perceive how much the relaxation and subsidence of the heart and arteries differ from their distension or diastole; and that the cause of the distension, relaxation, and constriction, is not one and the same; as contrary effects so must they rather acknowledge contrary causes; as different movements they must have different motors; just as all anatomists know that the flexion and extension of an extremity are accomplished by opposite antagonist muscles, and contrary or diverse motions are necessarily performed by contrary and diverse organs instituted by nature for the purpose. Neither do I find the efficient cause of the pulse aptly explained by this philosopher, when with Aristotle he assumes the cause of the systole to be the same as that of the diastole, viz., an effervescence of the blood due to a kind of ebullition. For the pulse is a succession of sudden strokes and quick percussions; but we know of no kind of fermentation or ebullition in which the matter rises and falls in the twinkling of an eye; the heaving is always gradual where the subsidence is notable. Besides, in the body of a living animal laid open, we can with our eyes perceive the ventricles of the heart both charged and distended by the contraction of the auricles, and more or less increased in size according to the charge; and farther, we can see that the distension of the heart is rather a violent motion, the effect of an impulsion, and not performed by any kind of attraction.

Some are of opinion that, as no kind of impulse of the nutritive juices is required in vegetables, but that these are attracted by the parts which require them, and flow in to take the place of what has been lost; so neither is there any necessity for an impulse in animals, the vegetative faculty in both working alike. But there is a difference between plants and animals. In animals, a constant supply of warmth is required to cherish the members, to maintain them in life by the vivifying heat, and to restore parts injured from without. It is not merely nutrition that has to be provided for.

So much for the circulation ; any impediment, or perversion, or excessive excitement of which, is followed by a host of dangerous diseases and remarkable symptoms : in connexion with the veins—varices, abscesses, pains, hemorrhoids, hemorrhages ; in connexion with the arteries—enlargements, phlegmons, severe and lancinating pains, aneurisms, sarcoses, fluxions, sudden attacks of suffocation, asthmas, stupors, apoplexies, and innumerable other affections. But this is not the place to enter on the consideration of these ; neither may I say under what circumstances and how speedily some of these diseases, that are even reputed incurable, are remedied and dispelled, as if by enchantment. I shall have much to put forth in my Medical Observations and Pathology, which, so far as I know, has as yet been observed by no one.

That I may afford you still more ample satisfaction, most learned Riolanus, as you do not think there is a circulation in the vessels of the mesentery, I shall conclude by proposing the following experiment : throw a ligature around the porta close to the liver, in a living animal, which is easily done. You will forthwith perceive the veins below the ligature swelling in the same way as those of the arm when the bleeding fillet is bound above the elbow ; a circumstance which will proclaim the course of the blood there. And as you still seem to think that the blood can regurgitate from the veins into the arteries by open anastomoses, let the vena cava be tied in a living animal near the divarication of the crural veins, and immediately afterwards let an artery be opened to give issue to the blood : you will soon observe the whole of the blood discharged from all the veins, that of the ascending cava among the number, with the single exception of the crural veins, which will continue full ; and this certainly could not happen were there any retrograde passage for the blood from the veins to the arteries by open anastomoses.

ANATOMICAL EXERCISES

ON

THE GENERATION OF ANIMALS;

TO WHICH ARE ADDED

ESSAYS ON PARTURITION; ON THE MEMBRANES, AND FLUIDS OF
THE UTERUS; AND ON CONCEPTION.

BY WILLIAM HARVEY,

DOCTOR OF PHYSIC, AND PROFESSOR OF ANATOMY AND SURGERY
IN THE COLLEGE OF PHYSICIANS OF LONDON.

LONDON, 1651.

To the learned and illustrious the President and Fellows
of the College of Physicians of London.

HARASSED with anxious, and in the end not much availing
cares, about Christmas last,[1] I sought to rid my spirit of the
cloud that oppressed it, by a visit to that great man, the chief
honour and ornament of our College, Dr. WILLIAM HARVEY,
then dwelling not far from the city.   I found him, Democritus
like, busy with the study of natural things, his countenance cheer-
ful, his mind serene, embracing all within its sphere.   I forthwith saluted him, and asked if all were well with him ?   " How
can it," said he, " whilst the Commonwealth is full of distractions, and I myself am still in the open sea?   And truly," he
continued, " did I not find solace in my studies, and a balm
for my spirit in the memory of my observations of former years,
I should feel little desire for longer life.   But so it has been,
that this life of obscurity, this vacation from public business,
which causes tedium and disgust to so many, has proved a
sovereign remedy to me."
    I answering said, " I can readily account for this : whilst
most men are learned through others' wits, and under cover of
a different diction and a new arrangement, vaunt themselves
on things that belong to the ancients, thou ever interrogatest
Nature herself concerning her mysteries.   And this line of
study as it is less likely to lead into error, so is it also more

---

[1] [This must have been Christmas, 1650, the year after the violent death of
the king.---ED.]

fertile in enjoyment, inasmuch as each particular point examined often leads to others which had not before been sur-
mised. You yourself, I well remember, informed me once that
you had never dissected any animal—and many and many a
one have you examined,—but that you discovered something un-
expected, something of which you were formerly uninformed."

" It is true," said he : " the examination of the bodies of
animals has always been my delight ; and I have thought that
we might thence not only obtain an insight into the lighter
mysteries of nature, but there perceive a kind of image or re-
flex of the omnipotent Creator himself. And though much has
already been made out by the learned men of former times, I
have still thought that much more remained behind, hidden by
the dusky night of nature, uninterrogated ; so that I have
oftentimes wondered and even laughed at those who have fancied that everything had been so consummately and absolutely
investigated by an Aristotle or a Galen, or some other mighty
name, that nothing could by possibility be added to their
knowledge. Nature, however, is the best and most faithful in-
terpreter of her own secrets ; and what she presents either more
briefly or obscurely in one department, that she explains more
fully and clearly in another. No one indeed has ever rightly
ascertained the use or function of a part who has not examined
its structure, situation, connexions by means of vessels, and
other accidents, in various animals, and carefully weighed and
considered all he has seen. The ancients, our authorities in
science, even as their knowledge of geography was limited by
the boundaries of Greece, so neither did their knowledge of
animals, vegetables, and other natural objects extend beyond
the confines of their country. But to us the whole earth lies
open, and the zeal of our travellers has made us familiar not
only with other countries and the manners and customs of their
inhabitants, but also with the animals, vegetables, and minerals that are met with in each. And truly there is no nation

so barbarous which has not discovered something for the general good, whether led to it by accident or compelled by necessity, which had been overlooked by more civilized communities. But shall we imagine that nothing can accrue to the wide domains of science from such advantages, or that all knowledge was exhausted by the first ages of the world? If we do, the blame very certainly attaches to our indolence, nowise to nature.

" To this there is another evil added : many persons, wholly without experience, from the presumed verisimilitude of a previous opinion, are often led by and by to speak of it boldly, as a matter that is certainly known ; whence it comes, that not only are they themselves deceived, but that they likewise lead other incautious persons into error."

Discoursing in this manner, and touching upon many topics besides with wonderful fluency and facility, as is his custom, I interposed by observing, " How free you yourself are from the fault you indicate all know who are acquainted with you ; and this is the reason wherefore the learned world, who are aware of your unwearied industry in the study of philosophy, are eagerly looking for your farther experiments."

" And would you be the man," said Harvey, smiling, " who should recommend me to quit the peaceful haven, where I now pass my life, and launch again upon the faithless sea?" You know full well what a storm my former lucubrations raised. Much better is it oftentimes to grow wise at home and in private, than by publishing what you have amassed with infinite labour, to stir up tempests that may rob you of peace and quiet for the rest of your days."

" True," said I ; " it is the usual reward of virtue to have received ill for having merited well. But the winds which raised those storms, like the north-western blast, which drowns itself in its own rain, have only drawn mischief on themselves."

Upon this he showed me his ' Exercises on the Generation of

Animals,' a work composed with vast labour and singular care; and having it in my hands, I exclaimed, " Now have I what I so much desired ! and unless you consent to make this work public, I must say that you will be wanting both to your own fame and to the public usefulness.   Nor let any fear of farther trouble in the matter induce you to withhold it longer : I gladly charge myself with the whole business of correcting the press."

Making many difficulties at first, urging, among other things, that his work must be held imperfect, as not containing his investigations on the generation of insects, I nevertheless prevailed at length, and he said to me, " I intrust these papers to your care with full authority either speedily to commit them to the press, or to suppress them till some future time."   Having returned him many thanks, I bade him adieu, and took my leave, feeling like another Jason laden with the golden fleece.   On returning home I forthwith proceeded to examine my prize in all its parts, and could not but wonder with myself that such a treasure should have lain so long concealed; and that whilst others produce their trifles and emptinesses with much ado, their messes twice, aye, an hundred times, heated up, our Harvey should set so little store by his admirable observations.   And indeed, so often as he has sent forth any of his discoveries to the world, he has not comported himself like those who, when they publish, would have us believe that an oak had spoken, and that they had merited the rarest honours,—a draught of hen's milk at the least.   Our Harvey rather seems as though discovery were natural to him, a thing of ease and of course, a matter of ordinary business; though he may nevertheless have expended infinite labour and study on his works.   And we have evidence of his singular candour in this, that he never hostilely attacks any previous writer, but ever courteously sets down and comments upon the opinions of each; and indeed he is wont to say, that it is argument of an indifferent cause when it is contended for with violence and distemper; and that truth scarce wants an advocate.

It would have been easy for our illustrious colleague to have woven the whole of this web from materials of his own; but to escape the charge of envy, he has rather chosen to take Aristotle and Fabricius of Aquapendente as his guides, and to appear as contributing but his portion to the general fabric. Of him, whose virtue, candour, and genius are so well known to you all, I shall say no more, lest I should seem to praise to his face one whose singular worth has exalted him beyond the reach of all praise. Of myself I shall only say, that I have done no more than perform the midwife's office in this business, ushering into the light this product of our colleague's genius as you see it, consummate and complete, but long delayed, and fearing perchance some envious blast: in other words, I have overlooked the press; and as our author writes a hand which no one without practice can easily read (a thing that is common among our men of letters), I have taken some pains to prevent the printer committing any very grave blunders through this—a point which I observe not to have been sufficiently attended to in the small work of his which lately appeared.[1]

Here then, my learned friends, you have the cause of my addressing you at this time, viz. that you may know that our Harvey presents an offering to the benefit of the republic of letters, to your honour, to his own eternal fame.

Farewell, and prosper.

GEORGE ENT.

[1] [Doubtless the Exercitatio de Circulatione Sanguinis ad Riolanum; 12mo, Cantab. 1649.—ED.]

INTRODUCTION.

It will not, I trust, be unwelcome to you, candid reader, if I yield to the wishes, I might even say the entreaties, of many, and in these Exercises on Animal Generation, lay before the student and lover of truth what I have observed on this subject from anatomical dissections, which turns out to be very different from anything that is delivered by authors, whether philosophers or physicians.

Physicians, following Galen, teach that from the semen of the male and female mingled in coition the offspring is produced, and resembles one or other, according to the *predominance* of this one or of that; and farther, that in virtue of the same predominance, it is either male or female. Sometimes they declare the semen masculinum as the *efficient cause*, and the semen femininum as supplying the *matter*; and sometimes, again, they advocate precisely the opposite doctrine. Aristotle, one of Nature's most diligent inquirers, however affirms the *principles* of generation to be the male and the female, she contributing the matter, he the form; and that immediately after the sexual act the vital principle and the first particle of the future foetus, viz. the heart, in animals that have red blood, are formed from the menstrual blood in the uterus.

But that these are erroneous and hasty conclusions is easily made to appear: like phantoms of darkness they suddenly vanish before the light of anatomical inquiry. Nor is any long refutation necessary where the truth can be seen with one's proper eyes; where the inquirer by simple inspection finds everything in conformity with reason; and where at the same time he is made to understand how unsafe, how base a thing it is to receive instruction from others' comments without examination of the objects themselves, the rather as the book of Nature lies so open and is so easy of consultation.

What I shall deliver in these my Exercises on Animal Generation I am anxious to make publicly known, not merely that posterity may there perceive the sure and obvious truth, but farther, and especially, that by exhibiting the method of investigation which I have followed, I may propose to the studious a new and, unless I mistake, a safer way to the attainment of knowledge.

For although it is a new and difficult road in studying nature, rather to question things themselves than, by turning over books, to discover the opinions of philosophers regarding them, still it must be acknowledged that it is the more open path to the secrets of natural philosophy, and that which is less likely to lead into error.

Nor is there any just cause wherefore the labour should deter any one, if he will but think that he himself only lives through the ceaseless working of his heart. Neither, indeed, would the way I propose be felt as so barren and lonely, but for the custom, or vice rather, of the age we live in, when men, inclined to idleness, prefer going wrong with the many, to becoming wise with the few through dint of toil and outlay of money. The ancient philosophers, whose industry even we admire, went a different way to work, and by their unwearied labour and variety of experiments, searching into the nature of things, have left us no doubtful light to guide us in our studies. In this way it is that almost everything we yet possess of note or credit in philosophy, has been transmitted to us through the industry of ancient Greece. But when we acquiesce in the discoveries of the ancients, and believe (which we are apt to do through indolence) that nothing farther remains to be known, we suffer the edge of our ingenuity to be taken off, and the lamp which they delivered to us to be extinguished. No one of a surety will allow that all truth was engrossed by the ancients, unless he be utterly ignorant (to pass by other arts for the present) of the many remarkable discoveries that have lately been made in anatomy, these having been principally achieved by individuals who, either intent upon some particular matter, fell upon the novelty by accident, or (and this is the more excellent way) who following the traces of nature with their own eyes, pursued her through devious but most assured ways till they reached her in the citadel of truth. And truly in such pursuits it is sweet not merely to toil, but even to grow weary, when the pains of discovering are amply compensated by the pleasures of discovery. Eager for novelty, we are wont to travel far into unknown countries, that with our own eyes we may witness what we have heard reported as having been seen by others, where, however, we for the most part find

———minuit præsentia famam :

that the presence lessens the repute. It were disgraceful, therefore, with this most spacious and admirable realm of nature before us, and where the reward ever exceeds the promise, did we take the reports of others upon trust, and go on coining crude problems out of these, and on them hanging knotty and captious and petty disputations. Nature is herself to be addressed; the paths she shows us are to be boldly trodden; for thus, and whilst we consult our proper senses, from inferior advancing to superior levels, shall we penetrate at length into the heart of her mystery.

Of.the Manner and Order of acquiring Knowledge.

Although there is but one road to science, that to wit,
in which we proceed from things more known to things less
known, from matters more manifest to matters more obscure;
and universals are principally known to us, science springing
by reasonings from universals to particulars; still the comprehen-
sion of universals by the understanding is based upon the perception of individual things by the senses.   Both of Aristotle's
propositions, therefore, are true: First, the one in his Physics,[1]
where he says, " The way is naturally prepared, from those
things that are more obvious and clear to us, to those things
that are more obvious and clear by nature.   For, indeed, the
same things are not both known to us and extant simply :
whence it is indispensable to proceed in this way, viz. from
those things that are of a more obscure nature, but to us are
more apparent, to those that are of a nature more obvious and
distinct.   Now those things are, in the first instance, more
perspicuous and manifest to us that are most confused in fact ;
whence it is necessary to proceed from universals to particulars ;
for the whole, according to the dictates of sense, is the more obvious ; and the universal is a certain whole."   And again, that
other in his Analytics,[2] where he thus expresses himself : " Singulars are to us more known, and are the first that exist according to the information of sense ; for, indeed, there is nothing in
the understanding which was not first in the sense.   And
although that reasoning is naturally prior and more known
which proceeds by syllogism, still is that more perspicuous to
us which is based on induction.   And therefore do we more
readily define singulars than universals, for there is more of

---

[1] Lib. i, c. 2, 3.   [2] Post. 2.

equivocation in universals : whence it is advisable from singulars to pass to universals."

All this agrees with what we have previously said, although at first blush it may seem contradictory ; inasmuch as universals are first imbibed from particulars by the senses, and in so far are only known to us as an universal is a certain whole and indistinct thing, and a whole is known to us according to sense. For though in all knowledge we begin from sense, because, as the philosopher quoted has it, sensible particulars are better known to sense, still the sensation itself is an universal thing. For, if you observe rightly, although in the external sense the object perceived is singular, as, for example, the colour which we call yellow in the eye, still when this impression comes to be made an abstraction, and to be judged of and understood by the internal sensorium, it is an universal. Whence it happens that several persons abstract several species, and conceive different notions, from viewing the same object at the same time. This is conspicuous among poets and painters, who, although they contemplate one and the same object in the same place at the same moment, and with all other circumstances agreeing, nevertheless regard and describe it variously, and as each has conceived or formed an idea of it in his imagination. In the same way, the painter having a certain portrait to delineate, if he draw the outline a thousand times, he will still give a different face, and each not only differing from the other, but from the original countenance ; with such slight variety, however, that looking at them singly, you shall conceive you have still the same portrait set before you, although, when set side by side, you perceive how different they are. Now the reason is this : that in vision, or the act of seeing itself, each particular is clear and distinct ; but the moment the object is removed, as it is by merely shutting the eyes, when it becomes an abstraction in the fancy, or is only retained in the memory, it appears obscure and indistinct ; neither is it any longer apprehended as a particular, but as a something that is common and universal. Seneca[1] explains this subtlety, according to Plato's views, in very elegant terms: " An idea," he says, " is an eternal copy of the things that have place in nature. I add an explanation of this definition, that the matter may be made plainer to you. I desire to take your portrait; I have you as the prototype of the picture, from which my mind takes a certain impression which it transfers to the canvass. The countenance, therefore, which teaches and directs me, and from which the imitation is sought, is the idea." A little farther on he proceeds: " I have but just made use of the image which a painter forms in his mind, by way of illustration. Now, if he would paint a likeness of Virgil, he forms an intuitive image of his subject: the idea is the face of Virgil, the type of his future work; and this which the artist conveys and transfers to his work is the resemblance or portrait. What difference is there? you ask: the one is the pattern or prototype, the other the form taken from the pattern and fixed in the work; the artist imitates the one, he creates the other. A statue has a certain expression of face; this is the Eidos, the species or representation; the prototype himself has a certain expression, which the statuary conceiving, transfers to his statue: this is the idea. Do you desire yet another illustration of the distinction? The Eidos is in the work; the idea without the work, and not only without the work, but it even existed before the work was begun." For the things that have formerly been noted, and that by use or wont have become firmly fixed in the mind of the artist, do, in fact, constitute art and the artistic faculty; art, indeed, is the reason of the work in the mind of the artist. On the same terms, therefore, as art is attained to, is all knowledge and science acquired; for as art is a habit with reference to things to be done, so is science a habit in respect of things

[1] Epist. 58.

to be known: as that proceeds from the imitation of types or forms, so this proceeds from the knowledge of natural things. Each has its origin in sense and experience, and it is impossible that there can rightly be either art or science without visible instance or example. In both, that which we perceive in sensible objects differs from the image itself which we retain in our imagination or memory. That is the type, idea, forma informans; this is the imitation, the Eidos, the abstract species. That is a thing natural, a real entity; this a representation or similitude, and a thing of the reason. That is occupied with the individual thing, and itself is single and particular; this is a certain universal and common thing. That in the artist and man of science is a sensible thing, clearer, more perfect; this a matter of reason and more obscure: for things perceived by sense are more assured and manifest than matters inferred by reason, inasmuch as the latter proceed from and are illustrated by the former. Finally, sensible things are of themselves and antecedent; things of intellect, however, are consequent, and arise from the former, and, indeed, we can in no way attain to them without the help of the others. And hence it is, that without the due admonition of the senses, without frequent observation and reiterated experiment, our mind goes astray after phantoms and appearances. Diligent observation is therefore requisite in every science, and the senses are frequently to be appealed to. We are, I say, to strive after personal experience, not to rely on the experience of others; without which, indeed, no one can properly become a student of any branch of natural science, nor show himself a competent judge of what I am about to say on the subject of generation; for without experience and skill in anatomy, he would not better understand me than could one born blind appreciate the nature and difference of colours, or one deaf from birth judge of sounds. I would, therefore, have you, gentle reader, to take nothing on trust from me concerning the generation of animals; I appeal to your own eyes as my witnesses and judge. For as all true science rests upon those principles which have their origin in the operation of the senses, particular care is to be taken that by repeated dissection the grounds of our present subject be fully established. If we do otherwise, we shall but come to empty and unstable opinions; solid and true science will escape us altogether: just as commonly happens to those who form their notions of distant countries and cities, or who pretend to get a knowledge of the parts of the human body, from drawings and engravings, which but too frequently present things under false and erroneous points of view. And so it is, that in the present age we have an abundance of writers and pretenders to knowledge, but very few who are really learned and philosophers.

Thus much have I thought good, gentle reader, to present to you, by way of preface, that understanding the nature of the assistance to which I have trusted, and the counsel by which I have been led in publishing these my observations and experiments; and that you yourself in passing over the same ground, may not merely be in a condition to judge between Aristotle and Galen, but, quitting subtleties and fanciful conjectures, embracing nature with your own eyes, that you may discover many things unknown to others, and of great importance.

Of the same matters, according to Aristotle.

There is no such thing as innate knowledge, according to Aristotle; neither opinion, nor art, nor understanding, nor speech, nor reason itself, inhere in us by nature and from our birth; but all of these, as well as the qualities and habitudes, which are believed to be spontaneous, and to lie under the control of our will, are to be regarded as among the number of those things that reach us from without according to nature:

such as the virtues and the vices, for which men are either praised and rewarded or reproved and punished. All our knowledge, therefore, of every kind has to be acquired. But this is not the place to inquire into the first principles of knowledge.

I believe, however, that it will not be useless if I premise a few words as to whence and how our knowledge reaches us, both with a view to rendering what I shall say on the subject of generation more readily intelligible, and of removing any doubts that may arise out of this opinion of the Stagirite,[1] who asserts that all doctrine and discipline based on reason are derived from antecedent knowledge; whence it seems to follow that there is either no first knowledge, or that this must be innate, a conclusion which is in contradiction with what has already been stated.

The doubt, however, is by and by resolved by Aristotle[2] himself, when he treats of the mode in which knowledge is acquired: for after he has taught that all certain knowledge is obtained through syllogism and demonstration, and made it manifest that every demonstrative syllogism proceeds from true and necessary first principles; he goes on to inquire how principles become known, and what the faculty is that knows; at the same time, too, he discusses the question, Whether habits, if not innate, are engendered; and whether, being innate, they lie concealed? " We have not," he says, " these habits; for it happens that they are concealed from those who acquire the most admirable kinds of knowledge through demonstration. If, however, we receive them, not having had them previously, how should we become informed, how learn from non-antecedent knowledge? It is obvious, therefore, that they are neither possessed, nor can they be engendered in the ignorant and those who are endowed with no habit. Whence it is essential that some faculty be possessed, not however any which were

---

[1] Analyt. post. lib. i, c. 1.   [2] Ib. lib. ii, cap. ult.

more excellent, more exquisite than they. Now it seems a thing common to all animals, that they have a congenital power of judging, which we call sense. Since sense is innate, then, the things perceived by sense remain in some animals; in others they do not remain. Those in whom they do not remain, however, have either no knowledge at all, or at least none beyond the simple perception of the things which do not remain; others, again, when they perceive, retain a certain something in their soul. Now, as there are many animals of this description, there is already a distinction between one animal and another; and to this extent, that in some there is reason from the memory of things; and in others there is none. Memory, therefore, as is said, follows from sense; but from repeated recollection of the same thing springs experience (for repeated acts of memory constitute a single experience). From experience, however, or from the whole and universal stored quietly in the mind, (one, to wit, in place of a multitude—because in the whole crowd of particulars there is one and the same universal,) is derived the principle of art and of science: of art, if it belong to production (i. e. action); of science, if it belong to that which is (i. e. the knowledge of entity). Consequently there are neither any definite habits that are innate, nor any habits that are formed from other and more known habits, but from sense."

From which words of Aristotle it plainly appears by what order or method any art or science is acquired, viz. The thing perceived by sense remains; from the permanence of the thing perceived results memory; from multiplied memory, experience; from experience, universal reason, definitions, and maxims or common axioms, the most certain principles of knowledge; for example, the same thing under like conditions cannot be and not be; every affirmation or negation is either true or false; and so on.

Wherefore, as we have said above, there is no perfect knowledge which can be entitled ours, that is innate; none but what has been obtained from experience, or derived in some way from our senses; all knowledge, at all events, is examined by these, approved by them, and finally presents itself to us firmly grounded upon some pre-existing knowledge which we possessed: because without memory there is no experience, which is nothing else than reiterated memory; in like manner memory cannot exist without endurance of the things perceived, and the thing perceived cannot remain where it has never been.

The supreme dictator in philosophy again and elsewhere expresses himself very elegantly in the same direction:[1] " All men desire by nature to know; the evidence of this is the pleasure they take in using their senses, among which the sight is that which is particularly preferred, because this especially serves us to acquire knowledge, and informs us of the greatest number of differences. Nature, therefore, endowed animals with sense; some of them, however, have no memory from the operations of their senses; others, again, have memory; and this is the reason wherefore some are more intelligent, and some more capable of receiving instruction than others, those, namely, that want recollection. Some show discretion independently of tuition: inasmuch as there are many that do not hear, such as bees and others of the same kind. But all animals which along with memory have the faculty of hearing are susceptible of education. Other creatures, again, live possessed of fancy and memory, but they have little store of experience; the human kind, however, have both art and reasoning. Now experience comes to man through memory; for many memories of the same thing have the force of a single experience: so that experience appears to be almost identical with certain kinds of art and science;[2] and, indeed, men acquire both art and science by experience: for experience, as Polus rightly remarks, begets art, inexperience is waited on by accident."

[1] Metaph. lib. i, c. 1.   [2] Plato in Gorgias.

11

By this he plainly tells us that no one can truly be entitled discreet or well-informed, who does not of his own experience, i. e. from repeated memory, frequent perception by sense,
and diligent observation, know that a thing is so in fact.
Without these, indeed, we only imagine or believe, and such
knowledge is rather to be accounted as belonging to others than
to us.   The method of investigating truth commonly pursued
at this time therefore is to be held as erroneous and almost
foolish, in which so many inquire what others have said, and
omit to ask whether the things themselves be actually so or
not; and single universal conclusions being deduced from several
premises, and analogies being thence shaped out, we have frequently mere verisimilitudes handed down to us instead of
positive truths.   Whence it comes that pretenders to knowledge and sophists, trimming up the discoveries of others,
changing the arrangement only, or the language, and adding
a few things of no importance, audaciously send them forth as
their own, and so render philosophy, which ought to be certain
and perspicuous, obscure and intricate.   For he who reads the
words of an author and fails, through his own senses, to obtain
images of the things that are conveyed in these words, derives
not true ideas, but false fancies and empty visions; whence
he conjures up shadows and chimeras, and his whole theory or
contemplation, which, however, he regards as knowledge, is
nothing more than a waking dream, or such a delirium as the
sick fancy engenders.

I therefore whisper in your ear, friendly reader, and recommend you to weigh carefully in the balance of exact experience all that I shall deliver in these Exercises on the Generation of Animals; I would not that you gave credit to aught
they contain save in so far as you find it confirmed and borne
out by the unquestionable testimony of your own senses.

The same course is even advised by Aristotle, who, after
having gone over a great many particulars about bees, says at

length :[1] "That the generation of bees takes place in this way appears both from reason and from those things that are seen to occur in their kind. Still all the incidents have not yet been sufficiently examined. And when the investigation shall be complete, then will sense be rather to be trusted than reason; reason, however, will also deserve credit, if the things demonstrated accord with the things that are perceived by sense."

Of the Method to be pursued in studying Generation.

Since in Animal Generation, (and, indeed, in all other subjects upon which information is desired,) inquiry must be begun from the causes, especially the material and efficient ones, it appears advisable to me to look back from the perfect animal, and to inquire by what process it has arisen and grown to maturity, to retrace our steps, as it were, from the goal to the starting place; so that when at last we can retreat no further, we shall feel assured that we have attained to the principles; at the same time we shall perceive from what primary matter, and from what efficient principle, and in what way from these the plastic force proceeds; as also what processes nature brings into play in the work. For primary and more remote matter, by abstraction and negation (being stripped of its garments as it were) becomes more conspicuous; and whatever is first formed or exists primarily in generation, is the material cause of everything that succeeds. For example, before a man attains to maturity, he was a boy, an infant, an embryo. And then it is indispensable to inquire further as to what he was in his mother's womb before he was an embryo or fœtus; whether made up of three bubbles, or a shapeless mass, or a conception or coagulum proceeding from the mingled seminal fluids of his parents, or

---

[1] De Gen. An. lib. iii, c. 10.

what else, as we have it delivered to us by writers. In like manner, before a fowl had attained to maturity or perfection, —because capable of engendering its like,—it was a chicken; previous to which it was an embryo or fœtus in the egg; and before this, Hieronymus Fabricius, of Aquapendente, has observed rudiments of the head, eyes, and spine. But when he asserts that the bones are formed before the muscles, heart, liver, lungs, and precordial parts, and contends that all the internal organs must exist before the external ones, he follows probabilities according to previous notions rather than inspection; and quitting the evidences of sense that rest on anatomy, he seeks refuge in reasonings upon mechanical principles; a procedure that is anything but becoming in a great anatomist, whose duty it was faithfully to narrate the changes he observed taking place day by day in the egg, up to the period when the fœtus is perfected; and this the rather as he expressly proposed to himself to write the history of the formation of the chick in the egg, and to exhibit in figures what happens in the course of each successive day. It would have been in harmony with such a design, I say, had we been informed, on the testimony of the senses, of what parts are formed first, together, or subsequently in the egg; and not had mere opinions or musty conjectures, and the instances of houses and ships, adduced in illustration of the order and mode of formation of the parts.

We, therefore, in conformity with the method proposed, shall show in the first place in the egg, and then in the conceptions of other animals, what parts are first, and what are subsequently formed by the great God of Nature with inimitable providence and intelligence, and most admirable order. Next we shall inquire into the primary matter out of which, and the efficient cause by which generation is accomplished, and also the order and economy of generation, as observed by us; that from thence, from its own work, we may have some certain information of the several faculties of the formative and vegetative soul, and of the nature of the soul itself, judging from its members or organs, and their functions.

This, indeed, cannot be done in all animals : first, because a sufficient number of several of these cannot be commanded; and again, because, from the small size of many, they escape our powers of vision. It must suffice, therefore, that this is done in some kinds which are more familiarly known to us, and that we refer all the rest to these as types or standards.

We have, therefore, selected those that may tend to render our experiments more undeniable, viz. the larger and more perfect animals, and that are easily within reach. For in the larger animals all things are more conspicuous; in the more perfect, they are also more distinct; and in those that we can command, and that live with us, everything is more readily examined : we have it in our power so often as we please to repeat our observations, and so to free them from all uncertainty and doubt. Now, among oviparous animals of this description, we have the common fowl, the goose, duck, pigeon; and then we have frogs, and serpents, and fishes ; crustacea, testacea, and mollusca; among insects, bees, wasps, butterflies, and silkworms; among viviparous creatures, we have sheep, goats, dogs, cats, deer, and oxen; lastly, we have the most perfect of all animals, man.

Having studied and made ourselves familiar with these, we may turn to the consideration of the more abstruse nature of the vegetative soul, and feel ourselves in a condition to under-stand the method, order, and causes of generation in animals generally ; for all animals resemble one or other of those above mentioned, and agree with them either generally or specifically, and are procreated in the same manner, or the mode of their generation at least is referrible by analogy to that of one or other of them. For Nature, perfect and divine, is ever in the same things harmonious with herself, and as her works either agree or differ, (viz. in genus, species, or some other proportion,) so is her agency in these (viz. generation or development) either the same or diverse. He who enters on this new and untrodden path, and out of the vast realm of Nature endeavours to find the truth by means of anatomical dissections and experiments, is met by such a multitude of facts, and these of so unusual an aspect, that he may find it more difficult to explain and describe to others the things he has seen, than he reckoned it labour to make his observations; so many things are encountered that require naming; such is the abundance of matter and the dearth of words. But if he would have recourse to metaphors, and by means of old and familiar terms would make known his ideas concerning the things he has newly discovered, the reader would have little chance of understanding him better than if they were riddles that were propounded; and of the thing itself, which he had never seen, he could have no conception. But then, to have recourse to new and unusual terms were less to bring a torch to lighten, than to darken things still more with a cloud: it were to attempt an explanation of a matter unknown by one still more unknown, and to impose a greater toil on the reader to understand the meaning of words than to comprehend the things themselves. And so it happens that Aristotle is believed by the inexperienced to be obscure in many places; and on this account, perhaps, Fabricius of Aquapendente rather intended to exhibit the chick in ovo in his figures than to explain its formation in words.

Wherefore, courteous reader, be not displeased with me, if, in illustrating the history of the egg, and in my account of the generation of the chick, I follow a new plan, and occasionally have recourse to unusual language. Think me not eager for vainglorious fame rather than anxious to lay before you observations that are true, and that are derived immediately from the nature of things. That you may not do me this injustice, I would have you know that I tread in the footsteps of those who have already thrown a light upon this subject, and that, wherever I can, I make use of their words. And foremost of all among the ancients I follow Aristotle; among the moderns, Fabricius of Aquapendente; the former as my leader, the latter as my informant of the way. For even as they who discover new lands, and first set foot on foreign shores, are wont to give them new names which mostly descend to posterity, so also do the discoverers of things and the earliest writers with perfect propriety give names to their discoveries. And now I seem to hear Galen admonishing us, that we should but agree about the things, and not dispute greatly about the words.

ANIMAL GENERATION.

Wherefore we begin with the history of the hen's egg.

Hieronymus Fabricius of Aquapendente, (whom, as I have said, I have chosen my informant of the way I am to follow,) in the beginning of his book on the Formation of the Ovum and Chick, has these words : " My purpose is to treat of the formation of the fœtus in every animal, setting out from that which proceeds from the egg : for this ought to take precedence of all discussion of the subject, both because from this it is not difficult to make out Aristotle's views of the matter, and because his treatise on the Formation of the Fœtus from the egg, is by far the fullest, and the subject is by much the most extensive and difficult."

We, however, commence with the history of the hen's egg as well for the reasons above assigned, as because we can thence obtain certain data which, as more familiar to us, will serve to throw light on the generation of other animals ; for as eggs cost little, and are always to be had, we have an opportunity from them of observing the first clear and unquestionable commencements of generation, how nature proceeds in the process, and with what admirable foresight she governs every part of the work.

Fabricius proceeds : " Now that the contemplation of the formation of the chick from the egg is of very ample scope, appears from this, that the greater number of animals are pro-

duced from ova. Passing by almost all insects and the whole
of the less perfect animals, which are obviously produced from
eggs, the greater number of the more perfect are also engendered from eggs." And then he goes on to particularize : " All
feathered creatures ; fishes likewise, with the single exception of
the whale tribes ; crustacea, testacea, and all mollusca ; among
land animals, reptiles, millepeds, and all creeping things ; and
among quadrupeds, the entire tribe of lizards."

We, however, maintain (and shall take care to show that it
is so), that all animals whatsoever, even the viviparous, and man
himself not excepted, are produced from ova ; that the first conception, from which the fœtus proceeds in all, is an ovum of
one description or another, as well as the seeds of all kinds of
plants. Empedocles,[1] therefore, spoke not improperly of the
oviparum genus arboreum, " the egg-bearing race of trees." The
history of the egg is therefore of the widest scope, inasmuch
as it illustrates generation of every description.

We shall, therefore, begin by showing where, whence, and
how eggs are produced ; and then inquire by what means and
order and successive steps the fœtus or chick is formed and perfected in and from the egg.

Fabricius has these additional words : " The fœtus of animals
is engendered in one case from an ovum, in another from the
seminal fluid, in a third from putrefaction ; whence some creatures are oviparous, others viviparous, and yet others, born of
putrefaction or by the spontaneous act of nature, automatically."

Such a division as this, however, does not satisfy me, inasmuch as all animals whatsoever may be said in a certain sense
to spring from ova, and in another certain sense from seminal
fluid ; and they are entitled oviparous, viviparous, or vermiparous, rather in respect of their mode of bringing forth than of
their first formation. Even the creatures that arise spontaneously are called automatic, not because they spring from putrefaction, but because they have their origin from accident, the
spontaneous act of nature, and are equivocally engendered, as it
is said, proceeding from parents unlike themselves. And, then,
certain other animals bring forth an egg or a worm as their
conception and semen, from which, after it has been exposed

---

[1] Arist. De Gen. Anim. lib. i, cap. 20.

abroad, a fœtus is produced; whence such animals are called oviparous or vermiparous. Viviparous animals are so entitled because they retain and cherish their conception in their interior, until from thence the fœtus comes forth into the light completely formed and alive.

Of the seat of generation.

" Nature," says Fabricius, " was first solicitous about the place [where generation should proceed], which she determined should be either within or without the animal: within she ordained the uterus; without, the ovum: in the uterus the blood and seminal fluid engendering; in the ovum, however, the fluids or elements of which it consists supplying pabulum for the production of the fœtus."

Now, whatever is procreated of the semen properly so called originates and is perfected either in the same place or in different places. All viviparous creatures derive their origin and have their completion in the uterus itself; but oviparous animals, as they have their beginning within their parents, and there become ova, so is it beyond their parents that they are perfected into the fœtal state. Among oviparous animals, however, there are some that retain their ova till such time as they are mature and perfect; such as all the feathered tribes, reptiles and serpents. Others, again, extrude their semina in a state still immature and imperfect, and it is without the body of the parent that increase, maturity, and perfection, are attained. Under this head we range frogs, many kinds of fishes, crustaceous, molluscous, and testaceous animals, the ova of which, when first extruded, are but beginnings, sketches, yelks which afterwards surround themselves with whites, and attracting, concocting, and attaching nutriment to themselves, are changed into perfect seeds or eggs. Such also are the semina of insects (called worms by Aristotle), which, imperfect on their extrusion and in the beginning, seek food for themselves, upon which they are nourished, and grow from a grub into a chrysalis: from an imperfect into a perfect egg or seed. Birds, however, and the rest of the oviparous tribes, lay perfect eggs; whence without the uterus the fœtus is engendered. And it was on this account that Fabricius admitted two seats of generation : one internal, the uterus ; another external, the ovum. But he would have had more reason, in my opinion, had he called the nest, or place where the eggs are laid, the external seat, that, to wit, in which the extruded seed or egg is cherished, matured, and perfected into a fœtus ; for it is from the differences of this seat that the generation of oviparous animals is principally distinguished. And it is, indeed, a thing most worthy of admiration to see these creatures selecting and preparing their nests with so much foresight, and fashioning, and furnishing, and concealing them with such inimitable art and ingenuity ; so that it seems imperative on us to admit in them a certain spark of the divine flame (as the poet said of bees) ; and, indeed, we can more readily admire than imitate their untaught art and sapience.

EXERCISE THE THIRD.

Of the upper part of the hen's uterus, or the ovary.

The uterus of the fowl is divided by Fabricius into the superior and inferior portions, and the superior portion he calls the ovary.

The ovary is situated immediately beneath the liver, close to the spine, over the descending aorta. In this situation, in the larger animals with red blood, the cœliac artery enters the mesentery, at the origin, namely, of the emulgent veins, or a little lower ; in the situation moreover in which in the other red-blooded and viviparous animals the vasa præparantia, tending to the testes, take their origin : in the same place at which the testes of the cock-bird are situated, there is the ovary of the hen discovered. For some animals carry their testicles externally ; others have them within the body, in the loins, in the space midway from the origins of the vasa præparantia. But the cock has his testicles at the very origin of these vessels, as if his spermatic fluid needed no preparation.

Aristotle[1] says that the ovum begins at the diaphragm ; " I, however," says Fabricius, " in my treatise on Respiration, have

---

[1] Hist. Anim. lib. vi, c. 2.

denied that the feathered kinds have any diaphragm. The difficulty is resolved by admitting that birds are not entirely destitute of a kind of diaphragm, inasmuch as they have a delicate membrane in the place of this septum, which Aristotle calls a cincture and septum. Still they have no diaphragm that is muscular, and that might aid respiration, like other animals. But, indeed, Aristotle did not know the muscles."

Thus is the prince of philosophers accused and excused in the same breath, his challenger being himself not free from error; because it is certain that Aristotle both knew the muscles, as I have elsewhere shown, and the membranes, which in birds are not only situated transversely in the direction of the cincture of the body, but extended in the line of the longitudinal direction of the belly, supplying the place of the diaphragm [of quadrupeds] and being subservient to respiration, as I have shown in the clearest manner in my disquisitions on the Respiration of Animals. And, passing over other particulars at this time, I shall only direct attention to the fact, that birds breathe with great freedom, and in singing also modulate their voice in the most admirable manner, their lungs all the while being so closely connected with their sides and ribs, that they can neither be dilated and rise, nor suffer contraction in any considerable degree.

The bronchia or ends of the trachea in birds, moreover, are perforate, and open into the abdomen (and this is an observation which I do not remember to have met with elsewhere), so that the air inspired is received into and stored up within the cells or cavities formed by the membranes mentioned above. In the same manner as fishes and serpents draw air into ample bladders situated in the abdomen, and there store it up, by which they are thought to swim more lightly; and as frogs and toads, when in the height of summer they respire more vigorously assume more than the usual quantity of air into their vesicular lungs, (whence they acquire so large a size,) which they afterwards freely expire, croaking all the while; so in the feathered tribes are the lungs rather the route and passage for respiration than its adequate instrument.

Now, had Fabricius seen this, he would never have denied that these membranes (with the assistance of the abdominal muscles at all events,) could subserve respiration and perform the office of the diaphragm, which, indeed, of itself, and without the assistance of the abdominal muscles, were incompetent to act as an instrument of respiration.   And, then, the diaphragm has another duty to perform in those creatures in whom it is muscular or fleshy, viz., to depress the stomach filled with food, and the intestines distended with flatus, so that the heart and lungs shall not be invaded, and life itself oppressed in its cita-del.   But as there was no danger of anything of this kind in birds, they have a membranous septum, perfectly well adapted to the purposes of respiration, so that they have very properly been said to have a diaphragm.   And were birds even entirely without anything in the shape of a diaphragm, still would Aristotle not be liable to criticism for speaking of the ova commencing at the septum transversum, because by this title he merely indicates the place where the diaphragm is usually met with in other animals.   In the same way we ourselves say that the ovary is situated at the origin of the spermatic vasa præparantia, although the hen has, in fact, no such vessels.

The perforations of the lungs discovered by me (and to which I merely direct attention in this place,) are neither obscure nor doubtful, but, in birds especially, sufficiently conspicuous, so that in the ostrich I found many conduits which readily admitted the points of my fingers.   In the turkey, fowl, and, indeed, almost all birds, you will find that a probe passed downwards by the trachea makes its way out of the lungs, and is disco-vered lying naked and exposed in one or another of the abdo-minal cells.   Air blown into the lungs of these creatures with a pair of bellows passes on with a certain force even into the most inferior of these cells.

We may even be permitted to ask, whether in man, whilst he lives, there is not a passage from openings of the same kind into the cavity of the thorax ?   For how else should the pus poured out in empyema and the blood extravasated in pleurisy make its escape ?   In penetrating wounds of the chest, the lungs themselves being uninjured, air often escapes by the wound ; or liquids thrown into the cavity of the thorax, are discharged with the expectoration.   But our views of this subject will be found fully expressed elsewhere, viz., in our disquisitions on the Causes, Uses, and Organs of Respiration.

I return to the ovary and the upper portion of the fowl's uterus, in which the rudiments of the eggs are produced. These, according to Aristotle,[1] in the first instance are small, and of a white colour; growing larger, they subsequently become of a paler and then of a deeper yellow.

The superior uterus of Fabricius, however, has no existence until after the hen has conceived, and contains the rudiments of ova within it; when it may be designated as a cluster of papulæ. And he therefore observes very properly, "The superior uterus is nothing more than an almost infinite congeries of yelks, which appear collected as it were into a single cluster, of a rounded form, and of every size, from that of a grain of mustard to that almost of a walnut or medlar. This multitude of vitelli is aggregated and conjoined very much in the manner of a bunch of grapes, for which reason I shall constantly speak of it as the vitellarium or raceme of yelks; a comparison which Aristotle himself made in speaking of the soft or scaleless fishes, when he says,[2] their ovary or roe is extruded agglutinated into a kind of raceme or bunch of grapes. And in the same way as in a bunch of grapes the several berries are seen to be of different sizes, some large, some small, some of very diminutive proportions, each hanging by its several peduncle, so do we find precisely the same thing in the vitellarium of the fowl."

In fishes, frogs, crustacea, and testacea, however, matters are otherwise arranged. The ovary or vitellary here contains ova of one uniform size only, which being extruded increase, attain maturity, and give birth to fœtuses simultaneously. But in the ovary of the common fowl, and almost all the rest of the oviparous tribes, the yelks are found in various stages of their growth, from dimensions that are scarcely visible up to the full size. Nevertheless the eggs of the fowl and other birds, (not otherwise than in those cases where the eggs are all engendered and laid at the same moment,) ripen their fœtuses under the influence of incubation in the same nest, and produce them perfect, nearly at the same time. In the family of the pigeons, however, (which lay and incubate no more than two eggs in the same nest,) I have observed that all the ova crowded together in the ovary, with the exception of a single pair, were of the same

---

[1] Hist. Animal. lib. vi, cap. 2. [2] De Gen. Anim. lib. iii, c. 8.

dimensions; this pair was very much larger than any of the others, and already prepared to descend into the second or lower uterus.   In these creatures, therefore, the number of young is great, not because of the multitude produced at a time, but of the frequency with which births take place, viz., every month. In the same way, among cartilaginous fishes, such as the skates, dog-fishes, &c., two eggs only come to maturity together, one of which descends from the right the other from the left corner of the uterus into the inferior portion, where they are cherished, and where they finally produce living fœtuses, precisely as happens among viviparous animals; in the ovary, nevertheless, there is almost infinite store of ova of various sizes—in the ray I have counted upwards of a hundred.

The ova of the other oviparous tribes are either perfected externally, as in the case of fishes, or they are concocted or matured, as in the instance of testacea, crustacea, and spiders. Testaceous animals lay their eggs amidst froth; the crustaceous tribes, such as the shrimp, crab, and lobster, bear them about with them, attached to certain appendages; and the spiders carry them about and cherish them, laid up in a kind of purse or basket, made of their web.   The beetle rolls its eggs in dung, using its hind legs in the operation, and buries them. Now, in all these creatures the quantity of eggs is almost incredibly great : in fishes they form two oblong bladders or follicles, as may be seen in the carp, herring, and smelt, in all of which, as there is no uterus, but merely an ovary present, so is this sometimes crowded with ova to such a degree, that it comes to surpass the body in bulk.

Of such ovaries of the mullet and carp, salted and pressed, and dried in the smoke, was prepared that article of food in such request among the Greeks and old Italians, (called botorcha by the latter, ᾠὰ τάριχα, i. e. salted eggs, by the former,) and very similar, we may presume, to the masses which we find in the insides of our smoked herrings, and to the compact granular red-coloured roe of our lobsters.   The article prepared from the salted roe of the sturgeon, which is called caviare, and resembles black soap, is still the delight of epicures.

In those fishes that are highly prolific such a quantity of eggs is engendered, that the whole abdomen can scarcely contain them, even when they are first produced, still less when they have grown to any size. In fishes, therefore, there is no part save the ovary dedicated to purposes of reproduction. The ova of these animals continue to grow without the body, and do not require the protection of an uterus for their evolution. And the ovary here appears to bear an analogy to the testicles or vesiculæ seminales, not only because it is found in the same place as the testes in the male, (the testes in the cock being situated, as we have said, close to the origin of the cœliac artery, near the waist, in the very same place as the ovary in the hen,) but because among fishes, in both sexes, as the time of spawning approaches, two follicles, alike in situation, size, and shape, are discovered, extending the whole length of the abdomen; which increase and become distended at the same period : in the male with a homogeneous milky spermatic matter, (whence the term milk or milt of fishes;) in the female with innumerable granules, which, from their diminutive size and close texture, in the beginning of the season, escape the powers of vision, and present themselves as constituting an uniform body, bearing the strongest resemblance to the milt of the male regularly coagulated. By and by they are seen in the guise of minute grains of sand, adhering together within their follicles.

In the smaller birds that lay but once a year, and a few eggs only, you will scarcely discover any ovary. Still, in the place where the testicles are situated in the male, there in the female, and not less obviously than the testicles of the male, you will perceive three or four vesicles (the number being in proportion to that of the eggs of which they are the rudiments), by way of ovary.

In the cornua of the uterus of snakes (which resemble the vasa deferentia in male animals), the first rudiments of the ova present themselves as globules strung upon a thread, in the same way as women's bracelets, or like a rosary composed of amber beads.

Those ova that are found in the ovary of the fowl consequently are not to be regarded as perfect eggs, but only as their rudiments; and they are so arranged on the cluster, they succeed each other in such an order and of such dimensions, that they are always ready for each day's laying. But none of the eggs in the ovary are surrounded with albumen; there the yelk exists alone, and each, as it enlarges, extricates itself from the

12

general congeries of smaller ones, in order that it may the more readily find space to grow. Fabricius, therefore, is right when he says,[1] " The yelks which are on the surface of the cluster are larger than those of the middle, which are surrounded as it were by the larger ones. The very smallest of all the ova are situated towards the centre." That is to say, those that grow acquire larger dimensions and become detached from the rest, and as this proceeds, the several yelks, besides their tunica propria, are invested with another from the ovary, which embraces them externally, and connects them with the base whence they spring. This coat is, therefore, entitled the peduncle by Fabricius, and its office is that of a foot-stalk, viz. to supply nourishment to the ovum, in the same way as fruit is nourished through the stalk by which it is connected with the tree. " For this peduncle is a hollow membranous bond of union, extending from the foundation of the cluster [the stroma of the ovary] to the yelk, coming into contact with which, it is dilated and expanded in the same way as the optic nerve in the eye, and covers the vitellus with an external tunic. This perchance was what Aristotle called the στόλον ὀμφαλοωδην, or umbilical appendix, and described as forming a kind of tube. This peduncle includes numerous vessels, which are distributed on all sides around the yelk.

So much is accurately related by Fabricius; but he errs when he says, " This tunic does not surround the entire vitellus, but only extends upon it a little beyond the middle, very much in the manner of an acorn within its cup; whence it comes that the outer portion of the yelk, which is not invested by the membrane in question, presents itself free from vessels, and to appearance naked." The membrane, nevertheless, surrounds the yelk completely; but on the outer aspect it is not very easily distinguished from the tunica propria, both of them being of extreme delicacy. Posteriorly, however, and where the yelk is turned towards the basis of the cluster, the tunic in question does not adhere to the vitellus, neither does it send any vessels to this part, but merely embraces it in the manner of a sac.

Each vitellus receives a distinct tunic from the ovarian basis; whence this is not to be regarded as the common uterus, since

[1] Op. cit. p. 3.

nothing is discovered here except the cluster or heap of ova, of many different sizes, proceeding from the same foundation.

Now, this foundation or basis is a body sui generis, arising on the spine of the feathered kinds, connected by means of large arteries and veins, and of a loose, porous, and spongy texture, in order that multitudes of ova may be produced from it, and that it may supply tunics to all; which tunics, when the yelks have grown to their full size, are distended by them, and then the tunics surround the vitelli, in the manner of sacks with narrower necks and more capacious bellies, very much like the flasks that are formed by the breath of the glass-blower.

Fabricius then proceeds: "The yelks, as they proceed from small beginnings, from the size of millet or mustard seeds, and are at first not only extremely small, but colourless, as Aristotle says, so do they increase by degrees, and, according to Aristotle, become first of a paler and then of a deeper yellow, until they have attained to the dimensions familiar to all." I, however, have observed ova vastly smaller than millet seeds, ova which, like papulæ or sudamina, or the finest grains of sand, (such as we have indicated as found in the roe of fishes,) almost escaped the powers of sight; their places, indeed, were only proclaimed by a kind of roughness of the membranes.

EXERCISE THE FOURTH.

Of the infundibulum.

The next succeeding portion of the uterus of the common fowl is called the infundibulum by Fabricius. It forms a kind of funnel or tube, extending downwards from the ovary, (which it everywhere embraces,) and becoming gradually wider, terminates in the superior produced portion of the uterus. This infundibulum yields a passage to the yelks when they have broken from their foot-stalks in their descent from the ovary into the second uterus (so it is styled by Fabricius). It resembles the tunica vaginalis in the scrotum, and is a most delicate membrane, very easily dilatable, fitted to receive the yelks that are daily cast loose, and to transmit them to the uterus mentioned.

Would you have an example of these structures? Figure to yourself a small plant, whose tuberous roots should represent the congeries of yelks; its stalk the infundibulum. Now, as the stalk of this plant dies in the winter and disappears, in like manner, when the fowl ceases to lay eggs, the whole ovary, with the infundibulum, withers, shrinks, and is annulled; the basis [stroma] and indication of the roots being still left.

This infundibulum seems only to discharge the office of a conduit, or tube of passage : the yelk is never observed sticking in it; but as the testes at times creep upwards through the tunicæ vaginales into the groins, and in some animals—the hare and the mole—even become concealed within the abdomen, and nevertheless again descend and show themselves externally, so are the vitelli transmitted through the infundibulum from the ovary into the uterus. Its office is served, and even its form is imitated, by the funnel which we make use of when we pour fluids from one vessel into another having a narrower mouth.

EXERCISE THE FIFTH.

Of the external portion of the uterus of the common fowl.

Fabricius pursues his account of the uterus after having described the ovary, and in such an inverse order, that he premises a description of the superior portion or appendage of the uterus before he approaches the uterus itself. He assigns to it three turns or spirals, with somewhat too much of precision or determinateness, and settles the respective situations of these spirals, which are nevertheless of uncertain seat. Here, too, he very unnecessarily repeats his definition of the infundibulum. I would, therefore, in this place, beg to be allowed to give my own account of the uterus of the fowl, according to the anatomical method, which I consider the more convenient, and proceeding from external to internal parts, in opposition to the method of Fabricius.

In the fowl stripped of its feathers, the fundament will be observed not contracted circularly, as in other animals, but forming a depressed orifice, slit transversely, and consisting of two lips lying over against each other, the superior of the two covering and concealing the inferior, which is puckered together. The superior labium, or velabrum, as it is called, arises from the root of the rump, and as the upper eyelid covers the eye, so does this cover the three orifices of the pudenda, viz. the anus, the uterus, and the ureters, which lie concealed under the velabrum as under a kind of prepuce; very much as in the pudenda of the woman we have the orifice of the vulva and the meatus urinarius concealed between the labia and the nymphæ. So that without the use of the knife, or a somewhat forcible retraction of the velabrum in the fowl, neither the orifice by which the fæces pass from the intestines, nor that by which the urine issues from the ureters, nor yet that by which the egg escapes from the uterus, can be perceived. And as the two excrementitious discharges (the urine and the fæces) are expelled together as from a common cloaca, the velabrum being raised at the time, and the respective outlets exposed; so, during intercourse, the hen on the approach of the cock uncovers the vulva, and prepares for his reception, a circumstance observed by Fabricius in the turkey hen when she is eager for the male. I have myself observed a female ostrich, when her attendant gently scratched her back, which seemed to excite the sexual appetite, to lie down on the ground, lift up the velabrum, and exhibit and protrude the vulva, seeing which the male, straightway inflamed with a like œstrum, mounted, one foot being kept firm on the ground, the other set upon the back of the prostrate female; the immense penis (you might imagine it a neat's tongue!) vibrated backwards and forwards, and the process of intercourse was accompanied with much ado in murmuring and noise—the heads of the creatures being at the same time frequently thrust out and retracted—and other indications of enjoyment. Nor is it peculiar to birds, but common to animals at large, that, wagging the tail and protruding the genital parts, they prepare for the access of the male. And, indeed, the tail in the majority of animals has almost the same office as the velabrum in the common fowl; unless it were raised or drawn aside, it would interfere with the discharge of the fæces and the access of the male.

In the female red-deer, fallow-deer, roe, and others of the more temperate animals, there is a corresponding protection to

their private parts, a membranous velabrum covering the vulva
and meatus urinarius, which must be raised before the penis of
the male can be introduced.

In animals that have a tail, moreover, parturition could not
take place unless this part were lifted up; and even the human
female is assisted in her labour by having the coccyx anointed
and drawn outwards with the finger.

A surgeon, a trustworthy man, and with whom I am upon
intimate terms, on his return from the East Indies informed
me, in perfect sincerity, that some inland and mountainous parts
of the island of Borneo are still inhabited by a race of caudate
human beings (a circumstance of which we also read in Pausa-
nias), one of whom, a virgin, who had only been captured with
great difficulty, for they live in the woods, he himself had seen,
with a tail, thick, fleshy, and a span in length, reflected between
the buttocks, and covering the anus and pudenda : so regularly
has nature willed to cover these parts.

To return. The structure of the velabrum in the fowl is like
that of the upper eyelid; that is to say, it is a fleshy and muscular fold of the skin, having fibres extending from the circumference on every side towards the centre; its inner surface, like
that of the eyelid and prepuce, being soft. Along its margin
also there is a semicircular tarsus, after the manner of that of the
eyelid; and in addition, between the skin and fleshy membrane,
an interposed cartilage, extending from the root of the rump,
the sickle-shaped tarsus being connected with it at right angles,
(very much as we observe a small tail comprehended between
the wing on either side, in bats). By this structure the velabrum is enabled more readily to open and close the foramina
pudendi that have been mentioned.

The velabrum being now raised and removed, certain foramina are brought into view, some of which are very distinct,
others more obscure. The more obvious are the anus and vulva,
or the outlet of the fæcal matters and the inlet to the uterus.
The more obscure are, first, that by which the urine is excreted
from the kidneys, and, second, the small orifice discovered by
Fabricius, " into which," he says, " the cock immits the spermatic fluid," a foramen, however, which neither Antony Ulm, a
careful dissector, has indicated in Aldrovandus, nor any one else
except Fabricius, so far as I know, has ever observed.

All these foramina are so close to one another that they seem almost to meet in a single cavity, which, as being common to the fæces and urine, may be called the cloaca. In this cavity, the urine, as it descends from the kidneys, is mingled with the feculent matters of the bowels, and the two are discharged together. Through this, too, the egg, as it is laid, forces itself a passage.

Now, the arrangements in this cavity are such, that both excrements descending into a common sac, the urine is made use of as a natural clyster for their evacuation. The cloaca is therefore thicker and more rugous than the intestine; and at the moment of laying and of coition, it is everted, (the velabrum which covers it being raised as I have already said,) the lower portion of the bowel being as it were prolapsed. At this moment all the foramina that terminate in the cloaca are conspicuous; on the return or reduction of the prolapsed portion, however, they are concealed, being all collected together as it were into the common purse or pouch.

The more conspicuous foramina, those, viz. of the anus and uterus, are situated, with reference to one another, differently in birds from what they are in other animals. In these the pudendum, or female genital part, is situated anteriorly between the rectum and bladder; in birds, however, the excrementitious outlet is placed anteriorly, so that the inlet to the uterus is situated between this and the rump.

The foramen, into which Fabricius believes the cock to inject his fluid, is discovered between the orifice of the vulva and the rump. I, however, deny any such use to this foramen; for in young chickens it is scarcely to be seen, and in adults it is present indifferently both in males and females. It is obvious, therefore, that it is both an extremely small and obscure orifice, and can have no such important function to perform: it will scarcely admit a fine needle or a bristle, and it ends in a blind cavity; neither have I ever been able to discover any spermatic fluid within it, although Fabricius asserts that this fluid is stored up there even for a whole year, and that all the eggs contained in the ovary may be thence fecundated, as it is afterwards stated.

All birds, serpents, oviparous quadrupeds, and likewise fishes, as may readily be seen in the carp, have kidneys and ureters through which the urine distils, a fact which was unknown to Aristotle and philosophers up to this time. In birds and serpents, which have spongy or largely vesicular lungs, the quantity of urine secreted is small, because they drink little, and that by sipping; there was, therefore, no occasion for an urinary bladder in these creatures: the renal secretion, as already stated, is accumulated in a common cavity or cloaca, along with the drier intestinal excrement. Nevertheless, I do find an urinary bladder in the carp and some other fishes.

In the common fowl the ureters descend from the kidneys, which are situated in long and ample cavities on either side of the back, to terminate in the common cavity or cloaca. Their terminations, however, are so obscure and so hidden by the margin of the cavity, that to discover them from without and pass a fine probe into them would be found impossible. Nor is this at all surprising, because in all, even the largest animals, the insertion of the ureters near the neck of the bladder is so tortuous and obscure, that although the urine distils freely from them into the bladder, and calculi even make their way out of them, still neither fluids nor air can be made to enter them by the use of any amount of force. On the other hand, in birds as well as other animals, a probe or a bristle passed downwards from the kidney towards the bladder by the ureters, readily makes its way into the cloaca or bladder.

These facts are particularly distinct in the ostrich, in which, besides the external orifice of the common cavity which the velabrum covers, I find another within the anus, having a round and constricted orifice, shutting in some sort in the manner of a sphincter.

Passing by these particulars, however, let us turn to others that bear more immediately upon our subject. The uterine outlet or vulva, then, or the passage from the common cavity to the uterus of the fowl, is a certain protuberance, soft, lax, wrinkled, and orbicular, resembling the orifice of the prepuce when closed, or appearing as if formed by a prolapse of the internal membrane of the uterus. Now this outlet is situated, as I have said, between the anus and rump, and slightly to the left of the middle line of the body, which Ulysses Aldrovandi imagines to be for the purpose of " facilitating intercourse, and the entrance of the genital organ of the cock." I have myself observed, however, repeatedly, that the hen turned the common orifice to the right or left indifferently, according to the side from which the cock approached her. Neither do I find any penis in the cock—neither, indeed, could Fabricius,—although in the goose and duck it is very conspicuous. But in its stead I discover an orifice in the cock, not otherwise than in the hen, although it is smaller and more contracted in her than in him ; and in the swan, goose, and duck the same thing also appears, the penis of the male goose and duck protruding through this orifice during intercourse.

In a black drake I noticed the penis of such a length that after intercourse it trailed on the ground, and a fowl following, pecked at it greedily, thinking it an earth-worm, as I imagine, so that it was retracted more quickly than usual.

In the male ostrich I have found within this pudendal orifice a very large glans, and the red body of the penis, as we discover them within the prepuce of the horse, resembling a deer's or a small neat's tongue in form and magnitude; and I have frequently observed this organ, rigid and somewhat hooked during the coitus, and when entered into the vulva of the female, held for some considerable time there without any movement : it was precisely as if the two creatures had been fastened together with a nail. Meantime, by the gesticulations of their heads and necks, and by their noises, they seemed to notify their nuptials, and to express the great degree of pleasure they experienced.

I have read in a treatise of Dr. Du Val, a learned physician of Rouen, that a certain hermaphrodite was referred to the surgeons and accoucheurs, that they might determine whether it were a man or a woman. They, from an examination of the genital organs, adjudged the party to be of the feminine gender, and a dress in accordance with this decision was ordered. By and by, however, the individual was accused of soliciting women, and of discharging the man's office ; and then it was found, that from a prepuce, as from the private parts of a woman, a penis protruded, and served to perform the male's business. I have myself occasionally seen the penis of a certain man so greatly shrunk in size, that, unless when excited, nothing was visible in the wrinkled prepuce above the scrotum but the extremity of the glans.

In the horse and some other animals, the principal and ample length of the member is protruded from its concealment. In the mole, too, which is a small animal, there is a remarkable retraction of the penis between the skin and muscles of the belly; and the vulva in the female of this creature is also longer and deeper than usual.

The cock, which is without a penis, performs copulation, as I imagine, in the same manner as the smaller birds, among which the process is rapidly executed, and by mere contact. The orifices of the male and female cloaca, which at the moment are protuberant externally, which, especially in the male, become tense and injected, like the glans penis, encounter, and coition is effected by a succession of salutes, not by any longer intromission of parts, for I do not think that the organs of the cock enter those of the hen at all.

In the copulation of horses, dogs, cats, and the like, the female presents her organ rigid and injected to the penis of the male. And this also takes place in birds which, if they be tame and suffer themselves to be handled, when inflamed with desire present their parts, which will then be found resisting and hard to the finger.

Birds are sometimes so lustful, that if you but stroke their backs gently with your hand, they will immediately lie down and expose and protrude their uterine orifice; and if this part be touched with the finger, they will not fail to proclaim their satisfaction. And that the females may thereby be made to lay eggs, as testified to by Aristotle,[1] I have myself found in the case of the blackbird, thrush, and others. I learned the fact, indeed, in former years by accident, and to my detriment; for my wife had a beautiful parrot, a great pet, learned and talkative enough, and so tame that it was allowed to roam at liberty about the house: when its mistress was absent it sought her everywhere; on her return it caressed her, and loudly proclaimed its joy; when called to it would answer; would fly to its mistress, and then seizing her clothes with beak and feet alternately, it climbed to her shoulder, whence creeping down the arm, it reached her hand, its usual seat. When ordered to speak or to sing, it would obey, although it were the night season and

---

[1] Hist. Anim. lib. vi, cap. 2.

quite dark. Full of play and lasciviousness, it would frequently sit in its mistress's lap, where it loved to have her scratch its head and stroke its back, upon which, fluttering with its wings and making a gentle noise, it testified the pleasure it experienced. I believed all this to proceed from his usual familiarity and love of being noticed ; for I always regarded the creature as a male, by reason of his proficiency in talking and singing. For among birds, the females rarely sing or challenge one another by their note ; the males alone solace their mates by their tuneful warblings, and call them to the rites of love. And it is on this account that Aristotle says,[1] " If partridges be placed over against the males, and the wind blow towards them from where the males sit, they are impregnated and conceive. They even for the most part conceive from the note of the male bird, if they be in season and full of desire. The flight of the male over them will also have the same effect, the male bird casting down a fertilizing influence upon the female." Now this happens especially in the spring season, whence the poet sings :[2]

> Earth teems in Spring, and craves the genial seed.
> The almighty father, Æther, then descends,
> In fertilizing showers, into the lap
> Of his rejoicing spouse, and mingling there
> In wide embrace sustains the progeny
> Innumerous that springs. The pathless woods
> Then ring with the wild bird's song, and flocks and herds
> Disport and spend the livelong day in love.

Not long after the caressings mentioned, the parrot, which had lived in health for many years, fell sick, and by and by being seized with repeated attacks of convulsions, seated in the lap of its mistress, it expired, grievously regretted. Having opened the body in search of the cause of death, I discovered an egg, nearly perfect, in the uterus, but in consequence of the want of a male, in a state of putrefaction ; and this, indeed, frequently happens among birds confined in cages, which show desire for the company of the male.

These and other instances induce me to believe that the

---

[1] Hist. Anim. lib. v, cap. 5, et lib. vi, cap. 2.   [2] Virgil, Georg. 2.

common fowl and the pheasant do not only solace their females with their crowing, but farther give them the faculty of producing eggs by its means; for when the cock crows in the night some of the hens perched near him bestir themselves, clapping their wings and shaking their heads; shuddering and gesticulating as they are wont to do after intercourse.

A certain bird, as large again as a swan, and which the Dutch call a cassowary, was imported no long time ago from the island of Java, in the East Indies, into Holland. Ulysses Aldrovandus[1] gives a figure of this bird, and informs us that it is called an emeu by the Indians. It is not a two-toed bird, like the ostrich, but has three toes on each foot, one of which is furnished with a spur of such length, strength, and hardness, that the creature can easily kick through a board two fingers' breadth in thickness. The cassowary defends itself by kicking forwards. In the body, legs, and thighs it resembles the ostrich; it has not a broad bill like the ostrich however, but one that is rounded and black. On its head, by way of crest, it has an orbicular protuberant horn. It has no tongue, and devours everything that is presented to it—stones, coals, even though alight, pieces of glass—all without distinction. Its feathers sprout in pairs from each particular quill, and are of a black colour, short and slender, approaching to hair or down in their characters. Its wings are very short and imperfect. The whole aspect of the creature is truculent, and it has numbers of red and blue wattles longitudinally disposed along the neck.

This bird remained for more than seven years in Holland, and was then sent, among other presents, by the illustrious Maurice Prince of Orange, to his serene majesty our King James, in whose gardens it continued to live for a period of upwards of five years. By and by, however, when a pair of ostriches, male and female, were brought to the same place, and the cassowary heard and saw these in a neighbouring inclosure, at their amours, unexpectedly it began to lay eggs, excited, as I imagine, through sympathy with the acts of an allied genus; I say unexpectedly, for all who saw the cassowary, judging from the weapons and ornaments, had regarded it as a male rather than a female. Of these eggs, one was laid entire, and this I

---

[1] Ornithol. lib. xx, p. 541.

opened, and found it perfect : the yelk surrounded by the white, the chalazæ attached on either side, and a small cavity in the blunt end ; there was also a cicatricula or macula alba present ; the shell was thick, hard, and strong; and having taken off the top, I had it formed into a cup, in the same way as ostrichs' eggs are commonly fashioned. This egg was somewhat less than that of an ostrich, and, as I have said, perfect in all respects. Undoubtedly, however, it was a sort of accidental egg, and, by reason of the absence of the male, unfruitful. I predicated the death of the cassowary as likely to happen soon when she began laying, moved to do so by what Aristotle says :[1] " Birds become diseased and die unless they produce fruitful eggs." And my prediction came true not long afterwards. On opening the body of the cassowary, I discovered an imperfect and putrid egg in the upper part of the uterus, as the cause of its untimely death, just as I had found the same thing in the parrot, and other instances besides.

Many birds, consequently, the more salacious they are, the more fruitful are they ; and occasionally, when abundantly fed, or from some other cause, they will even lay eggs without the access of the male. It rarely happens, however, that the eggs so produced are either perfected or laid; the birds are commonly soon seized with serious disorders, and at length die. The common fowl nevertheless not only conceives eggs, but lays them, quite perfect in appearance too; but they are always wind eggs, and incapable of producing a chick. In like manner many insects, among the number silkworms and butterflies, conceive eggs and lay them, without the access of the male, but they are still adventitious and barren. Fishes also do the same.

It is of the same significance in these animals when they conceive eggs, as it is in young women when their uterus grows hot, their menses flow, and their bosoms swell—in a word, when they become marriageable ; and who, if they continue too long unwedded, are seized with serious symptoms—hysterics, furor uterinus, &c. or fall into a cachectic state, and distemperatures of various kinds. All animals, indeed, grow savage when in heat, and unless they are suffered to enjoy one another, become

[1] Gen. Anim. lib. iii.

changed in disposition. In like manner women occasionally become insane through ungratified desire, and to such a height does the malady reach in some, that they are believed to be poisoned, or moon-struck, or possessed by a devil. And this would certainly occur more frequently than it does, without the influence of good nurture, respect for character, and the modesty that is innate in the sex, which all tend to tranquillize the inordinate passions of the mind.

EXERCISE THE SIXTH.

Of the uterus of the fowl.

The passage from the external uterine orifice to the internal parts and uterus itself, where the egg is perfected, is by that part which in other animals is called the vagina or vulva. In the fowl, however, this passage is so intricate, and its internal membrane is so loose and wrinkled, that although there is a ready passage from within outwards, and a large egg makes its way through all without much difficulty, still it scarcely seems likely that the penis of the male could penetrate or the spermatic fluid make its way through it; for I have found it impossible to introduce either a probe or a bristle; neither could Fabricius pass anything of the sort, and he says that he could not even inflate the uterus with air. Whence he was led I fancy to give an account of the uterus, proceeding from more internal to more external parts. Considering this structure of the uterus also, he denies that the spermatic fluid of the male can reach the cavity of the uterus, or go to constitute any part of the egg.[1] To this statement I most willingly subscribe; for, indeed, there is nothing in the fruitful egg which is not also in the barren one; there is nothing in the way of addition or change which indicates that the seminal fluid of the male has either made its way into the uterus, or come into contact with the egg. Moreover, although without the access of the cock all eggs laid are winded and barren, still through his influence, and long after inter-

---

[1] Op. cit. p. 31.

course, fruitful eggs are deposited, the rudiments or matter of which did not exist at the time of the communication.

With a view to explaining how the spermatic fluid of the cock renders eggs fecund, Fabricius says :[1] " Since the semen does not appear in the egg, and yet is thrown into the uterus by the cock, it may be asked why this is done if the fluid does not enter the egg ? Farther : if not present in the egg, how is that egg made fruitful by the spermatic fluid of the cock which it yet does not contain ? My opinion is that the semen of the cock thrown into the commencement of the uterus, produces an influence on the whole of the uterus, and at the same time renders fruitful the whole of the yelks, and finally of the perfect eggs which fall into it ; and this the semen effects by its peculiar property or irradiative spirituous substance, in the same manner as we see other animals rendered fruitful by the testicles and semen. For if any one will but bring to mind the incredible change that is produced by castration, when the heat, strength, and fecundity are lost, he will readily admit that what we have proposed may happen in reference to the single uterus of a fowl. But that it is in all respects true, and that the faculty of impregnating the whole of the ova, and also the uterus itself, proceeds from the semen of the cock, appears from the custom of those housewives who keep hens at home but no cock, that they commit their hens for a day or two to a neighbour's cock, and in this short space of time the whole of the eggs that will be laid for a certain season are rendered prolific. And this fact is confirmed by Aristotle,[2] who will have it that, among birds, one intercourse suffices to render almost all the eggs fruitful. For the fecundating influence of the seminal fluid, as it cannot exhale, so is it long retained in the uterus, to which it imparts the whole of its virtue ; nature herself stores it up, placing it in a cavity appended to the uterus, near the fundament, furnished with an entrance only, so that, being there laid up, its virtue is the better preserved and communicated to the entire uterus."

I, however, suspected the truth of the above views, all the more when I saw that the words of the philosopher referred to were not accurately quoted. Aristotle does not say that

---

[1] Op. cit. p. 37.   [2] De Gen. Anim. lib. iii, c. 1.

" Birds which have once copulated almost all continue to lay prolific eggs," but simply " almost all continue to lay eggs ;" the word " prolific" is an addition by Fabricius. But it is one thing to have birds conceiving eggs after intercourse, and another to say that these eggs are fruitful through this intercourse. And this is the more obvious from Aristotle's previous words, where he says, " Nor in the family of birds can those eggs even that are produced by intercourse acquire their full size unless the intercourse between the sexes be continued. And the reason is, that as the menstrual excretion in women is attracted by the intercourse of their husbands, (for the uterus, being warmed, draws the moisture, and the passages are opened,) so in birds it comes to pass that, as the menstruous discharge takes place very gradually, because of its being in small quantity, it cannot make its way externally, but is contained superiorly as high as the waist, and only distils down into the uterus itself. For the egg is increased by this, just as the fœtus of oviparous animals is nourished by that which reaches it through the umbilicus. For when once birds have copulated, almost all continue to lay eggs, but of small size and imperfect ;" and therefore unprolific, for the perfection of an egg is its being fertile. If, therefore, without continued intercourse, not even those eggs that were conceived in consequence of intercourse grow to their proper size, or, as Fabricius interprets it, are " perfected," much less are those eggs prolific which fowls continue to lay independently of intercourse with the male bird.

But lest any one should think that these words, " for the uterus warmed, draws, and the passages are opened," signify that the uterus can attract the semen masculinum into its cavity, let them be aware that the philosopher does not say that the uterus attracts the semen from without into its cavity, but that in females, from the veins and passages, opened by the heat of intercourse, the menstruous blood is attracted from its own body ; so in birds the blood is attracted to the uterus, warmed by repeated intercourse, whereby the eggs grow, as the fœtus of oviparous animals grows through the umbilicus.

But what Fabricius adds upon that cavity or bursa, in which he thinks the semen of the cock may be stored up for a whole year, has been already refuted by us, where we have stated that it contains no seminal fluid, and that it exists in the cock as well as in the hen. Wherefore, though I readily believed (if by fecundity we are to understand a greater number of larger eggs), that the hens of poor people, indifferently fed in all probability, will lay both fewer and smaller eggs unless they have the company of a cock; agreeably to what the philosopher quoted avers, viz.: "that hens which have once been trodden continue to lay larger, better, and a greater number of eggs through the whole of the year," (a result on which the abundance and the good quality of the food has unquestionably a great influence); still that hens should continue for a whole year to lay prolific eggs after a few addresses of the cock, appeared to me by no means probable: for, had a small number of contacts sufficed for the purposes of generation during so long a period, nature, which does nothing in vain, would have constituted the males among birds less salacious than they are; nor should we see the cock soliciting his hens so many times a day, even against their inclination.

We know that the hen, as soon as she quits the nest where she has just laid an egg, cackles loudly, and seems to entice the cock, who on his part crowing lustily, singles her out and straightway treads her, which surely nature had never permitted unless for purposes of procreation.

A male pheasant kept in an aviary was so inflamed with lust, that unless he had the company of several hen-birds, six at the least, he literally maltreated them, though his repeated addresses rather interfered with their breeding than promoted it. I have seen a single hen-pheasant shut up with a cock-bird (which she could in no way escape) so worn out, and her back so entirely stript of feathers through his reiterated assaults, that at length she died exhausted. In the body of this bird, however, I did not discover even the rudiments of eggs.

I have also observed a male duck, having none of his own kind with him, but associating with hens, inflamed with such desire that he would follow a pullet even for several hours, would seize her with his bill, and mounting at length upon the creature, worn out with fatigue, would compel her to submit to his pleasure.

The common cock, victorious in a battle, not only satisfies his desires upon the sultanas of the vanquished, but upon the body of his rival himself.

13

The females of some animals are likewise so libidinous that they excite their males by pecking or biting them gently about the head; they seem as if they whispered into their ears the sweets of love; and then they mount upon their backs and invite them by other arts to fruition: among the number may be mentioned pigeons and sparrows.

It did not therefore appear likely that a few treads, in the beginning of the year, should suffice to render fertile the whole of the eggs that are to be laid in its course.

Upon one occasion, however, in the spring season, by way of helping out Fabricius, and that I might have some certain data as to the time during which the fecundating influence of intercourse would continue, and the necessity of renewed communication, I had a couple of hens separated from the cock for four days, each of which laid three eggs, all of which were prolific. Another hen was secluded, and the egg she laid on the tenth day afterwards was fruitful. The egg which another laid on the twentieth day of her seclusion also produced a chick. It would therefore seem that intercourse, once or twice repeated, suffices to impregnate the whole bunch of yelks, the whole of the eggs that will be laid during a certain season.

I shall here relate another observation which I made at this time. When I returned two of the hens, which I had secluded for a time, to the cock, one of which was big with egg, the other having but just laid, the cock immediately ran to the latter and trod her greedily three or four times; the former he went round and round, tripping himself with his wing and seeming to salute her, and wish her joy of her return; but he soon returned to the other and trod her again and again, even compelling her to submit; the one big with egg, however, he always speedily forsook, and never solicited her to his pleasure. I wondered with myself by what signs he knew that intercourse would advantage one of these hens and prove unavailing to the other. But indeed it is not easy at any time to understand how male animals, even from a distance, know which females are in season and desirous of their company; whether it be by sight, or hearing, or smell, it is difficult to say. Some on merely hearing the voice of the female, or smelling at the place where she has made water, or even the ground over which she has passed, are straightway seized with desire and set off in pursuit to gratify it. But I shall have more to say on this subject in my treatise on the Loves, Lusts, and Sexual Acts of Animals. I return to the matter we have in hand.

Of the abdomen of the common fowl and of other birds.

From the external orifice proceeding through the vulva we come to the uterus of the fowl, in which the egg is perfected, surrounded with the white and covered with its shell. But before speaking of the situation and connections of this part it seems necessary to premise a few words on the particular anatomy of the abdomen of birds. For I have observed that the stomach, intestines, and other viscera of the feathered kinds were otherwise placed in the abdomen, and differently constituted, than they are in quadrupeds.

Almost all birds are provided with a double stomach ; one of which is the crop, the other the stomach, properly so called. In the former the food is stored and undergoes preparation, in the latter it is dissolved and converted into chyme.[1] The familiar names of the two stomachs of birds are the crop or craw, and the gizzard. In the crop the entire grain, &c. that is swallowed is moistened, macerated, and softened, and then it is sent on to the stomach that it may there be crushed and comminuted. For this end almost all the feathered tribes swallow sand, pebbles, and other hard substances, which they preserve in their stomachs, nothing of the sort being found in the crop. Now the stomach in birds consists of two extremely thick and powerful muscles (in the smaller birds they appear both fleshy and tendinous), so placed that, like a pair of millstones connected by means of hinges, they may grind and bruise the food ; the place of teeth, which birds want, being supplied by the stones which they swallow. In this way is the food reduced and turned into chyme[1] ; and then by compression (just as we

---

[1] [The word in the original is *chyle*, for which, in accordance with modern views, chyme is substituted.—ED.]

are wont, after having bruised an herb or a fruit, to squeeze out
the juice or pulp) the softer or more liquid part is forced out,
comes to the top, and is transferred to the commencement of
the intestinal canal; which in birds takes its rise from the upper
part of the stomach near the entrance of the œsophagus. That
this is the case in many genera of birds is obvious; for the
stones and other hard and rough substances which they have
swallowed, if long retained, become so smooth and polished that
they are unfit to comminute the food, when they are discharged.
Hence birds, when they select stones, try them with their
tongue, and, unless they find them rough, reject them. In the
stomach of both the ostrich and cassowary I found pieces of
iron and silver, and stones much worn down and almost reduced
to nothing; and this is the reason why the vulgar believe that
these creatures digest iron and are nourished by it.

If you apply the body of a hawk or an eagle, or other bird of
prey, whilst fasting, to your ear, you will hear a distinct noise,
occasioned by the rubbing, one against another, of the stones
contained in the stomach. For hawks do not swallow pebbles
with a view to cool their stomachs, as falconers commonly but
erroneously believe, but that the stones may serve for the com-
minution of their food; precisely as other birds, which have muscular stomachs, swallow pebbles, sand, or something else of the
same nature, to crush and grind the seeds upon which they live.

The stomach of birds, then, is situated within the cavity of
the abdomen, below the heart, lungs and liver: the crop, however, is without the body in some sort, being situated at the
lower part of the neck, over the os jugale or merry-thought. In
this bag, as I have said, the food is only macerated and softened;
and several birds regurgitate and give it to their young, in
some measure as quadrupeds feed their progeny with milk from
their breasts; this occurs in the whole family of the pigeons,
and also among rooks. Bees, too, when they have returned to
their hives, disgorge the honey which they have collected from
the flowers and concocted in their stomachs, and store it in
their waxen cells; and so also do hornets and wasps feed their
young. The bitch has likewise been seen to vomit the food
which she had eaten some time before, in a half-digested state,
and give it to her whelps: it is not, therefore, to be greatly

wondered at, if we see the poor women, who beg from door to door, when their milk fails, feeding their infants with food which they have chewed and reduced to a pulp in their own mouths.

The intestines commence in birds, as has been said, from the upper part of the stomach, and are folded up and down in the line of the longitudinal direction of the body, not transversely as in man. Immediately below the heart, about the waist, and where the diaphragm is situated in quadrupeds, for birds have no [muscular] diaphragm, we find the liver, of ample size, divided into two lobes situated one on either side (for birds have no spleen,) and filling the hypochondria. The stomach lies below the liver, and downwards from the stomach comes the mass of intestines, with numerous delicate membranes, full of air, interposed; the trachea opening in birds, as already stated, by several gaping orifices into membranous abdominal cells. The kidneys, which are of large size in birds, are of an oblong shape, look as if they were made up of fleshy vesicles, without cavities, and lie along the spine on either side, with the descending aorta and vena cava abdominalis adjacent; they further extend into and seem to lie buried within ample cavities of the ossa ilia. The ureters proceed from the anterior aspects of the kidneys, and run longitudinally towards the cloaca and podex, in which they terminate, and into which they pour the liquid excretion of the kidneys. This, however, is not in any great quantity in birds, because they drink little, and some of them, the eagle for example, not at all. Nor is the urine discharged separately and by itself, as in other animals; but, as we have said, it distils from the ureters into the common cloaca, which is also the recipient of the fæces, and the discharge of which it facilitates. The urine is also different in birds from what it is in other animals; for, as the urine in the generality of animals consists of two portions, one more serous and liquid, another thicker, which, in healthy subjects constitutes the hypostasis or sediment, and subsides when the urine becomes cold; so is it in birds, but the sedimentary portion is the more abundant, and is distinguished from the liquid by its white or silvery colour; nor is this sediment met with only in the cloaca, (where it abounds, indeed, and surrounds the fæces,) but in the whole course of the ureters, which are distinguished from the coverings of the kidneys by their white colour. Nor is it only in birds that

this abundant thicker renal secretion is seen; it is conspicuous
in serpents and other ovipara, particularly in those whose eggs
are covered with a harder or firmer membrane. And here, too,
is the thicker in larger proportion than the thinner and more
serous portion; its consistency being midway between thick
urine and stercoraceous excrement: so that, in its passage
through the ureters, it resembles coagulated or inspissated
milk; once discharged it soon concretes into a friable mass.

EXERCISE THE EIGHTH.

Of the situation and structure of the remaining parts of
the fowl's uterus.

Between the stomach and the liver, over the spine, and
where, in man and other animals the pancreas is situated;
between the trunk of the porta and the descending cava; at
the origin of the renal and spermatic arteries, and where the
cæliac artery plunges into the mesentery, there, in the fowl
and other birds, do the ovary and the cluster of yelks present
themselves; having in their front the trunk of the porta, the
gullet, and the orifice of the stomach: behind them, the vena
cava and the aorta descending along the spine; above the liver,
and beneath the stomach, lie adjacent. The infundibulum,
therefore, which is a most delicate membrane, descends from
the ovary longitudinally with the spine, between it and the
gizzard. And from the infundibulum (between the gizzard,
the intestines, the kidneys, and the loins,) the processus uteri
or superior portion of this organ descends with a great many
turnings and cells (like the colon and rectum in man), into the
uterus itself. Now the uterus, which is continuous with this
process, is situated below the gizzard, between the loins, the
kidneys, and the rectum, in the lower part of the abdomen,
close to the cloaca; so that the egg surrounded with its white,
which the uterus contains, is situated so low that, with the
fingers, it is easy to ascertain whether it be soft or hard, and
near the laying.

The uterus in the common fowl varies both in point of size

and of structure. In the fowl that is with egg, or that has lately laid, it is very different from what it is in the pullet, the uterus of which is fleshy and round, like an empty purse, and its cavity so insignificant that it would scarcely contain a bean; smooth externally, it is wrinkled and occupied by a few longitudinal plicæ internally: at first sight you might very well mistake it either for a large urinary bladder or for a second smaller stomach. In the gravid state, however, and in the fowl arrived at maturity (a fact which is indicated by the redder colour of the comb), the uterus is of much larger dimensions and far more fleshy; its plicæ are also larger and thicker, it in general approaches the size which we should judge necessary to receive an egg; it extends far upwards in the direction of the spinal column, and consists of numerous divisions or cells, formed by replications of the extended uterus, similar to those of the colon in quadrupeds and man. The inferior portion of the uterus, as the largest and thickest, and most fleshy of all, is strengthened by many plicæ of large size. Its configuration internally is oval, as if it were the mould of the egg. The ascending or produced portion of the uterus I designate the processus uteri: this part Fabricius calls the "uterus secundus," and says that it consists of three spiral turns or flexures; Ulyssus Aldrovandus, again, names it the "stomachum uteri." I must admit that in this part there are usually three turns to be observed; they are not, however, by any means so regular but that, as in the case of the cells of the colon, nature sometimes departs from her usual procedure here.

The uterus as it ascends higher, so does it become ever the thinner and more delicate, containing fewer and smaller plicæ, until at length going off into a mere membrane, and that of the most flimsy description, it constitutes the infundibulum; which, reaching as high as the waist or cincture of the body, embraces the entire ovary.

On this account, therefore, Fabricius describes the uterus as consisting of three portions; viz., the commencement, the middle, and the end. "The commencement," says he, "degenerating into a thin and most delicate membrane, forms an ample orifice, and bears a resemblance to an open-mouthed tube or funnel. The next portion (which I call the processus uteri), consisting of three transverse spiral turns, serves for the

supply of the albumen, and extends downwards to the most
inferior and capacious portion—the termination of the uterus—
in which the chalazæ, the two membranes, and the shell are
formed.[1]"

The whole substance of the uterus, particularly the parts
about the plicæ, both in its body and in its process, are covered
with numerous ramifications of blood-vessels, the majority of
which are arterial rather than venous branches.

The folds which appear oblique and transverse in the interior
of the uterus are fleshy substances; they have a fine white or
milky colour, and a sluggish fluid oozes from them, so that the
whole of the interior of the uterus, as well the body as the
process, is moistened with an abundance of thin albumen,
whereby the vitellus as it descends is increased, and the albumen
that is deposited around it is gradually perfected.

The uterus of the fowl is rarely found otherwise than containing an egg, either sticking in the spiral process or arrived
in the body of the organ. If you inflate this process when it is
empty it then presents itself as an oblique and contorted tube,
and rises like a turbinated shell or cone into a point. The
general arrangement of the spirals and folds composing the
uterus, is such as we have already observed it in the vulva:
there is a ready enough passage for the descending egg, but
scarce any return even for air blown in towards the superior
parts.

The processus uteri with its spirals, very small in the young
pullet, is so much diminished in the hen which has ceased laying,
that it shrinks into the most delicate description of membrane,
and then entirely disappears, so that no trace of it remains, any
more than of the ovary or infundibulum: nothing but a certain
glandular-looking and spongy mass appears in the place these
bodies occupied, which in a boiled fowl tastes sweet, and bears
some affinity to the pancreas and thymus of young mammiferous
animals, which, in the vernacular tongue, are called the sweetbread.

The uterus and the processus uteri are connected with the
back by means of a membranous attachment, which Fabricius
designates by the name of " mesometrium; because the second
uterus, together with this vascular and membranous body, may

[1] Fab. l. c. p. 17.

very fairly be compared with the intestines and the mesentery." For, as the intestine is bound down by the mesentery, so is this portion of the uterus attached to the spinal column by an oblong membranous process; lest by being too loose, and getting twisted, the passage of the yelks should be interfered with, instead of having a free and open transit afforded them as at present. The mesometrium also transmits numerous blood-vessels surcharged with blood, to each of the folds of the uterus. In its origin, substance, structure, use, and office, this part is therefore analogous to the mesentery. Moreover, from the fundus of the uterus lengthwise, and extending even to the infundibulum, there is a ligament bearing some resemblance to a tape-worm, similar to that which we notice in the upper part of the colon. It is as if a certain portion or stripe of the external tunic had been condensed and shortened in such a manner that the rest of the process is thrown into folds and cells: were you to draw a thread through a piece of intestine taken out of the body, and to tie this thread firmly on one side, you would cause the other side of the bowel to pucker up into wrinkles and cells; [even so is it with the uterus of the fowl.]

This then, in brief, is the structure of the uterus in the fowl that is laying eggs: fleshy, large, extensible both longitudinally and transversely, tortuous or winding in spirals and convolutions from the cloaca upwards, in the line of the vertebral column, and continued into the infundibulum.

EXERCISE THE NINTH.

Of the extrusion of the egg, or parturition of the fowl, in general.

The yelk, although only a minute speck in the ovary, gaining by degrees in depth of colour and increasing in size, gradually acquires the dimensions and characters that distinguish it at last. Cast loose from the cluster, it descends by the infundibulum, and, transmitted through the spirals and cells of the processus uteri, it becomes surrounded with albumen; and this, without in any place adhering to the uterus (as was rightly observed by Fabricius in opposition to Aristotle), or growing by means of any system of umbilical vessels; but as the eggs of

fishes and frogs, when extruded and laid in the water provide
and surround themselves with albumen, or as beans, vetches,
and other seeds and grains swell when moistened, and thence
supply nourishment to the germs that spring from them, so,
from the folds of the uterus that have been described, as from
an udder, or uterine placenta, an albuminous fluid exudes,
which the vitellus, in virtue of its inherent vegetative heat and
faculty, attracts and digests into the surrounding white. There
is, indeed, an abundance of fluid having the taste of albumen,
contained in the cavity of the uterus and entangled between the
folds that cover its interior. In this way does the yelk,
descending by degrees, become surrounded with albumen, until
at last, having in the extreme part of the uterus acquired a
covering of firmer membranes and a harder shell, it is perfected
and rendered fit for extrusion.

EXERCISE THE TENTH.

Of the increase and nutrition of the egg.

Let us hear Fabricius on these topics. He says : " As the
action of the stomach is to prepare the chyle, and that of
the testes to secrete the seminal fluid, (because in the stomach
chyle is discovered, and in the testes semen,) so we declare
the act of the uterus in birds to be the production of eggs,
because eggs are found there. But this, as it appears, is not
the only action of uteri; to it must be added the increase of the
egg, which succeeds immediately upon its production, and which
proceeds until it is perfected and attains its due size. For a
fowl does not naturally lay an egg until it is perfect and has
attained to its proper dimensions. The office of the uterus is,
therefore, the growth as well as the generation of the egg; but
growth implies and includes the idea of nutrition ; and, as
all generation is the act of two principles, one the agent,
another the matter, the agent in the production of eggs is
nothing else than the organs or instruments indicated, viz., the
compound uterus; and the matter nothing but the blood."

We, studious of brevity, and shunning all controversy, as in duty bound, as we readily admit that the office and use of the uterus is the procreation of the egg, so do we maintain the "adequate efficient," as it has been called, the immediate agent to inhere in the egg itself; and we assert farther, that the egg is both engendered and made to increase, not by the uterus, but by a certain natural principle peculiar to itself; and that this principle flows from the whole fowl into the rudiments of the vitellus, and whilst it was yet but a speck, and under the influence either of the calidum innatum or of nature, causes it to be nourished and to grow; just as there is a certain faculty in every particle of the body which secures its nutrition and growth.

As regards the manner in which the yelk is surrounded by the albumen, Aristotle appears to have believed [1] that in the sharp end of the egg (where he placed the commencement of the egg), whilst it was yet surrounded by soft membranes, there existed an umbilical canal, by which it was nourished; a view which Fabricius[2] challenges, denying that there is any such canal, or that the vitellus has any kind of connexion with the uterus. He farther lessens the doubt in regard to the albumen of the extruded egg, observing, that "the egg increases in a two-fold manner, inasmuch as the uterus consists of two portions, one superior, another inferior; and the egg itself consists of two matters—the yelk and the white. The yelk increases with a true growth, to wit, by means of the blood, which is sent to it through the veins whilst it is yet connected with the vitellarium. The albumen, however, increases and grows otherwise than the yelk; viz., not by means of the veins, nor by proper nutrition like the yelk, but, by juxtaposition, adhering to the vitellus as it is passing through the second uterus."

But my opinion is, that the egg increases everywhere in the same manner as the yelk does in the cluster; viz. by an inherent concocting principle; with this single difference, that in the ovary the nourishment is brought to it by means of vessels, whilst in the uterus it finds that which it imbibes already prepared for it. Juxtaposition of parts is equally necessary in every kind of nutrition and growth, and so also are concoction and distribution of the applied nutriment. Nor is one of these to be less accounted true nutrition than the other, inas-

[1] De Generat. Animal. lib. iii, cap. 2.   [2] Op cit. p. 11.

much as in both there is accession of new aliment, apposition, agglutination, and transmutation of particles. Nor can vetches or beans, when they attract moisture from the earth through their skins, imbibing it like sponges, be said with less propriety to be nourished than if they had obtained the needful moisture through the mouths of veins; and trees, when they absorb the dew and the rain through their bark, are as truly nourished as when they pump them in by their roots. With reference to the mode in which nutrition is effected, we have set down much in another place. It is another difficulty that occupies us at this time, viz., whether the yelk, whilst it is acquiring the white, does not make a certain separation and distinction in it; whether, in the course of the increase, a more earthy portion does not subside into the yelk or middle of the egg as towards the centre, which Aristotle believed, and another lighter portion surrounds this. For between the yelk which is still in the cluster, and the yelk which is found in the middle of a perfect egg, there is this principal difference, that although the former be of a yellow colour, still, in point of consistence, it rather resembles the white; and by boiling, it is, like the latter, thickened, compacted, inspissated, and becomes divisible into layers; whilst the yelk of the perfect egg is rendered friable by boiling, and is rather of an earthy consistency, not thick and gelatinous like albumen.

EXERCISE THE ELEVENTH.

Of the covering or shell of the egg.

It will now be proper, having spoken of the production of eggs, to treat of their parts and diversities. " An egg," says Fabricius, " consists of a yelk, the albumen, two chalazæ, three membranes, viz. one proper to the vitellus, two common to the entire egg, and a shell. To these two others are to be added, which, however, cannot be correctly reckoned among the parts of an egg; one of these is a small cavity in the blunt end of the egg, under the shell; the other is a very small white spot, a kind of round cicatricula connected with the surface of the yelk. The history of each of these parts and accidents must now be given more particularly, and we shall begin from without and proceed inwards.

" The external covering of the egg, called by Pliny the cortex and putamen, by Quintus Serenus the testa ovi, is a hard but thin, friable and porous covering, of different colours in different cases—white, light green, speckled, &c. All eggs are not furnished with a shell on their extrusion: the eggs of serpents have none; and some fowls occasionally, though rarely, lay eggs that are without shells. The shell, though everywhere hard, is not of uniform hardness; it is hardest towards the upper end." From this Fabricius[1] opines that we are to doubt as to the matter of which, and the season at which the shells of eggs are produced. Aristotle[2] and Pliny[3] affirm that the shell is not formed within the body of the fowl, but when the egg is laid; and that as it issues it sets by coming in contact with the air, the internal heat driving off moisture. And this, says Aristotle,[4] is so arranged to spare the animal pain, and to render the process of parturition more easy. An egg softened in vinegar is said to be easily pushed into a vessel with a narrow mouth.

Fabricius was long indisposed to this opinion, " because he had found an egg within the body of the fowl covered with a hard shell; and housewives are in the daily practice of trying the bellies of their hens with their fingers in order that they may know by the hardness whether the creatures are likely to lay that day or not." But by-and-by, when " he had been assured by women worthy of confidence, that the shells of eggs became hardened in their passage into the air, which dissipates a certain moisture diffused over the egg on its exit, fixing it in the shell not yet completely hardened;" and having afterwards " confirmed this by his own experience," he altered his opinion, and came to the conclusion, " that the egg surrounded with a shell, and having a consistency betwixt hard and soft, hardened notably at the moment of its extrusion, in consequence, according to Aristotle's views, of the concretion and dissipation of the thinner part of a certain viscid and tenacious humour, bedewed with which the egg is extruded; sticking to the recent shell this humour is dried up and hardened, the cold of the

---

[1] Loc. cit. p. 13.   [2] Hist. Anim. lib. vi, c. 2, et de Gen. Anim. lib. i, c. 8.
[3] Hist. Anim. lib. x, c. 52.   [4] De Gener. Anim. lib. iii, c. 2.

ambient air contributing somewhat to the effect. Of all this," he says, " you will readily be satisfied if you have a fowl in the house, and dexterously catch the egg in your hand as it is dropping."

I was myself long fettered by this statement of Aristotle, indeed until certain experience had assured me of its erroneousness; for I found the egg still contained in the uterus, almost always covered with a hard shell; and I once saw an egg taken from the body of a living fowl, and still warm, without a shell but covered with a tenacious moisture; this egg, however, did not acquire any hardness through the concretion or evaporation of the moisture in question, as Fabricius would have us believe, neither was it in any way changed by the cold of the surrounding air; but it retained the same degree of softness which it had had in the uterus.

I have also seen an egg just laid by a fowl, surrounded by a complete shell, and this shell covered externally with a soft and membranous skin, which however did not become hard. I have farther seen another hen's egg covered with a shell everywhere except at the extremity of the sharp end, where a certain small and soft projection remained, very likely such as was taken by Aristotle for the remains of an umbilicus.

Fabricius, therefore, appears to me to have wandered from the truth; nor was I ever so dexterous as to catch an egg in its exit, and discover it in the state between soft and hard. And this I confidently assert, that the shell is formed internally, or in the uterus, and not otherwise than all the other parts of the egg, viz. by the peculiar plastic power. A statement which I make all the more confidently because I have seen a very small egg covered with a shell, contained within another larger egg, perfect in all respects, and completely surrounded with a shell. An egg of this kind Fabricius calls an ovum centeninum; and our housewives ascribe it to the cock. This egg I showed to his serene Majesty King Charles, my most gracious master, in the presence of many persons. And the same year, in cutting up a large lemon, I found another perfect but very small lemon included within it, having a yellow rind like the other; and I hear that the same thing has frequently been seen in Italy.

It is a common mistake with those who pursue philosophical studies in these times, to seek for the cause of diversity of parts in diversity of the matter whence they arise. Thus medical men assert that the several parts of the body are both engendered and nourished by diverse matters, either the blood or the seminal fluid; viz. the softer parts, such as the flesh, by the thinner matter, the harder and more earthy parts, such as the bones, &c. by the firmer and thicker matter. But we have elsewhere refuted this too prevalent error. Nor do they err less who, with Democritus, compose all things of atoms; or with Empedocles, of elements. As if *generation* were nothing more than a separation, or aggregation, or disposition of things. It is not indeed to be denied, that when one thing is to be produced from another, all these are necessary, but generation itself is different from them all. I find Aristotle to be of this opinion; and it is my intention, by-and-by, to teach that out of the same albumen (which all allow to be uniform, not composed of diverse parts,) all the parts of the chick, bones, nails, feathers, flesh, &c. are produced and nourished. Moreover, they who philosophize in this way, assign a material cause [for generation], and deduce the causes of natural things either from the elements concurring spontaneously or accidentally, or from atoms variously arranged; they do not attain to that which is first in the operations of nature and in the generation and nutrition of animals; viz. they do not recognize that efficient cause and divinity of nature which works at all times with consummate art, and providence, and wisdom, and ever for a certain purpose, and to some good end; they derogate from the honour of the Divine Architect, who has not contrived the shell for the defence of the egg with less of skill and of foresight than he has composed all the other parts of the egg of the same matter, and produced it under the influence of the same formative faculty.

Although what has already been said be the fact, namely, that the egg, even whilst contained in the uterus, is provided with a hard shell, still the authority of Aristotle has always such weight with me that I never think of differing from him inconsiderately; and I therefore believe, and my observations bear me out in so much, that the shell does gain somewhat in solidity from the ambient air upon its extrusion; that the sluggish and slippery fluid with which it is moistened when laid, immediately becomes hardened on its exposure to the air. For the shell, whilst the egg is in the uterus, is much thinner and more transparent, and smoother on the surface; when laid, however, the shell is thicker, less translucid, and the surface is rough—it appears as if it were powdered over with a fine white dust which had but just adhered to it.

Let us, as we are upon this subject, expatiate a little :—

In the desert islands of the east coast of Scotland, such flights of almost every kind of sea-fowl congregate, that were I to state what I have heard from parties very worthy of credit, I fear I should be held guilty of telling greater stories than they who have committed themselves in regard to the Scottish geese produced, as they say, from the fruits of certain trees that had fallen into the sea. These geese the narrators themselves had never seen so produced; but I will here relate that which I have myself witnessed.

There is a small island which the Scots call the Bass Island (and speaking of this one will suffice for all), situated in the open ocean, not far from the shore, of the most abrupt and precipitous character, so that it rather resembles one huge rock or stone than an island, and indeed it is not more than a mile in circumference. The surface of this island in the months of May and June is almost completely covered with nests, eggs, and young birds, so that you can scarce find free footing anywhere; and then such is the density of the flight of the old birds above, that like a cloud they darken the sun and the sky; and such the screaming and din that you can scarce hear the voice of one who addresses you. If you turn your eyes below, and from your lofty stance and precipice regard the sea, there you perceive on all sides around an infinite variety of different kinds of sea-fowl swimming about in pursuit of their prey: the face of the ocean is very like that of a pool in the spring season, when it appears swarming with frogs; or to those sunny hills and cliffy mountains looked at from below, that are covered with numerous flocks of sheep and goats. If you sail round the island and look up, you see on every ledge and shelf, and recess, innumerable flocks of birds of almost every size and order; more numerous than the stars that appear in the unclouded moonless sky; and if you regard the flights that incessantly come and go you may imagine that it is a mighty swarm of bees you have before you. I should scarcely be credited did I name the revenue which was annually derived from the feathers, the eggs, and the old nests, which, as useful for firing, are all made objects of traffic by the proprietor; the sum he mentioned to me exceeds credibility. There was this particular feature which, as it refers to our subject, I shall mention, and also as it bears me out in my report of the multitudes of sea-fowl: the whole island appears of a brilliant white colour to those who approach it,—all the cliffs look as if they consisted of the whitest chalk; the true colour of the rock, however, is dusky and black. It is a friable white crust that is spread over all, which gives the island its whiteness and splendour, a crust, having the same consistency, colour, and nature as an egg-shell, which plasters everything with a hard, though friable and testaceous kind of covering. The lower part of the rock, laved by the ebbing and flowing tide, preserves its native colour, and clearly shows that the whiteness of the superior parts is due to the liquid excrements of the birds, which are voided along with the alvine fæces; which liquid excrements, white, hard, and brittle like the shell of the egg, cover the rock, and, under the influence of the cold of the air, incrust it. Now this is precisely the way in which Aristotle and Pliny will have it that the shell of the egg is formed. None of the birds are permanent occupants of the island, but visitors for purposes of procreation only, staying there for a few weeks, in lodgings, as it were, and until their young ones can take wing along with them. The white crust is so hard and solid, and adheres so intimately to the rock, that it might readily be mistaken for the natural soil of the place.

The liquid, white, and shining excrement is conveyed from the kidneys of birds by the ureters, into the common receptacle or cloaca; where it covers over the alvine fæces, and with them is discharged. It constitutes, in fact, the thicker portion of the urine of these creatures, and corresponds with that which, in our urine, we call the hypostase or sediment. We have already said something above on this topic, and have entered into it still more fully elsewhere. We always find an abundance of this white excrement in mews; where hawks besmear walls beside their perches, they cover them with a kind of gypseous crust, or make them look as if they were painted with white lead.

In the cloaca of a dead ostrich I found as much of this gypseous cement as would have filled the hand. And in like

14

manner the same substance abounds in tortoises and other oviparous animals; discharged from the body it soon concretes either into a friable crust, or into a powder which greatly resembles pulverized egg-shells, in consequence of the evaporation of its thinner part.

Among the many different kinds of birds which seek the Bass island for the sake of laying and incubating their eggs, and which have such variety of nests, one bird was pointed out to me which lays but one egg, and this it places upon the point of a rock, with nothing like a nest or bed beneath it, yet so firmly that the mother can go and return without injury to it; but if any one move it from its place, by no art can it be fixed or balanced again; left at liberty, it straightway rolls off and falls into the sea. The place, as I have said, is crusted over with a white cement, and the egg, when laid, is bedewed with a thick and viscid moisture, which setting speedily, the egg is soldered as it were, or agglutinated to the subjacent rock.

An instance of like rapid concretion may be seen any day at a statuary's, when he uses his cement of burnt alabaster or gypsum tempered with water; by means of which the likeness of one dead, or the cast of anything else may be speedily taken, and used as a mould.

There is also in like manner a certain earthy or solid something in almost all liquids, as, for example, tartar in wine, mud or sand in water, salt in lixivium, which, when the greater portion of the water has been dissipated, concretes and subsides; and so do I conceive the white sediment of birds to descend along with the urine from the kidneys into the cloaca, and there to cover over and incrust the egg, much as the pavement of a mews is plastered over by falcons, and every cliff of the aforementioned island by the birds that frequent it; much also as chamber utensils, and places where many persons make water, become covered with a yellow incrustation; that substance, in fact, concreting externally, of which calculi in the kidneys, bladder, and other parts are formed. I did formerly believe then, as I have said, persuaded especially by the authority of Aristotle and Pliny, that the shell of the hen's egg was formed of this white sediment, which abounds in all the oviparous animals whose eggs are laid with a hard shell, the matter concreting through contact with the air when the egg was laid. And so many additional observations have since strengthened this conclusion, that I can scarcely keep from believing that some part at least of the shell is thus produced.

Nevertheless, I would say with Fabricius : " Let all reasoning be silent when experience gainsays its conclusions." The too familiar vice of the present age is to obtrude as manifest truths, mere fancies, born of conjecture and superficial reasoning, altogether unsupported by the testimony of sense.

For I have very certainly discovered that the egg still contained in the uterus, in these countries at least, is covered with its shell; although Aristotle and Pliny assert the contrary, and Fabricius thinks that "it is not to be too obstinately gainsaid." In warmer places, perhaps, and where the fowls are stronger, the eggs may be extruded soft, and for the most part without shells. With us this very rarely happens. When I was at Venice in former years, Aromatarius, a learned physician, showed me a small leaf which had grown between the two valves of a peascod, whilst with us there is nothing more apparent in these pods than a small point where the germ is about to be produced. So much do a milder climate, a brighter sky, and a softer air, conduce to increase and rapidity of growth.

EXERCISE THE TWELFTH.

Of the remaining parts of the egg.

We have already spoken partially of the place where, the time when, and the manner how the remaining parts of the egg are engendered, and we shall have something more to add when we come to speak of their several uses.

" The albumen," says Fabricius,[1] " is the *ovi albus liquor* of Pliny, the *ovi candidum* of Celsus, the *ovi albor* of Palladius, the *ovi album et albumentum* of Apicius, the λευκὸν of the Greeks, the ὠοῦ λεύκωμα of Aristotle, the ὄρνιθος γάλα, or bird's milk of Anaxagoras. This is the cold, sluggish, white fluid of the egg, of different thickness at different places (thinner at the blunt and sharp ends, thicker in other situations,) and also in

[1] Loc. cit. p. 22.

variable quantity (for it is more abundant at the blunt end, less so at the sharp end, and still less so in the other parts of the egg), covering and surrounding the yelk on every side."

In the hen's egg, however, I have observed that there are not only differences in the albumen, but two albumens, each surrounded with its proper membrane. One of these is thinner, more liquid, and almost of the same consistence as that humour which, remaining among the folds of the uterus, we have called the matter and nourishment of the albumen; the other is thicker, more viscid, and rather whiter in its colour, and in old and stale eggs, and those that have been sat upon for some days, it is of a yellowish cast. As this second albumen everywhere surrounds the yelk, so is it, in like manner, itself surrounded by the more external fluid. That these two albumens are distinct appears from this, that if after having removed the shell you pierce the two outermost membranes, you will perceive the external albuminous liquid to make its escape, and the membranes to become collapsed and to sink down in the dish; the internal and thicker albumen, however, all the while retains its place and globular figure, inasmuch as it is bounded by its proper membrane, although this is of such tenuity that it entirely escapes detection by the eye; but if you then prick it, the second albumen will forthwith begin to flow out, and the mass will lose its globular shape; just as the water contained in a bladder escapes when it is punctured; in like manner the proper investing membrane of the vitellus being punctured, the yellow fluid of which it consists escapes, and the original globular form is destroyed.

"The vitellus," says Fabricius,[1] "is so called from the word vita, because the chick lives upon it; from its colour it is also spoken of as the yellow of the egg, having been called by the Greeks generally, χρυσὸν, by Hippocrates χλωρὸν, and by Aristotle ὦχρὸν and λεκυθὸν; the ancients, such as Suidas in Menander, called it νεοττὸν, i. e. the chick, because they believed the chick to be engendered from this part. It is the smoothest portion of the egg, and is contained within a most delicate membrane, immediately escaping if this be torn, and losing all figure; it is sustained in the middle of the egg; and in one egg

---

[1] Op. cit. p. 23.

is of a yellow colour, in another of a tint between white and yellow; it is quite round, of variable size, according to the size of the bird that lays the egg, and, according to Aristotle, of a deeper yellow in water birds, of a paler hue in land birds." The same author[1] also maintains that "the yellow and the white of an egg are of opposite natures, not only in colour but in qualities; for the yellow is inspissated by cold, which the white is not, but is rather rendered more liquid; and the white, on the contrary, is thickened by heat, which the yellow is not, unless it be burned or over-done, and it is more hardened and dried by boiling than by roasting." As in the macrocosm the earth is placed in the centre, and is surrounded by the water and the air, so is the yelk, the more earthy part of the egg, surrounded by two albuminous layers, one thicker, another thinner. And, indeed, Aristotle[2] says that, "if we put a number of yelks and whites together, and mix them in a pan, and then boil them with a slow and gentle fire, that the whole of the yelks will set into a globular mass in the middle, and appear surrounded by the whites." But many physicians have been of opinion that the white was the colder portion of the egg. Of these matters, however, more by and by.

The chalazæ, the treads or treadles (gralladura Ital.) are two in number in each egg, one in the blunt, another in the sharp end. The larger portion of them is contained in the white; but they are most intimately connected with the yelk, and with its membrane. They are two long-shaped bodies, firmer than the albumen and whiter; knotty, not without a certain transparency like hail, whence their name; each chalaza, in fact, is made up of several hailstones, as it seems, connected by means of albumen. One of them is larger than the other, and this extends from the yelk towards the blunt end of the egg; the other and smaller chalaza stretches from the yelk towards the sharp end of the egg. The larger is made up of two or three knots or seeming hailstones, at a trifling distance from one another, and of successively smaller size.

The chalazæ are found in the eggs of all birds, and in wind and unprolific as well as in perfect or prolific eggs, duly disposed in both their extremities. Whence the supposition

---

[1] Hist. Anim. lib. vi, cap. 2.   [2] Hist. Anim. et De Gen. Anim. lib. iii, c. 1.

among housewives that the chalazæ are the tread or spermatic fluid of the cock, and that the chick is generated from them is discovered to be a vulgar error.   But Fabricius himself, although he denies that they consist of the semen of the cock, still gives various reasons for maintaining that " they are the immediate matter which the cock fecundates, and from which the chick is produced ;" a notion which he seeks to prop by this feeble statement : " because in a boiled egg, the chalazæ are so contracted on themselves that they present the figure of a chick already formed and hatched." But it is not likely that several rudiments of a single fœtus should be wanted in one egg, neither has any one ever discovered the rudiments of the future chick save in the blunt end of the egg.   Moreover the chalazæ present no sensible difference in eggs that are fecundated by the intercourse of the two sexes, from those of eggs that are barren.   Our distinguished author is therefore mistaken in regard to the use of the chalazæ in the egg, as shall farther be made to appear by and by.

In the eggs of even the smallest birds there is a slender filament, the rudiments of the chalazæ, to be discovered ; and in those of the ostrich and cassowary I have found, in either end of the egg very thick chalazæ, of great length, and very white colour, made up of several globules gradually diminishing in size.

A small cavity is observed in the inside of an egg under the shell, at the blunt end ; sometimes exactly in the middle, at other times more to one side, almost exactly corresponding to the chalaza that lies below it.   The figure of this cavity is generally circular, though in the goose and duck it is not exactly so.   It is seen as a dark spot if you hold an egg opposite a candle in a dark place, and apply your hand edgeways over the blunt end.   In the egg just laid it is of small size,—about the size of the pupil of the human eye ; but it grows larger daily as the egg is older, and the air is warmer ; it is much increased after the first day of incubation ; as if by the exhalation of some of the more external and liquid albumen the remainder contracted, and left a larger cavity ; for the cavity in question is produced between the shell and the membrane which surrounds the whole of the fluids of the egg.   It is met with in all eggs ; I have discovered it, even in those that are still contained in the uterus, as soon as they had become invested with the shell.

They who are curious in such matters say that if this cavity be in the point or end of the egg it will produce a male, if towards the side, a female. This much is certain : if the cavity be small it indicates that the egg is fresh-laid; if large, that it is stale. But we shall have occasion anon to say more on this head.

There is a white and very small circle apparent in the investing membrane of the vitellus, which looks like an inbranded cicatrice, which Fabricius therefore calls cicatricula; but he makes little of this spot, and looks on it rather as an accident or blemish than as any essential part of the egg. The cicatricula in question is extremely small; not larger than a tiny lentil, or the pupil of a small bird's eye; white, flat, and circular. This part is also found in every egg, and even from its commencement in the vitellarium. Fabricius, therefore, is mistaken when he thinks that this spot is nothing more than the trace or cicatrice of the severed peduncle, by which the egg was in the first instance connected with the ovary. For the peduncle, as he himself admits, is hollow, and as it approaches the vitellus expands, so as to surround or embrace, and inclose the yelk in a kind of pouch : it is not connected with the yelk in the same way as the stalks of apples and other fruits are infixed, and so as to leave any cicatrice when the yelk is cast loose. And if you sometimes find two cicatriculæ in a large yelk, as Fabricius states, this might, perhaps, lead to the production of a monster and double fœtus, (as shall be afterwards shown), but would be no indication of the preexistence of a double peduncle. He is, however, immensely mistaken when he imagines that the cicatricula serves no purpose; for it is, in fact, the most important part of the whole egg, and that for whose sake all the others exist; it is that, in a word, from which the chick takes its rise. Parisanus, too, is in error, when he contends that this is the semen of the cock.

Of the diversities of eggs.

" The word ovum, or egg, is taken in a twofold sense, proper and improper. An ovum, properly so designated, I call that body to which the definition given by Aristotle[1] applies: An egg, says he, is that from part of which an animal is engendered, and the remainder of which is food for the animal so produced. But I hold that body to be improperly styled an egg which is defined by Aristotle[2] in the same place, to be that from the whole of which an animal is engendered; such as the eggs of ants, flies, spiders, some butterflies, and others of the tribe of extremely small eggs; which Aristotle almost always fears to commit himself by calling eggs, but which he rather styles vermiculi." What precedes is from Fabricius;[3] but we, whose purpose it is to treat especially of the generation of the hen's egg, have no intention to speak of the differences of all kinds of eggs; we shall limit ourselves to the diversities among hen's eggs.

The more recently laid are whiter than the staler, because by age, and especially by incubation, they become darker; the cavity in the blunt end of a stale egg is also larger than in a recent egg; eggs just laid are also somewhat rough to the feel from a quantity of white powder which covers the shell, but which is soon rubbed off, when the egg becomes smoother as well as darker. New-laid eggs, unbroken, if placed near a fire will sweat, and are much more palatable than those that have been kept for some time—they are, indeed, accounted a delicacy by some. [Fruitful] eggs, after two or three days' incubation, are still better flavoured than stale eggs; revived by the gentle warmth of the hen, they seem to return to the quality and entireness of the egg just laid. Farther, I have boiled an egg to hardness, after the fourteenth day of incubation, when the chick had already begun to get its feathers, when it occupied the middle of the egg, and nearly the whole of the yelk re-

---

[1] Hist. Anim. lib. i, cap. 5.   [2] Ibid. cap. 2.   [3] Op. cit. p. 19.

mained, in order that I might better distinguish the position of the chick : I found it lying, as it were, within a mould of the albumen, and the yelk possessed the same agreeable flavour and sweetness as that of the new-laid egg, boiled to the same degree of hardness. The yelk taken from the ovarium of a live fowl, and eaten immediately, tastes much sweeter raw than boiled.

Eggs also differ from one another in shape ; some are longer and more pointed, others rounder and blunter. According to Aristotle,[1] the long-shaped and pointed eggs produce females ; the blunt, on the contrary, yield males. Pliny,[2] however, maintains the opposite. " The rounder eggs," he says, " produce females, the others males ;" and with him Columella[3] agrees : " He who desires to have the greater number of his brood cocks, let him select the longest and sharpest eggs for incubation ; and on the contrary, when he would have the greater number females, let him choose the roundest eggs." The ground of Aristotle's opinion was this : because the rounder eggs are the hotter, and it is the property of heat to concentrate and determine, and that heat can do most which is most powerful. From the stronger and more perfect principle, therefore, proceeds the stronger and more perfect animal. Such is the male compared with the female, especially in the case of the common fowl. On the contrary, again, the smaller eggs are reckoned among the imperfect ones, and the smallest of all are regarded as entirely unproductive. It was on this account too that Aristotle, to secure the highest quality of eggs, recommends that the hens be frequently trodden. Barren and adventitious eggs, he asserts, are smaller and less savoury, because they are humid and imperfect. The differences indicated are to be understood as referring to the eggs of the same fowl; for when a certain hen goes on laying eggs of a certain character, they will all produce either males or females. If you understand this point otherwise, the guess as to males or females, from the indications given, would be extremely uncertain. Because different hens lay eggs that differ much in respect of size and figure: some habitually lay more oblong, others, rounder eggs, that do

---

[1] Hist. Anim. lib. vi, cap. 2.   [2] Lib. x, cap. 52 ; lib. ix.
[3] De Re Rust. cap. 5, Scalig. in loc.

not differ greatly one from another; and although I sometimes found diversities in the eggs of the same fowl, these were still so trifling in amount that they would have escaped any other than the practised eye. For as all the eggs of the same fowl acquire nearly the same figure, in the same womb or mould in which the shell is deposited, (much as the excrements are moulded into scybala in the cells of the colon,) it necessarily falls out that they greatly resemble one another; so that I myself, without much experience, could readily tell which hen in a small flock had laid a given egg, and they who have given much attention to the point, of course succeed much better. But that which we note every day among huntsmen is far more remarkable; for the more careful keepers who have large herds of stags or fallow deer under their charge, will very certainly tell to which herd the horns which they find in the woods or thickets belonged. A stupid and uneducated shepherd, having the charge of a numerous flock of sheep, has been known to become so familiar with the physiognomy of each, that if any one had strayed from the flock, though he could not count them, he could still say which one it was, give the particulars as to where it had been bought, or whence it had come. The master of this man, for the sake of trying him, once selected a particular lamb from among forty others in the same pen, and desired him to carry it to the ewe which was its dam, which he did forthwith. We have known huntsmen who, having only once seen a particular stag, or his horns, or even his print in the mud, (as a lion is known by his claws,) have afterwards been able to distinguish him by the same marks from every other; some, too, from the foot-prints of deer, seen for the first time, will draw inferences as to the size, and grease, and power of the stag which has left them; saying whether he were full of strength, or weary from having been hunted; and farther, whether the prints are those of a buck or a doe. I shall say thus much more: there are some who, in hunting, when there are some forty hounds upon the trace of the game, and all are giving tongue together, will nevertheless, and from a distance, tell which dog is at the head of the pack, which at the tail, which chases on the hot scent, which is running off at fault; whether the game is still running, or is at bay; whether the stag have run far, or have but just been raised from his lair. And all this amid the din of dogs, and men, and horns, and surrounded by an unknown and gloomy wood. We should not, therefore, be greatly surprised when we see those who have experience telling by what hen each particular egg in a number has been laid. I wish there were some equally ready way from the child of knowing the true father.

The principal difference between eggs, however, is their fecundity or barrenness—the distinction of fruitful eggs from hypenemic, adventitious, or wind eggs. Those eggs are called hypenemic, (as if the progeny of the wind,) that are produced without the concourse of the male, and are unfit for setting; although Varro[1] declares that the mares, in Lusitania, conceive by the wind. For zephyrus was held a fertilizing wind, whence its name, as if it were ζωηφερός, or life bringing. So that Virgil says:

> And Zephyrus, with warming breath resolves
> The bosom of the ground, and melting rains
> Are poured o'er all, and every field brings forth.

Hence the ancients, when with this wind blowing in the spring season, they saw their hens begin laying, without the concurrence of the cock, conceived that zephyrus, or the west wind, was the author of their fecundity. There are also what are called addle, and dog-day eggs, produced by interrupted incubation, and so called because eggs often rot in the dog-days, being deserted by the hens in consequence of the excessive heat; and also because at this season of the year thunder is frequent; and Aristotle[2] asserts that eggs die if it thunders whilst the hen is sitting.

Those eggs are regarded as prolific, which, no unfavorable circumstances intervening, under the influence of a gentle heat, produce chicks. And this they will do, not merely through the incubation of the mother, but of any other bird, if it be but of sufficient size to cherish and cover them, or by a gentle temperature obtained in any way whatever. "Eggs are hatched with the same celerity," says Aristotle,[3] "spontaneously in the ground, as by incubation. Wherefore in Egypt, it is the custom

---

[1] De Re Rust. lib. ii, cap. 1.
[2] Hist. Anim. lib. vi, cap. 2; Plin. Hist. Nat. lib. x, cap. 54.   [3] Ibid.

to bury them in dung, covered with earth.   And there was a tale in Syracuse, of a drunken fellow, who was accustomed to continue his potations until a number of eggs, placed under a mat bestrewed with earth, were hatched." The empress Livia, is also said to have carried an egg in her bosom until a chick was produced from it.   And in Egypt, and other countries, at the present time, chickens are reared from eggs placed in ovens. " The egg, therefore," as Fabricius[1] truly says, " is not only the uterus, and place where the generation of the chick proceeds, but it is that upon which its whole formation depends; and this the egg accomplishes as agent, as matter, as instrument, as place, and as all else that concurs."

For it is certain that the chick is formed by a principle inherent in the egg, and that nothing accrues to a perfect egg from incubation, beyond the warmth and protection; in the same way as to the chick when disclosed, the hen gives nothing more than her warmth and her care, by which she defends it from the cold and from injury, and directs it to its proper food. The grand desideratum, therefore, once the chickens are hatched, is that the hen lead them about, seek for and supply them with proper food, and cherish them under her wings. And this you will not easily supply by any kind of artifice.

Capons, and hybrids between the common fowl and the pheasant, produced in our aviaries, will incubate and hatch a set of eggs; but they never know how to take care of the brood—to lead them about properly, and to provide with adequate care for their nurture.

And here I would pause for a moment, (for I mean to treat of the matter more fully by and by,) to express my admiration of the perseverance and patience with which the females of almost every species of bird, sit upon the nest for so many days and nights incessantly, macerating their bodies, and almost destroying themselves from want of food; what dangers they will face in defence of their eggs, and when compelled to quit them for ever so short a time, through necessity, with what eagerness and haste they return to them again, and brood over them !   Ducks and geese, when they quit the nest for a few minutes, cover and conceal it with straw.   With what true

[1] Op. cit. p. 19.

magnanimity do these ill-furnished mothers defend their eggs! which, after all, perhaps, are mere wind or addle eggs, or not their own, or artificial eggs of chalk or ivory;—it is still the same, they defend all with equal courage. It is truly a remarkable love which birds display for inert and lifeless eggs; and their solicitude is repaid by no kind of advantage or enjoyment. Who does not wonder at the affection, or passion rather, of the clucking hen, which can only be extinguished by a drenching with cold water. In this state of her feeling she neglects everything,—her wings droop, her feathers are unpruned and ruffled, she wanders about restless and dissatisfied, disturbing other hens on their nests, seeking eggs everywhere, which she commences forthwith to incubate; nor will she be at peace until her desire has been gratified, until she has a brood to lead about with her, upon which she may expend her fervour, which she may cherish, feed, and defend. How pleasantly are we moved to laughter when we see the poor hen following to the water the supposititious brood of ducklings she has hatched, wandering restlessly round the pool, attempting to wade after them to her own imminent peril, and by her noises and various artifices striving to entice them back to the shore!

According to Aristotle,[1] barren eggs do not produce chicks because their fluids do not thicken under incubation, nor is the yelk or the white altered from its original constitution. But we shall revert to this subject in our general survey of generation.

Our housewives, that they may distinguish the eggs that are addled from those that will produce chicks, take them from the fourteenth to the sixteenth day of the incubation, and drop them softly into tepid water, when the spoilt ones sink, whilst the fruitful ones swim. If the included chick be well forward, and moves about with alacrity, the egg not only rolls over but even dances in the water. And if you apply the egg to your ear for several days before the hatching, you may hear the chick within kicking, scratching, and even chirping. When the hen that is sitting hears these noises, she turns the eggs and lays them otherwise than they were, until the chicks, getting into a comfortable position, become quiet; even as watchful

---

[1] Hist. Anim. lib. vi, cap. 2.

mothers are wont to treat their infants when they are restless and cry in their cradles.

Hens lay eggs in variable numbers : " Some hens," says the philosopher,[1] "except the two winter months, lay through the whole year; some of the better breeds will lay as many as sixty eggs before they show a disposition to sit; though these eggs are not so prolific as those of the commoner kinds.   The Adrianic hens are small, and lay every day, but they are ill-tempered, and often kill their young ones; they are particoloured in their plumage.   Some domestic fowls will even lay twice a day; and some, by reason of their great fecundity, die young."

In England some of the hens lay every day; but the more prolific commonly lay two days continuously and then miss a day : the first day the egg is laid in the morning, next day in the afternoon, and the third day there is a pause. Some hens have a habit of breaking their eggs and deserting their nests ; whether this be from disease or vice is not known.

Certain differences may also be observed in the incubation : some fowls only sit once, others twice, or thrice, or repeatedly. Florentius says, that in Alexandria, in Egypt, there are fowls called monosires, from which the fighting cocks are descended, which go on sitting for two or three periods, each successive brood being removed as it is hatched, and brought up apart. In this way the same hen will hatch forty, sixty, and even a greater number of chickens, at a single sitting.

Some eggs too, are larger, others smaller; a few extremely small; these, in Italy, are commonly called centenina; and our country folks still believe that such eggs are laid by the cock, and that were they set they would produce basilisks. " The vulgar," says Fabricius,[2] "think that this small egg is the last that will be laid, and that it comes as the hundredth in number, whence the name; that it has no yelk, though all the other parts are present—the chalazæ, the albumen, the membranes, and the shell.   And it seems probable that it is produced when all the other yelks have been fashioned into eggs, and no more remain in the vitellary ; on the other hand, however, a modicum of albumen remains, and out of this, it may be inferred, is the small egg in question produced."   To

---

[1] Hist. Anim. lib. vi, cap. 1.   [2] Op. cit. p. 10.

me, nevertheless, this does not appear likely; because it is certain that the whole ovary being removed, the uterus secundus also diminishes in size in the same proportion, and shrinks into a mere membrane, which contains neither any fluid nor any albumen. Fabricius proceeds: "The ova centenina are met with of two kinds : one of them being without a yelk, and this is the true centenine egg, because it is the last which the hen will lay at that particular season—she will now cease from laying for a time. The other is also a small egg, but it has a yelk, and will not prove the last which the hen will then lay, but is intermediate between those of the usual size that have preceded, and others that will follow. It is of small size because there has been a failure of the vegetative function, as happens to the peach, and other fruit, of which we see many of adequate size, but a few that are very diminutive." This may be in consequence of the inclemency of the weather, or the want of sun, or from defective nutriment in point either of quantity or quality. I should not readily allow, however, that the eggs last laid are always small.

Monstrous eggs are not wanting; "for the augurs," says Aristotle,[1] "held it portentous when eggs were laid that were all yellow; or when, on a fowl being laid open, eggs were found under the septum transversum, where the rudimentary eggs of the female usually appear, of the magnitude of perfect eggs.

To this head may be referred those eggs that produce twins, that have two yelks. Such an egg I lately found in the uterus of a fowl, perfect in all respects, and covered with a shell; the yelks, cicatriculæ, and thicker albuminous portions being all double, and the chalazæ present in two pairs : a single thinner albumen, however, surrounded all these, and this in its turn was included within the usual double common membrane, and single shell. For, indeed, although Aristotle says that fowls always lay some eggs of this kind, I shall hardly be induced to believe that this does not occur against the ordinary course of nature. And although twin chicks are produced from such eggs as I have ascertained in opposition to the opinion of Fabricius, who says that they produce chicks having four legs, or four wings and two heads, which, however, are not

---

[1] Aldrovand. Ornithol. lib. xiv, p. 260.

capable of living, but for the most part speedily die, either by reason of want of room or of air in the shell, or because the one proves a hinderance to the other and blights it; nor can it happen that both should be equally prepared for exclusion—that one should not prove an abortion.

Briefly and summarily the differences among eggs are principally of three kinds: some are prolific, some unprolific; some will produce males and some females; some are the produce of the two sexes of the same species, others of allied species and will produce hybrids, such as we see between the common hen and the pheasant, the progeny being referrible either to the first or to the last male that had connexion with the hen. Because, according to Aristotle,[1] "the egg, which receives its constitution by intercourse, passes from its own into another genus, if the hen be trodden when she carries either an adventitious egg or one that was conceived under the influence of another male, and this renewed intercourse take place before the yellow is changed into the white. So that hypenemic or wind eggs are made fruitful, and fruitful eggs receive the form of the male which has connexion last. But if the change has taken place into the white, it cannot happen either that the wind egg is turned into a fertile one, or that the egg which is contained in the uterus in virtue of a previous intercourse, shall be altered into the genus of the male which has the second communication." For the seminal fluid of the cock, as Scaliger wittily remarks, is like a testament, the last will or disposition in which is that which stands in force.

To these particulars it might perhaps be added, that some eggs are more strong and lusty than others, more full of life, if the expression may be used; though as there is a vital principle in the egg, so must there inhere the corresponding virtue that flows from it. For, as in other kinds of animals, some of the females are so replete with desire, so full of Venus, that they conceive from any and every intercourse, even once submitted to, and from a weakly male, and produce several young from the same embrace; others, on the contrary, are so torpid and sluggish, that unless they are assailed by a vigorous male, under the influence of strong desire, and that not once, but repeatedly, and for

---

[1] Hist. Anim. lib. vi, cap. 21.

a certain time, they continue barren. This is also the case with eggs, some of which, though they may have been conceived in consequence of intercourse, still remain unprolific unless perfected by repeated and continued connections. Whence it happens that some eggs are more speedily changed by incubation than others, exhibiting traces of the fœtus from the third day; others again, either become spoiled, or suffer transformation into the fœtus more slowly, exhibiting no indications of the future chick even up to the seventh day, as shall be made to appear by and by, in speaking of the generation of the chick from the egg.

Thus far have we discoursed of the uterus of the fowl, and its function; of the production of the hen's egg, and of its differences and peculiarities, from immediate observation; and from the instances quoted, conclusions may be drawn with reference to other oviparous animals.

We have now to pursue the history of the generation and formation of the fœtus from the egg. For indeed, as I have said above, the entire contemplation of the family of birds is comprehended in these two propositions: how is an egg engendered of a male and female; and by what process do males and females proceed from eggs?—the circle by which, under favour of nature, their kinds are continued to eternity.

Of the production of the chick from the egg of the hen.

Of the growth and generation of the hen's egg enough has already been said; and we have now to lay before the reader our observations on the procreation of the chick from the egg,—a duty which is equally difficult, and profitable, and pleasant. For in general the first processes of nature lie hid, as it were, in the depths of night, and by reason of their subtlety escape the keenest reason no less than the most piercing eye.

Nor in truth is it a much less arduous business to investigate the intimate mysteries and obscure beginnings of generation than to seek to discover the frame of the world at large, and the manner of its creation. The eternity of things is connected with the reciprocal interchange of generation and decay; and as the sun, now in the east and then in the west, completes the measure of time by his ceaseless revolutions, so are the fleeting things of mortal existence made eternal through incessant change, and kinds and species are perpetuated though individuals die.

The writers who have treated of this subject have almost all taken different paths; but having their minds preoccupied, they have hitherto gone to work to frame conclusions in consonance with the particular views they had adopted.

Aristotle,[1] among the ancients, and Hieron. Fabricius of Aquapendente, among the moderns, have written with so much accuracy on the generation and formation of the chick from the egg that little seems left for others to do. Ulyssus Aldrovandus,[2] nevertheless, described the formation of the chick in ovo; but he appears rather to have gone by the guidance of Aristotle than to have relied on his own experience. For Volcherus Coiter, living at this time in Bologna, and encouraged, as he tells us, by Aldrovandus, his master, opened incubated eggs every day, and illustrated many points besides those noted by Aldrovandus;[3] these discoveries, however, could scarcely have remained unknown to Aldrovandus. Æmilius Parisanus, a Venetian physician, having discarded the opinions of others, has also given a new account of the formation of the chick from the egg.

But since our observations lead us to conclude that many things of great consequence are very different from what they have hitherto been held to be, I shall myself give an account of what goes on in the egg from day to day, and what parts are there transmuted, directing my attention to the first days especially, when all is most obscure and confused, and difficult of observation, and in reference to which writers have more particularly drawn the sword against one another in defence of their several discordant observations, which, in sooth, they accommodate rather to their preconceived opinions respecting the material and efficient cause of animal generation than to simple truth.

What Aristotle says on the subject of the reproduction of

---

[1] Hist. Anim. lib. vi, cap. 2, 3.   [2] Ornithol. lib. xiv.
[3] Nobil. Exercit. lib. vi.

the chick in ovo is perfectly correct. Nevertheless, as if he had not himself seen the things he describes, but received them at second hand from another expert observer, he does not give the periods rightly; and then he is grievously mistaken in respect of the place in which the first rudiments of the egg are fashioned, stating this to be the sharp end, for which he is fairly challenged by Fabricius. Neither does he appear to have observed the commencement of the chick in the egg; nor could he have found the things which he says are necessary to all generation in the place which he assigns them. He will, for instance, have it that the white is the constituent matter (since nothing naturally can by possibility be produced from nothing.) And he did not sufficiently understand how the efficient cause (the seminal fluid of the cock,) acted without contact; nor how the egg could, of its own accord, without any inherent generative matter of the male, produce a chick.

Aldrovandus, adopting an error akin to that of Aristotle, says besides, that the yelk rises during the first days of the incubation into the sharp end of the egg, a proposition which no eyes but those of the blind would assent to; he thinks also that the chalazæ are the semen of the cock, and that the chick arises from them, though it is nourished both by the yelk and the white. In this he is obviously in opposition to Aristotle, who held that the chalazæ contributed nothing to the reproductive powers of the egg.

Volcherus Coiter is, on the whole, much more correct; and his statements are far more consonant with what the eye perceives. But his tale of the three globules is a fable. Neither did he rightly perceive the true commencement of the chick in ovo.

Hieronymus Fabricius contends that the chalazæ are not the sperma of the cock; but then he will have it that "from these, fecundated by the seminal fluid of the cock, as from the appropriate matter, the chick is incorporated." Fabricius observed the point of origin of the chick, the spot or cicatricula, namely, which presents itself upon the tunica propria of the yelk; but he regarded it as a cicatrice or scar left on the place where the peduncle had been attached; he viewed it as a blemish in the egg, not as any important part.

Parisanus completely refutes Fabricius's ideas of the chalazæ; but he himself obviously raves when he speaks of certain circles, and principal parts of the fœtus, viz., the liver and heart. He appears to have observed the commencement of the fœtus in ovo; but what it was he obviously did not know, when he says, "that the white point in the middle of the circles is the semen of the cock, from which the chick is produced."

Thus it comes to pass that every one, in adducing reasons for the formation of the chick in ovo, in accordance with preconceived opinions, has wandered from the truth. Some will have it that the semen or the blood is the matter whence the chick is engendered; others, that the semen is the agent or efficient cause of its formation. Yet to him who dispassionately views the question is it quite certain that there is no prepared matter present, nor any menstruous blood to be coagulated at the time of intercourse by the semen masculinum, as Aristotle will have it; neither does the chick originate in the egg from the seed of the male, nor from that of the female, nor from the two commingled.

EXERCISE THE FIFTEENTH.

The first examination of the egg; or of the effect of the first day's incubation upon the egg.

That we may be the more clearly informed of the effect which the first day's incubation produces upon the egg, we must set out by ascertaining what changes take place in an egg spontaneously, changes that distinguish a stale egg from one that is new-laid, when what is due to the incubation *per se* will first be clearly apprehended.

The space or cavity in the blunt end is present, as we have said, in every egg; but the staler the egg the larger does this hollow continually grow; and this is more especially the case when eggs are kept in a warm place, or when the weather is hot; the effect being due to the exhalation of a certain portion of the thinner albumen, as has been stated in the history of the egg. This cavity, as it increases, extends rather in the line of the length than of the breadth of the egg, and comes finally to be no longer orbicular.

The shell, already less transparent, becomes dingy.

The albumen grows thicker and more viscid, and acquires a straw or yellow colour.

The tunica propria of the vitellus becomes more lax, and appears wrinkled, for it seems that some even of this fluid is dissipated in the course of time.

The chalazæ are found in either end of every egg, in the same situation, and having the same consistence—whether the egg be recent or stale, fruitful or barren, it does not signify; by their means a firm connexion is established between the yelk and the white, and the two fluids preserve their relative positions. The chalazæ, indeed, are two mutually opposed supports or poles, and hinges of this microcosm; and are constructed as if made up of numerous coats of the albumen, twisted together at either end into a knotted rope, by which they are attached to the vitellus. And hence it happens that the yelk is separated from the white with difficulty, unless the chalazæ are either first divided with a knife or torn with the fingers; this done, the white immediately falls away from the yelk. It is by means of these hinges that the vitellus is both retained in the centre of the egg and preserved of its proper consistence. And they are so connected that the principal part, the cicatricula, to wit, always regards the same region of the egg, or its upper part, and is preserved equidistant from either end. For this spot or cicatricula is observed to be of the same consistence, dimensions, and colour, and in the same situation in the stale as in the new-laid egg. But as soon as the egg, under the influence of the gentle warmth of the incubating hen, or of warmth derived from another source, begins to pullulate, this spot forthwith dilates, and expands like the pupil of the eye, and from thence, as the grand centre of the egg, the latent plastic force breaks forth and germinates. This first commencement of the chick, however, so far as I am aware, has not yet been observed by any one.

On the second day of the incubation, after the egg has been exposed to warmth for twenty-four hours, under the hen, as the cavity in the blunt end has enlarged greatly and descended, so has the internal constitution of the egg also begun to be changed. The yelk, which had hitherto lain in the middle of the albumen, rises towards the blunt end, and its middle, where the cicatricula is situated, is lifted up and applied to the mem-

brane that bounds the empty space, so that the yelk now appears
to be connected with the cavity by means of the cicatricula; and
in the same measure as the yelk rises does the thicker portion
of the albumen sink into the sharp or lower end of the egg.
Whence it appears, as Fabricius rightly remarks, that Aristotle[1]
was either in error, or that there is a mistake in the codex,
when it is said, " In this time" (viz., between three and four
days, and as many nights,) the yelk is brought to the summit,
where the commencement of the egg is, and the egg is exposed
in this part," i. e. under the enlarged empty space. Now Aristotle[2] calls the principium ovi, or commencement of the egg, its
smaller end, which is last extruded.   But it is certain that the
yelk ascends towards the blunt end of the egg, and that the
cavity there enlarges.   And Aldrovandus is undoubtedly in
error when he speaks as if he had experience of the fact, and
says that the yelk rises to the sharp end. I will confess, nevertheless, that on the second or third day I have occasionally
observed the cicatricula expanded and the beginning of the
chick already laid, the yelk not having yet risen; this, however, happens rarely, and I am inclined to ascribe it to some
weakness in the egg.

On the second day of the incubation, or first day of inspection, the cicatricula in question is found to have enlarged to
the dimensions of a pea or lentil, and is divided into circles,
such as might be drawn with a pair of compasses, having an
extremely minute point for their centre.   It is very probable
that Aldrovandus observed this spot, for he says : " In the
midst of the yellow a certain whitish something makes its appearance, which was not noticed by Aristotle;" and also by
Coiter, when he expresses himself thus : " On the second day
there is in the middle of the yelk a part whiter than the rest;"
Parisanus, too, may have seen it; he observes : " In the course
of the second day I observe a white body of the size and form
of a middling lentil; and this is the semen of the cock covered
over with a white and most delicate tunic, which underlies the
two common membranes of the entire egg, but overlies the
tunica propria of the yelk."   I believe, however, that no one
has yet said that this cicatricula occurs in every egg, or has
acknowledged it to be the origin of the chick.

---

[1] Hist. Anim. lib. vi, cap. 3.   [2] Ibid. lib. iii, cap. 2.

Meantime the chalazæ or treadles will be seen to decline from either end of the egg towards its sides, this being occasioned by that alteration which we have noticed in the relative situations of the two fluids. The treadle from the blunt end descends somewhat; the one from the sharp end rises in the same proportion: as in a globe whose axis is set obliquely, one pole is as much depressed below the horizon as the other is raised above it.

The vitellus, too, particularly in the situation of the cica· tricula, begins to grow a little more diffluent than it was, and raises its tunica propria, (which we have found in stale eggs before incubation to be somewhat lax and wrinkled,) into a tumour; and it now appears to have recovered the same colour, consistency, and sweetness of taste that it had in the egg just laid.

Such is the process in the course of the first day that leads to the production of a new being, such the earliest trace of the future chick. Aldrovandus adds: "the albumen suffers no change," which is correct; but when he asserts that "the semen of the cock can be seen in it," he as manifestly errs. Resting on a most insufficient reason, he thought that the chalazæ were the semen of the cock, "because," forsooth, "the eggs that are without chalazæ are unfruitful." This I can very well believe; for these were then no proper eggs; for all eggs, wind eggs as well as those that are prolific, have chalazæ. But he, misled perhaps by the country women, who in Italian call the chalazæ *galladura*, fell into the vulgar error. Nor is Hieronymus Fabricius guilty of a less grave mistake when he exhibits the formation of the chick in a series of engravings, and contends that it is produced from the chalazæ; overlooking the fact that the chalazæ are present the whole of the time, and unchanged, though they have shifted their places; and that the commencement of the chick is to be sought for at a distance from them.

Second inspection of the egg.

The second day gone by, the circles of the cicatricula that have been mentioned, have become larger and more conspicuous, and may now be of the size of the nail of the ring-finger, sometimes even of that of the middle finger. By these rings the whole cicatricula is indistinctly divided into two, occasionally into three regions, which are frequently of different colours, and bear a strong resemblance to the cornea of the eye, both as respects dimensions, a certain degree of prominence, and the presence of a transparent and limpid fluid included within it. The centre of the cicatricula here stands for the pupil; but it is occupied with a certain white speck, and appears like the pupil of some small bird's eye obscured by a suffusion or cataract, as it is called. On this account we have called the entire object the oculum ovi, the eye of the egg.

Within the circles of the cicatricula, I say, there is contained a quantity of perfectly bright and transparent fluid, even purer than any crystalline humour; which, if it be viewed transversely and against the light, the whole spot will rather appear to be situated in the albumen than sunk into the membrane of the yelk, as before: it presents itself as a portion of the albumen dissolved and clarified, and included within a most delicate tunica propria. Hence I entitle this fluid the oculum seu colliquamentum album; it is as if a portion of the albumen, liquefied by the heat, shone apart, (which it does, unless disturbed by being shaken,) and formed a more spirituous and better digested fluid, separated from the rest of the albumen by a tunica propria, and situated between the two masses of liquid, the yelk and the albumen. It differs from the rest of the albumen by its clearness and transparency, as the water of a pellucid spring differs from that of a stagnant pool. The tunic which surrounds this fluid is so fragile and delicate that, unless the egg be handled with great care, it is apt to give way, when the pure spring is rendered turbid by a mixture of fluids.

I was long in doubt what I should conclude as to this

clear diffluent fluid, whether I should regard it as the innate heat, or radical moisture; as a matter prepared for the future fœtus, or a perfectly-concocted nourishment, such as dew is held to be among the secondary humours. For it is certain, as shall be afterwards shown, that the earliest rudiments of the fœtus are cast in its middle, that from this the chick derives its first nutriment, and even when of larger size continues to live amidst it.

This solution therefore increases rapidly in quantity, particularly in its internal region, which, as it expands, forces out and obliterates the external regions. This change is effected in the course of a single day, as is shown in the second figure of Fabricius. It is very much as it is with the eyes of those animals which have a very ample pupil, and see better by night than by day, such as owls, cats, and others, whose pupils expand very much in the dusk and dark, and, on the contrary, contract excessively in a brilliant light: one of these animals being taken quickly from a light into a shady place, the pupil is seen to enlarge in such wise that the coloured ring, called the iris, is very much diminished in size, and indeed almost entirely disappears.

Parisanus, falling upon these regions, is grossly mistaken when he speaks of " a honey-coloured, a white, a gray, and another white circle;" and says that " the fœtus is formed from the white middle point" (which, indeed, appears in these regions), and that " this is the semen of the cock." That he may exalt himself on a more notable subtlety he continues: " Before any redness is apparent in the body of the fœtus, two minute vesicles present themselves in it; in the beginning, however, neither of them is tinged with red;" one of these he would have us receive as the heart, the other as the liver. But in truth there is neither any vesicle present sooner than the redness of the blood is disclosed; nor does the embryo ever suddenly become red in the course of the first days of its existence; nor yet does any of these vesicles present us with a trace of the liver. Both of them belong, in fact, to the heart, prefiguring its ventricles and auricles, and palpitating, as we shall afterwards show, they respond reciprocally by their systoles and diastoles.

Aristotle[1] appears to have known this dissolved fluid, when he says : " A membrane, too, marked with sanguineous fibres, surrounds the white fluid at this time (the third day), arising from those orifices of the veins." Now the philosopher can neither be supposed by the words " white fluid," to refer to the albumen at large, because at this period the membrane of the white is not yet covered with veins; it is only the membrane of the dissolved fluid which appears with a few branches of veins distributed over it here and there. And because he says: " this membrane, too," as if he understood another than those which he had spoken of as investing the albumen and the yelk before incubation, and designated this one as first arising after the third day, and from the orifices of the veins.

Coiter seems also to have known of this dissolved fluid ; he says : " A certain portion of the albumen acquiring a white colour, another becoming thicker." The fluid in question is surrounded with its proper membrane, and is distinct and separate from the rest of the albumen before there is any appearance of blood. We shall have occasion, by and by, to speak of the singular importance of this fluid to the fœtuses of every animal. Whilst they float in it they are safe from suc- cussion and contusion, and other external injury of every kind; and they moreover are nourished by it. I once showed to their serene majesties the king and queen, an embryo, the size of a French-bean, which had been taken from the uterus of a doe; all its membranes were entire, and from its genital organs we could readily tell that it was a male. It was, in truth, a most agreeable natural spectacle ; the embryo perfect and elegant, floating in this pure, transparent, and crystalline fluid, invested with its pellucid tunica propria, as if in a glass vessel of the greatest purity, of the size of a pigeon's egg.

EXERCISE THE SEVENTEENTH.

The third inspection of the egg.

Having seen the second process or preparation of the egg, towards the production of the embryo which presents itself in

[1] Hist. Anim. lib. vi, cap. 3.

the course of the third day, we proceed to the Third Stage, which falls to be considered after the lapse of three days and as many nights. Aristotle[1] says : " Traces of generation commence in the egg of the hen after three days and three nights [of incubation] ;" for example, on Monday morning, if in the morning of the preceding Friday the egg has been put under the hen. This stage forms the subject of the third figure in Fabricius.

If the inspection of the egg be made on the fourth day, the metamorphosis is still greater, and the change likewise more wonderful and manifest with every hour in the course of the day. It is in this interval that the transition is made in the egg from the life of the plant to the life of the animal. For now the margin of the diffluent fluid looks red, and is purpurescent with a sanguineous line, and nearly in its centre there appears a leaping point, of the colour of blood, so small that at one moment, when it contracts, it almost entirely escapes the eye, and again, when it dilates, it shows like the smallest spark of fire. Such at the outset is animal life, which the plastic force of nature puts in motion from the most insignificant beginnings !

The above particulars you may perceive towards the close of the third day, with very great attention, and under favour of a bright light (as of the sun), or with the assistance of a magnifying glass. Without these aids you would strain your eyes in vain, so slender is the purple line, so slight is the motion of the palpitating point. But at the beginning of the fourth day you may readily, and at its close most readily, perceive the " palpitating bloody point, which already moves," says Aristotle, " like an animal, in the transparent liquid (which I call colliquamentum); and from this point two vascular branches proceed, full of blood, in a winding course" into the purpurescent circle and the investing membrane of the resolved liquid; distributing in their progress numerous fibrous offshoots, which all proceed from one original, like the branches and twigs of a tree from the same stem. Within the entering angle of this root, and in the middle of the resolved liquid, is placed the red palpitating point, which keeps order and rhythm in its pulsations, composed of [alternate] systoles and diastoles. In the diastole, when it has

[1] Hist. Anim. lib. vi, cap. 3.

imbibed a larger quantity of blood, it becomes enlarged, and starts into view; in the systole, however, subsiding instantaneously as if convulsed by the stroke, and expelling the blood, it vanishes from view.

Fabricius depicts this palpitating point in his third figure; and mistakes it—a thing which is extraordinary—for the body of the embryo; as if he had never seen it leaping or pulsating, or had not understood, or had entirely forgotten the passage in Aristotle. A still greater subject of amazement, however, is his total want of solicitude about his chalazæ all this while, although he had declared the rudiments of the embryo to be derived from them.

Ulyssus Aldrovandus,[1] writing from Bologna nearly at the same time, says: "There appears in the albumen, as it were, a minute palpitating point, which The Philosopher declares to be the heart. And I have unquestionably seen a venous trunk arising from this, from which two other branches proceeded; these are the blood-vessels, which he says extend to either investing membrane of the yelk and white. And I am myself entirely of his opinion, and believe these to be veins, and pulsatile, and to contain a purer kind of blood, adapted to the production of the principal parts of the body, the liver, to wit, the lungs, and others of the same description." Both of the vessels in question, however, are not veins, neither do they both pulsate; but one of them is an artery, another a vein, as we shall see by and by, when we shall farther show that these passages constitute the umbilical vessels of the embryo.

Volcher Coiter has these words: "The sanguineous point or globule, which was formerly found in the yelk, is now observed more in the albumen, and pulsates distinctly." He says, erroneously, "formerly found in the yelk;" for the point discovered in the vitellus is white, and does not pulsate; nor does the sanguineous point or globe appear to pulsate at the end of the second day of incubation. But the point which we have indicated in the middle of the circle, and as constituting its centre in connexion with the vitellus, disappears before that point which is characterized by Aristotle as palpitating, can be discerned; or, as I conceive, having turned red, begins to pulsate. For

[1] Ornithologia, lib. xiv, p. 217.

both points are situated in the centre of the resolved fluid, and near the root of the veins which thence arise; but they are never seen simultaneously: in the place of the white point there appears a red and palpitating point.

That portion of Coiter's sentence, however, where he says: "the punctus saliens is now seen in the albumen rather than in the yelk," is perfectly accurate. And, indeed, moved by these words, I have inquired whether the white point in question is turned into the blood-red point, inasmuch as both are nearly of the same size, and both make their appearance in the same situation. And I have, indeed, occasionally found an extremely delicate bright purple circle ending near the ruddy horizon surrounding the resolved liquid, in the centre of which there was the white point, but not the red and pulsating point apparent; for I have never observed these two points at one and the same time. It were certainly of great moment to determine: Whether or not the blood was extant before the pulse? and whether the pulsating point arose from the veins, or the veins from the pulsating point?

So far as my observations enable me to conclude, the blood has seemed to go before the pulse. This conclusion is supported by the following instance: on Wednesday evening I set three hen's eggs, and on Saturday evening, somewhat before the same hour, I found these eggs cold, as if forsaken by the hen: having opened one of them, notwithstanding, I found the rudiments of an embryo, viz., a red and sanguinolent line in the circumference; and in the centre, instead of a pulsating point, a white and bloodless point. By this indication I saw that the hen had left her nest no long time before; wherefore, catching her, and shutting her up in a box, I kept her upon the two remaining eggs, and several others, through the ensuing night. Next morning, very early, both of the eggs with which the experiment was begun, had revived, and in the centre there was the pulsating point, much smaller than the white point, from which, like a spark darting from a cloud, it made its appearance in the diastole; it seemed to me, therefore, that the red point emanated from the white point; that the punctum saliens was in some way engendered in that white point; that the punctum saliens, the blood being already extant, was either originally there produced, or there began to move. I have, indeed, repeatedly seen the punctum saliens when all but dead, and no longer giving any signs of motion, recover its pulsatile movements under the influence of renewed warmth.   In the order of generation, then, I conceive that the punctum and the blood first exist, and that pulsation only occurs subsequently.

This at all events is certain, that nothing whatever of the future fœtus is apparent on this day, save and except certain sanguineous lines, the punctum saliens, and those veins that all present themselves as emanating from a single trunk, (as this itself proceeds from the punctum saliens,) and are distributed in numerous branches over the whole of the colliquament or dissolved fluid.   These vessels afterwards constitute the umbilical vessels, by means of which, distributed far and wide, the fœtus as it grows obtains its nourishment from the albumen and vitellus.   You have a striking example of similar vessels and their branchings in the leaves of trees, the whole of the veins of which arise from the peduncle or foot-stalk, and from a single trunk are distributed to the rest of the leaf.

The entire including membrane of the colliquament traversed by blood-vessels, corresponds in form and dimensions with the two wings of a moth; and this, in fact, is the membrane which Aristotle[1] describes as "possessing sanguineous fibres, and at the same time containing a limpid fluid, proceeding from those mouths of the veins."

Towards the end of the fourth day, and the beginning of the fifth, the blood-red point, increased into a small and most delicate vesicle, is perceived to contain blood in its interior, which it propels by its contractions, and receives anew during its diastoles.

Up to this point I have not been able to perceive any difference in the vessels : the arteries are not distinguished from the veins, either by their coats or their pulsations.   I am therefore of opinion, that all the vessels may be spoken of indifferently under the name of veins, or, adopting Aristotle's[2] term, of venous canals.

"The punctum saliens," says Aristotle, "is already possessed of spontaneous motion, like an animal."   Because an animal is distinguished from that which is none, by the possession of

---

[1] Loc. supra cit.   [2] Ib.

sense and motion. When this point begins to move for the first time, consequently, we say well that it has assumed an animal nature; the egg, originally imbued with a vegetative soul, now becomes endowed in addition with a motive and sensitive force; from the vegetable it passes into the animal; and at the same time the living principle, which fashions the chick from the egg, and afterwards gives it the measure of intelligence it manifests, enters into the embryo. For, from the actions or manifestations, The Philosopher[1] concludes demonstratively, that the faculties or powers of acting are inherent, and through these the cause and principle of life, the soul, to wit, and the actions, inasmuch as manifestation is action.

I am myself farther satisfied from numerous experiments, that not only is motion inherent in the punctum saliens, which indeed no one denies, but sensation also. For on any the slightest touch, you may see the point variously commoved, and, as it were, irritated; just as sensitive bodies generally give indications of their proper sensations by their motions; and, the injury being repeated, the punctum becomes excited and disturbed in the rhythm and order of its pulsations. Thus do we conclude that in the sensitive-plant, and in zoophytes, there is inherent sensibility, because when touched they contract, as if they felt uncomfortable.

I have seen, I repeat, very frequently, and those who have been with me have seen this punctum, when touched with a needle, a probe, or a finger, and even when exposed to a higher temperature, or a severer cold, or subjected to any other molesting circumstance or thing, give various indications of sensibility, in the variety, force, and frequency of its pulsations. It is not to be questioned, therefore, that this punctum lives, moves, and feels like an animal.

An egg, moreover, too long exposed to the colder air, the punctum saliens beats more slowly and languidly; but the finger, or some other warmth being applied, it forthwith recovers its powers. And farther, after the punctum has gradually languished, and, replete with blood, has even ceased from all kind of motion, or other indication of life, still, on applying my warm finger, in no longer a time than is measured by twenty beats

[1] Liber de Anima.

of my pulse, lo! the little heart is revivified, erects itself anew, and, returning from Hades as it were, is restored to its former pulsations. The same thing happens through heat applied in any other way—that of the fire, or of hot water—as has been proved by myself and others again and again; so that it seemed as if it lay in our power to deliver the poor heart over to death, or to recall it to life at our will and pleasure.

What has now been stated, for the most part comes to pass on the fourth day from the commencement of the incubation— I say, for the most part,—because it is not invariably so, inasmuch as there is great diversity in the maturity of eggs, and some are more speedily perfected than others. As in trees laden with fruit, some, more forward and precocious, falls from the branches, and some, more crude and immature, still hangs firmly on the bough; so are some eggs less forward on the fifth day than others in the course of the third. This, that I might give it forth as a thing attested and certain, I have repeatedly ascertained in numerous eggs, incubated for the same length of time, and opened on the same day. Nor can I ascribe it to any difference of sex, or inclemency of weather, or neglect of incubation, or to any other cause but an inherent weakness of the egg itself, or some deficiency of the native heat.

Hypenemic or unfruitful eggs, begin to change at this time, as the critical day when they must show their disposition. As fertile eggs are changed by the inherent plastic force into colliquament (which afterwards passes into blood), so do wind-eggs now begin to change and to putrefy. I have, nevertheless, occasionally observed the spot or cicatricula to expand considerably even in hypenemic eggs, but never to rise into a cumulus, nor to become circumscribed by regularly disposed concentric circles. Sometimes I have even observed the vitellus to get somewhat clearer, and to become liquefied; but this was unequally; there were flocks, as if formed by sudden coagulation, swimming dispersed through it like clouds. And although such eggs could not yet be called putrid, nor were they offensive, still were they disposed to putrefaction; and, if continued under the hen, they soon arrived at this state, the rottenness commencing at the very spot where in fruitful eggs the reproductive germ appears.

The more perfect or forward eggs then, about the end of the fourth day, contain a double or bipartite pulsating vesicle, each portion reciprocating the other's motion, in such order and manner that whilst one is contracting, the other is distended with blood and ruddy in colour; but this last contracting anon forces out its charge of blood, and, an instant being interposed, the former rises again and repeats its pulse. And it is easy to perceive that the action of these vesicles is contraction, by which the blood is moved and propelled into the vessels.

"On the fourth day," says Aldrovandus,[1] "two puncta are perceived, both of which are in motion; these, undoubtedly, are the heart and the liver, viscera which Aristotle allowed to eggs incubated for three days."

The Philosopher,[2] however, nowhere says anything of the kind; neither, for the most part, are the viscera mentioned conspicuous before the tenth day. And I am indeed surprised that Aldrovandus should have taken one of these pulsating points for the liver, as if this viscus were ever moved in any such manner! It seems much better to believe that with the growth of the embryo one of the pulsating points is changed into the auricles, the other into the ventricles of the heart. For in the adult, the ventricles are filled in the same manner by the auricles, and by their contraction they are straightway emptied again, as we have shown in our treatise on the Motion of the Heart and Blood.

In more forward eggs, towards the end of the fourth day, I have occasionally found I know not what cause of obscurity intervening and preventing me from seeing these pulsating vesicles with the same distinctness as before; it was as if there had been a haze interposed between them and the eye. In a clearer light, nevertheless, and with the use of magnifying glasses, the observations of one day being further collated with those of the next succeeding day, it was discovered that the indistinctness was caused by the rudiments of the body, —a nebula concocted from part of the colliquament, or an effluvium concreting around the commencements of the veins.

Aldrovandus appears to have observed this: "On the fifth day," says he, "the punctum, which we have stated to be the

---

[1] Op cit. p. 217.   [2] De Generat. Animal. lib. iii, cap. 4.

heart, is no longer seen to move externally, but to be covered over and concealed; still its two meatus venosi are perceived more distinctly than before, one of them being, further, larger than the other." But our learned author was mistaken here; for this familiar divinity, the heart, enters into his mansion and shuts himself up in its inmost recesses a long time afterwards, and when the house is almost completely built. Aldrovandus also errs when he says, " by the vis insita of the veins, the remaining portion of the albumen acquires a straw colour," for this colour is observed in the thicker albumen of every spoilt egg, and it goes on increasing in depth from day to day as the egg grows staler, and this without any influence of the veins, the thinner portion only being dissipated.

But the embryo enlarging, as we say below, and the ramifications of the meatus venosi extending far and wide to the albumen and vitellus, portions of both of these fluids become liquefied, not indeed in the way Aldrovandus will have it, from some vis insita in the vessels, but from the heat of the blood which they contain. For into whatsoever part of either fluid the vessels in question extend, straightway liquefaction appears in their vicinity; and it is on this account that the yelk about this epoch appears double: its superior portion, which is in juxtaposition with the blunt end of the egg, has already become more diffluent than the rest, and appears like melted yellow wax in contrast with the other colder firmer portion; like bodies in general in a state of fusion, it also occupies a larger space. Now this superior portion, liquefied by the genial heat, is separated from the other liquids of the egg, but particularly the albumen, by a tunica propria of extreme tenuity. It therefore happens that if this most delicate, fragile, and invisible membrane be torn, immediately there ensues an admixture and confusion of the albumen and vitellus, by which everything is obscured. And such an accident is a frequent cause of failure in the reproductive power, (for the different fluids in question are possessed of opposite natures,) according to Aristotle,[1] in the place already so frequently referred to : "Eggs are spoiled and become addled in warm weather especially, and with good reason; for as wine grows sour in hot weather, the lees

---

[1] De Gener. Anim. lib. iii, c. 2.

becoming diffused through it, (which is the cause of its spoiling,) so do eggs perish when the yelk spoils, for the lees and the yelk are the more earthy portion in each. Wherefore wine is destroyed by an admixture with its dregs, and an egg by the diffusion of its yelk."[1] And here, too, we may not improperly refer to that passage[2] where he says : "When it thunders, the eggs that are under incubation are spoiled ;" for it must be a likely matter that a membrane so delicate should give way amidst a conflict of the elements. And perhaps it is because thunder is frequent about the dog days that eggs which are rotten have been called *cynosura ;* so that Columella rightly informs us that " the summer solstice, in the opinion of many, is not a good season for breeding chickens."

This at all events is certain, that eggs are very readily shaken and injured when the fowls are disturbed during incubation, at which time the fluids are liquefied and expanded, and their containing membranes are distended and extremely tender.

EXERCISE THE EIGHTEENTH.

The fourth inspection of the egg.

" In the course of the fifth day of incubation," says Aristotle,[3] " the body of the chick is first distinguished, of very small dimensions indeed, and white ; but the head conspicuous and the eyes extremely prominent, a state in which they afterwards continue long ; for they only grow smaller and shrink at a later period. In the lower portion of the body there is no rudimentary member corresponding with what is seen in the upper part. But of the channels which proceed from the heart, one now tends to the investing membrane, the other to the yelk; together they supply the office of an umbilical cord. The chick, therefore, derives its origin from the albumen, but it is afterwards nourished by the yelk, through the umbilicus."

These words of Aristotle appear to subdivide the entire generation of the chick into three stages or periods, viz. : from the

---

[1] Hist. Anim. lib. vi, c. 2.   [2] Ib. lib. viii, c. 5.   [3] Ib. lib. vi, c. 3.

first day of the incubation to the fifth ; from thence on to the tenth or fourteenth : and from this or that to the twentieth. It seems as if he had only given an account in his history of the circumstances he observed at these three epochs ; and it is then indeed that the greatest changes take place in the egg; as if these three critical seasons, or these three degrees in the process which leads from the perfect egg to the evolution of the chicken, were especially to be distinguished. On the fourth day the first particle of the embryo appears, viz. : the punctum saliens and the blood; and then the new being is incorporated. On the seventh day the chick is distinguished by its extremities, and begins to move. On the tenth it is feathered. About the twentieth it breathes, chirps, and endeavours to escape. The life of the egg, up to the fourth day, seems identical with that of plants, and can only be accounted as of a vegetative nature. From this onwards to the tenth day, however, like an animal, it is possessed by a sensitive and motive principle, with which it continues to increase, and is afterwards gradually perfected, becoming covered with feathers, furnished with a beak, nails, and all else that is necessary to its escape from the shell; emancipated from which, it enters at length on its own independent existence.

Of the incidents that happen after the fourth day, Aristotle enumerates three particularly, viz. : the construction of the body ; the distribution of the veins, which have already the office and nature of the umbilicus ; and the matter whence the embryo first arises, and is constituted and nourished.

In reference to the structure of the body, he speaks of its size and colour, of the parts which are most conspicuous in it, (the head and eyes,) and of the distinction of its extremities.

The body is indeed extremely minute, and of the form of the common maggot that gives birth to the fly ; it is of a white colour, too, like the maggot of the flesh-fly which we see cherished and nourished in putrid meat. He happily adds, " it is most remarkable for its head and eyes." For what first appears is homogeneous and indistinct, a kind of concretion or coagulation of the colliquament, like the jelly prepared from hartshorn ; it is a mere transparent cloud, and scarcely recognizable, save as it appears, divided, seemingly, into two parts, one of which is globular and much larger than the other ; this is the rudiment of the head, which first becomes visible on the fifth day, very soon after which the eyes are distinguishable, being from the first of large size and prominent, and marked off from the rest of the head and body by a certain circumfusion of black matter. Either of the eyes is larger than the whole of the rest of the head, in the same way as the head surpasses the remainder of the body in dimensions. The whiteness of the body, and prominence of the eyes, (which, as well as the brain, are filled internally with perfectly pellucid water, but externally are of a dark colour), continue for some time—up to the tenth day, and even longer; for, as we have seen, Aristotle says that " the eyes decrease at a late period, and contract to the proper proportion." But for my own part, I do not think that the eyes of birds ever contract in the same ratio which we observe between the head and eyes of a viviparous animal. For if you strip off the integuments from the head and eyes of a fowl or another bird, you will perceive one of the eyes to equal the entire brain in dimensions; in the woodcock and others, one of the eyes indeed is as large as the whole head, if you make abstraction of the bill. But this is common to all birds that the orbit or cavity which surrounds the eye is larger than the brain, a fact that is apparent in the cranium of every bird. Their eyes, however, are made to look smaller, because every part, except the pupil, is covered with skin and feathers; neither are they possessed of such a globular form as would cause them to project; they are of a flatter configuration, as in fishes.

" In the lower part of the body," says the philosopher, " we perceive the rudiments of no member corresponding with the superior members." And the thing is so in fact; for as the body at first appears to consist of little but head and eyes, so inferiorly there is neither any extremity,—wings, legs, sternum, rump,— nor any viscus apparent; the body indeed is still without any kind of proper form; in so far as I am able to perceive, it consists of a small mass adjacent to the vein, like the bent keel of a boat, like a maggot or an ant, without a vestige of ribs, wings, or feet, to which a globular and much more conspicuous mass is appended, the rudiment of the head, to wit, divided, as it seems, into three vesicles when regarded from either side, but in fact consisting of four cells, two of which, of great size and a black colour, are the rudiments of the eyes; of the remaining two

one being the brain, the other the cerebellum. All of these
are full of perfectly limpid water.   In the middle of the
blackness of the eye, the pupil is perceived shining like a transparent central spark or crystal.   I imagine that three of these
vesicles being particularly conspicuous, has been the cause of
indifferent observers falling into error.   For as they had learned
from the schoolmen that there was a triple dominion in the
animal body, and they believed that these principal parts, the
brain, the heart, and the liver, performed the highest functions
in the economy, they easily persuaded themselves that these
three vesicles were the rudiments and commencements of these
parts.   Coiter, however, as becomes an experienced anatomist,
affirms more truly that whilst he had observed the beak and
eyes from the seventh day of incubation, he could yet discover
nothing of the viscera.

But let us hear the philosopher further: " Of the conduits
which lead from the heart, one tends to the investing membrane,
another to the yelk, in order to perform the office of umbilicus."
The embryo having now taken shape, these veins do indeed
perform the function of the umbilical cord, the ramifications of
one of them proceeding to be distributed to the outer tunic
which invests the albumen, those of the other running for distribution to the vitellary membrane and its included fluid.
Whence it clearly appears that both of these fluids are alike
intended for the nourishment of the embryo.   And although
Aristotle says that "the chick has its commencement in the
albumen, and is nourished through the umbilicus by the yelk,"
he still does not say that the chick is formed from the albumen.
The embryo, in fact, is formed from that clear liquid which we
have spoken of under the name of the colliquament, and the
whole of what we have called the eye of the egg is contained
or included within the albumen.   Neither does our author say
that the whole and sole nutriment of the embryo reaches it
through the umbilicus.   My own observations lead me to interpret his words in this way: although the embryo of the fowl
begins to be formed in the albumen, nevertheless it is not nourished solely by that, but also by the yelk, to which one of the
two umbilical conduits pertains, and from whence it derives
nourishment in a more especial manner; for the albumen,
according to Aristotle's opinion, is the more concoct and purer

liquid, the yelk the more earthy and solid one, and, therefore, more apt to sustain the chick when it has once attained to greater consistency and strength; and further because, as shall be explained below, the yelk supplies the place of milk, and is the last part that is consumed, a residuary portion, even after the chick is born, and when it is following its mother, being still contained in its abdomen.

What has now been stated takes place from the fourth to the tenth day. I have yet to speak of the order and manner in which each of the particulars indicated transpires.

In the inspection made on the fifth day, we observed around the short vein which proceeds from the angle where the two alternately pulsating points are situated, something whiter and thicker, like a cloud, although still transparent, through which the vein just mentioned is seen obscurely, and as it were through a haze. The same thing I have occasionally seen in the more forward eggs in the course of the fourth day. Now this is the rudiment of the body, and from hour to hour it goes on increasing in compactness and solidity; both surrounding the afore-named vein, and being appended to it in the guise of a kind of globule. This globular rudiment far exceeds the coronal portion, as I shall call it, of the vermicular body; it is triangular in figure, being obscurely divided into three parts, like so many swelling buds of a tree. One of these is orbicular and larger than either of the other two; and it is darkened by most delicate filaments proceeding from the circumference to the centre; this appears to be the commencement of the ciliary body, and therefore proclaims that this is the part which is to undergo transformation into the eye. In its middle the minute pupil, shining like a bright point, as already stated, is conspicuous; and it was from this indication especially that I ventured to conjecture that the whole of the globular mass was the rudiment of the future head, and this black circle one of the eyes, having the other over against it; for the two are so situated that they can by no means be seen at once and together, one always lying over and concealing the other.

The first rudiment of the future body, which we have stated to sprout around the vein, acquires an oblong and somewhat bent figure, like the keel of a boat. It is of a mucaginous consistence, like the white mould that grows upon damp things excluded from the air. The vein to which this mucor attaches, as I have said, is the vena cava, descending along the spinal column, as my subsequent observations have satisfied me. And if you carefully note the order of contraction in the pulsating vesicles, you may see the one which contracts last impelling its blood into the root of this vein and distending it.

Thus there are two manifest contractions and two similar dilatations in the two vesicles which are seen moving and pulsating alternately; and the contraction of the one which precedes causes the distension or dilatation of the other; for the blood escapes from the cavity of the former vesicle, when it contracts, into that of the latter, which it fills, distends, and causes to pulsate; but this second vesicle, contracting in its turn, throws the blood, which it had received from the former vesicle, into the root of the vein aforesaid, and at the same time distends it.—I go on speaking of this vessel as a vein, though from its pulsation I hold it to be the aorta, because the veins are not yet distinguished from the arteries by any difference in the thickness of their respective coats.

After having contemplated these points with great care, and in many eggs, I remained for some time in suspense as to the opinion I should adopt; whether I should conclude that the concrete appended globular mass proceeded from the colliquament in which it swam, becoming a compacted and coagulated matter in the way that clouds are formed from invisible vapour condensed in the upper regions of the air; or believe that it took its rise from a certain effluvium exhaled from the sanguineous conduit mentioned, originating by diapedesis or transudation, and by deriving nourishment from thence, was enabled to increase? For the beginnings of even the greatest things are often extremely small, and, by reason of this minuteness, sufficiently obscure.

This much I think I have sufficiently determined at all events, viz. that the puncta salientia and meatus venosi, and the vena cava itself, are the parts that first exist; and that the globular mass mentioned afterwards grows to them. I am further certain that the blood is thrown from the punctum saliens into the vein, and that from this does the corpuscle in question grow, and by this is it nourished. The fungus or mucor first originates from an effluvium of the vein on which it appears, and it is thence nourished and made to increase; in the same way as mouldiness grows in moist places, in the dark corners of houses which long escape cleansing; or, like camphor upon cedar wood tables, and moss upon rocks and the bark of trees; lastly, as a kind of delicate down grows upon certain grubs.

Upon the same occasion I also debated with myself whether or not I should conclude, that with the coagulation of the colliquament accomplished, the rudiments of the head and body existed simultaneously with the punctum saliens and the blood, but in a pellucid state, and so delicate that they almost escaped the eye, until becoming inspissated into a fungus or mucor, they acquired a more opaque white colour, and then came into view; the blood meantime from its greater spissitude and purple colour being readily perceptible in the diaphanous colliquament. But now when I look at the thing more narrowly, I am of opinion that the blood exists before any particle of the body appears; that it is the first-born of all the parts of the embryo; that from it both the matter out of which the fœtus is embodied, and the nutriment by which it grows are derived; that it is in fine, if such thing there be, the primary generative particle. But wherefore I am led to adopt this idea shall afterwards be shown more at length when I come to treat of the primary genital part, of the innate heat, and the radical moisture; and, at the same time, conclude as to what we are to think of the vital principle (anima), from a great number of observations compared with one another.

About this period almost every hour makes a difference; every thing grows larger, more definite and distinct; the rate of change in the egg is rapid, and one change succeeds immediately upon the back of another. The cavity in the egg is now much larger, and the whole of its upper portion is empty; it is as if a fifth part of the egg had been removed.

The ramifications of the veins extend more widely, and are more numerous, not only in the colliquament as before, but they spread on one hand into the abumen, and on the other into the yelk, so that both of these fluids are everywhere covered over with blood-vessels. The upper portion of the yelk has now become much dissolved, so that it very obviously differs from the lower portion; there are now, as it were, two yelks, or two kinds of yelk; whilst the superior, like melted wax, is expanded and looks pellucid, the inferior has become more dense, and with the thicker portion of the albumen has subsided to the sharp end of the egg. The tunica propria of the upper portion of the yelk is so thin that it gives way on the slightest succussion, when there ensues admixture of the fluids, and, as we have said, interruption to the further progress of the process of generation.

And now it is that the rudiments of the embryo first become conspicuous, as may be seen in the fifth and sixth figure of Fabricius; the egg being put into fair water it will be easy to perceive what parts of the body are formed, what are still wanting. The embryo now presents itself in the form of a small worm or maggot, such as we encounter on the leaves of trees, in spots of their bark, in fruit, flowers, and elsewhere; but especially in the apples of the oak, in the centre of which, surrounded with a case, a limpid fluid is contained, which, gradually inspissated and congealed, acquires a most delicate outline, and finally assumes the form of a maggot; for some time, however, it remains motionless; but by and by, endowed with motion and sensation it becomes an animal, and subsequently it breaks forth and takes its flight as a fly.

Aristotle ascribes a similar mode of production to those creatures that are spontaneously engendered.[1] " Some are engendered of the dew," he says, "which falls upon the leaves." And by and by he adds, " butterflies are engendered from caterpillars, but these, in their turn, spring from green leaves, particularly that species of raphanus which is called cabbage. They are smaller than millet seeds at first, and then they grow into little worms; next, in the course of three days into caterpillars; after which they cease from motion, change their shape, and pass into chrysalides, when they are inclosed in a hard shell; although, if touched, they will still move. The shell after a long time cracks and gives way, and the winged animal, which we call a butterfly, emerges."

But our doctrine—and we shall prove it by and by—is, that all animal generation is effected in the same way; that all animals, even the most perfect, are produced from worms; a fact which Aristotle himself seems to have noted when he says:

---

[1] Hist. Anim. lib. v, c. 19.

"In all, nevertheless, even those that lay perfect eggs, the first conception grows whilst it is yet invisible; and this, too, is the nature of the worm."[1] For there is this difference between the generation of worms and of other animals, that the former acquire dimensions before they have any definite form or are distinguished into parts, in conformity with what the philosopher[2] says in the following sentence : " An animal is fashioned from an entire worm, not from any one particular part, as in the case of an egg, but the whole increases and becomes an articulated animal," i. e. in its growth it separates into parts.

It is indeed matter worthy of admiration, that the rudiments of all animals, particularly those possessed of red blood, such as the dog, horse, deer, ox, common fowl, snake, and even man himself, should so signally resemble a maggot in figure and consistence, that with the eye you can perceive no difference between them.

Towards the end of the fifth day or the beginning of the sixth, the head is divided into three vesicles : the first of these, which is also the largest, is rounded and black; this is the eye, in the centre of which the pupil can be distinguished like a crystalline point. Under this there lies a smaller vesicle, concealed in part, which represents the brain; and over this lies the third vesicle, like an added crest or rounded summit crowning the whole, from which the cerebellum is at length produced. In the whole of these there is nothing to be discovered but a little perfectly limpid water.

And now the rudiment of the body, which we have called the carina, distinctly proclaims itself to be the spinal column, to which sides soon begin to be added, and the wings and the lower extremities present themselves, projecting slightly from the body of the maggot. The venous conduits are, further, now clearly referrible to the umbilical vessels.

---

[1] De Gener. Animal. lib. iii, c. 9.   [2] Hist. Anim. lib. v, c. 19.

The fifth inspection of the egg.

On the sixth day the three cells of the head present themselves more distinctly, and the coats of the eyes are now apparent; the legs and the wings also bud forth, much in the way
in which, towards the end of June, we see tadpoles getting
their extremities, when they quit the water, and losing their
tails assume the form of frogs.

In the chick, the rump has still no other form than is conspicuous in animals at large, even in serpents; it is a round and
slender tail.   The substance of the heart now grows upon the
pulsating vesicle; and shortly afterwards the rudiments of the
liver and lungs are distinguished; the bill, too, makes its appearance at the same time.   Everything is of a pure white colour, especially the bill.   About the same epoch all the viscera
and the intestines are conspicuous.   But the heart takes
precedence of all the parts; and the lungs are visible before the
liver or brain.   The eyes, however, are seen first of all, by
reason of their large size and black colour.

And now, too, the embryo has a power of motion, and raises
its head and slightly twists itself, although there is still nothing
of the brain to be seen, but only a little limpid fluid inclosed
in a vesicle.   It is at length a perfect maggot, only differing
from a caterpillar in this, that when worms are set free from
their cells they creep about hither and thither and seek their
food, whilst the worm in the egg is stationary, and, surrounded
with its proper food, is furnished with aliment through the
umbilicus.

The viscera and intestines being now formed, and the fœtus
able to execute motions, the anterior portion of the body, without either thorax or abdomen, is perceived to be completely
open; so that the heart itself, the liver and the intestines, are
seen to hang pendulous externally.

Towards the end of this day and the beginning of the seventh,
the toes are distinguished, and the embryo already presents the
outlines of the chick, and opens its beak, and kicks with its

feet; in short, all the parts are sketched out, but the eyes, above all, are conspicuous. The viscera, on the contrary, are so indistinct, that Coiter affirms, that whilst he plainly saw the eyes and beak he could discover no viscus, even obscurely and confusedly shadowed forth.

The changes that take place from the beginning of the sixth to the end of the seventh day, occur for the major part in some eggs more quickly, in others a little more tardily. The coats of the eyes are now visible, but they only include a colourless and limpid fluid in their interior. The eyes themselves project somewhat beyond their orbits, and each of them does not less exceed the brain in size, than the head with which they are connected exceeds the whole of the rest of the body.

The vesicle, which like a ridge or crest expands beyond the confines of the brain, occupies the place of the cerebellum; and, like the other vesicles, is filled with a transparent fluid.

The brain is perceived to be obscurely bipartite, and refracts the light less than the cerebellum, though it is of a whiter colour. And as the heart is seen lying without the confines of the thorax, so likewise does the cerebellum protrude beyond the limits of the head.

If the head be removed, the vessels ascending to the brain may be observed as bloody points, with the use of a magnifying glass. And now, too, the rudiments of the spine begin to be first perceived distinct from the rest of the pulp, of a milky colour, but firmer consistence. So in the same way, and like flimsy threads of a spider's web, the ribs and other bones make their appearance in the guise of milky lines, amidst the pulp of the body; and the same thing appears more clearly in the formation of the larger oviparous animals. The heart, lungs, liver, and by way of intestines certain most delicate filaments, all present themselves of a white colour. The parenchyma of the liver is developed upon delicate fibrous stamens over the umbilical vein at the part where it enters, almost in the same manner as we have said that the rudiments of the body grow to the vein descending from the heart, or the vesicula pulsans. For in the same way as grapes grow upon the stalk of the bunch, buds upon twigs, and the ear upon the straw, does the liver adhere to the umbilical vein, and arise from it, even as fungi do from trees and excessive granulations from ulcers, or as sarcoses or morbid growths spring around the minute branches of conterminous arteries by which they are nourished, and occasionally attain to an excessive size.

Looking back upon this office of the arteries, or the circulation of the blood, I have occasionally and against all expectation completely cured enormous sarcoceles, by the simple means of dividing or tying the little artery that supplied them, and so preventing all access of nourishment or spirit to the part affected; by which it came to pass that the tumour, on the verge of mortification, was afterwards easily extirpated with the knife, or the searing iron. One man in particular (and this case I can confirm by the testimony of many respectable persons) had an enormous hernia carnosa, or sarcocosis of the scrotum, larger than a human head, and hanging as low as the knee; from its upper part a fleshy mass, of the thickness of the wrist, or such a rope as is used on ship-board, extended into the abdomen; and the evil had attained to such a height, that no one durst attempt the cure, either with the knife or any other means. Nevertheless, by the procedure above indicated, I succeeded in completely removing this huge excrescence which distended the scrotum, and involved the testicle in its middle; this latter organ, with its vas præparans and vas deferens, and other parts which descend in the tunica vaginalis, being left all the while safe and uninjured. But this cure, as well as various others, accomplished in opposition to vulgar opinion and by unusual procedures, I shall relate at greater length in my Medical Observations, if God grant me longer life.

I mention such cases with a view of more clearly showing that the liver grows upon the vessels, and is only developed some time after the appearance of the blood; that its parenchyma is derived from the arteries whence the matter is effused, and that for a while it remains white and bloodless, like various other parts of the body. Now in the same manner and order precisely as the chick is developed from the egg, is the generation of man and other animals accomplished.

Whence it appears that the doctrine which makes the liver the author and fashioner of the blood, is altogether groundless, although both formerly and at the present time this view obtained universal assent; this was the reason wherefore the liver was reckoned as among the principal and first-formed organs of the body. This viscus indeed was so highly dignified that it was thought to be produced in the very beginning, and simultaneously with the heart, from the seminal fluid of the mother; and the medical fable of the three vesicles or three kids, as they were called, was eagerly defended. Among the number of modern abettors of such views, Parisanus has of late with confidence enough, but little skill, been singing to the old measure. These good people do not consider that the vesicles are in motion in the egg, that the heart is palpitating and the blood present and perfectly concocted, before any sign or vestige of the liver appears. The blood is much rather to be accounted the efficient cause of the liver, than this the author of the blood : for the liver is engendered after the blood, and from it, being adnate to the vessels that contain it.

But neither can I agree with the Aristotelians, who maintain that the heart is the author of the blood; for its parenchyma or proper substance arises some little time after the blood, and is superadded to the pulsating vesicles. I am, however, in much doubt as to whether the pulsating vesicle or point, or the blood itself be the older; whether it be the fluid contained, or the containing sacs. It is obvious, nevertheless, that that which contains is formed for the sake of that which is contained, and is, therefore, made later. And this much, upon the faithful testimony of our eyes, is certain, that the first particle and prime basis of the body are the veins, to which all the other parts are posthumous and superadded. But upon this point we shall say more by and by.

Meantime we may be permitted to smile at that factitious division of the parts into spermatic and sanguineous; as if any part were produced immediately from the seminal fluid, and all did not spring from the same source !

I return to our subject. The colliquament now extends over more than half the egg. The heart, hanging outwards, is at some short distance from the body. And if you look attentively you may perceive some of the umbilical vessels pulsating.

The sixth inspection.

Everything is still more distinct upon the seventh day, and the rudiments of several of the particular parts are now conspicuous, viz., the wings, legs, genital organs, divisions for the toes, thighs, ilia, &c. The embryo now moves and kicks, and the form of the perfect chick is recognizable; from this time forward, indeed, nothing is superadded; the very delicate parts only increase in size. The more the parts grow the more is the albumen consumed, and the external membranes united come to be of the nature of the secundines, and ever more and more closely represent the umbilical cord. Wherefore I conceive that, from the seventh, we may at once pass on to the tenth day, nothing of any moment occurring in this interval which is not particularly noted by other writers, especially by Aristotle.

It happens, nevertheless, that when a number of eggs are examined together, some are found more precocious and forward, having everything more distinct; others, again, are more sluggish, and these have the parts less apparent. The season of the year, the place where the incubation is carried on, the sedulousness with which it is performed, and other accidents, have undoubtedly great influence on this diversity of result. I remember on one occasion, on the seventh day to have seen the cavity in the blunt end enlarged in a sluggish egg, the colliquament covered with veins, the vermicular embryo in its middle, the rudiments of the eyes, and all the rest as it is met with in the generality of eggs on the fifth day; but the pulsatory vesicles were not yet apparent, nor was the trunk or root of the veins from which we have said that they originate, yet to be discovered. I therefore regarded this egg as of a feeble nature and left behind, as possessed of an inadequate reproductive faculty, and near to its death; all the more when I observed its colliquament less pellucid and refractive than usual, and the vessels not of such a bright red colour as wont. When the vital spirit is about to escape, that part which is first influenced in generation and earliest attracts attention is also the first that fails and disappears.

The inspection after the tenth day.

All that presents itself on the tenth day is so accurately described by Aristotle that scarcely anything remains for us to add. Now his opinion, according to my interpretation of it, is this, viz., that "on the tenth day the entire chick is conspicuous,"[1] being pellucid and white in every part except the eyes and the venous ramifications. " The head at this time is larger than the whole of the rest of the body; and eyes larger than the head are connected with it," (adhering, and being in some sort appended to the head,) " but having as yet no pupils," (perfectly formed pupils must here be understood, for it is not difficult to make out the distinct tunics of the eye at this epoch;) " the eyes, if removed at this time, will be found as large as beans and black, and if they be incised, a clear humour flows out, cold, and refracting the light powerfully, but nothing else," i. e., in the whole head there is nothing but the limpid water which has been mentioned. Such is the state of matters from the seventh to the tenth day, as we have said above. " At the same time," he continues, " the viscera also appear, and all that appertains to the abdomen and intestines," viz., the substance of the heart, the lungs, liver, &c., all of a white colour, mucilaginous, pulpy, without any kind of consistency. " The veins, too, that issue from the heart are already in connexion with the umbilicus, from which one vein extends to the membrane that includes the vitellus, which has now become more liquid and diffluent than it was originally ; another to the membrane which surrounds everything," (i. e., the tunica colliquamenti,) " and embraces the fœtus, the vitellus and the interjacent fluid. For the embryo increasing somewhat, one portion of the vitellus is

---

[1] Hist. Anim. lib. vi, cap. 3.

superior, another inferior; but the albumen in the middle is liquid, and still extends under the inferior portion of the vitellus, as it did previously." Thus far Aristotle.

And now the arteries are seen distinctly accompanying the veins, both those that proceed to the albumen and those that are distributed to the vitellus. The vitellus also at this time liquefies still more and becomes more diffluent, not entirely, indeed, but, as already said, that portion of it which is uppermost; neither do the branches of the veins proceed to every part of the vitellus alike, but only to that part which we have spoken of as resembling melted wax. The veins that are distributed to the albumen have, in like manner, arteries accompanying them. The larger portion of the albumen now dissolves into a clear fluid, the colliquament, which surrounds the embryo that swims in its middle, and comes between the two portions of the vitellus, viz., the superior and the inferior; underneath all (in the sharp end of the egg), the thicker and more viscid portion of the albumen is contained. The superior portion of the yelk already appears more liquid and diffluent than the inferior; and wherever the branches of the veins extend, there the matter seems suddenly to swell and become more diffluent.

"On the tenth day," continues our author, "the albumen subsides, having now become a small tenacious, viscid, and yellowish mass"—so much of it, that is to say, as has not passed into the state of colliquament.

For already the larger portion of the white has become dissolved, and has even passed into the body of the embryo, viz., the whole of the thinner albumen, and the greater portion of the thicker. The yelk, on the contrary, rather looks larger than it did in the beginning. Whence it clearly appears that the yelk has not as yet served for the nutrition of the embryo, but is reserved to perform this office by and by. In so far as we can conjecture from the course and distribution of the veins, the embryo from the commencement is nourished by the colliquament; upon this blood-vessels are first distributed, and then they spread over the membrane of the thinner albumen, next over the thicker albumen, and finally over the vitellus. The thicker albumen serves for nutriment after the thinner; the vitellus is drawn upon last of all.

The delicate embryo, consequently, whilst it is yet in the vermicular state, is nourished with the thinnest and best concocted aliment, the colliquament and thinner albumen; but when it is older it has food supplied to it more in harmony with its age and strength.

Aristotle describes the relative situation of the several parts in the following words : " In the anterior and posterior part, the membrane of the egg lies under the shell,—I do not mean the membrane of the shell itself, but one under this, in which there is contained a clear fluid"—the colliquament; "then the chick and the membrane including it, which keeps it distinct from the fluid around it." But here I suspect that there is an error in the text; for as the author himself indicates the thing, it ought rather to stand thus: "then the chick, enveloped in a membrane, continues or swims in the clear fluid ;" which membrane is not exterior to the one that immediately lines the shell, but another lying under this; which, when the first or external albumen is consumed, and the remainder of the thicker albumen is depressed into the sharp end of the egg, of two membranes forms a single tunic that now begins to present itself like the secundine called the chorion. And Aristotle says well, " there is a clear fluid contained in it," by which words he does not mean the albumen, but the colliquament derived from the albumen, and in which the embryo swims ; for the albumen that remains subsides into the small end of the egg.

EXERCISE THE TWENTY-SECOND.

The inspection after the fourteenth day.

From the seventh to the fourteenth day everything has grown and become more conspicuous. The heart and all the other viscera have now become concealed within the abdomen of the embryo, and the parts that formerly were seen naked and projecting externally, can now only be perceived when the thorax and abdomen are laid open. The chick too now begins to be covered with feathers, the roots of which are first perceived as black points. The pupils of the eyes are distinguished; the eyelids appear, as does also the membrana nictitans in the greater canthus of the eye, a membane which is proper to birds, and which they use for cleansing the eyeball. The convolutions of the brain farther make their appearance; the cerebellum is included within the skull; and the tail acquires the characteristic shape of the bird's rump.

After the fourteenth day the viscera, which up to this time have been white, gradually begin to assume a flesh or reddish colour. The heart, having now entered the penetralia of the thorax and been covered with the sternum, inhabits the dwelling place which itself had formed. The cerebrum and cerebellum acquire solidity under the dome of the skull; the stomach and intestines, however, are not yet included within the abdomen, but, connected with the parts within, hang pendulous externally.

Of the two vessels that proceed from the abdomen to the umbilicus, near the anus, one is an artery, as its pulse proclaims, and arises from the arteria magna or aorta, the other is a vein, and extends from the vitellus by the side of the intestines to the vena portæ, situated in the concave part of the liver. The other trunk of the umbilical vessels, collecting its branches from the albumen, passes the convexity of the liver, and enters the vena cava near the base of the heart.

As all these things go on becoming clearer from day to day, so the greater portion of the albumen is also gradually consumed; this, however, is nowise the case with the vitellus, which remains almost entire up to this time, and indeed is seen of the same size as it was the first day.

In the course of the following days five umbilical vessels are conspicuous; one of these is the great vein, arising from the cava above the liver, and distributing its branches to the albumen; two other veins proceed from the porta, both having the same origin, and run to the two portions of the vitellus, which we have but just described; and these are accompanied by two arteries arising one on either side from the lumbars.

The chick now occupies a larger space in the egg than all the rest of the matter included in it, and begins to be covered with feathers; the larger the embryo grows, the smaller is the quantity of albumen that is present. It is also worthy of observation, that the membrane of the colliquament which we have said unites with the external investing membrane, and constitutes the secundine or chorion, now includes the whole of the vitellus in one, and becoming contracted, draws the vitellus along with the intestines towards the chick, conjoins them with its body, and incloses them as it were in a thick sac. Everything that was previously extremely delicate and transparent, becomes more opaque and fleshy as the sac contracts, which at length, like a hernial tumour of the scrotum, includes and supports both the intestines and the yelk; contracting every day in a greater and greater degree, it comes finally to constitute the abdomen of the chick. You will find the yelk, about the eighteenth day, lying [in its bag] among the intestines, the belly at large being lax; yet are the parts not so firmly fixed but that the intestines (as in the case of a scrotal hernia), along with the vitellus, can be pushed up into the belly, or forced out of it as it were into a pouch. I have occasionally seen the vitellus prolapsed in this way from the abdominal cavity of a pigeon, which had been prematurely excluded from the shell in the summer season.

The chick at this epoch looks big-bellied and as if it were affected with a hernia, as I have said. And now the colliquament, which was at first in large quantity, gradually grows turbid, suffers change, and is consumed, so that the chick comes to lie bent over the vitellus. At the same period, before the liver assumes its sanguineous colour, and performs the business of what is called the second concoction, the bile, which is commonly believed to be separated as an excretion by the power of the liver, is seen of a green colour between the lobes of that organ. In the cavity of the stomach there is a limpid fluid contained, obviously of the same appearance and taste as the colliquament in which the fœtus swims; this passing on by the intestines, gradually changes its colour, and is converted into chyle; and finally in the lower portion of the bowels an excrementitious matter is encountered, of the same character as that which is met with in the lower intestines of chicks already excluded from the egg. When the chick is further advanced you may even see this fluid concocted and coagulated; just as in those animals that feed on milk, a coagulum is formed, which afterwards separates into serum and firmer curd.

When the albumen is almost all removed, and only a very small quantity of the colliquament is left, for several days before the exclusion, the chick no longer swims, but, as I have said, bends over the vitellus ; and rolled up into a round ball, with the head for the most part placed between the right thigh and wing, it is seen with its beak, nails, feathers, and all other parts complete. Sometimes it sleeps, and sometimes it wakes, and moving about it breathes and chirps. If you apply the egg to your ear, you will hear the chick within making a noise, kicking, and unquestionably chirping; according to Aristotle, he now also uses his eyes. If you cautiously drop the egg into warm water, it will swim, and the chick within, aroused by the warmth, will leap, and, as I have already said, cause the egg to tumble about. And it is by this means that our country folks distinguish prolific from unproductive eggs which sink when put into water.

When the albumen is entirely gone, just before the exclusion, the umbilical vessel, which we have described as distributed to the albumen, is obliterated; or as Aristotle says,[1] "that umbilicus which proceeds to the external secundines is detached from the animal and dies; but the one which leads to the vitellus becomes connected with the small intestine of the chick."

The excrement that is first formed in the intestines is white and turbid, like softened egg-shell; and some of the same matter may be found contained in the secundines. The philosopher admits this when he says : "At the same time, too, the chick discharges a large quantity of excrement into the outer membrane; and there are white excrements within the abdomen, as well as those that have been evacuated."

Time running on, very shortly before the exclusion, light green fæces are formed, similar to those which the chick discharges when excluded from the egg. In the crop, too, we can discover a portion of the colliquament which has been swallowed; and in the stomach some curd or coagulum.

Up to this time the liver has not yet acquired its. purple or blood-red colour, but has a tint verging from white into yellow, such as the liver of fishes presents. The lungs, however, are of a florid red.

---

[1] Hist. Anim. lib. vi, cap. 3.

The yelk is now contained in the abdomen among the intestines : and this is the case not merely whilst the chick is in the egg, but even after its exclusion, and when it is running about following its mother in search of food. So that what Aristotle frequently asserts appears to be absolutely true, viz., that the yelk is destined for the food of the chick ; and the chick does certainly use it for food, included in his interior as it is, during the few first days after his exclusion, and until such time as his bill gains the hardness requisite to break and prepare his food, and his stomach the strength necessary to digest it. And, indeed, the yelk of the egg is very analogous to milk. Aristotle gives us his support in this opinion in the place already so frequently referred to :[1] " The chick now lies over much of the yellow, which at last diminishes, and, in process of time, disappears entirely, being all taken into the body of the bird, where it is stored, so that on the tenth day after the exclusion of the chick, if the belly be laid open, you will still find a little of the yelk upon the intestines." I have myself found certain remains of the yelk even upon the thirteenth day ; and if the argument derivable from the duct of the umbilical veins which we have described as terminating in the porta of the liver by one or another trunk, be of any avail, the chick is already nourished almost in the same manner as it is subsequently, the sustenance being attracted from the yelk by the umbilical vessels, in the same way as chyle is by and by transmitted by the mesenteric veins from the intestines. For the vessels terminate in either case in the porta of the liver, to which the nourishment attracted in the same way is in like manner transmitted. It is not necessary, therefore, to have recourse to any lacteal vessels of the mesentery, which, in the feathered tribes, are nowhere to be distinguished.

Let me be permitted here to add what I have frequently found : With a view to discovering more distinctly the relative situations of the embryo and the fluids, I have boiled an egg hard, from the fourteenth day of the incubation up to the day when the exclusion would have taken place, the major part of the albumen being already consumed, and the vitellus divided.

[1] Hist. Anim. lib. vi, cap. 3.

Breaking the shell, and regarding the position of the chick, I found both the remains of the albumen and the two portions of the vitellus (which we have said are divided by the colliquation induced by the gentle heat), possessing the consistency, colour, taste, and other qualities which distinguish the yelks of unincubated eggs similarly boiled. I have, therefore, frequently asked myself how it came to pass that unprolific eggs set under a hen are made to putrefy and become offensive by the same extraneous heat which produces no such effect upon prolific eggs, both of the fluids of which remain sweet and unchanged, although they have an embryo in the midst of them, (and this even containing some small quantity of excrementitious matter within it,) so that did any one eat the yelk of such an egg in the dark, he would not distinguish it from that of a fresh egg which had never been sat upon.

EXERCISE THE TWENTY-THIRD.

Of the exclusion of the chick, or the birth from the egg.

The egg is, as we have said, a kind of exposed uterus, and place in which the embryo is fashioned: for it performs the office of the uterus and enfolds the chick until the due time of its exclusion arrives, when the creature is born perfect. Oviparous animals consequently are not distinguished from viviparous by the circumstance of the one bringing forth their young alive, and the other not doing so; for the chick not only lives and moves within the egg, but even breathes and chirps whilst there; and, when it escapes from the shell, enjoys a more perfect existence than the fœtus of animals in general. Oviparous and viviparous animals rather differ in their modes of bringing forth; the uterus or place in which the embryo is formed being within the animal in viviparous tribes, where it is cherished and brought to maturity, whilst in oviparous tribes the uterus, or egg, is exposed or without the animal, which, nevertheless, by sitting on it does not cherish it less truly than if it were still contained within the body.

For though the mother occasionally quits her eggs on various errands, it is only for a short season; she still has such affection for them that she speedily returns, covers them over, cherishes them beneath her breast and carefully defends them; and this on to the twenty-first or twenty-second day, when the chicks, in search of freer air, break the shell and emerge into the light.

Now we must not overlook a mistake of Fabricius, and almost every one else in regard to this exclusion or birth of the chick. Let us hear Fabricius.[1]

"The chick wants air sooner than food, for it has still some store of nourishment within it; in which case the chick, by his chirping, gives a sign to his mother of the necessity of breaking the shell, which he himself cannot accomplish by reason of the hardness of the shell and the softness of his beak, to say nothing of the distance of the shell from the beak, and of the position of the head under the wing. The chick, nevertheless, is already so strong, and the cavity in the egg is so ample, and the air contained within it so abundant, that the breathing becomes free and the creature can emit the sounds that are proper to it; these can be readily heard by a bystander, and were recognized both by Pliny and Aristotle,[2] and perchance have something of the nature of a petition in their tone. For the hen hearing the chirping of the chick within, and knowing thereby the necessity of now breaking the shell in order that the chick may enjoy the air which has become needful to it, or if you will, you may say, that desiring to see her dear offspring, she breaks the shell with her beak, which is not hard to do, for the part over the hollow, long deprived of moisture, and exposed to the heat of incubation, has become dry and brittle. The chirping of the chick is consequently the first and principal indication of the creature desiring to make its escape, and of its requiring air. This the hen perceives so nicely, that if she hears the chirping to be low and internal, she straightway turns the egg over with her feet, that she may break the shell at the place whence the voice proceeds without detriment to the chick.

[1] Op. cit. p. 59.
[2] Plin. lib. x, cap. 53. Arist. Hist. Anim. lib. vi, cap. 3.

Hippocrates adds,[1] "Another indication or reason of the chick's desiring to escape from the shell, is that when it wants food it moves vigorously, in search of a larger supply, by which the membrane around it is torn, and the mother breaking the shell at the place where she hears the chick moving most lustily, permits it to escape."

All this is stated pleasantly and well by Fabricius; but there is nothing of solid reason in the tale. For I have found by experience that it is the chick himself and not the hen that breaks open the shell, and this fact is every way in conformity with reason. For how else should the eggs that are hatched in dunghills and ovens, as in Egypt and other countries, be broken in due season, where there is no mother present to attend to the voice of the supplicating chick, and to bring assistance to the petitioner? And how again are the eggs of sea and land tortoises, of fishes, silkworms, serpents, and even ostriches to be chipped? The embryos in these have either no voice with which they can notify their desire for deliverance, or the eggs are buried in the sand or slime where no chirping or noise could be heard. The chick therefore is born spontaneously, and makes its escape from the eggshell through its own efforts. That this is the case appears from unquestionable arguments: when the shell is first chipped, the opening is much smaller than accords with the beak of the mother; but it corresponds exactly to the size of the bill of the chick, and you may always see the shell chipped at the same distance from the extremity of the egg, and the broken pieces, especially those that yield to the first blows, projecting regularly outwards in the form of a circlet. But as any one on looking at a broken pane of glass can readily determine whether the force came from without or from within, by the direction of the fragments that still adhere, so in the chipped egg it is easy to perceive, by the projection of the pieces around the entire circlet, that the breaking force comes from within. And I myself and many others with me besides, hearing the chick scraping against the shell with its feet, have actually seen it perforate this part with its beak, and extend the fracture in a circle like a coronet. I have further

[1] In lib. de nat. pueri.

seen the chick raise up the top of the shell upon its head and remove it.

We have gone at length into some of these matters, as thinking that they were not without all speculative interest, as we shall show by and by. The arguments of Fabricius are easily answered. For I admit that the chick in ovo produces sounds, and these perchance may even have something of the implorative in their nature; but it does not therefore follow that the shell is broken by the mother. Neither is the bill of the chick so soft, nor yet so far from the shell, that it cannot pierce through its prison walls, particularly when we see that the shell, for the reasons assigned, is extremely brittle. Neither does the chick always keep its head under its wing, so as to be thereby prevented from breaking the shell, but only when it sleeps or has died. For the creature wakes at intervals and scrapes and kicks, and struggles, pressing against the shell, tearing the investing membranes, and chirps, (and that this is done whilst petitioning for assistance I willingly concede,) all of which things may readily be heard by any one who will use his ears. And the hen listening attentively when she hears the chirping deep within the egg does not break the shell, but she turns the egg with her feet and gives the chick within another and a more commodious position. But there is no occasion to suppose that the chick by his chirping informs his mother of the propriety of breaking the shell, or seeks deliverance from it. For very frequently for two days before the exclusion you may hear the chick chirping within the shell. Neither is the mother, when she turns the egg, looking for the proper place to break it; but as the child when uncomfortably laid in his cradle is restless and whimpers and cries, and his fond mother turns him this way and that, and rocks him till he is composed again, so does the hen when she hears the chick restless and chirping within the egg, and feels it, when hatched, moving uneasily about in the nest, immediately raise herself and observe that she is not pressing on it with her weight, or keeping it too warm, or the like, and then with her bill and her feet she moves and turns the egg until the chick within is again at its ease and quiet.

Of twin-bearing eggs.

Twin-bearing eggs are such as produce twin chickens, and according to Aristotle,[1] "are possessed of two yelks, which, in some are separated by a layer of thin albumen, that they may less encroach on one another; in others, however, there is nothing of the sort, and then the two yelks are in contact."

I have frequently seen twin eggs, each of the yelks in which was surrounded by an albumen, with common and proper membranes surrounding them. I have also met with eggs having two yelks connate, as it were, both of which were embraced by a single and common albumen.

"Some fowls" says Aristotle,[2] "always produce twins, in which the particulars relating to the yelk that have been stated are clearly perceived. A certain fowl laid within two of twenty eggs, all of which, except those that were unprolific, produced twins. Of the twins, however, one was always larger, the other smaller, and the smaller chick was frequently deformed in addition."

With us twin eggs are occasionally produced, and twin chicks too, although very rarely, are engendered. I have never myself, however, seen both of these chicks live and thrive; one of them either died within the egg or at the time of the exclusion. And this the words of Aristotle prepare us to expect, when he says " one of the two is larger, the other smaller ;" this is as much as to say that one of them is stronger and of greater age, the other weaker and less prepared for quitting the shell: my own opinion therefore is, that the two yelks are of different origins and maturity. It is therefore scarcely possible but that the stronger and more advanced chick, if the egg be broken and it emerge into the light, will cause the blight and abortion of the other. But if the stronger bird do not chip the shell, he himself is threatened with a present danger, viz. want of air.

---

[1] Hist. Anim. lib. vi, cap. 3.   [2] Ibid.

At the exclusion from the shell, consequently, certain death hangs over one or other, if not over both.

Fabricius either not observing the above words of Aristotle, or neglecting them, says : " If an egg have now and then two yelks, it engenders a chick having four legs or wings, and two heads—a monster, in short; never two chicks distinct from one another, and that can be spoken of as a pair ; there is but one trunk, to which are appended two heads, &c."

Whence we may infer that he himself had never seen nor heard from credible persons that such eggs produce two pullets, and therefore that he agrees with me in regarding such eggs as rare, and in holding that they never produce two chicks both alike capable of living.

I am surprised nevertheless that, with the authority of Aristotle before him, he should have said that "two chicks, distinct and separate, are *never* produced from such eggs," but always a monster ; the rather as he thinks that the embryo is engendered from the chalazæ as from the appropriate matter, and he could not but see that there are four chalazæ in every twin-egg.

I should rather imagine that when two vitelli are included by the same albumeu in a twin-egg, and are so intimately associated that their cicatriculæ, when they are resolved together, constitute a single eye or colliquament, may engender a monstrous embryo with four feet, two heads, &c., because I see nothing to hinder this ; and such a production do I conceive to have been engendered by the egg of which Fabricius speaks.

But where two yelks have existed separately, parted by their several membranes, and furnished with chalazæ, albumens, and all else requisite to the generation of the chick, I hold that we must conclude, with Aristotle, that such an egg, as it has all the parts of two eggs except the shell, so does it also possess the faculty or faculties of as many ; and unless it be a wind or barren egg, that it will for the most part produce two embryos, and but rarely a single monstrous individual.

Certain Deductions from the preceding History of the Egg.

Such is the history of the hen's egg; in which we have spoken
of its production, and of its action or faculty to engender a
chick, at too great length, it may appear to those who do not
see the end and object of such painstaking, of such careful observation. Wherefore I think it advisable here to state what
fruits may follow our industry, and in the words of the learned
Lord Verulam, to "enter upon our second vintage." Certain
theorems, therefore, will have to be gathered from the history
given; some of which will be quite certain, some questionable
and requiring further sifting, and some paradoxical and opposed
to popular persuasion. Some of these, moreover, will have reference to the male, some to the female, several to the egg, and
finally, a few to the formation of the chick. When these have
been carefully discussed seriatim, we shall be in a condition to
judge with greater certainty and facility of the generation of
all other animals.

Of the nature of the egg.

Of the theorems that refer to the egg, some teach us what it
is, some show its mode of formation, and others tell of the parts
which compose it.

It is certain, in the first place, that one egg produces one
chick only. Although the egg be in a certain sense an external
uterus, still it most rarely engenders several embryos, but by
far the most frequently produces no more than a single pullet.
And when an egg produces two chicks, which it does sometimes,
still is this egg to be reputed not single but double, and as
possessed of the nature and parts of two eggs.

For an egg is to be viewed as a conception proceeding from

the male and the female, equally endued with the virtue of either, and constituting an unity from which a single animal is engendered.

Nor is it the beginning only, but the fruit and conclusion likewise. It is the beginning as regards the being to be engendered; the fruit in respect of the two parents : at once the end proposed in their engendering, and the origin of the chick that is to be. "But the seed and the fruit," according to Aristotle,[1] "differ from one another in the relations of prior and posterior; for the fruit is that which comes of another, the seed is that from which this other comes: were it otherwise, both would be the same."

The egg also seems to be a certain mean; not merely in so far as it is beginning and end, but as it is the common work of the two sexes and is compounded by both; containing within itself the matter and the plastic power, it has the virtue of both, by which it produces a fœtus that resembles the one as well as the other. It is farther a mean between the animate and the inanimate world; for neither is it wholly endowed with life, nor is it entirely without vitality. It is still farther the mid-passage or transition stage between parents and offspring, between those who are, or were, and those who are about to be; it is the hinge and pivot upon which the whole generation of the bird revolves. The egg is the terminus from which all fowls, male and female, have sprung, and to which all their lives tend, — it is the result which nature has proposed to herself in their being. And thus it comes that individuals in procreating their like for the sake of their species, endure for ever. The egg, I say, is a period or portion of this eternity; for it were hard to say whether an egg exists for the sake of the chick that it engenders, or the pullet exists for the sake of the egg which it is to engender. Which of these was the prior, whether with reference to time or nature,— the egg or the pullet? This question, when we come to speak of the generation of animals in general, we shall discuss at length.

The egg, moreover,—and this is especially to be noted,— corresponds in its proportions with the seeds of plants, and has all the same conditions as these, so that it is to be regarded, not without reason, as the seed or sperma of the common fowl,

---

[1] De Gen. Anim. lib. i, cap. 13.

in the same way as the seeds of plants are justly entitled their eggs, not only as being the *matter* or that from which, but the *efficient* or that by which the pullet is engendered.　　In which finally no part of the future offspring exists *de facto*, but in which all parts inhere *in potentia*.

The seed, properly so called, differs however from the *geniture*, which by Aristotle is defined to be " that which, proceeding from the generator, is the cause, that which first obtains the principle of generation; in those, to wit, whom nature destined to copulate.　　But the seed is that which proceeds from these two in their connection : and such is the seed of all vegetables, and of some animals, in which the sexes are not distinct; like that which is first produced by male and female commingled, a kind of promiscuous conception, or animal; for this already possesses what is required of both."

The egg consequently is a natural body endowed with animal virtues, viz. principles of motion and rest, of transmutation and conservation; it is, moreover, a body which, under favorable circumstances, has the capacity to pass into an animal form; heavy bodies indeed do not sink more naturally, nor light ones float, when they are unimpeded, than do seeds and eggs in virtue of their inherent capacity become changed into vegetables and animals.　　So that the seed and the egg are alike the fruit and final result of the things of which they are the beginning and efficient cause.

For a single pullet there is a single egg; and so Aristotle[1] says : " from one seed one body is engendered; for example, from a single grain of wheat one plant; from a single egg one animal; for a twin-egg is, in fact, two eggs."

And Fabricius[2] with truth observes : " The egg is not only an exposed uterus, and place of generation, but that also on which the whole reproduction of the pullet depends, and which the egg achieves as agent, as matter, as instrument, as seat, and all else, if more there be, that is needful to generation."　　He shows it to be an organ because it consists of several parts, and this, from the statement of Galen, who will have the very essence of an organ to be that " it consist of several parts, all of

---

[1] Gen. Anim. lib. i, cap. 20.　　　　　　[2] Loc. cit. p. 47.

which conspire to one and the same action though diverse in faculty and use; for some are principal instruments in the action; some are indispensable to it,—without them it could not take place; some secure its better performance; and some, in fine, are extant for the safety and preservation of everything else." He also shows it to be an *agent*, when from Aristotle and Galen he lays down the two actions of the egg, viz.: "the generation of the chick, and the growth and nutrition of the pullet." At the conclusion he expresses himself clearly in these words : " In the works of nature we see conjunct and one, the artificer, the instrument, and the matter; the liver, for instance, is both the agent and the instrument for the production of the blood; and so every part of the body ; Aristotle,[1] therefore, said well that the moving powers were not easily distinguished from the instruments. In artificial things, indeed, the artificer and the instrument are distinct, as much so as the workman and his hammer, the painter and his pencil. And the reason adduced by Galen[2] is this : that in things made by art the artificer is without the work; in natural things, again, the artificer is within it, conjunct with the instruments, and pervading the whole organization."

To this I add these perspicuous words of Aristotle.[3] " Of extant things some are consistent with nature, others with other causes. Animals and their parts, and plants, and simple bodies, as earth, fire, air, and water, consist with nature, and are allowed universally to do so; but these bodies differ entirely from those that do not consist with nature. For whatsoever consists with nature is seen to have within itself a principle of motion and of rest, now according to place, now according to increment and decrement, and again according to change. A couch or litter, a garment, and other things of the same description, however designated, inasmuch as they are made by art, have no inherent faculty of change; but inasmuch as they are made of [wood, or] earth, or stone, [or of wool, silk, or linen,] or of mixtures of these, they have such a faculty. As if nature were a certain principle and cause wherefore that should move and be at rest in which she inheres originally, independently, and not by accident. I say, particularly, *not by accident*, because it might happen that one being a physician should himself be the cause

[1] De Gener. Anim. lib. ii, cap. 4.   [2] De form. fœt.   [3] Phys. lib. i, cap. 1.

of his own good health; but he is not familiar with medicine in
the same respect as he has worked his own cure; it happens
simply that the man who here recovers his health is a physician.   It therefore occasionally happens, that these two things
are distinct and separate.   But it is not otherwise with everything besides that is of art : none of these has in itself a principle
of performance or action, though some of them have such a
principle in other things and beyond themselves, such as a
house, and aught else that is made with hands; and some have
even such a principle inherent, but not *per se* and independently:
everything, for example, may by accident become a cause to itself. Nature is therefore, as stated [that which has an inherent principle of motion]; and those things have nature within
them which possess this principle. Now all such are substances;
for nature is always some subject, and inheres in the subject."

These things I have spoken of at length, and even quoted
the words of the writers appealed to, that it might thence appear
first, that all I attribute to the egg is actually there, viz. :
matter, organ, efficient cause, place, and everything else requisite to the generation of the chick; and next and more especially,
that the truth in regard to the following very difficult questions might be made clearly to appear, viz.: Which and what
principle is it whence motion and generation proceed ?   By
what virtue does the semen act, according to Aristotle ? What
is it that renders the semen itself fruitful ? (for the philosopher
will have it that nature in all natural bodies is the innate principle of motion and of rest, and not any second accident.)
Whether is that which in the egg is cause, artificer, and principle
of generation and of all the vital and vegetative operations—
conservation, nutrition, growth—innate or superadded ? and
whether does it inhere primarily, of itself, and as a kind of
nature, or intervene by accident, as the physician in curing diseases ? Whether is that which transforms the egg into a pullet
inherent or acquired, or is it already conceived in the ovary, and
does it nourish, augment, and perfect the egg there ?

What is it besides that preserves the egg sweet after it is laid?
What is it that renders an egg fruitful—is it to be called soul, or
a portion of the soul, or something belonging to the soul, or something having a soul, or is it intelligence, or, finally, is it Divinity?
seeing that it acts to a definite end, and orders all with in-

imitable providence and art, and yet in an incomprehensible manner, always obtaining what is best both for simple being and for well-being, for protection also and for ornament. And all this not only in the fruitful egg which it fecundates, but in the hypenemic egg which it nourishes, causes to increase, and preserves. Nay, it is not merely the vitellus in the vitellarium or egg-bed, but the smallest speck whence the yelk is produced, of no greater size than a millet or a mustard-seed, that it nourishes and makes to grow, and finally envelopes with albumen, and furnishes with chalazæ, and surrounds with membranes and a shell. For it is probable that even the barren egg, whilst it is included within the fowl and is connected with her, is nourished and preserved by its internal and inherent principle, and made to increase (not otherwise than the eggs of fishes and frogs, exposed externally, increase and are perfected), and to be tranformed from a small speck into a yelk, and transferred from the ovary to the uterus (though it have no connexion with the uterus), there to be endued with albumen, and at length to be completed with its chalazæ, membranes, and shell. But what that may be in the hypenemic egg as well as in the fruitful one, which in a similar manner and from the same causes or principles produces the same effects; whether it be the same soul, or the same part of the soul, or something else inherent in both, must be worthy of inquiry : it seems probable, however, that the same things should proceed from similar causes.

Although the egg whilst it is being produced is contained within the fowl, and is connected with the ovary of the mother by a pedicle, and is nourished by blood-vessels, it is not therefore to be spoken of as a part of the mother; nor is it to be held as living and vegetating through her vital principle, but by a virtue peculiar to itself and an internal principle; just as fungi, and mosses, and the misletoe, which although they adhere to vegetables and are nourished by the same sap as their leaves and germs, still form no part of these vegetables, nor are they ever so esteemed. Aristotle, with a view to meeting these difficulties, concedes a vegetative soul to the egg, even to the hypenemic one. He says :[1] " Females, too, and all things that live are endowed with the vegetative virtue of the soul, as has

---

[1] Gener. Anim. lib. iii, cap. 7.

been often said; and therefore this [hypenemic] egg is perfect as the conception of a plant, but imperfect as that of an animal." And he inculcates the same doctrine elsewhere,[1] when he asks: " In what manner or sense are hypenemic eggs said to live? For they cannot do so in the same sense as fruitful eggs, otherwise a living thing might be engendered by their agency.   Nor do they comport themselves like wood or stone; because these perish by a kind of corruption, as having formerly had life in a certain manner.   It is positive, therefore, that hypenemic eggs have a certain kind of soul potentially; but what? of necessity that ultimate soul, which is the appanage of vegetables; for this equally inheres in all things, in animals as well as vegetables."

But it is not the same soul that is found in hypenemic as in fruitful eggs; otherwise would a pullet be indifferently produced from both; but how and in what respects the soul attached to each is different from the other, Aristotle does not sufficiently explain, when he inquires :[2] " Wherefore are all the parts of an egg present in the hypenemic egg, and it still incapable of producing a chick? because," he replies, " it is requisite that it have a sensitive soul."   As if in fruitful eggs, besides the vegetative soul, there were a sensitive soul present.   Unless you understand the vegetative soul as inhering *actually* in the fruitful egg, which contains the sensitive soul within it *potentially;* whence the animal, and the sensible parts of the animal are subsequently produced.   But neither do writers satisfactorily untie this knot, nor set the mind of the inquirer free from the difficulties that entangle him.   For he sees that the egg is a true animal seed, according to this sentence of the Stagyrite :[3] " In those things endowed with life, in which the male and female sexes are not distinct, the seed is already present as a conception.   I entitle *conception* the first mixture from the male and female (the analogue of the vegetable seed therefore). Wherefore from one seed there is engendered one body, as from one egg one animal."

It appears, consequently, that for one egg there is one soul or vital principle.[4]   But whether is this that of the mother, or that

---

[1] Gener. Anim. lib. ii, cap. 4.   [2] Ibid. lib. ii, cap. 4.   [3] Ibid. lib. i, cap. 20.
[4] [The word *anima* of the original, which is translated *soul* above, I shall in what follows generally render *vital principle*. Ed.]

of the father, or a mixture of the two? And here the greatest difficulties are occasioned by those eggs that are produced by the concurrence of animals of different species, as, for example, of the common fowl and pheasant. In such an egg, I ask, is it the vital principle of the father or that of the mother, which inheres? or is it a mixture of the two? But how can vital principles be mingled, if the vital principle (as form) be act and substance, which it is, according to Aristotle? For no one will deny, whatever it be ultimately which in the fruitful egg is the beginning and cause of the effects we witness, that it is a substance susceptible of divers powers, forces, or faculties, and even conditions,—virtues, vices, health and sickness. For some eggs are esteemed to be longer, others shorter lived; some engender chickens endowed with the qualities and health of body that distinguished their parents, others produce young that are predisposed to disease. Nor is it to be said that this is from any fault of the mother, seeing that the diseases of the father or male parent are transferred to the progeny, although he contributes nothing to the matter of the egg; the procreative or plastic force which renders the egg fruitful alone proceeding from the male; none of its parts being contributed by him. For the semen which is emitted by the male during intercourse does by no means enter the uterus of the female, in which the egg is perfected; nor can it, indeed, (as I first announced, and Fabricius agrees with me,) by any manner or way get into the inner recesses of that organ, much less ascend as high as the ovary, near the waist or middle of the body, so that besides its peculiar virtue it might impart a portion of matter to the numerous ova whose rudiments are there contained. For we know, and are assured by unquestionable experience, that several ova are fecundated by one and the same connexion,— not those only that are met with in the uterus and ovary, but those likewise that are in some sort not yet begun, as we shall state by and by, and indeed, as we have already had occasion to assert in our history.

If, therefore, an egg be rendered fruitful by its proper vital principle, or be endowed with its own inherent fecundating force, whence or whereby either a common fowl, or a hybrid betwixt the fowl and the pheasant is produced, and that either male or female, like the father or the mother, healthy or diseased; we must infallibly conclude that the egg, even when contained in the ovary, does not live by the vital principle of the mother, but is, like the youth who comes of age, made independent even from its first appearance; as the acorn taken from the oak, and the seeds of plants in general, are no longer to be considered parts of the tree or herb that has supported them, but things made in their own right, and which already enjoy life in virtue of a proper and inherent vegetative power.

But if we now admit that there is a living principle in a fertile egg, it may become matter of discussion whether it is the same living principle which already inheres in the egg that will inhere in the future chick, or whether it is a different one that actuates each ? For it is matter of necessity that we admit the inherence of a certain principle which constitutes and causes the egg to grow, and which farther engenders and makes the chick to increase. We have to inquire, therefore, whether the animating principle of the egg and of the chick be one and the same, or several and different ? And then, were several vital principles recognized, some appertaining to the egg, others to the chick, we should next have to inquire : whence and at what epoch the animating principle of the chick entered it? and what is it in the egg which causes the cicatricula to dilate before the advent of the living principle; which draws the eye of the vitellus upwards, as stated, and produces the colliquament, changes the constitution of the fluids of the egg, and preordains everything for the construction of the future chick before there is even a vestige of it to be seen? Or whence shall we say the aliment fit for the embryo is derived, and by which it is nourished and made to grow, before it is yet in being ? For these acts are seen to be the work of the vegetative soul of the embryo, and have reference to the coming pullet, ensuring its nutrition and growth. And again, when the embryo is begun, or the chick is half formed, what is it which constitutes that embryo or that chick one and continuous and connex with the liquids of the egg ? What nourishes and makes the chick to grow, and preserves the fluids that are fit for its nutrition from putrefaction, and prepares, and liquefies, and concocts them ?

If the vital principle be the act of the organic body possessing life *in potentia,* it seems incredible that this principle can inhere in the chick before something in the shape of an organized body is extant. Nor is it more credible that the vital principle of the egg and chick can be identical, if the vital principle be conservative of that only to which it belongs; but the egg and the chick are different things, and manifest dissimilar and even opposite vital acts, in so much so that one appears to be produced by the destruction of the other. Or should we perchance maintain that the same principle and cause of life inheres in both, in the pullet half fashioned, to wit, and the egg half consumed, as if it were one and a simple act of the same body; or as if from parts producing one natural body, one soul or vital principle also arose, which was all in all, as is commonly said, and all in each particular part? Just as with leaves and fruit conspicuous on the stem of a tree, wherever a division is made we still say that the principle or first cause of the slip and of the whole tree is the same; the leaves and the fruit are, as it were, the form and end, the trunk of the tree the beginning. So too in a line, wherever a division is made, this will become the end or boundary of the part behind it, the commencement of the part before it. And the same thing is seen to obtain in respect of quality and motion, that is to say, in every kind of transmutation and generation.

So much at this time upon these topics, which will by and by engage us at greater length, when we come to speak of the nature of the living principle of the embryos of animals in general; of its being; of its accession in respect of the how and the when; and how it is all in all, and all in each particular part, the same and yet different. Points which we shall determine from numerous observations.

EXERCISE THE TWENTY-SEVENTH.

The egg is not the product of the uterus, but of the vital principle.

" As we have said," says Fabricius,[1] " that the action of the stomach was to convert the food into chyle, and the action of the

[1] Op. cit. p. 8.

testicles to produce semen, because in the stomach we find
chyle, in the testes semen, so do we definitely assert that the
.egg is the product of the uterus of birds, because it is found in
this part.   The organ and seat of the generation of eggs is,
therefore, intimately known and obvious to us.   And farther,
inasmuch as there are two uteri in birds, one superior and the
other inferior, and these are considerably different from one
another, and consequently perform different offices, it is in like
manner clear what particular action is to be ascribed to each.
The superior is devoted to the production of the yelk, the inferior to that of the albumen and remaining parts, or of the perfect egg, as lies obvious to sense; for in the superior uterus
we never find aught beyond a multitude of yelks, nor in the
inferior uterus, other than entire and perfect eggs.   But these
are not all the functions of the uteri as it appears, but the
following are farther to be noted and enumerated, viz.: the increase of the egg, which succeeds immediately upon its production, and proceeds until it is perfected and acquires its
proper dimensions.   For the fowl does not naturally lay an egg
until it has become complete and has acquired its due dimensions.   The actions of the uteri are consequently the increase as
well as the engenderment of the egg; but increase supposes and
includes nutrition, as is obvious.   And since all generation is the
effect of the concurrence of two, viz., the agent and the matter,
the agent in the generation of an egg is nothing else than the
instruments or organs aforesaid, to wit, the double uterus; and
the matter is nothing but the blood."

Now whilst I admit the action of the uterus to be in a
manner the generation of the egg, I by no means allow that the
egg is nourished and increased by this organ.   And this, both
for the reasons already alleged by us when we treated of the
vital principle of the egg, which is that which nourishes it, and
also because it appears little likely (according to Aristotle,[1] it is
impossible,) that all the internal parts of the egg, in all their
dimensions, should be fashioned and made to increase by an
external agent, such as the uterus is with reference to the
egg; for how, I beseech you, can that which is extrinsic ar-

---

[1] Gener. Anim. lib. ii, cap. 1.

range the natural matter in things that are internal, and supply
fresh matter according to the several dimensions in the place
of that which has been lost ?   How can anything be affected
or moved by that which does not touch it ?   Wherefore, without question, the same things happen in the engenderment of
eggs which take place in the beginning of all living things
whatsoever, viz.: they are primarily constituted by external and
preexisting beings; but so soon as they are endowed with life,
they suffice for their own nourishment and increase, and this
in virtue of peculiar inherent forces, innate, implanted from the
beginning.

What has already been said of the vital principle appears
clearly to proclaim that the egg is neither the work of the
uterus, nor governed by that organ; for it is manifest that the
vegetative principle inheres even in the hypenemic egg, inasmuch as we have seen that this egg is nourished and is preserved, increases and vegetates, all of which acts are indications of
the presence of the principle mentioned.   But neither from the
mother nor the uterus can this principle proceed, seeing that
the egg has no connexion or union with them, but is free and
unconnected, like a son emancipated from pupillage, rolling
round within the cavity of the uterus and perfecting itself, even
as the seeds of plants are perfected in the bosom of the earth,
viz., by an internal vegetative principle, which can be nothing
else than the vegetative soul.

And it will appear all the more certain that it is possessed
of a soul or vital principle, if we consider by what compact,
what moving power, the round and ample yelk, detached from
the cluster of the ovary, descends through the infundibulum—
a most slender tube composed of a singularly delicate membrane,
and possessed of no motory fibres—and opening a path for itself,
approaches the uterus through such a number of straits, arrived
in which it continues to be nourished, and grows and is surrounded with albumen.   Now as there is no motory organ discoverable either in the ovary which expels the vitellus, or in the
infundibulum which transmits, or in the uterus which attracts
it, and as the egg is not connected with the uterus, nor yet
with the ovary by means of vessels, nor hangs from either by
an umbilical cord, as Fabricius truly states, and demonstrates

most satisfactorily, what remains for us contemplating such great and important processes but that we exclaim with the poet: [1]

'Tis innate soul sustains; and mind infused
Through every part, that actuates the mass.

And although the rudiments of eggs, which we have said are mere specks, and have compared to millet seeds in size, are connected with the ovary by means of veins and arteries, in the same manner as seeds are attached to plants, and consequently seem to be part and parcel of the fowl, and to live and be nourished after the manner of her other parts, it is nevertheless manifest, that seeds once separated from the plants which have produced them, are no longer regarded as parts of these, but like children come of age and freed from leading-strings, they are maintained and governed by their own inherent capacities.

But of this matter we shall speak more fully, when we come to treat of the soul or living principle of the embryo in general, and of the excellence and divine nature of the vegetative soul from a survey of its operations, all of which are carried on with such foresight, art, and divine intelligence; which, indeed, surpass our powers of understanding not less than Deity surpasses man, and are allowed, by common consent, to be so wonderful that their ineffable lustre is in no way to be penetrated by the dull edge of our apprehension.

What shall we say of the animalcules which are engendered in our bodies, and which no one doubts are ruled and made to vegetate by a peculiar vital principle (anima)? of this kind are lumbrici, ascarides, lice, nits, syrones, acari, &c.; or what of the worms which are produced from plants and their fruits, as from gall-nuts, the dog-rose, and various others? "For in almost all dry things growing moist, or moist things becoming dry, an animal may be engendered." [2] It certainly cannot be that the living principles of the animals which arise in gall-nuts existed in the oak, although these animals live attached to the oak, and derive their sustenance from its juices. In like manner it is credible that the rudiments of eggs exist in the ovarian cluster by their proper vital principle, not by that of the mother, although they are connected with her body by means of arteries

---

[1] Æneïd. vi.   [2] Arist. Hist. Anim. lib. v, cap. 32.

and veins, and are nourished by the same food as herself. Because, as we have stated in our history, all the vitellary specks do not increase together, like the grapes of a bunch, or the corns of an ear of wheat, as if they were pervaded by one common actuating force or concocting and forming cause; they come on one after another, as if they grew by their own peculiar energy, each that is most in advance severing itself from the rest, changing its colour and consistence, and from a white speck becoming a yelk, in regular and determinate sequence. And what is more particularly astonishing is that which we witness among pigeons and certain other birds, where two yelks only come to maturity upon the ovarian cluster together, one of which, for the major part, produces a male, the other a female, an abundance of other vitellary specks remaining stationary in the ovary, until the term comes round for two more to increase and make ready for a new birth. It is as if each successive pair received fertility from the repeated addresses of the male; as if the two became possessed of the vital principle together; which, once infused, they forthwith increase spontaneously, and govern themselves, living of their own not through their mother's right. And, in sooth, what else can you conceive working, disposing, selecting, and perfecting, as respects this pair of vitellary papulæ and none others, but a peculiar vital principle? And although they attract nourishment from the mother, they still do so no otherwise than as plants draw food from the ground, or as the embryo obtains it from the albumen and vitellus.

Lastly, since the papula existing in the ovary receives fecundity from the access of the male, and this of such a kind that it passes into the form and likeness of the concurring male, whether he were a common cock or a pheasant, and there is as great diversity in the papulæ as there are males of different kinds; what shall we hold as inherent in the papulæ themselves, by whose virtue they are distinguished from one another and from the mother? Undoubtedly it must be the vital principle by which they are distinguished both from each other and from the mother.

It is in a similar manner that fungi and parasitic plants live upon trees. And besides, we in our own bodies frequently suffer from cancers, sarcoses, melicerides, and other tumours of the same description, which are nourished and grow as it seems by their own inherent vegetative principle, the true or natural parts of the body meantime shrinking and perishing. And this apparently because these tumours attract all the nourishment to themselves, and defraud the other parts of the body of their nutritious juices or proper genius. Whence the familiar names of phagedæna and lupus; and Hippocrates, by the words το θεῖον, perhaps understood those diseases which arise from poison or contagion; as if in these there was a certain vitality and divine principle inherent, by which they increase and through contagion generate similar diseases even in other bodies. Aristotle[1] therefore says: " all things are full of soul ;" and elsewhere he seems to think that " even the winds have a kind of life, and a birth and a death." [2] But there is no doubt that the vitellus, when it is once cast loose and freed from all connexion with the fowl, during its passage through the infundibulum and its stay in the cavity of the uterus, attracts a sluggish moisture to itself, which it absorbs, and by which it is nourished; there too it surrounds itself with albumen, furnishes itself with membranes and a shell, and finally perfects itself. All of which things, rightly weighed, we must needs conclude that it is possessed by a proper vital principle (anima).

EXERCISE THE TWENTY-EIGHTH.

The egg is not produced without the hen.

Leaving points that are doubtful, and disquisitions bearing upon the general question, we now approach more definite and obvious matters.

And first, it is manifest that a fruitful egg cannot be produced without the concurrence of a cock and hen: without the hen no egg can be formed ; without the cock it cannot become fruitful. But this view is opposed to the opinion of those who derive the origin of animals from the slime of the ground. And truly when we see that the numerous parts concurring in

---

[1] De Gen. Anim. lib. iii, cap. 2.   [2] Ibid. lib. iv, cap. 10.

the act of generation,—the testes and vasa deferentia in the male, the ovarium and uterus and blood-vessels supplying them in the female—are all contrived with such signal art and forethought, and everything requisite to reproduction in a determinate direction—situation, form, temperature,—arranged so admirably, it seems certain, as nature does nothing in vain, nor works in any round-about way when a shorter path lies open to her, that an egg can be produced in no other manner than that in which we now see it engendered, viz., by the concurring act of the cock and hen. Neither, in like manner, in the present constitution of things, can a cock or hen ever be produced otherwise than from an egg. Thus the cock and the hen exist for the sake of the egg, and the egg, in the same way, is their antecedent cause; it were therefore reasonable to ask, with Plutarch, which of these was the prior, the egg or the fowl? Now the fowl is prior by nature, but the egg is prior in time; for that which is the more excellent is naturally first; but that from which a certain thing is produced must be reputed first in respect of time. Or we may say: this egg is older than that fowl (the fowl having been produced from it); and, on the contrary, this fowl existed before that egg (which she has laid). And this is the round that makes the race of the common fowl eternal; now pullet, now egg, the series is continued in perpetuity; from frail and perishing individuals an immortal species is engendered. By these, and means like to these, do we see many inferior or terrestrial things brought to emulate the perpetuity of superior or celestial things.

And whether we say, or do not say, that the vital principle (anima) inheres in the egg, it still plainly appears, from the circuit indicated, that there must be some principle influencing this revolution from the fowl to the egg and from the egg back to the fowl, which gives them perpetuity. Now this, according to Aristotle's views,[1] is analogous to the element of the stars; and is that which makes parents engender, and gives fertility to their ova; and the same principle, Proteus like, is present under a different form, in the parents as in the eggs. For, as the same intelligence or spirit which incessantly actuates the mighty mass of the universe, and compels the same sun from

---

[1] De Gener. Anim. lib. ii, cap. 3.

the rising to the setting, in his passage over the various regions
of the earth, so also is there a vis enthea, a divine principle inherent in our common poultry, showing itself now as the plastic,
now as the nutritive, and now as the augmentative force, though
it is always and at all times present as the conservative and
vegetative force, and now assumes the form of the fowl, now that
of the egg; but the same virtue continues to inhere in either to
eternity.   And although some animals arise spontaneously, or
as is commonly said from putrefaction, and some are produced
from the female alone, for Pliny[1] says: "in some genera, as in
certain fishes, there are no males, every one taken being found
full of roe;" still whatever is produced from a perfect egg is so
in virtue of the indispensable concurrence of male and female.
Aristotle[2] consequently says: "the grand principles of generation
must be held to be the male and the female;" the first two principles of the egg are therefore the male and the female ; and the
common point or conception of these is the egg, which combines
the virtues of both parents. We cannot, in fact, conceive an egg
without the concurrence of a male and female fowl, any more
than we can conceive fruit to be produced without a tree. We
therefore see individuals, males as well as females, existing for
the sake of preparing eggs, that the species may be perennial,
though their authors pass away. And it is indeed obvious, that
the parents are no longer youthful, or beautiful, or lusty, and
fitted to enjoy life, than whilst they possess the power of producing and fecundating eggs, and, by the medium of these, of
engendering their like. But when they have accomplished this
grand purpose of nature, they have already attained to the
height, the ακμη of their being,—the final end of their existence
has been accomplished; after this, effete and useless, they begin
to wither, and, as if cast off and forsaken of nature and the
Deity, they grow old, and, a-weary of their lives, they hasten
to their end.   How different the males when they make themselves up for intercourse, and swelling with desire are excited by
the venereal impulse! It is surprising to see with what passion
they are inflamed; and then how trimly they are feathered, how
vainglorious they show themselves, how proud of their strength,
and how pugnacious they prove ! But, the grand business of life
accomplished, how suddenly, with failing strength and pristine

[1] Hist. Natur. lib. ix, cap. 16.   [2] De Gen. Anim. lib. i, cap. 2.

fervour quenched, do they take in their swelling sails, and, from late pugnacity, grow timid and desponding ! Even during the season of jocund masking in Venus's domains, male animals in general are depressed by intercourse, and become submissive and pusillanimous, as if reminded that in imparting life to others, they were contributing to their own destruction. The cock alone, replete with spirit and fecundity, still shows himself alert and gay; clapping his wings, and crowing triumphantly, he sings the nuptial song at each of his new espousals ! yet even he, after some length of time in Venus's service, begins to fail ; like the veteran soldier, he by and by craves discharge from active duty. And the hen, too, like the tree that is past bearing, becomes effete, and is finally exhausted.

EXERCISE THE TWENTY-NINTH.

Of the manner, according to Aristotle, in which a perfect and fruitful egg is produced by the male and female fowl.

Shortly before we said that a fruitful egg is not engendered spontaneously, that it is not produced save by a hen, and by her only through the concurrence of the cock. This agrees with the matter of the following sentence of Aristotle :[1] " The principles of generation have particular reference to male and female ; the male as supplying the original of motion and reproduction ; the female as furnishing the matter."

In our view, however, an egg is a true generative seed, analogous to the seed of a plant; the original conception arising between the two parents, and being the mixed fruit or product of both. For as the egg is not formed without the hen, so is it not made fruitful without the concurrence of the cock.

We have therefore to inquire how the egg is produced by the hen and is fertilized by the cock; for we have seen that hypenemic eggs, and these animated too, are engendered by the hen, but that they are not prolific without the intercourse of the cock. The male and the female consequently, both set their mark

---

[1] De Gen. Anim. lib. i, cap. 2.

upon a fruitful egg; but not, I believe, in the way in which
Aristotle imagines, viz.: that the male concurs in the motion and
commencement of generation only, the female supplying nothing
but the matter, because the contrary of this is obvious in hypenemic eggs. And although it be true as he says: "That male and
female differ in respect of reason, because the faculty of each is
different, and, in respect of sense, because certain parts differ
likewise. The difference according to reason boasts this distinction, that the male has the power of engendering in
another; the female has only the power of engendering in herself; whereby it comes that that which is engendered is produced, this being contained in that which engenders. But as
males and females are distinguished by certain faculties and
functions, and as an instrument is indispensable to every office,
and the parts of the body are adapted as instruments of the
functions, it was necessary that certain parts should be set aside
for purposes of procreation and coition, and these differing from
one another, whereby the male differs from the female."

It does not, however, follow from thence, that what he appears inclined to infer is correct, where he says: "The male is
the efficient agent, and by the motion of his generative virtue
(genitura), creates what is intended from the matter contained
in the female; for the female always supplies the matter, the
male the power of creation, and this it is which constitutes one
male, another female. The body and the bulk, therefore, are
necessarily supplied by the female; nothing of the kind is required from the male; for it is not even requisite that the instrument, nor the efficient agent itself, be present in the thing
that is produced. The body, then, proceeds from the female,
the vital principle (anima) from the male; for the essence of
every body is its vital principle (anima)." But an egg, and
that animated, is engendered by the pullet without the concurrence of the male; whence it appears that the hen too, or the
female, may be the efficient agent, and that all creative force or
vital power (anima) is not derived exclusively from the male.
This view indeed appears to be supported by the instance
quoted by Aristotle himself, for he says:[1] "Those animals not
of the same species, which copulate, (which those animals do

---

[1] Op. cit. lib. ii, cap. 4.

that correspond in their seasons of heat and times of uterogestation, and do not differ greatly in their size,) produce their first
young like themselves, but partaking of the species of both parents;
of this description is the progeny of the fox and dog, of the partridge and common fowl, &c.; but in the course of time from
diversity results diversity, and the progeny of these different
parents at length acquires the form of the female; in the same
way as foreign seed is changed at last in conformity with the
nature of the soil, which supplies matter and body to the seed."

From this it appears, that in the generation of the partridge
with the common fowl it is not the male alone that is efficient,
but the female also; inasmuch as it is not the male form only,
but one common or subordinate that appears in the hybrid, as
like the female as it is like the male in vital endowment (anima),
and bodily form. But the vital endowment (anima) is that
which is the true form and species of an animal.

Farther, the female seems even to have a superior claim to
be considered the efficient cause: "In the course of time," says the
philosopher, " the progeny of different species assumes the form
of the female ;" as if the semen or influence of the male were
the less powerful; as if the species impressed by him disappeared
with the lapse of time, and were expelled by a more powerful
efficient cause. And the instance from the soil confirms this
still farther : " for foreign seeds are changed at length according
to the nature of the soil." Whence it seems probable that the
female is actually of more moment in generation than the male;
for, " in the world at large it is admitted that the earth is to
nature as the female or mother, whilst climate, the sun, and
other things of the same description, are spoken of by the names
of generator and father."[1] The earth, too, spontaneously engenders many things without seed ; and among animals, certain
females, but females only, procreate of themselves and without
the concurrence of the male : hens, for example, lay hypenemic
eggs ; but males, without the intervention of females, engender
nothing.

By the same arguments, indeed, by which the male is maintained to be the principle and prime ' efficient ' in generation, it
would seem that the female might be confirmed in the preroga-

[1] Op. cit. lib. i, cap. 2.

19

tive of ἐνεργείᾳ or efficiency. For is not that to be accounted efficient in which the reason of the embryo and the form of the work appear; whose obvious resemblance is perceived in the embryo, and which, as first existing, calls forth the other? Since, therefore, the form, cause, and similitude inhere in the female not less—and it might even be said that they inhere more—than in the male, and as she also exists previously as prime mover, let us conclude for certain that the female is equally efficient in the work of generation as the male.

And although Aristotle[1] says well and truly, "that the conception or egg receives no part of its body from the male, but only its form, species, and vital endowment (anima), and from the female its body solely, and its dimensions," it is not yet made sufficiently to appear that the female, besides the matter, does not in some measure contribute form, species, and vital endowment (anima). This indeed is obvious in the hen which engenders eggs without the concurrence of a male; in the same way as trees and herbs, in which there is no distinction of sexes, produce their seeds. For Aristotle himself admits,[2] that even the hypenemic egg is endowed with a vital principle (anima). The female must therefore be esteemed the efficient cause of the egg.

Admitting that the hypenemic egg is possessed of a certain vital principle, still it is not prolific; so that it must further be confessed that the hen of herself is not the efficient cause of a perfect egg, but that she is made so in virtue of an authority, if I may use the word, or power required of the cock. For the egg, unless prolific, can with no kind of propriety be accounted perfect; it only obtains perfection from the male, or rather from the female, as it were upon precept from the male; as if the hen received the art and reason, the form and laws of the future embryo from his address. And so in like manner the female fowl, like to a fruitful tree, is made fertile by coition; by this is she empowered not only to lay eggs, but these perfect and prolific eggs. For although the hen have as yet no rudiments of eggs prepared in her ovary, nevertheless, made fertile by the intercourse of the male, she by and by not only produces them there, but lays them, teeming with life, and apt to produce

---

[1] Op. cit. lib. ii, cap. 4.   [2] Ibid.

embryos. And here that practice of the poor folks finds its application : " Having hens at home, but no cock, they commit their females to a neighbour's male for a day or two ; and from this short sojourn the fecundity of the whole of the eggs that will be laid during the current season is secured."[1] Not only are those eggs which are still nothing more than yelk and have no albumen, or which exist only as most minute specks in the ovary, but eggs not yet extant, that will be conceived long afterwards, rendered fertile by the same property.

EXERCISE THE THIRTIETH.

Of the uses of this disquisition on fecundity.

This disquisition on the inherent qualities of the egg and the cause of its fecundity, is alike in point of difficulty and subtlety, but of the highest importance. For it was imperative on us to inquire what there was in the conception, what in the semen masculinum, and what in the female fowl, which render these fertile; and what there is in the fruitful cock which makes him differ from a bird that is barren. Is the cause identical with that which we have called the vital principle (anima) in the embryo, or it is a certain portion of the vegetative principle? Because, in order to apprehend the entire cause of generation, it is of much moment that the first cause be understood; for science is based upon causes, especially first causes, known. Nor is this inquiry less important in enabling us to understand the nature of the vital principle (anima). These questions, indeed, rightly apprehended, not only are Aristotle's opinions of the causes of generation refuted or corrected, but all that has been written against him is easily understood.

We ask, therefore, whether it is the same thing or something different, which in the rudimentary ovum, yelk, egg, cock and hen, or her uterus, confers fruitfulness? In like manner in what respect does this something agree or differ in each? Still farther, is it a substance whence the fecundating virtue flows?—

---

[1] Fabricius, op. cit. p. 37.

it appears susceptible of powers, faculties, and accidents. Likewise, is it corporeal also? for that which engenders mixture appears to be mixed :—the progeny has a common resemblance to the mother and father, and exhibits a doubtful nature when animals of dissimilar species, such as the pheasant and common fowl, engender ; that, too, appears to be corporeal which suffers from without, and to such an extent that not only are weakly embryos procreated, but even deformed and diseased ones, obnoxious to the vices as well as to the virtues of their progenitors.

With respect to these several particulars we may farther be permitted to doubt whether that which confers fecundity is engendered or accrues from without? Whether, to wit, it is transfused from the egg to the embryo and chick, from the hen to the egg, from the cock to the hen? For there appears to be something that is transferred or transfused, something, namely, which from the cock is transfused into the hen, and from her is given to the uterus, to the ovary, to the egg ; something which passing from the seed to the plant, is rendered again by the plant to the seed, and imparts fecundity. Because there is this common to all things which are perpetuated by generation, that they derive their origin from seed. But the semen, the conception, and the egg, are all of the same essential kind, and that which confers fertility on these is one and the same, or of like nature ; and this indeed is divine, the analogue of heaven, possessed of art, intelligence, foresight. This is plainly to be seen from its admirable operations, artifices, and wisdom, where nothing is vain, or inconsiderate, or accidental, but all conduces to some good end.

Of the general principles and science of this subject we shall treat more at length in the proper place ; we have now said as much incidentally as seems necessary, the occasion having presented itself along with our consideration of the hen's egg, namely, how many things inhere which induce fertility, and how this is induced, and whether it is an affection, a habit, a power, or a faculty; whether it is to be regarded as a form and substance, as a something contained generally, or only in some particular part—since it is quite certain that a hypenemic egg is a perfect egg in so far as each sensible particular is concerned, and yet is barren ; the uterus in like manner, and the hen and the cock are all perfect ; yet are they severally sterile, as being without that which confers fecundity. All of these matters we shall advert to after we have shown what and how two principles, male and female, concur in the production of the egg and the process of generation, and in what way both may be regarded as efficient causes and parents of the egg.

The egg is not produced by the cock and hen in the way Aristotle would have it.

It is certain, as we have said, that a fruitful egg is not produced without the concurrence of the cock and hen; but this is not done in the way that Aristotle thought, viz. by the cock as prime and sole ' agent,' the hen only furnishing the ' matter.' Neither do I agree with him when he says :[1] " When the semen masculinum enters the female uterus, it coagulates the purest portion of the catamenia ;" and shortly afterwards : " but when the catamenia of the female has set in the uterus, it forms, with the semen masculinum, a coagulum like that of milk ; for curd is milk containing vital heat, which attracts like particles around it, and combines and coagulates them ; and the semen of the male (genitura) bears the same affinity to the nature of the catamenia. For milk and the menstrual discharge are of the same nature. When coagulation has taken place, then an earthy humour is excreted and is drawn around, and the earthy portion drying up, the membranes are produced both as matter of necessity, and also for a certain purpose. And these things take place in the same manner in all creatures, both oviparous and viviparous."

But the business in the generation of an egg is very different from this; for neither does the semen, or rather the ' geniture,' proceeding from the male in the act of intercourse, enter the uterus in any way, nor has the hen, after she conceives, any particle of excrementitious matter, even of the purest kind, or any blood in her uterus which might be fashioned or perfected by the discharge of the male. Neither are the parts of the egg,

---

[1] De Gen. Anim. lib. ii, cap. 4.

the membranes, to wit, and the fluids, produced by any kind of
coagulation; neither is there any thing like curdled milk to be
discovered in the uterus, as must be obvious from the foregoing
exercises.   It follows, therefore, and from thence, that neither
does the conception, whence the animal springs, as the herb arises
from a fruitful seed, comport itself in the manner Aristotle
imagined, since this takes place in viviparous animals in the
same way as the egg is formed in oviparous animals, as he himself avows, and as shall be demonstrated by and by in our observations.   Because it is certain that eggs of every description—prolific and barren—are engendered and formed by the
hen singly, but that fecundity accrues from the male alone ;—
the cock, I say, contributes neither form nor matter to the egg,
but that only by which it becomes fertile and fit to engender a
chick.   And this faculty the cock confers by his semen (genitura), emitted in the act of intercourse, not only on the egg
that is already begun, or is already formed, but on the uterus
and ovary, and even on the body of the fowl herself, in such
wise that eggs which have yet to be produced, eggs, none of the
matter of which yet exists either in the ovary or in any other
part of the body, are thence produced possessed of fecundity.

EXERCISE THE THIRTY-SECOND.

Nor in the manner imagined by physicians.

Conception, according to the opinion of medical men, takes
place in the following way : during intercourse the male and
female dissolve in one voluptuous sensation, and eject their
seminal fluids (genituræ) into the cavity of the uterus, where
that which each contributes is mingled with that which the
other supplies, the mixture having from both equally the faculty
of action and the force of matter; and according to the predominance of this or of that geniture does the progeny turn out male
or female.   It is farther imagined that immediately after the
intercourse, the active and passive principles cooperating, something of the conception is formed in the uterus.   For contrary
to the Aristotelians, they maintain that the male is no more the

efficient cause of generation than the female, but some mixture
of the two; and that neither the menstrual blood nor its purest
part is the prime matter of the conception, but the spermatic
fluid; whence the first particles or their rudiments are spoken
of as spermatic, these at an after period being nourished and
made to increase through the blood.

But it is obvious that neither is the egg engendered by the
cock and hen in this way; for the hen in the act of intercourse
emits no semen from which an egg might be formed; nor can
aught like a seminal fluid of the hen be demonstrated at any
time; and indeed the animal is destitute of the organs essential
to its preparation, the testes and vasa spermatica. And though
the hen have an effective force in common with the cock (as
must be manifest from what precedes), and it is a mixture of
some sort that renders an egg fruitful, still this does not happen
according to the predominance of the genitures, or the manner
of their mixture, for it is certain, and Fabricius admits it, that
the semen of the cock does not reach the cavity of the uterus;
neither is there any trace of the egg to be discovered in the
uterus immediately after intercourse, and as its consequence,
although Aristotle himself repeatedly avers that there is, asserting that "something of the conception forthwith ensues."
But I shall by and by demonstrate that neither does any such
imaginary mixture of seminal fluids take place in any animal,
nor that immediately upon intercourse, even of a fruitful kind,
is there anything in the shape of semen or blood, or of the
rudiments of an embryo present or demonstrable in the cavity
of the uterus. Nothing is found in the egg or embryo which
leads us to suppose that the semen masculinum is either there
contained or mingled. The vulgar notion of the chalazæ being
the tread of the cock is a sheer mistake; and I am surprised,
since there are two of them, one in either end of the egg, that
no one has yet been found to maintain that this was the cock's
seed, that the hen's. But this popular error is at once answered
by the fact that the chalazæ are present with the same characters
in every egg, whether it be fertile or barren.

The male and the female are alike efficient in the business of generation.

The medical writers with propriety maintain, in opposition to the Aristotelians, that both sexes have the power of acting as efficient causes in the business of generation; inasmuch as the being engendered is a mixture of the two which engender: both form and likeness of body, and species are mixed, as we see in the hybrid between the partridge and common fowl. And it does indeed seem consonant with reason to hold that they are the efficient causes of conception whose mixture appears in the thing produced.

Aristotle entertaining this opinion says :[1] " In some animals it is manifest that such as the generator is, such is the engendered; not, however, the same and identical, not one numerically, but one specifically, as in natural things. A man engenders a man, if there be nothing preternatural in the way, as a horse [upon an ass] engenders a mule, and other similar instances. For the mule is common to the horse and the ass; it is not spoken of as an allied kind; yet may horse and ass both be there conjoined in a hybrid state." He says farther in the same place: " It is enough that the generator generate, and prove the cause that the species be found in the matter: for such and such an entire species is still found associated with such and such flesh and bones—here it is Gallias, there it is Socrates."

Wherefore if such an entire form, as a mule, be a mixture of two, viz.: a horse and an ass, the horse does not suffice to produce this form of a mule in the ' matter;' but, as the entire form is mixed, so another efficient cause is contributed by the ass and added to that supplied by the horse. That, therefore, which produces a mule compounded of two, must itself be an ' adequate efficient,' and mixed, if only ' univocal.' For example, this woman and that man engender this Socrates; not in so far as they are both human beings, and of one and the same

---

[1] Metaphys. lib. vii, cap. 8.

species, but in so far as this man and that woman in these bones and muscles constitute human forms, of both of which, if Socrates be a certain mixture, a compound of both, that by which he is made must needs be a mixed univocal compound of the two; i. e. a mixed efficient of a mixed effect. And therefore it is that the male and female by themselves, and separately, are not genetic, but become so united *in coitu,* and made one animal as it were; whence, from the two as one, is produced and educed that which is the true efficient proximate cause of conception.

The medical writers also, in directing their attention to the particulars of human generation alone, come to conclusions on generation at large; and the spermatic fluid proceeding from the parents *in coitu* has in all probability been taken by them for true seed, analogous to the seeds of plants. It is not without reason, therefore, that they imagine the mixed efficient cause of the future offspring to be constituted by a mixture of the seminal matters of each parent. And then they go on to assert that the mixture proceeding immediately from intercourse is deposited in the uterus and forms the rudiments of the conception. That things are very different, however, is made manifest by our preceding history of the egg, which is a true conception.

EXERCISE THE THIRTY-FOURTH.

Of the matter of the egg, in opposition to the Aristotelians and the medical writers.

The position taken up by the medical writers against the Aristotelians, viz., that the blood is not the first element in a conception, is clearly shown from the generation of the egg to be well chosen: neither during intercourse, nor before nor after it, is there a drop of blood contained in the uterus of the fowl; neither are the rudiments of eggs red, but white. Many animals also conceive in whose uteri, if they be suddenly laid open after intercourse, no blood can be demonstrated.

But when they contend that the maternal blood is the food of the fœtus in utero, especially of its more sanguineous parts,

as they style them, and that the fœtus from the outset is as it
were a portion of the mother, being nourished and growing
through her blood, and vegetating through her spirit; so that
neither does the heart pulsate, nor the liver compose blood, nor
any part of the fœtus perform any kind of independent office,
but everything is carried on through the mother's means, they in
their turn are as certainly mistaken, and argue from erroneous
observations.   For the embryo in the egg boasts of its own
blood, formed from the fluids contained within the egg ; and its
heart is seen to pulsate from the very beginning : it borrows nothing in the shape either of blood or spirits from the hen, for
the purpose of forming its so called sanguineous parts and its
feathers ; as most clearly appears to any one who looks on with
an unbiassed mind.   From observations afterwards to be communicated, I believe indeed that it will be held as sufficiently
proven that even the fœtus of viviparous animals still contained
in the uterus is not nourished by the blood of the mother and
does not vegetate through her spirit; but boasts of its own peculiar vital principle and powers, and its own blood, like the chick
in ovo.

With reference to the matter which the embryo obtains from
its male and female parent, however, and the way and manner
of generation as commonly discoursed of in the schools, viz.: that
conception is produced or becomes prolific from mixture of the
genitures and their mutual action and passion, as also of the
seminal fluid of the female, and the parts which are spoken of
as sanguineous and spermatic, numerous and striking observations afterwards to be related have compelled me to adopt
opinions at variance with all such views. At this time I shall only
say that I am greatly surprised how physicians, particularly those
among them who are conversant with anatomy, should pretend
to support their opinions by means of two arguments especially,
which rightly understood, seem rather to prove the opposite ;
viz., from the shock and resolution of the forces and the effusion
of fluid which women at the moment of the sexual orgasm
frequently experience, they argue that all women pour out a
seminal fluid, and that this is necessary to generation.

But passing over the fact that the females of all the lower
animals, and all women, do not experience any such emission
of fluid, and that conception is nowise impossible in cases where

it does not take place, for I have known several, who without anything of the kind were sufficiently prolific, and even some who after experiencing such an emission and having had great enjoyment, nevertheless appeared to have lost somewhat of their wonted fecundity; and then an infinite number of instances might be quoted of women who, although they have great satisfaction in intercourse, still emit nothing, and yet conceive; passing over these facts, I say, I cannot but express surprise at those especially, who, conceiving such an emission on the part of the female necessary to conception, have not adverted to the fact that the fluid emitted is discharged, cast out, and is particularly abundant about the clitoris and orifice of the vulva; that it is seldom poured out within the vulva, never within the uterus, and so as to be mingled with the semen of the male; moreover, it is of a mere serous or ichorous consistency, like urine, by no means thick and apparently unctuous, like the spermatic matter of the male. But how shall we suppose that to be of use internally which is discharged externally? Or shall we say that this humour, as if bidding the uterus farewell, is taken to the verge of the vulva, that it may be then recalled with greater favour by the uterus?

The other argument is drawn from the genital organs of women, the testes, to wit, and vasa spermatica, præparantia et deferentia, which are held to serve for the preparation of the spermatic fluid. I, for my part, greatly wonder how any one can believe that from parts so imperfect and obscure, a fluid like the semen, so elaborate, concoct and vivifying, can ever be produced, endowed with force and spirit and generative influence adequate to overcome that of the male; for this is implied in the discussion concerning the predominance of the male or the female, as to which of them is to become the agent and efficient cause, which the matter and pathic principle. How should such a fluid get the better of another concocted under the influence of a heat so fostering, of vessels so elaborate, and endowed with such vital energy?—how should such a fluid as the male semen be made to play the part of mere matter?—But of these things more hereafter.

Meantime it is certain that the egg of the hen is not engendered from any such discharge of fluid during sexual intercourse, although after connexion, and brimful of satisfaction, she shakes herself for joy, and, as if already possessed of the richest treasure, as if gifted by supreme Jove the preserver with the blessing of fecundity, she sets to work to prune and ornament herself. The pigeon, particularly that kind which comes to us from Africa, expresses the satisfaction she feels from intercourse in a remarkable manner; she leaps, spreads her tail, and sweeps the ground with its extremity, she pecks and prunes her feathers—all her actions are as if she felt raised to the summit of felicity by the gift of fruitfulness.

We have said that the primary matter of the egg does not consist of blood as Aristotle would have it, neither does it proceed from any mixture of the male and female seminal fluids. Whence it truly originates we have already stated in part in our history; and we shall by and by have occasion to speak of the subject more at length when we come to treat generally of the matter from which every conception is originally produced.

In how far is the fowl efficient in the generation of the egg, according to Aristotle? And wherefore is the concurrence of the male required?

It has been already stated that the cock and hen are the two principles in the generation of the egg, although of the manner in which they are so I am of a different opinion from Aristotle and medical authorities. From the production of the egg we have clearly shown that the female as well as the male was efficient, and that she had within her a principle whence motion and the faculty of forming flowed; although in the sexual act the male neither confers the matter, nor does the female eject any semen whence the egg is constituted. It is consequently manifest, in some animals at least, that nature has not, on account of the distinction into male and female, established it as a law that the one, as agent, should confer form, the other, as passive, supply matter, as Aristotle apprehended; nor yet that during intercourse each should contribute a seminal fluid, by the mixture of which a conception or ovum should be produced, as physicians commonly suppose.

Now since everything that has been delivered by the ancients on generation is comprehended in these two opinions, it appears to have escaped every one up to this time, first, why the hen by herself does not generate, like vegetables, but requires a male to be associated with her in the work; and then how the conception or ovum is procreated by the male and the female together, or what either of them contributes to the process, and for what end intercourse was established.

Aristotle, in opposition to the entire tenor of his hypothesis, viz. that the male is to be regarded as the agent, the female as supplying the matter only, when he sees that eggs are actually produced by hens without the concurrence of the male, is compelled to admit that the female is likewise efficient; he was farther not ignorant of the fact that an egg even when extruded could preserve itself, nourish itself, increase in size and produce an embryo, as happens with the eggs of fishes; and he has besides accorded a vital principle to an egg, even to a hypenemic one. But he endeavours to explain to what extent a female is efficient, and how a hypenemic egg is endowed with a vital principle, in the passage where he says[1] : " Hypenemic eggs admit of generation to a certain point; for that they can ever go the length of producing an animal is impossible, this being the work of the senses [the sensible soul]. But females and all things that live, as already repeatedly stated, possess the vegetative soul. Wherefore the hypenemic egg as a vegetable is perfect, but as an animal it is imperfect." By this he seems to insinuate that the hypenemic egg is possessed of a vegetative soul, inasmuch as this is inherent in all things that live, and an egg is alive. In like manner he ascribes to the hen the power of creating and of conferring the vegetative soul ; because all females acquire this virtue, so that a hypenemic egg in so far as it lives as a vegetable is perfect, in so far as it is an animal however it is imperfect. As if a male were not required that a conception or ovum should be produced, and produced perfect ; but that from this ovum an animal should be engendered. Not, I say, that an egg be produced as perfect in all respects as is the conception of a vegetable; but

[1] De Gener. Anim. lib. iii, c. 7.

that it should be imbued with the animal principle. The egg, consequently, is formed by the hen, but it is made prolific by the cock.

Aristotle adds in the same place: "There is a distinction of sexes through the whole class of birds. And therefore it happens that the hen perfects her egg, not yet influenced by the intercourse of the male, in so far as it is a plant; but as it is not a plant, there she does not perfect it: nor does anything come of it which engenders. For neither has it arisen simply, like the seed of a plant, nor like an animal conception, by intercourse." He is here speaking of the wind egg; by and by he adds: "But those eggs that are conceived through intercourse are already characterized in a portion of the albumen: such eggs become fruitful through the male which first copulated, for they are then supplied with both principles."

By this he seems to confess that the female is also effective in the work of generation, or is possessed of the faculty of engendering; because in every female there inheres a vegetative soul, whose faculty it is to engender. And, therefore, when he is speaking of the differences between the male and female, he still acknowledges both as generative; for he says: "We call that animal male which engenders in another, female that which engenders in itself." From his own showing, therefore, both engender; and as there is a vegetative soul inherent in both, so is there also its faculty of generation. But how they differ has already been shown in the History of the Egg: the hen generates of herself without the concurrence of the cock, as a plant out of itself produces fruit; but it is a wind egg that is thus produced: it is not made fruitful without the concurrence of the cock either preceding or succeeding. The female generates, then, but it is only up to a certain mark, and the concurrence of the male is requisite that this faculty of engendering be made complete, that she may not only lay an egg, but such an egg as will, under favorable circumstances, produce a pullet. The male appears to be ordained by nature to supply this deficiency in the generative powers of the female, as will be clearly shown by and by, and that that which the female of herself cannot accomplish, viz. the production of a fruitful egg, may be supplied and made good by the act of the male, who imparts this virtue to the fowl or the egg.

EXERCISE THE THIRTY-SIXTH.

The perfect hen's egg is of two colours.

Every egg, then, is not perfect; but some are to be held imperfect because they have not yet attained their true dimensions, which they only receive when extruded; others are imperfect because they are yet unprolific, and only acquire a fertilizing faculty from without, such are the eggs of fishes. Other eggs again are held imperfect by Aristotle, because they are of one colour only, inasmuch as perfect eggs consist of yelk and albumen, and are of two colours, as if better concocted, more distinct in their parts, endowed with higher heat. The eggs that are called centenine or hundredth eggs, and which Fabricius[1] will have it are engendered of certain remainders of albumen, are of one colour only, and by reason of their deficiency of heat and their weakness, are regarded as imperfect. Of all eggs, there are none more perfect than those of the hen, which are produced complete in all their fluids and appendages, of proper size and fruitful.

Aristotle assigns the following reason wherefore some eggs are of two colours, others of one hue only :[2] " In the hotter animals those things from which the principles of their origin are derived, are distinct and separate from those which furnish their nutrition; now the one of these is white, the other is yellow." As if the chick derived its origin from the albumen and was nourished by the vitellus alone. In the same place he proceeds thus : " That part which is hot contributes properly to the form in the constitution of the extremities; but the part that is more earthy, and is further removed, supplies material for the trunk. Whence in eggs of two colours the animal derives its origin from the white, for the commencement of animal existence is in the white; but the nourishment is obtained from the yellow." He consequently thinks that this is the reason why these fluids are distinct, and why eggs are produced of two colours.

---

[1] Op cit. p. 10.   [2] De Generat. Animal. lib. iii, cap. 1.

Now these ideas are partly true, partly false. It is not true, for instance, that the embryo of the common fowl is first formed from the albumen and then nourished by the vitellus; for, from the history of the formation of the chick in ovo, from the course of the umbilical vessels and the distribution of their branches, which undoubtedly serve for obtaining nourishment, it obviously appears that the constituent matter, and the nutriment are supplied to the chick from its first formation by the yelk, as well as the white; the fluid which we have called the colliquament seems farther to be supplied, not less by the vitellus than the albumen; a certain portion of both the fluids seems, in fact, to be resolved. And then the spot, by the expansion of which the colliquament is formed in the first instance, and which we have called the eye, appears to be impressed upon the membrane of the vitellus.

The distinction into yellow and white, however, seems to be a thing necessary : these matters, as they are undoubtedly of different natures, appear also to serve different offices; they are therefore completely separate in the perfect egg, one of them being more the other less immediately akin to proper alimentary matter; by the one the fœtus is nourished from the very beginning, by the other it is nourished at a later period. For it is certain, as Fabricius asserts, and as we afterwards maintain, that both of them are truly nutritious, the albumen as well as the vitellus, the albumen being the first that is consumed. I therefore agree with Aristotle against the physicians, that the albumen is the purer portion of the egg, the better concocted, the more highly elaborated; and, therefore, whilst the egg is getting perfected in the uterus, is the albumen as the hotter portion poured around in the circumference, the yelk or more earthy portion subsiding to the centre. For the albumen appears to contain the larger quantity of animal heat, and so to be nutriment of a more immediate kind. For like reasons it is probable that the albumen is purer and better concocted externally than it is internally.

When medical writers affirm that the yelk is the hotter and more nutritious portion of the egg, this I imagine is meant as it affords food to us, not as it is found to supply the wants of the chick in ovo. This, indeed, is obvious from the history of the formation of the chick, by which the thin albumen is absorbed and used up sooner than the thick, as if it formed the more appropriate aliment, and were more readily transmuted into the substance of the embryo, of the chick that is to be. The yelk, therefore, appears to be a more distant or ultimate aliment than the albumen, the whole of which has been used up before any notable portion of the vitellus is consumed. The yelk, indeed, is still found inclosed within the abdomen of the chick after its exclusion from the shell, as if it were destined to serve the new being in lieu of milk for its sustenance.

Eggs, consisting of white and yellow, are therefore more perfect, as more distinct in constitution, and elaborated by a higher temperature. For in the egg there must be included, not only the matter of the chick but also its first nutriment; and what is provided for a perfect animal, must, itself, be perfect and highly elaborated; as that is, in fact, which consists of different parts, some of which, as already stated, are prior and purer, and so more easy of digestion; others posterior, and therefore more difficult of transmutation into the substance of the chick. Now the yelk and albumen differ from one another by such kinds of distinction. Perfect eggs are, consequently, of two colours : they consist of albumen and yelk, as if these constituted fluids of easier or more difficult digestion, adapted to the different ages and vigour of the chick.

EXERCISE THE THIRTY-SEVENTH.

Of the manner in which the egg is increased by the albumen.

From the history it appears that the rudiments of the eggs in the ovary are of very small size, mere specks, smaller than millet seeds, white and replete with watery fluid : these specks, however, by and by, become yelks, and then surround themselves with albumen.

Aristotle seems to think that the albumen is generated in the way of secretion from the vitellus. It may be well to add his words :[1] " The sex," he says, " is not the cause of the double

---

[1] De Gener. Animal. lib. iii, cap. 1.

colour, as if the white were derived from the male, the yellow from the female; both are furnished by the female. But one of them is hot, the other is cold. Now these two portions are distinct in animals, fraught with much heat; in those that are not so fraught the eggs are not thus distinct. And this is the reason why the conceptions of these are of one colour. But the semen of the male alone sets the conception; therefore is the conception of the bird small and white in the first instance; but in the course of time, and when there is a larger infusion of blood, it becomes entirely yellow; and, last of all, when the heat declines, the white portion, as a humour of equal temperature surrounds it on every side. For the white portion of the egg is, by its nature, moist, and includes animal heat in itself; and it is for this reason that it is seen in the circumference, the yellow and earthy portion remaining in the interior."

Fabricius,[1] however, thinks that "the albumen only adheres to the vitellus by juxtaposition. For while the yelk is rolled through the second uterus and gradually descends, it also gradually assumes to itself the albumen which is there produced, and made ready, that it may be applied to the yelk; until the yelk having passed the middle spirals and reached the last of them, already surrounded with the albumen, it now surrounds itself with the membranes and shell." Fabricius will therefore have it that the egg increases in a two-fold manner: "partly by means of the veins, as concerns the vitellus, and partly by an appositive increase, as regards the albumen." And, among other reasons, this was perchance one for the above opinion: that when an egg is boiled hard the albumen is readily split into layers lying one over another. But this also occurs to the yelk still connected with the ovary, when boiled hard.

Wherefore, taught by experience, I rather incline to the opinion of Aristotle; for the albumen is not merely perceived as added in the way Fabricius will have it, but fashioned also, distinguished by chalazæ and membranes, and divided into two different portions; and all this in virtue of the inherence of the same vegetative vital principle by which the egg is more conspicuously divided into two distinct substances—a yelk and

[1] Op. cit. p. 12.

a white. For the same faculty that presides over the formation of the egg in general, presides over the constitution of each of its parts in particular. Neither is it altogether true that the yelk is first formed and the albumen added to it afterwards; for what is seen in the ovary is not the vitellus of the egg, but rather a compound containing the two liquids mingled together. It has the colour of the vitellus, indeed, but in point of consistence it is more like the albumen; and when boiled hard it is not friable like the proper yelk, but, like the white, is concreted, jelly-like, and seen to be composed of thin lamellæ; and it has a kind of white papula, or spot, in the middle.

Aristotle seems to derive this separation from the dissimilar nature of the yelk and white; for he says,[1] as we have already stated, that if a number of eggs be thrown into a pan and boiled, in such wise that the heat shall not be quicker than the separation of the eggs, (citatior quam ovorum distinctio,) the same thing will take place in the mass of eggs which occurs in the individual egg : the whole of the yelks will set in the middle, the whites round about them.

This I have myself frequently found to be true on making the trial, and it is open to any one to repeat the experiment; let him only beat yelks and whites together, put the mixture into a dutch oven, or between two plates over the fire, and having added some butter, cause it to set slowly into a cake, he will find the albumen covering over the yelks situated at the bottom.

EXERCISE THE THIRTY-EIGHTH.

Of what the cock and hen severally contribute to the production of the egg.

Both cock and hen are to be reputed parents of the chick ; for both are necessary principles of an egg, and we have proved both to be alike its efficient : the hen fashions the egg, the cock makes it fertile. Both, consequently, are instruments

---

[1] Fabricius, op. cit. p. 12.

of the plastic virtue by which this species of animal is perpetuated.

But as in some species there appears to be no occasion for males, females sufficing of themselves to continue the kind; so do we discover no males among these, but females only, containing the fertile rudiments of eggs in their interior; in other species, again, none but males are discovered which procreate and preserve their kinds by emitting something into the mud, or earth, or water. In such instances nature appears to have been content with a single sex, which she has used as an instrument adequate to procreation.

Another class of animals has a generative fluid fortuitously, as it were, and without any distinction of sex; the origin of such animals is spontaneous. But "as some things are made by art, and some depend on accident, health for example,"[1] so also some semen of animals is not produced by the act of an individual agent, as in the case of a man engendered by a man; but in some sort univocally, as in those instances where the rudiments and matter, produced by accident, are susceptible of taking on the same motions as seminal matter, as in "animals which do not proceed from coitus, but arise spontaneously, and have such an origin as insects which engender worms."[2] For as mechanics perform some operations with their unaided hands, and others not without the assistance of particular tools; and as the more excellent and varied and curious works of art require a greater variety in the form and size of the tools to bring them to perfection, inasmuch as a greater number of motions and a larger amount of subordinate means are required to bring more worthy labours to a successful issue—art imitating nature here as everywhere else, so also does nature make use of a larger number and variety of forces and instruments as necessary to the procreation of the more perfect animals. For the sun, or Heaven, or whatever name is used to designate that which is understood as the common generator or parent of all animated things, engenders some of themselves, by accident, without an instrument, as it were, and equivocally; and others through the concurrence of a single individual, as in those instances where an animal is produced from another animal of the same genus

---

[1] Arist. Phys. lib. i, cap. 1.　　　　[2] Ib. lib. ii, cap. 3.

which supplies both matter and form to the being engendered; so in like manner in the generation of the most perfect animals where principles are distinguished, and the seminal elements of animated beings are divided, a new creation is not effected save by the concurrence of male and female, or by two necessary instruments. Our hen's egg is of this kind; to its production in the perfect state the cock and the hen are necessary. The hen engenders in herself, and therefore does she supply place and matter, nutriment and warmth; but the cock confers fecundity; for the male, as Aristotle says,[1] always perfects generation, secures the presence of a sensitive vital principle, and from such an egg an animal is engendered.

To the cock, therefore, as well as to the hen, are given the organs requisite to the function with which he is intrusted; in the hen all the genital parts are adapted to receive and contain, as in the cock they are calculated to give and immit, or prepare that which transfers fecundity to the female, he engendering, as it were, in another, not in himself.

When we anatomize the organs appropriated to generation, therefore, we readily distinguish what each sex contributes in the process; for a knowledge of the instruments here leads us by a direct path to a knowledge of their functions.

EXERCISE THE THIRTY-NINTH.

Of the cock and the particulars most remarkable in his constitution.

The cock, as stated, is the prime efficient of the perfect or fruitful hen's egg, and the chief cause of generation : without the male no chick would ever be produced from an egg, and in many ovipara not even would any egg be produced. It is, therefore, imperative on us that we look narrowly into his offices and uses, and inquire particularly what he contributes to the egg and chick, both in the act of intercourse and at other times.

[1] Op. cit.

It is certain that the cock in coition emits his 'geniture,' commonly called semen, from his sexual parts, although he has no penis, as I maintain ; because his testes and long and ample vasa deferentia are full of this fluid.   But whether it issues in jets, with a kind of spirituous briskness and repeatedly as in the hotter viviparous animals, or not, I have not been able to ascertain.   But as I do not find any vesiculæ containing semen, from which, made brisk and raised into a froth by the spirits, it might be emitted ; nor any penis through whose narrower orifice it might be forcibly ejaculated, and so strike upon the interior of the hen ; and particularly when I see the act of intercourse so rapidly performed between them; I am disposed to believe that the parts of the hen are merely moistened with a very small quantity of seminal fluid, only as much as will adhere to the orifice of the pudenda, and that the prolific fluid is not emitted by any sudden ejaculation ; so that whilst among animals repeated ejaculations take place during the same connection, among birds, which are not delayed with any complexity of venereal apparatus, the same object is effected by repeated con- nections.   Animals that are long in connection, copulate rarely ; and this is the case with the swan and ostrich among birds. The cock, therefore, as he cannot stay long in his connections, supplies by dint of repeated treadings the reiterated ejaculations of the single intercourse in other animals ; and as he has neither penis nor glans, still the extremities of the vasa deferentia, inflated with spirits when he treads, become turgid in the manner of a glans penis, and the orifice of the uterus of the hen, compressed by them, her cloaca being exposed for the oc- casion, is anointed with genital fluid, which consequently does not require a penis for its intromission.

We have said, however, that such was the virtue of the semen of the cock, that not only did it render the uterus, the egg in utero, and the vitelline germ in the ovary, but the whole hen prolific, so that even the germs of vitelli, yet to be produced, were impregnated.

Fabricius has well observed, that the quantity of spermatic fluid contained in the testes and vasa deferentia of the cock was large ; not that the hen requires much to fecundate each of her eggs, but that the cock may have a supply for the large number of hens he serves and for his repeated addresses to them.

The shortness and straight course of the spermatic vessels in the cock also assist the rapid emission of the spermatic fluid: anything that must pass through lengthened and tortuous conduits of course escapes more slowly and requires a greater exercise of the impelling power or spirit to force it away.

Among male animals there is none that is more active or more haughty and erect, or that has stronger powers of digestion than the cock, which turns the larger portion of his food into semen; hence it is that he requires so many wives,—ten or even a dozen. For there are some animals, single males of which suffice for several females, as we see among deer, cattle, &c.; and there are others, of which the females are so prurient that they are scarcely satisfied with several males, such as the bitch and the wolf; whence prostitutes were called *lupæ* or wolves, as making their persons common; and stews were entitled *lupanaria*. Whilst some animals, of a more chaste disposition, live, as it were, in the conjugal estate, so that the male is married to a single female only, and both take part in providing for the wants of the family; for since nature requires that the male supply the deficiencies of the female in the work of generation, and as she alone in many cases does not suffice to cherish and feed and protect the young, the male is added to the wife that he may take part in the burthen of bringing up the offspring. Partridges lead a wedded life, because the females alone cannot incubate such a number of eggs as they lay, (so that they are said, by some, to make two nests,) nor to bring up such a family as by and by appears without assistance. The male pigeon also assists in building the nest, takes his turn in incubating the eggs, and is active in feeding the young. In the same way many other instances of conjugal life among the lower animals might be quoted, and indeed we shall have occasion to refer to several in what yet remains to be said.

Those males, among animals, which serve several females, such as the cock, have an abundant secretion of seminal fluid, and are provided with long and ample vasa deferentia. And at whatever time or season the clustered rudimentary papulæ in the ovary come to maturity and require fecundation, that they may go on to be turned into perfect eggs, the males will then be found to have an abundance of seminal fluid, and the testicles

to enlarge and become conspicuous in the very situation to
which they transfer their fecundating influence, viz. the præcordia.   This is remarkable in fishes, birds, and the whole race
of oviparous animals; the males of which teem with fecundating
seminal fluid at the same precise seasons as the females become
full of eggs.

Whatever parts of the hen, therefore, are destined by nature
for purposes of generation, viz. the ovary, the infundibulum,
the processus uteri, the uterus itself, and the pudenda; as also
the situation of these parts, their structure, dimensions, temperature, and all that follows this; all these, I say, are either
subordinate to the production and growth of the egg, or to intercourse and the reception of fecundity from the male; or, for
the sake of parturition, to which they conduce either as principal and convenient means, or as means necessary, and without which what is done could not be accomplished; for nothing
in nature's works is fashioned either carelessly or in vain.   In
the same way all the parts in the cock are fashioned subordinate
to the preparation or concoction of the spermatic fluid, and its
transference to the hen.

Now those males that are so vigorously constituted as to
serve several females are larger and handsomer, and in the
matter of spirit and arms excel their females in a far greater
degree than the males of those that live attached to a single
female.   Neither the male partridge, nor the crow, nor the
pigeon, is distinguished from the female bird in the same decided way as the cock from his hens, the stag from his does, &c.

The cock, therefore, as he is gayer in his plumage, better
armed, more courageous and pugnacious, so is he replete with
semen, and so apt for repeated intercourse, that unless he have
a number of wives he distresses them by his frequent assaults;
he not only invites but compels them to his pleasure, and leaping
upon them at inconvenient and improper seasons, (even when
they are engaged in the business of incubation) and wearing
off the feathers from their backs, he truly does them an injury.
I have occasionally seen hens so torn and worn by the ferocious
addresses of the cock, that with their backs stript of feathers
and laid bare in places, even to the bone, they languished
miserably for a time and then died.   The same thing also
occurs among pheasants, turkeys, and other species.

Of the hen.

There are two instruments and two first causes of generation, the male and the female—for to the hen seems to belong the formation of the egg, as to the cock the fertilizing principle. In the act of intercourse, then, of these two, that which renders the egg fruitful is either transmitted from the male to the female, or by means of coition is generated in the hen. The nature of this principle, however, is no less difficult to ascertain than are the particulars of its communication, whether, for instance, we suppose such communication to take place with the whole system of the hen, or simply with her womb, or with the egg already formed, or further, with all the eggs now commencing and hereafter about to commence their existence in the ovary. For it is probable, from what I have formerly mentioned, and also from the experiment of Fabricius,[1] that but a few acts of intercourse, and the consorting of the hen with the cock for some days, are sufficient to fecundate her, or at least her womb, during the whole year. And so far I can myself affirm, from my own observation, to wit, that the twentieth egg laid by a hen, after separation from the cock, has proved prolific. So that, in like manner as it is well known that, from the seed of male fishes shed into the water, a large mass of ova is impregnated, and that in dogs, pigs, and other animals, a small number of acts of intercourse suffice for the procreation of many young ones, (some even think it well established, that if a bitch have connexion more than three or four times, her fruitfulness is impaired, and that more females than males are then engendered), so may the cock, by a few treadings, render prolific not only the egg in the womb, but also the whole ovarium, and, as has been often said, the hen herself. Nay, what is more remarkable, and indeed wonderful, it is said that in Persia,[2] on cutting open the female mouse, the young ones still contained in the belly are already pregnant; in other words, they are

---

[1] Op. cit. p. 31.   [2] Arist. Hist. Anim. lib. vi, c. 37.

mothers before they are born! as if the male rendered not only
the female fruitful, but also impregnated the young which she
had conceived; in the same way as our cock fertilizes not
merely the hen, but also the eggs which are about to be produced by her.

But this is confidently denied by those physicians who assert
that conception is produced from a mixture of the seed of each
sex. And hence Fabricius,[1] although he affirms that the seed of
the cock ejected in coition never does, nor can, enter the cavity
of the womb, where the egg is formed, or takes its increase, and
though he plainly sees that the eggs when first commencing in
the ovarium are, no less than those which exist in the womb,
fecundated by the same act of coition, and that of these no part
could arise from the semen of the cock, yet has he supposed
that this semen, as if it must needs be present and permanent,
is contained during the entire year in the "bursa" of the
fruitful hen, and reserved in a "foramen cæcum." This opinion we have already rejected, as well because that cavity is
found in the male and female equally, as because neither
there, nor anywhere else in the hen, have we been able to discover this stagnant semen of the cock; as soon as it has performed its office, and impressed a prolific power on the female,
it either escapes out of the body, or is dissolved, or is turned
into vapour and vanishes. And although Galen,[2] and all
physicians with him, oppose by various reasonings this dissolving
of the semen, yet, if they carefully trace the anatomical arrangement of the genital parts, and at the same time weigh other
proofs of the strongest kind, they must confess that the semen
of the male, as it is derived from the testicles through the vasa
deferentia, and as it is contained in the vesiculæ seminales,
is not prolific unless it be rendered spiritual and effervesce into
a frothy nature by the incitement of intercourse or desire.
For it is not, as Aristotle[3] bears witness, its bodily form, or
fire, or any such faculty, that renders the semen prolific, but
the spirit which is contained in it, and the nature which inheres
in it, bearing a proportion to the element of the stars. Wherefore, though we should allow with Fabricius that the semen is
retained in the "bursa," yet, when that prolific effervescence or

---

[1] Op. cit. pp. 38, 39.   [2] Arist. de Gen. Anim. lib. ii, cap. 3.   [3] Ibid.

spirit had been spent, it would forthwith be useless and sterile. Hence, too, physicians may learn that the semen of the male is the architect of the progeny, not because the first conception is embodied out of it, but because it is spiritual and effervescent, as if swelling with a fertilising spirit, and a preternatural influence. For otherwise the story of Averrhöes, of the woman who conceived in a bath, might bear an appearance of truth. But of these things more in their proper place.

In the same manner then as the egg is formed from the hen, so is it probable, that from the *females* of other animals, as will hereafter be shown, the first conceptions take both material and form; and that, too, some little time after the semen of the male has been introduced, and has disappeared again. For the cock does not confer any fecundity on the hen, or her eggs, by the simple emission of his semen, but only in so far as that fluid has a prolific quality, and is imbued with a plastic power; that is to say, is spiritual, operative, and analogous to the essence of the stars. The male, therefore, is no more to be considered the first principle, from which conceptions and the embryo arise, because he is capable of secreting and emitting semen, than is the female, which creates an egg without his assistance. But it is on this consideration rather that he is entitled to his prerogative, that he introduces his semen, imbued as it is with the spirit and the virtue of a divine agent, such as, in a moment of time, performs its functions, and conveys fertility. For, as we see things suddenly set on fire and blasted by a spark struck from a flint, or the lightning flashing from a cloud, so equally does the seed of the male instantly affect the female which it has touched with a kind of contagion, and transfer to her its prolific quality, by which it renders fruitful in a moment, not only the eggs, but the uterus also, and the hen herself. For an inflammable material is not set on fire by the contact of flame more quickly, than is the hen made pregnant by intercourse with the cock. But what it is that is transferred from him to her, we shall afterwards find occasion to speak of, when we treat this matter specially and at greater length.

In the meantime we must remark, that, if it be derived from the soul, (for whatever is fruitful is probably endowed also with a soul; and we have said before, that the egg, in

Aristotle's opinion, as well as the seeds of plants, has a vegetative soul,) that soul, or at all events the vegetative one, must be
communicated as a graft, and transferred from the male to the
female, from the female to the egg, from the egg to the fœtus;
or else be generated in each of these successively by the contagion of coition.

The subject, nevertheless, seems full of ambiguity; and so
Aristotle, although he allows that the semen of the male has
such great virtue, that a single emission of it suffices for fecundating very many eggs at the same time, yet, lest this admission should seem to gainsay the efficacy of frequent repetitions
of intercourse, he further says,[1] "In birds, not even those eggs
which arise through intercourse can greatly increase in size,
unless the intercourse be continued; and the reason of this is,
that, as in women, the menstrual excretion is drawn downwards
by sexual intercourse, (for the uterus, becoming warm, attracts
moisture, and its pores are opened,) so also does it happen with
birds, in which the menstrual excrement, because it accumulates gradually, and is retained above the cincture, and cannot
escape, from being in small quantity, only passes off when it has
reached the uterus itself.   For by this is the egg increased, as
is the fœtus of the viviparous animal by that which flows through
the umbilicus.   For almost all birds, after but a single act of
intercourse, continue to produce eggs, but they are small."

Now, so far perhaps would the opinion of Aristotle be correct, that more and larger eggs are procured by frequently-
repeated intercourse; because, as he says, there may be "a flow
of more fruitful material to the womb, when warmed by the
heat of coition;" not however that frequent coition must necessarily take place in order to render the eggs that are laid prolific.
For experience, as we have said, teaches the contrary, and the
reason which he alleges does not seem convincing; since the
rudiments of eggs are not formed in the uterus from menstrual
blood, which is found in no part of the hen, but in the ovary,
where no blood pre-exists, and originate as well without, as
along with the intercourse of the cock.

The hen, as well as all other females, supplies matter, nutrition, and place to the conception.   The matter, whence the

[1] De Gen. Anim. lib. iii, cap. 1.

rudiments of all eggs are produced in the ovary and take their increase, seems to be the very same from which all the other parts of the hen, namely, the fleshy, nervous, and bony structures, as well as the head and the rest of the members, are nourished and grow. Nourishment is in fact conveyed to each single papula and yelk contained in the ovary by means of vessels, in the same way precisely as to all the other parts of the hen. But the place where the egg is provided with membranes, and perfected by the addition of the chalazæ and shell, is the uterus.

But that the hen neither emits any semen during intercourse, nor sheds any blood into the cavity of the uterus, and that the egg is not formed in the mode in which Aristotle supposed a conception to arise, nor, as physicians imagine, from a mixture of the seminal fluids; as also that the semen of the cock does not penetrate into, nor is attracted towards, the cavity of the uterus of the hen, is all made manifestly clear by this one observation, namely, that after intercourse there is nothing more to be found in the uterus, than there was before the act. And when this shall have been afterwards clearly established and demonstrated to be true of all kinds of animals, which conceive in a uterus, it will at the same time be equally evident, that what has hitherto been handed down to us from all antiquity on the generation of animals, is erroneous; that the fœtus is not constituted of the semen either of the male or female, nor of a mixture of the two, nor of the menstrual blood, but that in all animals, as well in the prolific conception as after it, the same series of phenomena occur as in the generation of the chick from the egg, and as in the production of plants from the seeds of their several kinds. For, besides that, it appears the male is not required as being in himself agent, workman, and efficient cause; nor the female, as if she supplied the matter; but that each, male as well as female, may be said to be in some sort the operative and parent; and the fœtus, as a mixture of both, is created a mixed resemblance and kind. Nor is that true which Aristotle often affirms, and physicians take for granted, namely, that immediately after intercourse, something either of the fœtus or the conception may be found in the uterus, (for instance, the heart, the " three bullæ," or some other principal part,) at any rate *something*—

a coagulum, some mixture of the spermatic substances, or other things of the like kind.   On the contrary, it is not till long after intercourse that the eggs and conception first commence their existence, among the greater number of animals, and these the most perfect ones; I mean in the cases where the females have been fruitful and have become pregnant.   And that the female is prolific, before any conception is contained in the uterus, there are many indications, as will be hereafter set forth in the history of viviparous animals : the breasts enlarge, the uterus begins to swell, and by other symptoms a change of the whole system is discerned.

But the hen, though she have for the most part the rudiments of eggs in her before intercourse, which are afterwards by this act rendered fruitful, and there be, therefore, something in her immediately after coition, yet even when she, as in the case of other animals, has as yet no eggs ready prepared in the ovary, or has at the time of the intercourse got rid of all she had, yet does she by and by, even after some lapse of time, as if in possession of both principles or the powers of both sexes, generate eggs by herself after the manner of plants; and these (I speak from experience) not barren, but prolific.

Nay, what is more, if you remove all the eggs from beneath a hen that has been fecundated and is now sitting, (after having already laid all her eggs, and no more remain in the ovary,) she will begin to lay again; and the eggs thus laid will be prolific, and have both principles inherent in them.

EXERCISE THE FORTY-FIRST.

Of the sense in which the hen may be called the "prime efficient:" and of her parturition.

It has already been said, that the hen is the efficient cause of generation, or an instrument of Nature in this work, not indeed immediately, or of herself; but when rendered prolific by commission from, and in virtue of the male.   But as the male is considered by Aristotle to be the first principle of generation on his own merits, because the first impulse toward generation proceeds from him, so may the hen in some measure be put down as the first cause of generation ; inasmuch as the male is undoubtedly inflamed to venery by the presence of the female. " The female fish," says Pliny,[1] " will follow the male at the season of intercourse, and strike his belly with her nose ; at the spawning time the male will do the like to the female." I have myself at times seen male fishes in shoals following a female that was on the point of spawning, in the same way as dogs pursue a bitch, that they might sprinkle the ova just laid with their milk or seed. But this is particularly to be remarked in the more wanton and lascivious females, who stir up the dormant fires of Cupid, and inspire a silent love ; hence it is that the common cock, so soon as he sees one of his own hens that has been absent for ever so short time, or any other stranger-hen, forthwith feels the sting of desire, and treads her. Moreover, victorious in a battle, although wounded and tired from the fight, he straightway sets about treading the wives of his vanquished foe one after another. And that he may further feed the flame of love thus kindled in his breast, by various gesticulations, incitements, and caresses, often crowing the while, calling his hens to him, approaching and walking round them, and tripping himself with his wings, he entices his females to intercourse as by a kind of fascination. Such are the arts of the male ; but sometimes a certain sullenness of the female, and an apparent disinclination on her part, contribute not a little to arouse the ardour of the male and stimulate his languishing desire, so that he fills her more quickly and more copiously with prolific spirit. But of allurements of this kind, and in what degree they promote conception, we shall speak more hereafter. For, if you carefully weigh the works of nature, you will find that nothing in them was made in vain, but that all things were ordered with a purpose and for the sake of some good end.

Almost all females, though they have pleasure in the act of intercourse and impregnation, suffer pain in parturition. But the reverse is the case with the hen, who loudly complains during intercourse and struggles against it ; but in parturition,

[1] Hist. Nat. lib. ix, cap. 50.

although the egg be very large in comparison with the body and the orifice of the uterus, and it does nothing to further its exit, (as is customary with the young of viviparous animals,) yet she brings forth easily and without pain, and immediately afterwards commences her exultations; and with her loud cackling calls the cock as it seems to share in her triumph.

But, although many rudiments of eggs are found in the hen's ovary, of various sizes and in different stages, so that some are larger and nearer to maturity than others, yet all of them appear to be fecundated, or to receive the prolific faculty from the tread of the cock at the same time and in the same degree. And though a considerable time elapse (namely, thirty or more days) before the common hen or hen-partridge lay all the eggs which she has conceived, yet in a stated time after the mother has begun to sit upon them (say twenty or two and twenty days) all the young are hatched nearly at the same time; nor are they less perfect than if they had commenced their origin simultaneously, from the period of one and the same conception, as the whelps of bitches do.

And while we are here, and while I think how small are the prolific germs of eggs, mere papulæ and exudations less than millet-seeds, and contemplate the full proportions of the cock that springs from thence, his fine spirit, and his handsome plumage, I cannot but express my admiration that such strength should be reposed in the nature of things in such insignificant elements, and that it has pleased the omnipotent Creator out of the smallest beginnings to exhibit some of his greatest works. From a minute and scarce perceptible papula springs the hen, or the cock, a proud and magnificent creature. From a small seed springs a mighty tree; from the minute gemmule or apex of the acorn, how wide does the gnarled oak at length extend his arms, how loftily does he lift his branches to the sky, how deeply do his roots strike down into the ground! "It is in truth a great miracle of nature," says Pliny,[1] "that from so small an origin is produced a material that resists the axe, and that supplies beams, masts, and battering-rams. Such is the strength, such the power of nature!" But in the seeds of all plants there is a gemmule or bud of such a kind, so

---

[1] Lib. xvii, cap. 10.

small that if the top only, a very point, be lost, all hope of propagation is immediately destroyed; in so small a particle does all the plastic power of the future tree seem lodged ! The provident ant by gnawing off this little particle stores safely in her subterraneous hoard the grain and other seeds she gathers, and ingeniously guards against their growing : "The cypress," adds Pliny, in the same place, "bears a seed that is greatly sought after by the ant ; which makes us still further wonder, that the birth of mighty trees should be consumed in the food of so small an animal." But on these points we shall say more when we show that many animals, especially insects, arise and are propagated from elements and seeds so small as to be invisible, (like atoms flying in the air,) scattered and dispersed here and there by the winds; and yet these animals are supposed to have arisen spontaneously, or from decomposition, because their ova are nowhere to be found. These considerations, however, may furnish arguments to that school of philosophy which teaches that all things are produced from nothing ; and indeed there is hardly any ascertainable proportion between the rudiment and the full growth of any animal.

Nor should we so much wonder what it is in the cock that preserves and governs so perfect and beautiful an animal, and is the first cause of that entity which we call the soul ; but much more, what it is in the egg, aye, in the germ of the egg, of so great virtue as to produce such an animal, and raise him to the very summit of excellence. Nor are we only to admire the greatness of the artificer that aids in the production of so noble a work, but chiefly the " contagion " of intercourse, an act which is so momentary ! What is it, for instance, that passes from the male into the female, from the female into the egg, from the egg into the chick ? What is this transitory thing, which is neither to be found remaining, nor touching, nor contained, as far as the senses inform us, and yet works with the highest intelligence and foresight, beyond all art ; and which, even after it has vanished, renders the egg prolific, not because it now touches, but because it formerly did so, and that not merely in the case of the perfect and completed egg, but of the imperfect and commencing one when it was yet but a speck ; aye, and makes the hen herself fruitful before she has yet produced any germs of eggs, and this too so suddenly, as

21

if it were said by the Almighty, "Let there be progeny," and straight it is so?

Let physicians, therefore, cease to wonder at what always excites their astonishment, namely, the manner in which epidemic, contagious, and pestilential diseases scatter their seeds, and are propagated to a distance through the air, or by some 'fomes' producing diseases like themselves, in bodies of a different nature, and in a hidden fashion silently multiplying themselves by a kind of generation, until they become so fatal, and with the permission of the Deity spread destruction far and wide among man and beast; since they will find far greater wonders than these taking place daily in the generation of animals. For agents in greater number and of more efficiency are required in the construction and preservation of an animal, than for its destruction; since the things that are difficult and slow of growth, decay with ease and rapidity. Seneca[1] observes, with his usual elegance, "How long a time is needed for conception to be carried out to parturition! with what labour and tenderness is an infant reared! to what diligent and continued nutrition must the body be subject, to arrive at adolescence! but by what a nothing is it destroyed! It takes an age to establish cities, an hour to destroy them. By great watching are all things established and made to flourish, quickly and of a sudden do they fall in pieces. That which becomes by long growth a forest, quickly, in the smallest interval of time, and by a spark, is reduced to ashes." Nor is even a spark necessary, since by the solar rays transmitted through a small piece of glass and concentrated to a focus, fire may be immediately produced, and the largest things be set in flames. So easy is every thing to nature's majesty, who uses her strength sparingly, and dispenses it with caution and foresight for the commencement of her works by imperceptible additions, but hastens to decay with suddenness and in full career. In the generation of things is seen the most excellent, the eternal and almighty God, the divinity of nature, worthy to be looked up to with reverence; but all mortal things run to destruction of their own accord in a thousand ways.

---

[1] Nat. Quæst. lib. iii, cap. 27.

Of the manner in which the generation of the chick takes place from the egg.

Hitherto we have considered the egg as the fruit and end; it still remains for us to treat of it as the seed and beginning. " We must now inquire," says Fabricius[1], " how the generation of the chick results from the egg, setting out from that principle of Aristotle and Galen, which is, even conceded by all, to wit, that all things which are made in this life, are manifestly made by these three: workers, instruments, and matter.

But since in natural phenomena, the work is not extrinsic, but is included in the matter, or the instruments, he concludes that we must take cognizance only of the agent and the matter.

As we are here about to shew in what manner the chick arises from the egg, however, I think it may be of advantage for me to preface this, by showing the number of modes in which one thing may be said to be made from another.

For so it will appear, more clearly and distinctly, after which of these generation takes place in the egg, and what are the right conclusions in regard to its matter, its instruments, and efficient cause.

Aristotle[2] has laid down that there are four modes in which one thing is made from another: "first, when we say that from day night is made, or from a boy a man, since one is after the other; secondly, when we say that a statue is made from brass, or a bed from wood, or any thing else from a certain material, so that the whole consists of something, which is inherent and made into a form; thirdly, as when from a musical man is made an unmusical one, or from a healthy, a sick one, or contraries in any way: fourthly, as Epicharmus exaggerates it, as of calumnies, cursing; of cursing, fighting. But all these are to be referred to that from whence the movement took its rise; for the calumny is a certain portion of the whole

---

[1] Op. cit. p. 28.   [2] De Gen. Anim. lib. i, cap. 18.

quarrel. Since then these are the methods in which one thing is made from another, it is clear that the seed is in one of two of these. For that which is born arises out of it, either as from matter, or as from the prime mover. For it is not, ' as this is after that,' in the same way as after the Panathenœa navigation; nor as ' one contrary from another;' for in such case, a thing would be born out of its contrary, because it is in a state of decay, and there must be something else as subject matter."

By these words, Aristotle rightly infers, that the semen proceeding from the male, is the efficient or instrumental cause of the embryo; since it is no part of what is born, either in the first or third manner; (namely, as one thing is after another, or as it is out of its contrary;) nor does it arise from the subject matter.

But then, as he adds, in the same place, "that which comes out of the male in coition, is not with truth and propriety called semen, but rather geniture; and it is different from the seed properly so called. For that is called the geniture which, proceeding from the generant, is the cause which first promotes the beginning of generation. I mean in those creatures, which nature designed to have connection; but the seed is that which derives its origin from the intercourse of the two (i. e. of the male and female); such is the seed of all plants; and of some animals in which the sex is not distinct; it is the produce, as it were, of the male and female mixed together originally, like a kind of promiscuous conception;" and such as we have formerly in our history declared the egg to be, which is called both fruit and seed. For the seed and the fruit are distinct from each other, and in the relation of antecedent and consequent; the fruit is that which is out of something else, the seed is that out of which something else comes; otherwise both were the same.

It remains then, to inquire, in how many of the aforesaid ways the fœtus may arise, not indeed from the geniture of the male, but out of the true seed, or out of the egg or conception, which is in reality the seed of animals.

In how many ways the chick may be said to be formed from the egg.

It is admitted, then, that the fœtus is formed from a prolific egg, as out of the proper matter, and as it were by the requisite agency, and that the same egg stands for both causes of the chick. For inasmuch as it derives its origin from the hen, and is considered as a fruit, it is the matter : but, in so far as it contains in its whole structure the prolific and plastic faculty infused by the male, it is called the efficient cause of the chick.

Moreover, not only as Fabricius supposed, are these, namely, the agent and the instrument, inseparably joined in one and the same egg, but it is also necessary, that the aliment by which the chick is nourished, be present in the same place. Indeed, in the prolific egg, these four are found together, to wit, the agent, the instrument, the matter, and the aliment, as we have shown in our history.

Wherefore, we say, that the chick is formed from the prolific egg in all the aforesaid ways, namely, as from matter, by an efficient, and by an instrument ; and moreover, as a man grows out of a boy, as the whole is made up of its parts, and as a thing grows from its nutriment; a contrary thing springs from a contrary.

For after incubation is begun, as soon as by the internal motive principle a certain clear liquid which we have called the eye of the egg is produced, we say that that liquid is made as it were out of a contrary ; in the same way as we suppose the chyle through concoction to be formed out of its contraries, (namely, crude articles of food,) and in the same way as we are said to be nourished by contraries ; so, from the albumen is formed and augmented that to which we have given the names of the eye and the colliquament ; and in the same manner, from that clear fluid do the blood and pulsating vesicle, the first particles of the chick, receive their being, nutrition, and growth. The nutriment, I say, is by the powers of an inherent and innate heat, assimilated by means of concoction, as it were out of a contrary. For the crude and unconcocted are contrary to the concocted and assimilated, as the unmusical man is to the musical, and the sick to the sound man.

And when the blood is engendered from the clear colliquament, or a clear fluid is produced from the white or the yelk, there is generation as regards the former, corruption as regards the latter; a transmutation, namely, is made from the extremes of contraries, the subject-matter all the while remaining the same. To explain: by the breaking up of the first form of the white, the colliquament is produced; and from the consumption of this colliquament follows the form of the blood, in the same way precisely as food is converted into the substance of the thing fed.

It is thus, then, that the chick is said to be made out of the egg, as it were by a contrary; for in the nutrition and growth of the chick in the egg, white and yelk are equally broken up and consumed, and finally the whole substance of the egg. It is clear, therefore, that the chick is formed from the egg, as it were by a contrary, namely the aliment, and as if by an abstraction, and from a non-entity. For the first particle of the chick, viz. : the blood or punctum saliens, is constituted out of something which is not blood, and altogether its contrary, the same subject-matter always remaining.

The chick too is made from the egg, as a man is made from a boy. For in the same way, as out of plants seeds arise, and out of seeds, buds, sprouts, stems, flowers, and fruits ; so also out of the egg, the seed of the hen is produced, the dilatation of the cicatricula and the colliquament, the blood and the heart, as the first particle of the fœtus or fruit; and all this, in the same way as the day from the night, the summer from the spring, a man from a boy—one follows or comes after the other. So that, in the same way as fruits arise after flowers on the same stem, so likewise is the colliquament formed after the egg, the blood after this, as from the primogeneous humour, the chick after the blood, and out of it, as the whole out of a part ; in the same way, as by Epicharmus's exaggeration, out of calumnies comes cursing, and out of cursing fighting. For the blood first begins its existence with the punctum saliens, and at the same time, seems to be as well a part of the chick, and a kind of efficient or instrument of its generation, inseparable, as Fabricius thinks, from the agent. But how the egg may be called the efficient and instrument of generation, has partly been explained already, and will be illustrated more copiously by what we shall presently say.

So much has been fully established in our history, that the punctum pulsans and the blood, in the course of their growth, attach round themselves the rest of the body, and all the other members of the chick, just as the yelk in the uterus, after being evolved from the ovary, surrounds itself with the white; and this not without concoction and nutrition. Now the common instrument of all vegetative operations, is, in the opinion of all men, an internal heat or calidum innatum, or a spirit diffused through the whole, and in that spirit a soul or faculty of a soul. The egg, therefore, beyond all doubt, has its own operative soul, which is all in the whole, and all in each individual part, and contains within itself a spirit or animal heat, the immediate instrument of that soul. To one who should ask then, how the chick is made from the egg, we answer: after all the ways recited by Aristotle, and devised by others, in which it is possible for one thing to be made from another.

EXERCISE THE FORTY-FOURTH.

Fabricius is mistaken with regard to the matter of the generation of the chick in ovo.

As I proposed to myself at the outset, I continue to follow Fabricius as pointing out the way; and we shall, therefore, consider the three things which he says are to be particularly regarded in the generation of the chick, viz.: the agent, the matter, and the nourishment of the embryo. These must needs be all contained in the egg; he proposes various doubts or questions, and quotes the opinions of the most weighty authorities in regard to them, these opinions being frequently discordant.   The first difficulty is in reference to the matter and nourishment of the chick.   Hippocrates,[1] Anaxagoras, Alcmaeon, Menander, and the ancient philosophers, all thought that the chick was engendered from the vitellus, and was nourished by the albumen.   Aristotle,[2] however, and after him, Pliny,[3] maintained, on the contrary, that the chick was incorporated from the albumen, and nourished by the vitellus.   But Fabricius himself, will have it that neither the white nor yelk forms the matter of the chick ; he strives to combat both of the preceding opinions, and teaches that the white and the yellow alike do no more than nourish the chick. One of his arguments, amongst a great number of others which I think are less to be acquiesced in, appears to me to have some force.   The branches of the umbilical vessels, he says, through which the embryo undoubtedly imbibes its nourishment, are distributed to the albumen and the vitellus alike, and both of these fluids diminish as the chick grows.   And it is on this ground, that Fabricius in confirmation of his opinion, says[4] : "Of the bodies constituting the egg, and adapted to forward the generation of the chick, there are only three, the albumen, the vitellus, and the chalazæ ; now the albumen and vitellus are the nourishment of the chick ; so that the chalazæ alone remain as matter from which it can be produced."

Nevertheless, that the excellent Fabricius is in error here, we have demonstrated above in our history.   For after the chick is already almost perfected, and its head and its eyes are distinctly visible, the chalazæ can readily be found entire, far from the embryo, and pushed from the apices towards the sides: the office of these bodies, as Fabricius himself admits, is that of ligaments, and to preserve the vitellus in its proper position within the albumen.   Nor is that true, which Fabricius adds in confirmation of his opinion, namely, that the chalazæ are situated in the direction of the blunt part of the egg.   For after even a single day's incubation, the relative positions of the fluids of the egg are changed, the yelk being drawn upwards, and the chalazæ on either hand removed, as we have already had occasion to say.

[1] Lib. de Nat. Pueri.

[2] Hist. Anim. lib. vi, cap. 3, et de Gen. Anim. lib. iii, cap. 1 & 2.

[3] Lib. x, cap. 53.   [4] Op. cit. p. 34.

He is also mistaken when he speaks of the chalazæ, as proper parts of the egg. The egg consists in fact but of white and yelk ; the chalazæ as well as the membranes, are mere appendages of the albumen and vitellus. The chalazæ, in particular, are the extremities of certain membranes, twisted and knotted ; they are produced in the same way as a rope is formed by the contortion of its component filaments, and exist for the purpose of more certainly securing the several elements of the egg in their respective places.

Fabricius, therefore, reasons ill when he says, that " the chalazæ are found in the part of the egg where the embryo is produced, wherefore it is engendered from them ;" for even on his own showing, this could never take place, he admitting that the chalazæ are extant in either extremity of the egg, whilst the chick never makes its appearance save at the blunt end ; in which, moreover, at the first commencement of generation, no chalaza can be seen. Farther, if you examine the matter in a fresh egg, you will find the superior chalaza not immediately under the blunt end or its cavity, but declined somewhat to the side ; not to that side, however, where the cavity is extending, but rather to the opposite side. Still farther, from what has preceded, it is obvious that the relative positions of the fluids of the egg are altered immediately that incubation is begun : the eye increased by the colliquament is drawn up towards the cavity in the blunt end of the egg, whence the white and the chalaza are on either hand withdrawn to the side. For the macula or cicatricula which before incubation was situated midway between the two ends, now increased into the eye of the egg, adjoins the cavity in the blunt end, and whilst one of the chalazæ is depressed from the blunt end, the other is raised from the sharp end, in the same way as the poles of a globe are situated when the axis is set obliquely ; the greater portion of the albumen, particularly that which is thicker, subsides at the same time, into the sharp end.

Neither is it correct to say, that the chalazæ bear a resemblance in length and configuration to the chick on its first formation, and that the number of their nodules corresponds with the number of the principal parts of the embryo ; a statement which gives Fabricius an opportunity of adducing an argument connected with the *matter* of the chick, based on the similarity of its consistency to that of the chalazæ. But the red mass (which Fabricius regarded as the liver) is neither situated in nor near the chalaza, but in the middle of the clear colliquament; and it is not any rudiment of the liver but of the heart alone. Neither does his view square with the example he quotes of the tadpole, " of which," he says, " there is nothing to be seen but the head and the tail, that is to say, the head and spine, without a trace of upper or lower extremities." And he adds, " he who has seen a chalaza, and this kind of conception, in so far as the body is concerned, will believe that in the former, he has already seen the latter." I, however, have frequently dissected the tadpole, and have found the belly of large size, and containing intestines and liver and heart pulsating; I have also distinguished the head and the eyes. The part which Fabricius takes for the head, is the rounded mass [or entire body] of the tadpole, whence the creature is called 'gyrinus,' from its circular form. It has a tail with which it swims, but is without legs. About the epoch of the summer solstice, it loses the tail, when the extremities begin to sprout. Nothing however occurs in the nature of a division of the embryo pullet into the head and spine, which should induce us to regard it as produced from the chalazæ, and in the same manner as the tadpole.

The position and fame of Fabricius, however, a man exceedingly well skilled in anatomy, do not allow me to push this refutation farther. Nor indeed, is there any necessity so to do, seeing that the thing is so clearly exhibited in our history.

Our author concludes, by stating that his opinion is of great antiquity, and was in vogue even in the times of Aristotle.

For my own part, nevertheless, I regard the view of Ulysses· Aldrovandus as the older, he maintaining, that the chalazæ are the spermatic fluid of the cock, from which and through which alike the chick is engendered.

Neither notion, however, is founded on fact, but is the popular error of all times : the chalazæ, treads, or treadles, as our English name implies, are still regarded by the country folks as the semen of the cock.

" The treadles (grandines)," says Aldrovandus; " are the spermatic fluid of the cock, because no fertile egg is without them." But neither is any unprolific egg without these parts, a fact which Aldrovandus was either ignorant of or concealed. Fabricius admits this fact; but though he has denied that the semen of the male penetrates to the uterus or is ever found in the egg, he nevertheless, contends, that the chalazæ alone of all the parts of the egg are impregnated with the prolific power of the egg, and are the repositories of the fecundating influence; and this, with the fact staring him in the face all the while, that there is no perceptible difference between the chalazæ of a prolific and an unprolific egg. And when he admits, that the mere rudiments of eggs in the ovary, as well as the vitelli that are surrounded with albumen, become fecundated through the intercourse of the cock, I conceive that this must have been the cause of the error committed by so distinguished an individual. It was the current opinion, as I have said oftener than once, both among philosophers and physicians, that the matter of the embryo in animal generation, was the geniture, either of the male, or of the female, or resulted from a mixture of the two, and that from this, deposited in the uterus, like a seed in the ground, which produces a plant, the animal was engendered. Aristotle, himself, is not very far from the same view, when he maintains the menstrual blood of the female to be the seed, which the semen of the male coagulates, and so composes the conception.

The error which we have announced, having been admitted by all in former times, as a matter of certainty, it it not to be wondered at, that various erroneous opinions based on each man's conjecture, should have emanated from it. They, however, are wholly mistaken, who fancy that anything in the shape of a ' prepared or fit matter ' must necessarily remain in the uterus after intercourse, from which the fœtus is produced, or the first conception is formed, or that anything is immediately fashioned in the uterine cavity that corresponds to the seed of a plant deposited in the bosom of the ground. For it is quite certain, that in the uterus of the fowl, and the same thing is true of the uterus of every other female animal, there is nothing discoverable after intercourse more than there was before it.

It appears, consequently, that Fabricius erred when he said :[1] " In the same way as a viviparous animal is incorpo-

<hr>

[1] Op. sup. cit. p. 35.

rated from a small quantity of seminal matter, whilst the matter which is taken up as food and nourishment is very large; so a small chalaza suffices for the generation of a chick, and the rest of the matter contained in the egg goes to it in the shape of nutriment." From which it is obvious, that he sought for some such ' prepared matter ' in the egg, whence the chick should be incorporated; mainly, as it seems, that he might not be found in contradiction with Aristotle's definition of an egg,[1] viz.: as " that from part of which an animal is engendered; and the remainder of which is food for the thing engendered." This of Fabricius, therefore, has the look of a valid argument, namely, " Since there are only three parts in the egg,—the albumen, the vitellus, and the chalazæ; and the two former alone supply aliment; it necessarily follows, that the chalazæ alone are the matter from which the chick is constituted."

Thus, our learned anatomist, blinded by a popular error, seeking in the egg for some particular matter fitted to engender the chick distinct from the rest of the contents of the egg, has gone astray. And so it happens to all, who forsaking the light, which the frequent dissection of bodies, and familiar converse with nature supplies, expect that they are to understand from conjecture, and arguments founded on probabilities, or the authority of writers, the things or the facts which they ought themselves to behold with their own eyes, to perceive with their proper senses. It is not wonderful, therefore, when we see that we have so many errors accredited by general consent, handed down to us from remote antiquity, that men otherwise of great ingenuity, should be egregiously deceived, which they may very well be, when they are satisfied with taking their knowledge from books, and keeping their memory stored with the notions of learned men. They who philosophise in this way, by tradition, if I may so say, know no better than the books they keep by them.

In the egg then, as we have said, there is no distinct part or prepared matter present, from which the fœtus is formed; but in the same way as the apex or gemmule protrudes in a seed; so in the egg, there is a macula or cicatricula, which

---

[1] Hist. Anim. lib. iii, cap. 8.

endowed with plastic power, grows into the eye of the egg and the colliquament, from which and in which the primordial or rudimentary parts of the chick, the blood, to wit, and the punctum saliens are engendered, nourished, and augmented, until the perfect chick is developed. Neither is Aristotle's definition of an egg correct, as a body from part of which an embryo is formed, and by part of which it is nourished, unless the philosopher is to be understood in the following manner : The egg is a body, from part of which the chick arises, not as from a special matter, but as a man grows out of a boy ; or an egg is a perfect conception from which the chick is said to be partly constituted, partly nourished ; or to conclude, an egg is a body, the fluids of which serve both for the matter and the nourishment of the parts of the fœtus. In this sense, indeed, Aristotle[1] teaches us that the matter of the human fœtus is the menstrual blood; " which (when poured into the uterus by the veins) nature employs to a new purpose ; viz., that of generation, and that a future being may arise, such as the one from which it springs ; for potentially it is already such as is the body whose secretion it is, namely, the mother."

EXERCISE THE FORTY-FIFTH.

What is the material of the chick, and how it is formed in the egg ?

Since, then, we are of opinion, that for the acquisition of truth, we cannot rely on the theories of others, whether these rest on mere assertions, or even may have been confirmed by plausible arguments, except there be added thereto a diligent course of observation ; we propose to show, by clearly-arranged remarks derived from the book of nature, what is the material of the fœtus, and in what manner it thence takes its origin. We have seen that one thing is made out of another (tanquam ex materia) in two ways, and this as well in works of art, as in those of nature, and more particularly in the generation of animals.

[1] De Gen. Anim. lib. ii, cap. 4.

One of these ways, viz., when the object is made out of something pre-existing, is exemplified by the formation of a bed out of wood, or a statue from stone ; in which case, the whole material of the future piece of work has already been in existence, before it is finished into form, or any part of the work is yet begun; the second method is, when the material is both made and brought into form at the same time. Just then as the works of art are accomplished in two manners, one, in which the workman cuts the material already prepared, divides it, and rejects what is superfluous, till he leaves it in the desired shape (as is the custom of the statuary) ; the other, as when the potter educes a form out of clay by the addition of parts, or increasing its mass, and giving it a figure, at the same time that he provides the material, which he prepares, adapts, and applies to his work ; (and in this point of view, the form may be said rather to have been *made* than *educed ;*) so exactly is it with regard to the generation of animals.

Some, out of a material previously concocted, and that has already attained its bulk, receive their forms and transfigurations ; and all their parts are fashioned simultaneously, each with its distinctive characteristic, by the process called metamorphosis, and in this way a perfect animal is at once born ; on the other hand, there are some in which one part is made before another, and then from the same material, afterwards receive at once nutrition, bulk, and form : that is to say, they have some parts made before, some after others, and these are at the same time increased in size and altered in form. The structure of these animals commences from some one part as its nucleus and origin, by the instrumentality of which the rest of the limbs are joined on, and this we say takes place by the method of epigenesis, namely, by degrees, part after part ; and this is, in preference to the other mode, generation properly so called.

In the former of the ways mentioned, the generation of insects is effected where by metamorphosis a worm is born from an egg ; or out of a putrescent material, the drying of a moist substance or the moistening of a dry one, rudiments are created, from which, as from a caterpillar grown to its full size, or from an aurelia, springs a butterfly or fly already of a proper size, which never attains to any larger growth after it is first born; this is called metamorphosis. But the more perfect animals with red blood are made by epigenesis, or the superaddition of parts. In the former, chance or hazard seems the principal promoter of generation, and there, the form is due to the potency of a preexisting material; and the first cause of generation is 'matter,' rather than 'an external efficient;' whence it happens too that these animals are less perfect, less preservative of their own races, and less abiding, than the red-blooded terrestrial or aquatic animals, which owe their immortality to one constant source, viz. the perpetuation of the same species; of this circumstance we assign the first cause to nature and the vegetative faculty.

Some animals then are born of their own accord, concocted out of matter spontaneously, or by chance, as Aristotle seems to assert, when he speaks of animals whose matter is capable of receiving an impulse from itself, viz. the same impulse given by hazard, as is attributable to the seed, in the generation of other animals. And the same thing happens in art, as in the generation of animals. Some things, which are the result of art, are so likewise of chance, as good health; others always owe their existence to art; for instance, a house. Bees, wasps, butterflies, and whatever is generated from caterpillars by metamorphosis, are said to have sprung from chance, and therefore to be not preservative of their own race; the contrary is the case with the lion and the cock; they owe their existence as it were to nature or an operative faculty of a divine quality, and require for their propagation an identity of species, rather than any supply of fitting material.

In the generation by metamorphosis forms are created as if by the impression of a seal, or, as if they were adjusted in a mould; in truth the whole material is transformed. But an animal which is created by epigenesis attracts, prepares, elaborates, and makes use of the material, all at the same time; the processes of formation and growth are simultaneous. In the former the plastic force cuts up, and distributes, and reduces into limbs the same homogeneous material; and makes out of a homogeneous material organs which are dissimilar. But in the latter, while it creates in succession parts which are differently and variously distributed, it requires and makes a material which is also various in its nature, and variously distributed, and such as is now adapted to the formation of one part, now of another; on which account we believe the perfect hen's-egg to be constituted of various parts.

Now it appears clear from my history, that the generation of the chick from the egg is the result of epigenesis, rather than of metamorphosis, and that all its parts are not fashioned simultaneously, but emerge in their due succession and order; it appears, too, that its form proceeds simultaneously with its growth, and its growth with its form; also that the generation of some parts supervenes on others previously existing, from which they become distinct; lastly, that its origin, growth, and consummation are brought about by the method of nutrition; and that at length the fœtus is thus produced. For the formative faculty of the chick rather acquires and prepares its own material for itself than only finds it when prepared, and the chick seems to be formed and to receive its growth from no other than itself. And, as all things receive their growth from the same power by which they are created, so likewise should we believe, that by the same power by which the chick is preserved, and caused to grow from the commencement, (whether that may have been the soul or a faculty of the soul,) by that power, I say, is it also created. For the same efficient and conservative faculty is found in the egg as in the chick; and of the same material of which it constitutes the first particle of the chick, out of the very same does it nourish, increase, and superadd all the other parts. Lastly, in generation by metamorphosis the whole is distributed and separated *into* parts; but in that by epigenesis the whole is put together *out of* parts in a certain order, and constituted *from* them.

Wherefore Fabricius was in error when he looked for the material of the chick, (as a distinct part of the egg, from which its body was formed,) as if the chick were created by metamorphosis, or a transformation of the material in mass; and as if all, or at least the principal parts of the body sprang from the same material, and, to use his own words, were incorporated simultaneously. [He is, therefore, of course opposed to the notion] of the chick being formed by epigenesis, in which a certain order is observed according to the dignity and the use of parts, where at first a small foundation is, as it were, laid, which, in the course of growth, has at one and the same time distinct structures formed and its figure established, and acquires an additional birth of parts afterwards, each in its own order; in the same way, for instance, as the bud bursting from the top of the acorn, in the course of its growth, has its parts separately taking the form of root, wood, pith, bark, boughs, branches, leaves, flowers, and fruit, until at length out comes a perfect tree; just so is it with the creation of the chick in the egg: the little cicatrix, or small spot, the foundation of the future structure, grows into the eye and is at the same time separated into the colliquament; in the centre of which the punctum sanguineum pulsans commences its being, together with the ramification of the veins; to these is presently added the nebula, and the first concretion of the future body; this also, in proportion as its bulk increases, is gradually divided and distinguished into parts, which however do not all emerge at the same time, but one after the other, and each in its proper order. To conclude, then: in the generation of those animals which are created by epigenesis, and are formed in parts, (as the chick in the egg,) we need not seek one material for the incorporation of the fœtus, another for its commencing nutrition and growth; for it receives such nutrition and growth from the same material out of which it is made; and, vice versâ, the chick in the egg is constituted out of the materials of its nutrition and growth. And an animal which is capable of nutrition is of the same potency as one which is augmentative, as we shall afterwards show; and they differ only, as Aristotle says, in their distinctness of being; in all other respects they are alike. For, in so far as anything is convertible into a substance, it is nutritious, and under certain conditions it is augmentative: in virtue of its repairing a loss of substance, it is called nutriment, in virtue of its being added, where there is no such loss of substance, it is called increment. Now the material of the chick, in the processes of generation, nutrition, and augmentation is equally to be considered as aliment and increment. We say simply that anything is generated, when no part of it has pre-existed; we speak of its being nourished and growing when it has already existed. The part of the fœtus which is first formed is said to be begotten or born; all substitutions or additions are called adnascent, or aggenerate.

22

In all there is the same transmutation or generation from the same to the same ; as concerns a part, this is performed by the process of nutrition and augmentation, but as regards the whole, by simple generation; in other respects the same processes occur equally. For from the same source from which the material first takes its existence, from that source also does it gain nutriment and increase. Moreover, from what we shall presently say, it will be made clear that all the parts of the body are nourished by a common nutritious juice ; for, as all plants arise from one and the same common nutriment, (whether it be dew or a moisture from the earth,) altered and concocted in a diversity of manners, by which they are also nourished and grow ; so likewise to identical fluids of the egg, namely, the albumen and the yelk, do the whole chick and each of its parts owe their birth and growth.

We will explain, also, what are the animals whose generation takes place by metamorphosis, and of what kind is the pre-existent material of insects which take their origin from a worm or a caterpillar ; a material from which, by transmutation alone, all their parts are simultaneously constituted and embodied, and a perfect animal is born ; likewise, to what animals any constant order in the successive generation of their parts attaches, as is the case with such as are at first born in an imperfect condition, and afterwards grow to maturity and perfection ; and this happens to all those that are born from an egg. As in these the processes of growth and formation are carried on at the same time, and a separation and distinction of parts takes place in a regularly observed order, so in their case is there no immediate pre-existing material present, for the incorporation of the fœtus, (such as the mixture of the semina of the male and female is generally thought to be, or the menstrual blood, or some very small portion of the egg,) but as soon as ever the material is created and prepared, so soon are growth and form commenced; the nutriment is immediately accompanied by the presence of that which it has to feed. And this kind of generation is the result of epigenesis as the man proceeds from the boy; the edifice of the body, to wit, is raised on the punctum saliens as a foundation; as a ship is made from a keel, and as a potter makes a vessel, as the carpenter forms a footstool out of a piece of

wood, or a statuary his statue from a block of marble. For out
of the same material from which the first part of the chick or
its smallest particle springs, from the very same is the whole
chick born; whence the first little drop of blood, thence
also proceeds its whole mass by means of generation in the
egg; nor is there any difference between the elements which
constitute and form the limbs or organs of the body, and those
out of which all their similar parts, to wit, the skin, the flesh,
veins, membranes, nerves, cartilages, and bones, derive their
origin. For the part which was at first soft and fleshy, afterwards, in the course of its growth, and without any change in
the matter of nutrition, becomes a nerve, a ligament, a tendon;
what was a simple membrane becomes an investing tunic; what
had been cartilage is afterwards found to be a spinous process
of bone, all variously diversified out of the same similar material. For a similar organic body (which the vulgar believe to
consist of the elements) is not created out of elements at first
existing separately, and then put together, united, and altered;
nor is it put together out of constituent parts; but, from a transmutation of it when in a mixed state, another compound is
created: to take an instance, from the colliquament the blood
is formed, from the blood the structure of the body arises,
which appears to be homogeneous in the beginning, and resembles the spermatic jelly; but from this the parts are
at first delineated by an obscure division, and afterwards become separate and distinct organs.

Those parts, I say, are not made similar by any successive
union of dissimilar and heterogeneous elements, but spring out
of a similar material through the process of generation, have
their different elements assigned to them by the same process,
and are made dissimilar. Just as if the whole chick was created by a command to this effect, of the Divine Architect: "let
there be a similar colourless mass, and let it be divided into
parts and made to increase, and in the meantime, while it is
growing, let there be a separation and delineation of parts;
and let this part be harder, and denser, and more glistening,
that be softer and more coloured," and it was so. Now it is in
this very manner that the structure of the chick in the egg
goes on day by day; all its parts are formed, nourished, and
augmented out of the same material. First, from the spine

arise the sides, and the bones are distinguishable from the flesh by minute lines of extreme whiteness; in the head three bullæ are perceived, full of crystalline fluid, which correspond to the brain, the cerebellum, and one eye, easily observable by a black speck; the substance which at first appears a milky coagulum, afterwards gradually becomes cartilaginous, has spinous processes attached to it, and ends in being completely osseous; what was at first of a mucous nature and colourless, is converted at length into red flesh and parenchyma; what was at one time limpid and perfectly pure water, presently assumes the form of brain, cerebellum, and eyes. For there is a greater and more divine mystery in the generation of animals, than the simple collecting together, alteration, and composition of a whole out of parts would seem to imply; inasmuch as here the whole has a separate constitution and existence before its parts, the mixture before the elements. But of this more at another time, when we come to specify the causes of these things.

EXERCISE THE FORTY-SIXTH.

Of the efficient cause of the generation of the chick and fœtus.

We have thus far spoken of the matter from which the chick in ovo is generated. We have still with Fabricius to say a few words on the efficient cause of the chick. As this subject is surrounded with difficulties, however; as writers nowhere else dispute more virulently or more wordily, and Aristotle himself in explaining the matter is singularly intricate and perplexed, and as various questions that can by no means be lightly treated do in fact present themselves for consideration, I conceive that I shall be undertaking a task worthy of the toil if, as I have done in the disquisition on the "matter," I set out here by stating in how many ways anything can be said to be "efficient" or "effective." We shall thus obtain a clearer idea of what it is which we are to inquire after under the name of "efficient," and further, what estimate we are to form of the ideas of writers upon this subject; it will at the same time appear from our observations what is truly and properly to be called " an efficient."

Aristotle [1] defines an efficient cause to be that " whence is derived the first principle of change or quiescence; as a counsel, a father; and simply as doing that which is done; the transmute of the thing transmuted." In the generation of animals accordingly many and various kinds of cause inducing motion are brought forward; sometimes an accident or quality is assigned; and so animal heat and the formative faculty are called efficient causes. Sometimes it is an external substance, previously existing, in which inheres the plastic force or formative faculty that is designated in the same way; as the cock or his seminal fluid, by the influence of which the chick is procreated from the egg. Occasionally it is some internal substance, self-existent, such as spirit, or innate heat. And again, it is some other substance, such as form, or nature, or soul, or some portion of the vegetative soul, that is regarded as the efficient, such a principle as we have already declared to inhere in the egg.

Besides, since one thing whence motion proceeds is nearer and another more remote, it sometimes happens that the media between the prime efficient and the thing last effected, and instruments are regarded as efficient causes; subordinate conclusions, likewise, or the principles of subsequents, are reckoned among the number of efficient causes; in this way some parts are themselves spoken of as genital parts, such as the heart, whence Aristotle affirms that all the rest of the body is produced; a statement which we have found borne out by our history. The heart, I repeat, or at all events its rudimentary parts, namely, the vesicle and pulsating point, construct the rest of the body as their future dwelling-place; when erected it enters and conceals itself within its habitation, which it vivifies and governs, and applying the ribs and sternum as a defence, it walls itself about. And there it abides, the household divinity, first seat of the soul, prime receptacle of the innate heat, perennial centre of animal action; source and origin of all the faculties; only solace in adversity!

Moreover, since the " efficient " is so styled with reference

---

[1] Metaph. lib. v, cap. 2; et Phys. lib. ii, tit. 28.

to the effect, as some parts produced by epigenesis are posterior in order to other parts, and are different from antecedent parts,—as effects differ, so does it seem probable that efficients also vary : from things that produce different operations, different motions likewise proceed. Thus physicians in their physiologies assign certain organs as the agents of chylification, others of sanguification, others of generation, &c.; and anatomists speak of the ossific, carnific, and neurific faculties, which they conceive produce bones, flesh, and nerves.

But in the generation of the chick, of several actions differing not a little from one another, it is certain that the efficient causes must also differ; those that present themselves to us as accidental efficients of generation must nevertheless be necessary, seeing, that unless they are associated or intervene, nothing is effected; those, to wit, are rightly held " efficients " which, whilst they remove external hinderances, either cherish the conception, or stimulate and turn mere potentiality into positive action. Under this head we should arrange incubation, the proper temperature of the air and the place, the spring season, the approach of the sun in the circle of the zodiac; in like manner the preparing causes which lead the vitellus to rise, make the macula to dilate, and the fluids in the egg to liquefy, are all properly held " efficients."

Further, to the number of efficient causes are to be reckoned the generative and architectonic faculties, styled parts by Fabricius, viz., the immutative, the concoctive, the formative, the augmentative, as also the effective causes of certain accidentals, viz., that which constitutes the pullet male or female, like the father or the mother, taking after the form of the first or last male having connection with the mother; that too whence the offspring is an animal; whether perfect or defective; robust and healthy, or diseased; longer or shorter lived; keeping up the characters of the race or degenerating from them; a monster, an hybrid, &c.

Lastly, when we were discussing the efficient causes of the fœtus, we were not inattentive to its admirable structure, to the functions and uses of all its parts and members; neither did we overlook the foresight, the art, the intelligence, the divine inspiration with which all things were ordained and skilfully continued for the ends of life. It is not enough that we inquire what is the "efficient," the architect, the adviser, but that we likewise venerate and adore the omnipotent Creator and preserver of a work, which has been well entitled a microcosm. We also ask whence this divine something comes, when it arrives, and where it resides in the egg; this something which is analogous to the essence of the stars, and is near akin to art and intelligence, and the vicar of the Almighty Creator?

From what precedes it will be apparent how difficult it were to enumerate all the efficient causes of the chick; it is indispensable, indeed, in the complete investigation of this subject to refer to a general disquisition; we could not from the single generation of the chick in ovo, and without clearer light derived from investigations extended to other animals, venture on conclusions that should be applicable to the whole animal creation. And this all the more, since Aristotle himself has enumerated such a variety of efficient principles of animals; for he at one time adduces the ' male'[1] as the principal efficient cause, as that, to wit, in which the reason of the engendered chick resides, according to the axiom;[2] " all things are made by the same ' univocal :' " at another time he takes ' the male semen ;'[3] or, ' the nature of the male emitting semen :'[4] sometimes it is ' that which inheres in the semen,'[5] ' which causes seeds to be prolific, spirit, to wit, and nature in that spirit corresponding in its qualities to the essence of the stars :' elsewhere he says it is ' heat ;'[6] ' moderate heat ;'[7] ' a certain and proportionate degree of heat ;'[8] ' the heat in the blood ;'[9] ' the heat of the ambient air;' ' the winds ;'[10] 'the sun;' 'the heavens;' ' Jupiter ;' ' the soul ;' and, somewhere, nature is spoken of by him as ' the principle of motion and rest.'

Aristotle[11] concludes the discussion on the efficient cause by declaring it " extremely doubtful" whether it be " anything extrinsic; or something inherent in the geniture or semen; and whether it be any part of the soul, or the soul itself, or something having a soul ?"

---

[1] Metaphys. lib. i, c. 2 ; lib. iv, c. 1.

[2] Ib. lib. vii, cap. x.

[3] De Part. Anim. lib. i, cap. 1.

[4] De Gen. Anim. lib. i,   20.

[5] Ibid. lib. ii, cap. 3.

[6] Ibid. lib. v, cap. 3.

[7] De Gen. Anim. lib. iv, cap. 2.

[8] Ibid. lib. iv, cap. 4.

[9] De Part. Anim. lib. ii, cap. 2.

[10] De Gen. Anim. lib. iv, cap. 2; et De Gen. et cor. lib. ii, tit. 30.

[11] De Gen. Anim. lib. ii. cap. 1.

To escape from such a labyrinth of " efficient causes," it were necessary to be furnished with Ariadne's thread, composed from observations on almost every animal that lives; on this account the subject is deferred till we come to our more general disquisition. Meantime we shall recount the particulars which either manifestly appear in the special history of the chick from the egg, or which differ from the ideas usually entertained, or that seem to demand further inquiry.

Of the manner in which the efficient cause of the chick acts, according to Aristotle.

It is universally allowed, that the male is the primary efficient cause in generation, on the ground that in him the species or form resides; and it is further affirmed, that the emission of his ' geniture' during coition, is the cause both of the existence and the fertility of the egg. But none of the philosophers nor physicians, ancient or modern, have sufficiently explained in what manner the seed of the cock produced a chick from the egg; nor have they solved the question proposed by Aristotle. Nor, indeed, is Aristotle himself much more explanatory, when he says, " that the male contributes not in respect of quantity, but of quality, and is the origin of action; but that it is the female which brings the material." And a little after, " It is not every male that emits seed, and in those which do so, this is no part of the fœtus; just as in the case of a carpenter, nothing is translated from him to the substance of the wood which he uses, nor does any part of the artist's skill reside in the work when completed; but a form and appearance are given by his operation to the matter; and the soul, which originates the idea of forms, and the skill to imitate them, moves the hands, or other limb, whatever it may be, by a motion of a certain quality; or from diversity proceeds difference; or from similarity proceeds resemblance. But the hands and instruments move the material. So the nature of a male, which emits semen, uses that semen as an instrument, and an act having motion; as in works of art the instruments are moved, for in them, in some sort, the motion of the art exists."

By these words he seems to imply, that generation is owing to the motion of a certain quality. Just as in art, though the first cause (the "ratio operis") be in the mind of the artist, yet afterwards, the work is effected by the movement of the hands or other instruments; and although the first cause be removed (as in automatons,) yet is it in some sort said to move what it now does not touch, but once has touched, so long as motion continues in the instrument.

Also in the next book, he says : " When the semen of the male has arrived as far as the uterus of the female, it arranges and coagulates the purest part of the excrement (meaning the menstrual blood existing in the uterus) ; and, by a motion of this kind, changes the material, which has been prepared in the uterus, till it forms part of the chick ; and this, hereafter, although the semen after the performance of this motion disappears, exists as part of the fœtus, and becomes animate (as the heart,) and regulates its own powers and growth, as a son emancipated from his father, and having his own establishment. And so it is necessary that there be some commencing principle, from which afterwards the order of the limbs may be delineated, and a proper disposition made of those things that concern the absolution of the animal ; a principle, which may be the source of growth and motion to all the other parts ; the origin of all, both similar and dissimilar parts, and the source of their ultimate aliment. For that which is already an animal grows, but the ultimate aliment of an animal is the blood, or something corresponding to the blood, whose vessels and receptacles are the veins ; wherefore, the heart is the origin of the veins. But veins, like roots, spread to the uterus, and through these the fœtus derives its nourishment. The heart too, being the beginning of all nature and the containing end, ought to be made first ; as if it were a genital part by its own nature, which, as the original of all the other parts, and of the whole animal, and of sense, must needs be the first ; and by its heat, (since all the parts are in the material *potentially*,) when once the beginning of the motion has taken place, all that follows is excited, just as in spontaneous miracles; and the parts are commenced, not by change of place, but by alteration in softness, hardness, temperature, and the other differences observed in similar parts, these being now actually made, which had before existed only potentially."

This is, in nearly so many words, the opinion of Aristotle, which supposes that the fœtus is formed from the seed by motion, although it is not at present in communication with the fœtus, but simply has been so at a former time: his reasonings are, indeed, ingenious, and carefully put together, and from what we see in the order of the generation of parts, not improbable. For the heart, with the channel of the veins, is first noticed as an animate principle, in which motion and sense reside; or, as it were, an emancipated son, and a genital part, whence the order of the members is delineated, whence all things pertaining to the completion of the animal are disposed, and which has all the attributes bestowed upon it by Aristotle.

But it seems impossible, that the heart should be formed in the egg by the seed of the male, when that seed neither exists in the egg, nor touches it, nor ever has touched it; because the seed does not enter the uterus where the egg is, (as is allowed by Fabricius,) nor is in any way attracted by it; nay, even the maternal blood is not in the egg, nor any other prepared matter, out of which the seed of the male may form this genital part, the author of all the others. For it is not immediately after coition, while the seed still remains within the body, and is in communication, that any part of the chick exists in the egg, but after many days, when incubation has taken place. Moreover, in fishes, when the geniture of the male does nothing but touch the eggs externally, and does not enter into them, it is not likely that it performs any more ample functions when the agency is external, than does the seed of the cock in the already formed eggs of the hen. Besides, since immediately after coition no trace of the egg as yet exists, but it is afterwards generated by the hen herself (I am speaking of the prolific egg); when now the seed of the cock is departed and vanished, there is no probability that the fœtus is formed in that egg by the aforesaid seed, through means of one or any number of successive motions.

Nor indeed does the difference between prolific and unprolific or wind eggs consist herein, that the former contained the seed of the male, as Aldrovandus supposed; nor has it been noticed that anything has been formed and coagulated in the egg by the seed of the male, nor has any sensible transmutation been discovered (for indeed, there is no sensible difference between the fertile and the wind egg); and yet a prolific egg, conceived long after coition, has in itself the faculties of both sexes; viz., the capability of being both formed itself, and of forming a chick; as if, according to the idea of Aristotle, it had derived its origin from the coition of the two, and their mutual endeavours towards the same end; and compelled by the force of this argument, as mentioned above, when speaking of the generation of the ovum, he has endowed the egg with a vital principle (anima.) If such really exist, then, without doubt it would be the origin and efficient of all the natural phenomena which take place in the egg. For if we consider the structure of the chick, displaying, as it does, so much art, so divine an intelligence and foresight; when we see the eyes adapted for vision, the bill for taking food, the feet for walking, the wings for flying, and similarly the rest of its parts, each to its own end, we must conclude, whatever the power be which creates such an animal out of an egg, that it is either the soul, or part of the soul, or something having a soul, or something existing previous to, and more excellent than the soul, operating with intelligence and foresight.

From the generation of the chick, it is also manifest that, whatever may have been its principle of life or first vegetative cause, this cause itself first existed in the heart. Now, if this be the soul of the chicken, it is equally clear, that that soul must have existed in the punctum saliens and the blood; since we there discover motion and sense; for the heart moves and leaps like an animal. But if a soul exists in the punctum saliens, forming, nourishing, and augmenting the rest of the body, in the manner which we have pointed out in our history, then it, without doubt, flows from the heart, as from a fountain-head, into the whole body. Likewise, if the existence of the vital principle (anima) in the egg, or, as Aristotle supposes, if the vegetative part of the soul be the cause of its fertility, it must follow that the punctum saliens, or animate genital part, proceeds from the vital principle (anima) of the egg, (for nothing is its own author,) and that the said vital principle (anima) passes from the egg into the punctum saliens, presently into the heart, and thence into the chick.

Moreover, if the egg have a prolific virtue, and a vegetative soul, by which the chick is constructed, and if it owe them, as is allowed on all hands, to the semen of the cock; it is clear that this semen is also endowed with an active principle (anima.) For such is Aristotle's opinion, when he expresses himself as follows: "As to whether the semen has a vital principle (anima) or not, the same reasoning must be adduced which we have employed in the consideration of other parts. For no active principle (anima) can exist, except in that thing whose vital principle it is; nor can there be any part which is not partaker of the vital principle, except it be equivocally, as the eye of a dead man. We must, therefore, allow, both that the semen has an active principle (anima) and is potential."

Now from these premises, it follows that the male is the primary efficient in which the ratio and forma reside, which produces a seed or rather a prolific geniture, and imparts it, imbued as it is with an anima vegetativa (with which also the rest of its parts are endowed) to the female. The introduction of this geniture begets such a movement in the material of the hen, that the production of an animate egg is the result, and from thence too the first particle of the chick is animated, and afterwards the whole chick. And so, according to Aristotle, either the same soul passes, by means of some metempsychosis, from the cock into his geniture, from the geniture into the material of the female, thence into the egg, and from the egg into the chick; or else, it is raised up in each of the subsequent things by its respective antecedent; namely, in the seed of the male by the male himself, in the egg by the seed, last in the chick by the egg, as light is derived from light.

The efficient, therefore, which we look for in the egg, to explain the birth of the chick, is the vital principle (anima); and therefore, the vital principle of the egg; for, according to Aristotle, a soul does not exist except in that thing whose soul it is.

But it is manifest, that the seed of the male is not the efficient of the chick; neither as an instrument capable of forming the chick by its motion, as Aristotle would have it, nor as an animate substance transferring its vitality (anima) to the chick. For in the egg there is no semen, neither does any touch it, nor has ever done so; ("and it is impossible that that which does not touch should move, or that anything should be affected by that which does not move it,") and therefore the vitality of the semen ought not to be said to exist in it; and although the vital principle may be the efficient in the egg, yet it would not appear to result more from the cock or his semen, than from the hen.

Nor, indeed, is it transferred by any metempsychosis or translation from the cock and his semen into the egg, and thence into the chick. For how can this translation be carried on into the eggs that are yet to exist, and to be conceived after intercourse? unless either some animate semen be in the mean time working in some part of the hen; or the vital principle only have been translated without the seed, in order to be infused into any egg which might thereafter be produced; but neither of these alternatives is true. For in no part of the hen is the semen to be found; nor is it possible that the hen after coition should be possessed of a double vital principle, to wit, her own, and that of the future eggs and chicks; since "the living principle or soul is said to be nowhere but in that thing whose soul it is," much less can one or more vital principles lie hidden in the hen, to be afterwards subservient to the future eggs and chicks in their order, as they are produced.

We have adduced these passages out of Aristotle in order to set forth his opinion of the manner in which the seed of the cock produces the chick from the egg; and thereby throw at least some light on this difficult question. But whereas the said passages do not explain the mode in which this is accomplished, nor even solve the doubts proposed by himself, it appears that we are still sticking in the same mud, and caught in the same perplexities (concerning the efficient cause of the fœtus in the generation of animals;) indeed, so far from Aristotle's arguments rendering this question more clear, they appear on the contrary to involve it in more and greater doubts.

Wherefore it is no wonder that the most excellent philosopher was in perplexity on this head, and that he has admitted so great a variety of efficient causes, and at one time has been compelled to resort to automatons, coagulation, art, instruments, and motions, for illustrations; at another time to an 'anima' in the egg, and in the seed of the male. Moreover, when he seems positively and definitively to determine what it is in each seed, whether of plants or animals, which render the same fertile, he repudiates heat and fire as improper agents; nor does he admit any faculty of a similar quality; nor can he find anything in the seed which should be fit for that office; but he is driven to acknowledge something incorporeal, and coming from foreign sources, which he supposes (like art, or the mind) to form the fœtus with intelligence and foresight, and to institute and ordain all its parts for its welfare. He takes refuge, I say, in a thing which is obscure and not recognizable by us; namely, in a spirit contained in the seed, and in a frothy body, and in the nature in that spirit, corresponding in proportion to the elements of the stars. But what that is, he has nowhere informed us.

The opinion of Fabricius on the efficient cause of the chick is refuted.

As I have chosen Aristotle, the most eminent among the ancient philosophers, and Fabricius of Aquapendente, one of the foremost anatomists of modern times, as my especial guides and sources of information on the subject of animal generation, when I find that I can make nothing of Aristotle upon a particular topic, I straightway turn to Fabricius; and now I desire to know what he thought of the efficient cause of generation.

I find that he endeavours to satisfy three doubts or difficulties involved in this subject: First, What is the 'efficient' of the chick? This he answers, by saying, the semen of the male. Secondly, How does this appear in the egg, and in what way does the semen of the cock fecundate the egg? Thirdly and lastly, In what order are the parts of the chick engendered?

As to the first query, it appears from our observations, that the cock and his seminal fluid are verily the 'efficient,' but not the 'adequate' cause of generation; that the hen comes in here as something. In this place, therefore, we are principally to inquire how the semen of the cock fecundates the egg otherwise unprolific, and secures the engenderment of a chick from it?

But let us hear Fabricius :[1] "Those things differ," he observes, "that are produced from eggs, from those that originate from semen, in this, that oviparous animals have the matter from which the embryo is incorporated distinct and separate from the agent; whilst viviparous animals have the efficient cause and the matter associate and concorporate. For the 'agent' in the oviparous animal is the semen of the male, in the fowl the semen of the cock, which neither is nor can be in the egg; the 'matter,' again, is the chalazæ from which the fœtus is incorporated. These two differ widely from one another; for the chalazæ are added after the vitellus is formed, whilst it is passing through the second uterus, and are an accession to the internal egg; the semen galli, on the contrary, is stored near the fundament, is separated from the chalazæ by a great interval, and nevertheless by its irradiating faculty, fecundates both the whole egg and the uterus. Now in the viviparous animal, the semen is both 'matter' and 'agent,' the two consisting and being conjoined in the same body."

Our author appears to have introduced this distinction between oviparous and viviparous animals, that he might spare, or at all events, that he might not directly shock or upset the notions of medical writers on the generation of man, they teaching that the seminal fluids of either sex, projected together in intercourse, are mingled; that as one or other preponderates, this becomes the 'efficient,' that stands in lieu of the 'matter;' and that the two together, tending to the same end, amalgamate into the 'conception' of the viviparous animal.

But when he finds that neither in the egg nor uterus of the fowl is there any semen or blood, and avows his belief that nothing is emitted by the male in intercourse, that can by possibility reach the uterus of the female, nor in the egg discovers a trace of aught supplied by the male, he is compelled

[1] Op. cit. p. 38.

to doubt how the semen, which is nowhere to be detected, which is neither mixed with the 'geniture' of the female, nor yet is added to it, nor touches it, can fecundate the egg, or constitute the chick. And this all the more urgently, when he has stated that a few connections in the beginning of the season suffice to secure the fecundity of all the eggs that will be laid in its course. For how should it seem otherwise than impossible that from the semen galli communicated in the spring, but now long vanished, lost or consumed, the eggs that continue to be laid through the summer and autumn, should still be rendered fruitful and fit to produce pullets?

It is that he may meet such a difficulty half way, that he coins the difference which has been noticed. By way of bolstering up his views, he farther adduces three additional considerations:—First, since the semen galli is neither extant in the egg, nor was ever present in the uterus, nor is added as 'material cause' as in viviparous animals, he has chosen to make it resident for a whole year in the body of the hen. And then that he may have a fit receptacle or storehouse for the fecundating fluid, he finds a blind sac near the inlet to the uterus, in which he says the cock deposits his semen, wherein, as in a treasury, it is stored, and from which all the eggs are fecundated. Lastly, although the semen in that bursa comes into contact neither with the uterus, nor the egg, nor the ovary, whereby it might fecundate the egg, or secure the generation of a chick, he says, nevertheless, that from thence, a certain spiritual substance or irradiation penetrates to the egg, fecundates its chalazæ, and from these produces a chick. By this affirmation, however, he appears to support the opinion of Aristotle, namely, that the female supplies the 'matter' in generation, the male the 'efficient force;' and to oppose the postulate of medical writers about the mixture of seminal fluids, for the sake of which, nevertheless, as I have said, he seems to have laid down his distinction between oviparous and viviparous animals. To give an air of greater likelihood to this notion of his, he goes on to enumerate the changes which the semen, not yet emitted, but laid up in the testes and vesiculæ seminales of animals, occasions.

But besides the fact that all this does not bear upon the

question, for the principal element under discussion is, not how the semen galli renders the egg prolific, but rather, how does the semen galli fashion and construct the chick from the egg ? Almost everything he adduces in support of his view appears either false or open to suspicion, as is obvious, from the facts stated in our history; for neither is the blind cavity situated at the root of the uropygium or coccyx of the fowl, which he entitles " bursa," destined as a receptacle for the semen of the cock, nor can any semen be discovered there, as we have said ; but the cavity is encountered in the male as well as in the female fowl.

Our authority nowhere explains what he understands by a " spiritual substance," and an " irradiation ;" nor what he means by " a substance through whose virtue the egg is vivified :" he does not say whether it is any " corporeal " or " formal " substance, which by " irradiation " proceeds from the semen laid up in the bursa, and, (what is especially required,) constructs a pullet from the egg.

In my opinion, Fabricius does no more here than say : " It produces the chick because it irradiates the egg; and forms because it vivifies ;" he attempts to explain or illustrate the exceedingly obscure subject of the formation of a living being by means still more obscure. For the same doubt remains untouched, how, to wit, the semen of the cock without contact, an " external efficient " at best, separate in point of place, and existing in the bursa, can form the internal parts of the fœtus in ovo,—the heart, liver, lungs, intestines, &c., out of the chalazæ by " irradiation." Unless, indeed, our author will have it that all takes place at the dictum as it were of a creator seated on his throne, and speaking the words : Let such things be ! namely, bones for support, muscles for motion, special organs for sense, members for action, viscera for concoction and the like, and all ordered for an end and purpose with foresight, and understanding and art. But Fabricius nowhere demonstrates that the semen has any such virtue, nowhere explains the manner in which without so much as contact the semen can effect such things; particularly when we see that the egg incubated by a bird of another kind than that which laid it, or cherished in any other way, or in dung,

23

or in an oven, far from the bursa of the parent hen, is still quickened and made to produce an embryo.

The same difficulty still remains, I say : how or in what way is the semen of the cock the " efficient" of the chick ? It is in no wise removed by invoking the irradiation of a spiritual substance. For did we even admit that the semen was stored in the bursa, and that it incorporated the embryo from the chalazæ by metamorphosis and irradiation, we should not be the less deeply immersed in the difficulty of accounting for the formation of all the internal parts of the chick. But these notions have already been sufficiently refuted by us.

Wherefore, in investigating the efficient cause of the chick, we must look for it as inhering in the egg, not as concealed in the bursa; and it must be such, that although the egg have long been laid, be miles removed from the hen that produced it, and be set under another hen than its parent, even under a bird of a different kind, such as a turkey or guineafowl, or merely among hot sand or dung, or in an oven constructed for the purpose, as is done in Egypt, it will still cause the egg to produce a creature of the same species as its parents, like them, both male and female, and if the parents were of different kinds, of a hybrid species, and having a mixed resemblance.

The knot therefore remains untied, neither Aristotle nor Fabricius having succeeded even in loosening it, namely: how the semen of the male or of the cock forms a pullet from an egg, or is to be termed the " efficient" of the chick, especially when it is neither present in, nor in contact with, nor added to the egg. And although almost all assert that the male and his semen are the efficient cause of the chick, still it must be admitted, that no one has yet sufficiently explained how it is so, particularly in our common hen's egg.

The inquiry into the efficient cause of the chick is one of great difficulty.

The discussion of the efficient cause of the chick is, as we have said, sufficiently difficult, and all the more in consequence of the various titles by which it has been designated. Aristotle, indeed, recites several efficient causes of animals, and numerous controversies have arisen on the subject among writers, (these having been particularly hot between medical authors and Aristotelians,) who have come into the arena with various explanations, both of the nature of the efficient cause and of the mode of its operation.

And indeed the Omnipotent Creator is nowhere more conspicuous in his works, nowhere is his divinity more loudly proclaimed, than in the structure of animals. And though all know and admit that the offspring derives its origin from male and female, that an egg is engendered by a cock and a hen, and that a pullet proceeds from an egg, still we are not informed either by the medical schools or the sagacious Aristotle, as to the manner in which the cock or his semen fashions the chick from the egg. For from what we have had occasion to say of the generation of oviparous and other animals, it is sufficiently obvious that neither is the opinion of the medical authorities admissible, who derive generation from the admixture of the seminal fluids of the two sexes, nor that of Aristotle, who holds the semen masculinum for the efficient, and the menstrual blood for the material cause of procreation. For neither in the act of intercourse nor shortly after it, is aught transferred to the cavity of the uterus, from which as matter any part of the fœtus is immediately constituted. Neither does the "geniture" proceeding from the male in the act of union (whether it be animated or an inanimate instrument) enter the uterus; neither is it attracted into this organ; neither is it stored up within the fowl; but it is either dissipated or escapes.

Neither is there anything contained in the uterus immediately after intercourse, which, proceeding from the male, or
from the female, or from both, can be regarded as the matter
or rudiment of the future fœtus. Neither is the semen galli
stored and retained in the bursa Fabricii of the hen or elsewhere, that from thence, as by the irradiation of some spiritual substance, or by contact, the egg may be fashioned or
the chick constituted from the egg. Neither has the hen
any other semen save papulæ, yelks, and eggs. These observations of ours, therefore, render the subject of generation
one of greater difficulty than ever, inasmuch as all the pre-
sumptions upon which the two old opinions repose are totally
overthrown. The fact is especial, as we shall afterwards
demonstrate, that all animals are alike engendered from eggs;
and in the act of intercourse, whether of man or the lower
quadrupeds, there is no seminal fluid, proceeding from the
male or the female, thrown into the uterus or attracted by
this organ; there is nothing to be discovered within its cavity,
either before intercourse, during the act, or immediately after
it, which can be regarded as the matter of the future fœtus,
or as its efficient cause, or as its commencement.

Daniel Sennert, a man of learning and a close observer of
nature, having first passed the reasonings of a host of others
under review, approaches the subject himself; and concludes
that the vital principle inheres in the semen and is almost
identical with that which resides in the future offspring. So
that Sennert does not hesitate to aver that the rational soul
of man is present in his seminal fluid, and by a parity of
reasoning that the egg possesses the animating principle of the
pullet; that the vital principle is transported to the uterus of
the female with the semen of the male, and that from the
seminal fluids of either conjoined, not mixed (for mixture, he
says, is applied to things of different species), and endowed
with soul or the vital principle a perfect animal emerges. And
therefore, he says, the semen of either parent is required,
whether to the constitution of the ovum or of the embryo.
And having said so much, he seems to think that he has overcome all difficulties, and has delivered a certain and perspicuous
truth.

But in order that we should concede a soul or vital principle

(anima) to the egg, and that combined from the souls of the
parents, these being occasionally of different species, the horse
and the ass, the common fowl and the pheasant, for example,
this vital principle not being a mixture but only an union; and
allow the pullet to be produced in the manner of the seeds of
plants, by the same efficient principle by which the perfect
animal is afterwards preserved through the rest of its life, so
that it would be absurd to say that the fœtus grew by one
vital principle without the uterus or ovum, and by another
within the uterus or ovum—did we grant all this, I say
(although it is invalid and undeserving faith), our history of
generation from the egg, nevertheless, upsets the foundations
of the doctrine, and shows it to be entirely false; namely, that
the egg is produced from the semen of the cock and hen, or
that any seminal fluid from either one or other is carried to
the uterus, or that the embryo or any particle of it is fashioned
from any seminal fluid transported to the uterus, or that the
semen galli, as efficient cause and plastic agent, is anywhere
stored up or reserved within the body of the hen to serve when
attracted into the uterus, as the matter and nourishment
whence the fœtus which it has produced should continue to
grow. The conditions are wanting which he himself admits,
after Aristotle, to be necessary, viz., that the embryo be constituted by that which is actual and preexists, and the chick by
that which is present and exists in the place where the chick
is first formed and increases; further, that it be produced by
that which is accomplished immediately and conjunctly, and is
the same by which the chick is preserved and grows through
the whole of its life. For the semen galli (and whether it is
viewed as animate or inanimate is of no moment) is nowise
present and conjunct either in the egg or in the uterus; neither
in the matter from which the chick is fashioned, nor yet in the
chick itself already begun, and as contributing either to its
formation or perfection.

He dreams, too, when he seeks illustrations of his opinions
on an animated semen from such instances as the seeds of
plants and acorns; because he does not perceive the difference alleged by Aristotle[1] between the " geniture" admitted in

---

[1] De Gener. Anim. lib. ii, cap. 1.

intercourse and the first conception engendered by both parents; neither does he observe on the egg produced originally in the cluster of the vitellarium, and without any geniture, whether proceeding from the male or the female, translated to the uterus. Neither does he understand that the uterus is, even after intercourse, completely empty of matter of every kind, whether transmitted by the parents, or produced by the intercourse, or transmuted in any way whatever. Neither had he read, or at all events he does not refer to the experiment of Fabricius, namely, that a hen is rendered so prolific by a few treads of the cock, that she will continue to lay fruitful eggs for the rest of the year, although in the interval she receives no new accessions of semen for the fecundation of each egg as it is laid, neither does she retain any of the seminal fluid which she received so long ago.

So much is certain, and disputed by no one, that animals, all those at least that proceed from the intercourse of male and female, are the offspring of this intercourse, and that they are procreated as it seems by a kind of contagion, much in the same way as medical men observe contagious diseases, such as leprosy, lues venera, plague, phthisis, to creep through the ranks of mortal men, and by mere extrinsic contact to excite diseases similar to themselves in other bodies; nay, contact is not necessary; a mere halitus or miasm suffices, and that at a distance and by an inanimate medium, and with nothing sensibly altered: that is to say, where the contagion first touches, there it generates an "univocal" like itself, neither touching nor existing in fact, neither being present nor conjunct, but solely because it formerly touched. Such virtue and efficacy is found in contagions. And the same thing perchance occurs in the generation of animals. For the eggs of fishes, which come spontaneously to their full size extrinsically, and without any addition of male seminal fluid, and are therefore indubitably possessed of vitality without it, merely sprinkled and touched with the milt of the male, produce young fishes. The semen of the male, I say, is not intromitted in such wise as to perform the part of "agent" in each particular egg, or to fashion the body, or to introduce vitality (anima); the ova are only fecundated by a kind of contagion. Whence Aristotle calls the milt of the male fish, or the genital fluid diffused in water, at one time "the genital and fœtific fluid," at another, "the vital virus." For he says[1]: "The male fish sprinkles the ova with his genital semen, and from the ova that are touched by this vital virus young fishes are engendered."

Let it then be admitted as matter of certainty that the embryo is produced by contagion. But a great difficulty immediately arises, when we ask : how, in what way is this contagion the author of so great a work ? By what condition do parents through it engender offspring like themselves, or how does the semen masculinum produce an " univocal" like the male whence it flowed ? When it disappears after the contact, and is naught in act ulteriorly, either by virtue of contact or presence, but is corrupt and has become a nonentity, how, I ask, does a nonentity act ? How does a thing which is not in contact fashion another thing like itself ? How does a thing which is dead itself impart life to something else, and that only because at a former period it was in contact ?

For the reasoning of Aristotle[2] appears to be false, or at all events defective, where he contends " That generation cannot take place without an active and a passive principle; and that those things can neither act nor prove passive which do not touch ; but that those things come into mutual contact which, whilst they are of different sizes, and are in different places, have their extremes together."

But when it clearly appears that contagion from noncontingents, and things not having their extremities together, produce ill effects on animals, wherefore should not the same law avail in respect of their life and generation ? There is an " efficient" in the egg which, by its plastic virtue (for the male has only touched though he no longer touches, nor are there any extremes together), produces and fashions the fœtus in its kind and likeness. And through so many media or instruments is this power, the agent of fecundity, transmitted or required that neither by any movement of instruments as in works of art, nor by the instance of the automaton quoted by Aristotle, nor of our clocks, nor of the kingdom in which the mandate of the sovereign is everywhere of avail, nor yet by the

---

[1] Hist. Animal. lib. vi, cap. 13. [2] De Gen. et cor. lib. i, cap. 6.

introduction of a vital principle or soul into the semen or
" geniture," can the aforementioned doctrine be defended.

And hence have arisen all the controversies and problems
concerning the attraction of the magnet and of amber; on
sympathy and antipathy; on poisons and the contagion of
pestilential diseases ; on alexipharmics and medicines which
prove curative or injurious through some hidden or rather unknown property, all of which seem to come into play independently of contact.   And above all on what it is in generation
which, in virtue of a momentary contact—nay, not even of
contact, save through several media—forms the parts of the
chick from the egg by epigenesis in a certain order, and produces an " univocal" and like itself, and that entirely because it
was in contact at a former period.   How, I ask again, does
that which is not present, and which only enjoyed extrinsic
contact, come to constitute and order all the members of the
chick in the egg exposed without the body of the parent, and
often at a long interval after it is laid ? how does it confer life
or soul, and a species compounded of those of the concurring
generants?   Inasmuch as nothing, it seems, can reproduce
itself in another's likeness.

EXERCISE THE FIFTIETH.

Of the efficient cause of animals, and its conditions.

That we may proceed in our subject, therefore, and penetrate so far into the knowledge of the efficient cause of animal
generation as seems needful in this place, we must begin by
observing what instruments or media are devoted to it.   And
here we come at once to the distinction into male and female ;
seminal fluid and ovum, and its primordium.   For some males,
as well as some females, are barren, or but little prolific; and
the seed of the male is at one time more, at another time less
prolific; because the semen masculinum stored up in the
vesiculæ seminales is esteemed unfruitful, unless it is raised

into froth by the spirits and ejected with force. And even then perchance it is not endowed with equal fecundating force at all times. Neither are all the germs of yelks in the ovary, nor all the eggs in the uterus made fertile at the same instant.

Now I call that fruitful which, unless impeded by some extrinsic cause, attains by its inherent force to its destined end, and brings about the consequence for the sake of which it is ordained. Thus the cock is called fruitful which has his hens more frequently and surely pregnant, the eggs they lay being at the same time perfect and proper for incubation.

The hen in like manner is esteemed fruitful which has the faculty of producing eggs, or of receiving and long retaining the virtue of prolific conception from the cock. The cluster of germs and the ovary itself are regarded as prolific when the germs are numerous and of good size.

The egg in the same way is fruitful which differs from a subventaneous or hypenemic egg, and which, cherished by incubation, or in any other way, does not fail to produce a chick.

Such an efficient cause consequently is required for the chick, as shall impart the virtue of fecundity to it, and secure it the power of acting as an efficient cause in its turn. Because that, or its analogue at least, by means of which they become prolific, is present in all animals. And the inquiry is the same in each case, when we ask what it is in the egg which renders it prolific, and distinguishes it from a wind egg; what in the vitellary germ and ovary; what in the female; what, finally, in the semen and the cock himself? What, moreover, it is in the blood and punctum saliens, or first formed particle of the chick, whence all the other parts arise with their appropriate structures and arrangements ; what in the embryo or chick itself whereby it becomes more or less robust and agile, attains to maturity with greater or less rapidity, and lives with various degrees of health, for a longer or shorter period?

Nor is the inquiry very different which goes to ascertain what sex the male and the female, or the cock and the hen, confer upon the prolific egg; and what proceeds from each that contributes to the perfection or resemblance of the chick, viz., whether the egg, the conception, the matter,

and the nutriment proceed from the mother, and the plastic
virtue from the father; or rather a certain contagion im-
mitted during intercourse, or produced and received from him,
which in the body of the hen, or in the eggs, either perma-
nently excites the matter of the eggs, or attracts nourishment
from the female, and concocts and distributes it first for the
growth of the eggs, and then for the production of the chicks;
finally, whether from the male proceeds all that has reference
to form and life and fecundity, from the female, again, all that
is of matter, constitution, place, and nourishment? For among
animals where the sexes are distinct, matters are so arranged,
that since the female alone is inadequate to engender an embryo and to nourish and protect the young, a male is associated
with her by nature, as the superior and more worthy progenitor,
as the consort of her labour, and the means of supplying her
deficiencies; in the case of the hen, of correcting by his contagion
the inferiority of the hypenemic eggs which she produces, and
so rendering them prolific. For as the pullet, engendered of an
egg, is indebted to that egg for his body, vitality, and principal
or generative part, so and in like manner does the egg receive
all that is in it from the female, the female in her turn being
dependent on the male for her fecundity which is conferred
in coition.

And here we have an opportunity of inquiring, whether the
male be the first and principal cause of the generation of the
offspring; or whether the male along with the female are the
mediate and instrumental causes of nature itself, or of the first
and supreme generator? And such an inquiry is both becoming and necessary, for perfect science of every kind depends on a knowledge of causes. To the full understanding
of generation, therefore, it is incumbent on us to mount from
the final to the first and supreme efficient cause, and to hold
each and every cause in especial regard.

We shall have occasion to define that which is the first and
supreme efficient cause of the chick in ovo by and by, when
we treat of that which constitutes the efficient cause [of gene-
ration] among animals in general. Here, meantime, we shall
see what its nature may be.

The first condition, then, of the primary efficient cause of
generation, properly so called, is, as we have said, that it be

the prime and principal fertilizer, whence all mediate causes receive the fecundity imparted. For example, the chick is derived from the punctum saliens in the egg, not only as regards the body, but also, and this especially, as respects the life (anima): the punctum saliens, or heart, is derived from the egg, the egg from the hen, and the hen has her fecundity from the cock.

Another condition of the prime efficient is discovered from the work achieved, viz., the chick, because that is the prime efficient in which the reason of the effect is principally displayed. But since every generative efficient engenders another like itself, and the offspring is of a mixed nature, the prime efficient must also be a certain mixed something.

Now, I maintain that the offspring is of a mixed nature, inasmuch as a mixture of both parents appears plainly in it, in the form and lineaments, and each particular part of its body, in its colour, mother-marks, disposition to diseases, and other accidents. In mental constitution, also, and its manifestations, such as manners, docility, voice, and gait, a similar temperament is discoverable. For as we say of a certain mixture, that it is composed of elements, because their qualities or virtues, such as heat, cold, dryness, and moisture, are there discovered associated in a certain similar compound body, so, in like manner, the work of the father and mother is to be discerned both in the body and mental character of the offspring, and in all else that follows or accompanies temperament. In the mule, for instance, the body and disposition, the temper and voice, of both parents (of the horse and the ass, e. g.) are mingled; and so, also, in the hybrid between the pheasant and the fowl, in that between the wolf and the dog, &c., corresponding traits are conspicuous.

When, therefore, the chick shows his resemblance to both parents, and is a mixed effect, the primary genital cause (which it resembles) must needs be mixed. Wherefore that which fashions the chick in the egg is of a mixed nature, a certain something mixed or compounded, and the work of both parents. And if any kind of contagion, engendered under the influence of sexual intercourse, in which the male and female mingle and form but one body, either originates or remains in the body of the female, that, too, must be of a mixed nature or power, whence, subsequently, a fertile egg will be produced, endowed with plastic powers, the consequence of a mixed nature, or of a mixed efficient instrument, from which a chick, also of a mixed nature, will be produced.

I have used the word *contagion* above, because Aristotle's view is contradicted by all experience, viz., that a certain part of the embryo is immediately made by intercourse. Neither is it true, as some of the moderns assert, that the vital principle (anima) of the future chick is present in the egg; for that cannot be the vital principle of the chick which inheres in no part of its body. Neither can the living principle be said either to be left or to be originated by intercourse; otherwise in every pregnant woman there would be two vital principles (animæ) present. Wherefore, until it shall have been determined what the efficient cause of the egg is, what it is of mixed nature that must remain immediately upon intercourse, we may be permitted to speak of it under the title of a Contagion.

But where this contagion lies hid in the female after intercourse, and how it is communicated and given to the egg, demands quite a special inquiry, and we shall have occasion to treat of the matter when we come to discuss the conception of females in general. It will suffice, meantime, if we say that the same law applies to the prime efficient—in which inheres the reason of the future offspring—as to the offspring; as this is of a mixed nature, the nature of its cause must also be mixed; and it must either proceed equally from both parents, or from something else which is employed by both concurrently as instruments, animated, co-operating, mixed, and in the sexual act coalescing unto one. And this is the third condition of the prime efficient, that it either imparts motion to all the intermediate instruments in succession, or uses them in some other way, but comes not itself into play. Whence the origin of the doubt that has arisen, whether, in the generation of the chick, the cock were the true prime efficient, or whether there were not another prior, superior to him? For, indeed, all things seem to derive their origin from a celestial influence, and to follow the movements of the sun and moon. But we shall be able to speak more positively of this matter after we have shown what we understand by the "instrument," or "instrumental efficient cause," and how it is subdivided.

Instrumental efficients, then, are of different kinds : some, according to Aristotle, are factive, others active ; some have no capacity any way unless conjoined with another prior efficient, as the hand, foot, genital organs, &c. with the rest of the body; others have an influence even when separate and distinct, as the seminal fluid and the ovum. Some instruments, again, have neither motion nor action beyond those that are imparted to them by the prime efficient ; and others have peculiar inherent principles of action, to which nature indeed allows no motion in the business of generation, though she still uses their faculties, and prescribes them laws or limits in their operations, not otherwise than the cook makes use of fire in cooking, and the physician of herbs and drugs in curing diseases.

Sennert, that he may uphold the opinion he had espoused of the vital principle (anima) being present in the semen, and the formative faculty of the chick being extant in the egg, asserts that not only is the egg, but the semen of the cock, endowed with the living principle of the future chick. Moreover, he distinctly denies that there is any separate instrumental efficient ; and says, that that only ought to be entitled " instrument" which is conjoined with the prime efficient ; and that only " instrumental efficient," which has no motion or action save that which is imparted to it by the prime efficient, or which is continuously and successively received, and in virtue of which it acts. And on this ground he rejects the example of projectiles, which have received force from the projecting agent, and, separated from it, act nevertheless ; as if swords and spears were properly to be called warlike weapons, but arrows and bullets to be refused this title. He also rejects the argument derived from the republic, denying thereby that magistrates, counsellors, or ministers, are instruments of government ; although Aristotle regards a counsel as an efficient, and in express terms calls a minister an instrument.[1] Sennert likewise denies the example of automata ; and says and gainsays much besides, with a view to confirming himself in his position, that the semen and the egg are possessed of a living principle (anima), and are not mediate or instrumental, but principal agents. Sennert, nevertheless, as it were compelled by the force of

---

[1] Polit. lib. i, cap. 4.

truth, lays down such conditions for a principal agent, as fully and effectually contradict all that he had said before. He tells us, for instance, that "whatever produces a work or an effect more noble than itself, or an effect unlike itself, is not a principal efficient, but an instrumental cause;" granting which, who would not infer that the semen and the egg were instruments? seeing that the pullet is an effect more noble than the egg, and every way unlike either this or the spermatic fluid. Wherefore, when the learned Sennert denies the semen and the egg to be instruments or organs, because they are distinct from the prime agents, he takes his position upon a false basis; because, as the prime generator procreates offspring by various means or media, the medium being here conjunct, as the hand of the workman is with his body, there separate and distinct, as is the arrow let loose from the bow, it is still to be regarded as an instrument.

From the conditions now enumerated of an instrumental cause, it seems to follow that the prime efficient in the generation of the chick is the cock, or, at all events, the cock and hen, because the resulting pullet resembles these; nor can it be held more noble than they, which are its prime efficients or parents. I shall, therefore, add another condition of the prime efficient, whence it may, perhaps, appear that the male is not the prime, but only the instrumeutal, cause of the chick; viz., that the prime efficient in the formation of the chick makes use of artifice, and foresight, and wisdom, and goodness, and intelligence, which far surpass the powers of our rational soul to comprehend, inasmuch as all things are disposed and perfected in harmony with the purpose of the future work, and that there be action to a determinate end; so that every, even the smallest, part of the chick is fashioned for the sake of a special use and end, and with respect not merely to the rearing of the fabric, but also to its well-being, and elegance and preservation. But the male or his semen is not such either in the act of kind or after it, that art, intelligence, and foresight can be ascribed to him or it.

The proper inference from these premises appears to be that the male, as well as his seminal fluid, is the efficient instrument; and the female not less than the egg she lays the same. Wherefore, we have to seek refuge in a prior, superior, and more excellent cause, to which, with all propriety, are ascribed foresight, intelligence, goodness, and skill, and which is by so much more excellent than its effect or work, as the architect is more worthy than the pile he rears, as the king is more exalted than his minister, as the workman is better than his hands or tools.

The male and female, therefore, will come to be regarded as merely the efficient instruments, subservient in all respects to the Supreme Creator, or father of all things. In this sense, consequently, it is well said that the sun and moon engender man; because, with the advent and secession of the sun, come spring and autumn, seasons which mostly correspond with the generation and decay of animated beings. So that the great leader in philosophy says:[1] "The first motion [of the sphere?] is not the cause of generation and destruction; it is the motion of the ecliptic that is so, this being both continuous and having two movements; for, if future generation and corruption are to be eternal, it is necessary that something likewise move eternally, that interchanges do not fail, that of the two actions one only do not occur. The cause of the perpetuity [of animal species?] is, therefore, the law of the universe; and the obliquity [of the ecliptic?] is the cause of the approach and accession, [of the sun?] and of his being now nearer, now more remote: when he quits us, and removes to a distance, it is then that decay and corruption intervene; and, in like manner, when he approaches, it is then that he engenders; and if, as he frequently approaches, he engenders; so, because he frequently recedes, does he cause corruption; for the causes of contraries are contrary."

All things, therefore, grow and flourish in spring, (on the approach of the sun, that is to say, he being the common parent and producer, or at all events the immediate and universal instrument of the Creator in the work of reproduction); and this is true not of plants only but of animals also; nor less of those that come spontaneously, than of those that are propagated by the consentient act of male and female. It is as if, with the advent of this glorious luminary, Venus the bountiful descended from heaven, waited on by Cupid and a cohort of graces, and prompted all living things by the bland incitement

[1] De Generat. et corr. lib. ii, cap. 10.

of love to secure the perpetuity of their kinds.   Or (and it is
thus that we have it in the mythology) it is as if the genital
organs of Saturn, cast into the sea at this season, raised a foam,
whence sprung Aphrodite.   For, in the generation of animals,
as the poet says, " superat tener omnibus humor,"—a gentle
moisture all pervades,—and the genitals froth and are replete
with semen.

The cock and the hen are especially fertile in the spring ; as
if the sun, or heaven, or nature, or the soul of the world, or the
omnipotent God—for all these names signify the same thing—
were a cause in generation superior and more divine than they ;
and thus it is that the sun and man, i.e. the sun through man
as the instrument, engender man.   In the same way the preserver of all things, and the male among birds, give birth to the
egg, from whence the chick, the perfect bird, is made eternal
in its kind by the approach and recession of the god of day,
who, by the divine will and pleasure, or by fate, serves for the
generation of all that lives.

Let us conclude, therefore, that the male, although a prior
and more excellent efficient than the female, is still no more
than an instrumental efficient, and that he, not less than the
female, must refer his fecundity or faculty of engendering as
received from the approaching sun ; and, consequently, that
the skill and foresight, which are apparent in his work, are
not to be held as proceeding from him but from God ; inasmuch as the male in the act of kind neither uses counsel nor
understanding ; neither does man engender the rational part
of his soul, but only the vegetative faculty ; which is not regarded as any principal or more divine faculty of the soul, but
one only of a lower order.

Since, then, there is not less of skill and prescience manifested in the structure of the chick than in the creation of man
and the universe at large, it is imperative even in the generation of man to admit an efficient cause, superior to, and more
excellent than man himself : otherwise the vegetative faculty,
or that part of the soul or living principle which fashions and
preserves a man, would have to be accounted far more excellent
and divine, and held to bear a closer resemblance to God than
the rational portion of the soul, whose excellence, nevertheless,
we extol over all the faculties of all animals, and esteem as

that which has right and empire in them, and to which all created things are made subservient. Or we should else have to own that in the works of nature there was neither prudence, nor art, nor understanding; but that these appeared to us, who are wont to judge of the divine things of nature after our own poor arts and faculties, or to contrast them with examples due to ourselves; as if the active principles of nature produced their effects in the same way as we are used to produce our artificial works, by counsel, to wit, or discipline acquired through the mind or understanding.

But nature, the principle of motion and rest in all things in which it inheres, and the vegetative soul, the prime efficient cause of all generation, move by no acquired faculty which might be designated by the title of skill or foresight, as in our undertakings; but operate in conformity with determinate laws like fate or special commandments—in the same way and manner as light things rise and heavy things descend. The vegetative faculty of parents, to wit, engenders in the same way, and the semen finally arrives at the form of the fœtus, as the spider weaves her web, as birds build nests, incubate their eggs, and cherish their young, or as bees and ants construct dwellings, and lay up stores for their future wants; all of which is done naturally and from a connate genius or disposition; by no means from forecast, instruction, or reason. That which in us is the principle or cause of artificial operations, and is called art, intellect, or foresight, in the natural operations of the lower animals is nature, which is αὐτοδίδακτος, self-taught, instilled by no one; what in them is innate or connate, is with us acquired. On this account it is, that they who refer all to art and artifice are to be held indifferent judges of nature or natural things; and, indeed, it is wiser to act in the opposite way, and selecting standards in nature to judge of things made by art according to them. For all the arts are but imitations of nature in one way or another; as our reason or understanding is a derivative from the Divine intelligence, manifested in his works; and when perfected by habit, like another adventitious and acquired soul, gaining some semblance of the Supreme and Divine agent, it produces somewhat similar effects.

Wherefore, according to my opinion, he takes the right and pious view of the matter, who derives all generation from the same eternal and omnipotent Deity, on whose nod the universe itself depends.   Nor do I think that we are greatly to dispute about the name by which this first agent is to be called or worshipped; whether it be God, Nature, or the Soul of the universe,—whatever the name employed,—all still intend by it that which is the beginning and the end of all things; which exists from eternity and is almighty; which is author or creator, and, by means of changing generations, the preserver and perpetuator of the fleeting things of mortal life; which is omnipresent, not less in the single and several operations of natural things, than in the infinite universe; which, by his deity or providence, his art and mind divine, engenders all things, whether they arise spontaneously without any adequate efficient, or are the work of male and female associated together, or of a single sex, or of other intermediate instruments, here more numerous, there fewer, whether they be univocal, or are equivocally or accidentally produced : all natural bodies are both the work and the instruments of that Supreme Good, some of them being mere natural bodies, such as heat, spirit, air, the temperature of the air, matters in putrefaction, &c., or they are at once natural and animated bodies; for he also makes use of the motions, or forces, or vital principles of animals in some certain way, to the perfection of the universe and the procreation of the several kinds of animated beings.

From what has now been said, we are apprized to a certain extent of the share which the male has in the business of generation.   The cock confers that upon the egg, which, from unprolific, makes it prolific, this being identical with that which the fruit of vegetables receives from the fervour of the summer sun, which secures to them maturity, and to their seeds fertility; and not different from that which fertilizes things spontaneously engendered, and brings caterpillars from worms, aurelias from caterpillars, from aurelias moths, butterflies, bees, &c.

In this way is the sun, by his approach, both the beginning of motion and transmutation in the coming fruit, and the end, also, inasmuch as he is the author of the fertility of its included seed : and, as early spring is the prime efficient of leaves and flowers and fruits, so is summer, in its strength, the cause of final perfection in the ripeness and fecundity of the seed.   With a view to strengthen this position, I shall add this one from among a large number of observations. Some persons in these countries cultivate orange trees with singular care and economy, and the fruit of these trees, which, in the course of the first year, will grow to the size of the point of the thumb, comes to maturity the following summer. This fruit is perfect in all respects, save and except that it is without pips or seeds.

Pondering upon this with myself, I thought that I had here an example of the barren egg, which is produced by the hen without the concurrence of the cock, and which comprises everything that is visible in a fruitful egg, but is still destitute of germinant seed; as if it were the same thing that was imparted by the cock, in virtue of which a wind-egg becomes a fruitful egg, which in warmer countries is dispensed by the sun, and causes the fruit of the orange tree to be produced replete with prolific seed. It is as if the summer in England sufficed for the production of the fruit only, as the hen for the production of the egg, but like the female fowl was impotent as a pro-genetrix; whilst in other countries enjoying the sun's light in larger proportion, the summer acquired the characters of the male, and perfected the work of generation.

Thus far have we treated this subject by the way, that, from the instance of the egg, we might learn what conditions were required in the prime efficient in the generation of animals;— for it is certain, that in the egg there is an agent,—as there is also in every conception and germ,—which is not merely infused by the mother, but is first communicated in coitu by the father, by means of his spermatic fluid; and which is itself primarily endowed with such virtue by heaven and the sun, or the Supreme Creator. It is equally manifest, that this agent, existing in every egg and seed, is so imbued with the qualities of the parents, that it builds up the offspring in their likeness, not in its own; and this mingled also as proceeding from both united in copulation. Now, as all this proceeds with the most consummate foresight and intelligence, the presence of the Deity therein is clearly proclaimed.

But we shall have to speak at greater length upon this subject, when we strive to show what it is that remains with the female immediately after intercourse, and where it is stored; at the same time that we explain—since there is nothing visible in the cavity of the uterus after intercourse—what that prolific contagion or prime conception is; whether it is corporeal and laid up within the female, or is incorporeal; whether the conception of the uterus be of the same nature or not with the conceptions of the brain, and fecundity be acquired in the same way as knowledge—a conclusion, in favour of which there is no lack of arguments; or, as motion and the animal operations, which we call appetites, derive their origin from the conceptions of the brain, may not the natural motions and the operations of the vegetative principle, and particularly generation, depend on the conception of the uterus? And then we have to inquire how this prolific contagion is of a mixed nature, and is imparted by the male to the female, and by her is transferred to the ovum? Finally, how the contagious principle of all diseases and preternatural affections spreads insensibly, and is propagated?

EXERCISE THE FIFTY-FIRST.

Of the order of generation; and, first, of the primary genital particle.

It will be our business, by and by, when we come to treat of the matter in especial, to show what happens to the female from a fruitful embrace; what it is that remains with her after this, and which we have still spoken of under the name of contagion, by which, as by a kind of infection, she conceives, and an embryo subsequently begins to grow of its own accord. Meantime, we shall discourse of those things that manifestly appear in connexion with the organs of generation which seem most worthy of particular comment.

And first, since it appears certain that the chick is produced by epigenesis, or addition of the parts that successively arise, we shall inquire what part is formed first, before any of the rest appear, and what may be observed of this and its particular mode of generation.

What Aristotle [1] says of the generation of the more perfect

---

[1] De Gen. Anim. lib. ii, cap. 1.

animals, is confirmed and made manifest by all that passes in the egg, viz. : that all the parts are not formed at once and together, but in succession, one after another; and that there first exists a particular genital particle, in virtue of which, as from a beginning, all the other parts proceed. As in the seeds of plants, in beans and acorns, to quote particular instances, we see the gemmula or apex, protruding, the commencement of the entire prospective herb or tree. "And this particle is like a child emancipated, placed independently, a principle existing of itself, from whence the series of members is subsequently thrown out, and to which belongs all that is to conduce to the perfection of the future animal." [1] Since, therefore, "No part engenders itself, but, after it is engendered, concurs in its own growth, it is indispensable that the part first arise which contains within itself the principle of increase; for whether it be a plant or an animal, still has it within itself the power of vegetation or nutrition;" [2] and at the same time distinguishes and fashions each particular part in its several order; and hence, in this same primogenate particle, there is a primary vital principle inherent, which is the author and original of sense and motion, and every manifestation of life.

That, therefore, is the principal particle whence vital spirit and native heat accrue to all other parts, in which the calidum innatum sive implantatum of physicians first shows itself, and the household deity or perennial fire is maintained; whence life proceeds to the body in general, and to each of its parts in particular; whence nourishment, growth, aid, and solace flow; lastly, where life first begins in the being that is born, and last fails in that which dies.

All this is certainly true as regards the first engendered part, and appears manifestly in the formation of the chick from the egg. I am therefore of opinion that we are to reject the views of certain physicians, indifferent philosophers, who will have it that three principal and primogenate parts arise together, viz. : the brain, the heart, and the liver; neither can I agree with Aristotle himself, who maintains that the heart is the first engendered and animated part; for I think that the privilege of priority belongs to the blood alone; the blood being that

---

[1] De Gen. Anim. lib. ii, cap. i.   [2] Ibid. cap. 4.

which is first seen of the newly engendered being, not only in the chick in ovo, but in the embryo of every animal whatsoever, as shall plainly be made to appear at a later stage of our inquiry.

There appears at first, I say, a red-coloured pulsating point or vesicle, with lines or canals extending from it, containing blood in their interior, and, in so far as we are enabled to perceive from the most careful examination, the blood is produced before the punctum saliens is formed, and is farther endowed with vital heat before it is put in motion by a pulse; so that as pulsation commences in it and from it, so, in the last struggle of mortal agony, does motion also end there. I have indeed ascertained by numerous experiments instituted upon the egg, as well as upon other subjects, that the blood is the element of the body in which, so long as the vital heat has not entirely departed, the power of returning to life is continued.

And since the pulsating vesicle and the sanguineous tubes extending thence are visible before anything else, I hold it as consonant with reason to believe that the blood is prior to its receptacles, the thing contained, to wit, to its container, inasmuch as this is made subservient to that. The vascular ramifications and the veins, therefore, after these the pulsating vesicle, and, finally, the heart, as being every one of them organs destined to receive and contain the blood, are, in all likelihood, constructed for the express purpose of impelling and distributing it, and the blood is, consequently, the principal portion of the body.

This conclusion is favoured by numerous observations; particularly by the fact that some animals, and these red-blooded, too, live for long periods without any pulse; some even lie concealed through the whole winter, and yet escape alive, though their heart had ceased from motion of every kind, and their lungs no longer played; they had lain in fact like those who lie half dead in a state of asphyxia from syncope, leipothymia, or the hysterical passion.

Emboldened by what I have observed both in studying the egg, and whilst engaged in the dissection of living animals, I maintain, against Aristotle, that the blood is the prime part that is engendered, and the heart the mere organ destined for its circulation. The function of the heart is the propulsion of the blood, as clearly appears in all animals furnished with red blood; and the office of the pulsating vesicle in the generation of the chick ab ovo, as well as in the embryos of mammiferous animals, is not different, a fact which I have repeatedly demonstrated to others, showing the vesicula pulsans as a feeble glancing spark, contracting in its action, now forcing out the blood which was contained in it, and again relaxing and receiving a fresh supply.

The supremacy of the blood farther appears from this, that the pulse is derived from it; for, as there are two parts in a pulsation, viz.: distension or relaxation, and contraction, or diastole and systole, and, as distension is the prior of these two motions, it is manifest that this motion proceeds from the blood; the contraction, again, from the vesicula pulsans of the embryo in ovo, from the heart in the pullet, in virtue of its own fibres, as an instrument destined for this particular end. Certain it is, that the vesicle in question, as also the auricle of the heart at a later period, whence the pulsation begins, is excited to the motion of contraction by the distending blood. The diastole, I say, takes place from the blood swelling, as it were, in consequence of containing an inherent spirit, so that the opinion of Aristotle in regard to the pulsation of the heart,—namely, that it takes place by a kind of ebullition,—is not without some mixture of truth; for what we witness every day in milk heated over the fire, and in beer that is brisk with fermentation, comes into play in the pulse of the heart; in which the blood, swelling with a sort of fermentation, is alternately distended and repressed; the same thing that takes place in the liquids mentioned through an external agent, namely adventitious heat, is effected in the blood by an intimate heat, or an innate spirit; and this, too, is regulated in conformity with nature by the vital principle (anima), and is continued to the benefit of animated beings.

The pulse, then, is produced by a double agent: first, the blood undergoes distension or dilatation, and secondly, the vesicular membrane of the embryo in the egg, the auricles and ventricles in the extruded chick, effect the constriction. By these alternating motions associated, is the blood impelled through the whole body, and the life of animals is thereby continued.

Nor is the blood to be styled the primigenial and principal

portion of the body, because the pulse has its commencement in and through it; but also because animal heat originates in it, and the vital spirit is associated with it, and it constitutes the vital principle itself, (ipsa anima); for wheresoever the immediate and principal instrument of the vegetative faculty is first discovered, there also does it seem likely will the living principle be found to reside, and thence take its rise; seeing that the life is inseparable from spirit and innate heat.

For "however distinct are the artist and the instrument in things made by art," as Fabricius [1] well reminds us, "in the works of nature they are still conjoined and one. Thus the stomach is the author and the organ of chylopoesis." In like manner are the vital principle and its instrument immediately conjoined; and so, in whatever part of the body heat and motion have their origin, in this also must life take its rise, in this be last extinguished; and no one, I presume, will doubt that there are the lares and penates of life enshrined, that there the vital principle (anima) itself has its seat.

The life, therefore, resides in the blood, (as we are also informed in our sacred writings,) [2] because in it life and the soul first show themselves, and last become extinct. For I have frequently found, from the dissection of living animals, as I have said, that the heart of an animal that was dying, that was dead, and had ceased to breathe, still continued to pulsate for a time, and retained its vitality. The ventricles failing and coming to a stand, the motion still goes on in the auricles, and finally in the right auricle alone; and even when all motion has ceased, there the blood may still be seen affected with a kind of undulation and obscure palpitation or tremor, the last evidence of life. Every one, indeed, may perceive that the blood—this author of pulsation and life,—longest retains its heat; for when this is gone, and it is no longer blood, but gore, so is there, then, no hope of a return to life. But, truly, as has been stated, both in the chick in ovo and in the moribund animal, if you but apply some gentle stimulus either to the punctum saliens or to the right auricle of the heart after the failure of all pulsation, forthwith you will see motion, pulsation, and life restored to the blood—provided always, be it

[1] Op. Eup. cit. p. 28.   [2] Leviticus xvii, 11, 14.

understood, that the innate heat and vital spirit have not been wholly lost.

From this it clearly appears that the blood is the generative part, the fountain of life, the first to live, the last to die, and the primary seat of the soul; the element in which, as in a fountain head, the heat first and most abounds and flourishes; from whose influxive heat all the other parts of the body are cherished, and obtain their life; for the heat, the companion of the blood, flows through and cherishes and preserves the whole body, as I formerly demonstrated in my work on the motion of the blood.

And since blood is found in every particle of the body, so that you can nowhere prick with a needle, nor make the slightest scratch, but blood will instantly appear, it seems as if, without this fluid, the parts could neither have heat nor life. So that the blood, being in ever so trifling a degree concentrated and fixed,—Hippocrates called the state ἀπόληψις τῶν φλεβῶν —stasis of the veins,—as in lipothymia, alarm, exposure to severe cold, and on the accession of a febrile paroxysm, the whole body is observed to become cold and torpid, and, overspread with pallor and livor, to languish. But the blood, recalled by stimulants, by exercise, by certain emotions of the mind, such as joy or anger, suddenly all is hot, and flushed, and vigorous, and beautiful again.

Therefore it is that the red and sanguine parts, such as the flesh, are alone spoken of as hot, and the white and bloodless parts, on the contrary, such as the tendons and ligaments, are designated as cold. And as red-blooded animals excel exsanguine creatures, so also, in our estimate of the parts, are those which are more liberally furnished with native heat and blood, held more excellent than all the others. The liver, spleen, kidneys, lungs, and heart itself,—parts which are especially entitled viscera,— if you will but squeeze out all the blood they contain, become pale and fall within the category of cold parts. The heart itself, I say, receives influxive heat and life along with the blood that reaches it, through the coronary arteries; and only so long as the blood has access to it. Neither can the liver perform its office without the influence of the blood and heat it receives through the cœliac artery; for there is no influx of heat without an afflux of blood by the arteries, and this is the reason wherefore, when parts are first produced, and before they have taken upon them the performance of their respective duties, they all look bloodless and pale, in consequence of which they were formerly regarded as spermatic by physicians and anatomists, and in generation it was usual to say that several days were passed in the milk.   The liver, lungs, and substance of the heart itself, when they first appear, are extremely white; and, indeed, the cone of the heart and the walls of the ventricles are still seen to be white, when the auricles, replete with crimson blood, are red, and the coronary vein is purple with its stream.   In like manner, the parenchyma of the liver is white, when its veins and their branches are red with blood; nor does it perform any duty until it is penetrated with blood.

The blood, in a word, so flows around and penetrates the whole body, and imparts heat and life conjoined to all its parts, that the vital principle, having its first and chief seat there, may truly be held as resident in the blood; in this way, in common parlance, it comes to be all in all, and all in each particular part.

But so little is it true, as Aristotle and the medical writers assert, that the liver and the heart are the authors and compounders of the blood, that the contrary even appears most obviously from the formation of the chick in ovo, viz.: that the blood is much rather the fashioner of the heart and liver; a fact, which physicians themselves appear unintentionally to confirm, when they speak of the parenchyma of the liver as a kind of effusion of blood, as if it were nothing more than so much blood coagulated there.   But the blood must exist before it can either be shed or coagulated; and experience palpably demonstrates that the thing is so, seeing that the blood is already present before there is a vestige either of the body or of any viscus; and that in circumstances where none of the mother's blood can by possibility reach the embryo, an event which is vulgarly held to occur among viviparous animals.

The liver of fishes is always perceived of a white colour, though their veins are of a deep purple or black; and our fowls, the fatter they become, the smaller and paler grows the liver.   Cachectic maidens, and those who labour under chlorosis, are not only pale and blanched in their bodies generally, but in their livers as well, a manifest indication of a want of blood in their system.   The liver, therefore, receives both its heat and colour from the blood; the blood is in no wise derived from the liver.

From what has now been said, then, it appears that the blood is the first engendered part, whence the living principle in the first instance gleams forth, and from which the first animated particle of the embryo is formed; that it is the source and origin of all other parts, both similar and dissimilar, which thence obtain their vital heat and become subservient to it in its duties. But the heart is contrived for the sole purpose of ministering between the veins and the arteries—of receiving blood from the veins, and, by its ceaseless contractions, of propelling it to all parts of the body through the arteries.

This fact is made particularly striking, when we find that neither is there a heart found in every animal, neither does it necessarily and in every instance pulsate at all times where it is encountered; the blood, however, or a fluid which stands in lieu of it, is never wanting.

EXERCISE THE FIFTY-SECOND.

Of the blood as prime element in the body.

It is unquestionable, then, and obvious to sense, that the blood is the first formed, and therefore the genital part of the embryo, and that it has all the attributes which have been ascribed to it in the preceding exercise. It is both the author and preserver of the body; it is the principal element moreover, and that in which the vital principle (anima) has its dwelling-place. Because, as already said, before there is any particle of the body obvious to sight, the blood is already extant, has already increased in quantity, " and palpitates within the veins," as Aristotle expresses it,[1] " being moved hither and thither, and being the only humour that is distributed to every part of the animal body. The blood, moreover, is that alone which lives and is possessed of heat whilst life continues."

And further, from its various motions in acceleration or re-

---

[1] Hist. Anim. lib. iii, cap. 19.

tardation, in turbulence and strength, or debility, it is manifest that the blood perceives things that tend to injure by irritating, or to benefit by cherishing it. We therefore conclude that the blood lives of itself, and supplies its own nourishment; and that it depends in nowise upon any other part of the body, which is either prior to itself or of greater excellence and worth. On the contrary, the whole body, as posthumous to it, as added and appended as it were to it, depends on the blood, though this is not the place to prove the fact; I shall only say, with Aristotle,[1] that "The nature of the blood is the undoubted cause wherefore many things happen among animals, both as regards their tempers and their capacities." To the blood, therefore, we may refer as the cause not only of life in general, —inasmuch as there is no other inherent or influxive heat that may be the immediate instrument of the living principle except the blood,—but also of longer or shorter life, of sleep and watching, of genius or aptitude, strength, &c. " For through its tenuity and purity," says Aristotle in the same place, " animals are made wiser and have more noble senses; and in like manner they are more timid and courageous, or passionate and furious, as their blood is more dilute, or replete with dense fibres."

Nor is the blood the author of life only, but, according to its diversities, the cause of health and disease likewise: so that poisons, which come from without, such as poisoned wounds, unless they infect the blood, occasion no mischief. Life and death, therefore, flow for us from the same spring. " If the blood becomes too diffluent," says Aristotle,[2] " we fall sick; for it sometimes resolves itself into such a sanguinolent serum, that the body is covered with a bloody sweat; and if there be too great a loss of blood, life is gone." And, indeed, not only do the parts of the body at all times become torpid when blood is lost, but if the loss be excessive, the animal necessarily dies. I do not think it requisite to quote any particular experiment in confirmation of these views: the whole subject would require to be treated specially.

The admirable circulation of the blood originally discovered by me, I have lived to see admitted by almost all; nor has

---

[1] De Part. Anim. lib. ii, cap. 4.   [2] Hist. Anim. lib. iii, cap. 19.

aught as yet been urged against it by any one which has seemed greatly to require an answer. Wherefore I imagine that I shall perform a task not less new and useful than agreeable to philosophers and medical men, if I here briefly discourse of the causes and uses of the circulation, and expose other obscure matters respecting the blood; if I show, for instance, how much it concerns our welfare that by a wholesome and regulated diet we keep our blood pure and sweet. When I have accomplished this it will no longer, I trust, seem so improbable and absurd to any one as it did to Aristotle[1] in former times, that the blood should be viewed as the familiar divinity, as the soul itself of the body, which was the opinion of Critias and others, who maintained that the prime faculty of the living principle (anima) was to feel, and that this faculty inhered in the body in virtue of the nature of the blood. Thales, Diogenes, Heraclitus, Alcmæon, and others, held the blood to be the soul, because, by its nature, it had a faculty of motion.

Now that both sense and motion are in the blood is obvious from many indications, although Aristotle[2] denies the fact. And, indeed, when we see him, yielding to the force of truth, brought to admit that there is a vital principle even in the hypenemic egg; and in the spermatic fluid and blood a " certain divine something corresponding with the element of the stars," and that it is vicarious of the Almighty Creator; and if the moderns be correct in their views when they say that the seminal fluid of animals emitted in coitu is alive, wherefore should we not, with like reason, affirm that there is a vital principle in the blood, and that when this is first ingested and nourished and moved, the vital spark is first struck and enkindled? Unquestionably the blood is that in which the vegetative and sensitive operations first proclaim themselves; that in which heat, the primary and immediate instrument of life, is innate; that which is the common bond between soul and body, and the vehicle by which life is conveyed into every particle of the organized being.

Besides, if it be matter of such difficulty to understand the spermatic fluid as we have found it, to fathom how through it the formation of the body is made to begin and proceed with

---

[1] De Anima, lib. i, cap. 2.
[2] De Hist. Anim. lib. i, cap. 19; et de Part. Anim. lib. ii, cap. 3.

such foresight, art, and divine intelligence, wherefore should we not, with equal propriety, admit an exalted nature in the blood, and think at least as highly of it as we have been led to do of the semen?—the rather, as this fluid is itself produced from the blood, as appears from the history of the egg; and the whole organized body not only derives its origin, as from a genital part, but even appears to owe its preservation to the blood.

We have, indeed, already said so much incidentally above, intending to speak on the subject more particularly at another time.   Nor do I think that we are here to dispute whether it is strictly correct to speak of the blood as a *part;* some deny the propriety of such language, moved especially by the consideration that it is not sensible, and that it flows into all parts of the body to supply them with nourishment.   For myself, however, I have discovered not a few things connected with the manner of generation which differ essentially from those motions which philosophers and medical writers generally either admit or reject.   At this time I say no more on this point; but though I admit the blood to be without sensation, it does not follow that it should not form a portion, and even a very principal portion, of a body which is endowed with sensibility. For neither does the brain nor the spinal marrow, nor the crystalline or the vitreous humour of the eye, feel anything, though, by the common consent of all, philosophers and physicians alike, these are parts of the body.   Aristotle placed the blood among the partes similares; Hippocrates, as the animal body according to him is made up of containing, contained, and impelling parts, of course reckoned the blood among the number of parts contained.

But we shall have more to say on this topic when we treat of that wherein a part consists, and how many kinds of parts there are.   Meantime, I cannot be silent on the remarkable fact, that the heart itself, this most distinguished member in the body, appears to be insensible.

A young nobleman, eldest son of the Viscount Montgomery, when a child, had a severe fall, attended with fracture of the ribs of the left side.   The consequence of this was a suppurating abscess, which went on discharging abundantly for a long time, from an immense gap in his side; this I had from himself and other credible persons who were witnesses.   Between the 18th and 19th years of his age, this young nobleman, having travelled through France and Italy, came to London, having at this time a very large open cavity in his side, through which the lungs, as it was believed, could both be seen and touched. When this circumstance was told as something miraculous to his Serene Majesty King Charles, he straightway sent me to wait on the young man, that I might ascertain the true state of the case. And what did I find? A young man, well grown, of good complexion, and apparently possessed of an excellent constitution, so that I thought the whole story must be a fable. Having saluted him according to custom, however, and informed him of the king's expressed desire that I should wait upon him, he immediately showed me everything, and laid open his left side for my inspection, by removing a plate which he wore there by way of defence against accidental blows and other external injuries. I found a large open space in the chest, into which I could readily introduce three of my fingers and my thumb; which done, I straightway perceived a certain protuberant fleshy part, affected with an alternating extrusive and intrusive movement; this part I touched gently. Amazed with the novelty of such a state, I examined everything again and again, and when I had satisfied myself, I saw that it was a case of old and extensive ulcer, beyond the reach of art, but brought by a miracle to a kind of cure, the interior being invested with a membrane, and the edges protected with a tough skin. But the fleshy part, (which I at first sight took for a mass of granulations, and others had always regarded as a portion of the lung,) from its pulsating motions and the rhythm they observed with the pulse,—when the fingers of one of my hands were applied to it, those of the other to the artery at the wrist—as well as from their discordance with the respiratory movements, I saw was no portion of the lung that I was handling, but the apex of the heart! covered over with a layer of fungous flesh by way of external defence, as commonly happens in old foul ulcers. The servant of this young man was in the habit daily of cleansing the cavity from its accumulated sordes by means of injections of tepid water; after which the plate was applied, and, with this in its place, the young man felt adequate to any exercise or expedition, and, in short, he led a pleasant life in perfect safety.

Instead of a verbal answer, therefore, I carried the young man himself to the king, that his majesty might with his own eyes behold this wonderful case : that, in a man alive and well, he might, without detriment to the individual, observe the movement of the heart, and, with his proper hand even touch the ventricles as they contracted. And his most excellent majesty, as well as myself, acknowledged that the heart was without the sense of touch ; for the youth never knew when we touched his heart, except by the sight or the sensation he had through the external integument.

We also particularly observed the movements of the heart, viz. : that in the diastole it was retracted and withdrawn ; whilst in the systole it emerged and protruded ; and the systole of the heart took place at the moment the diastole or pulse in the wrist was perceived ; to conclude, the heart struck the walls of the chest, and became prominent at the time it bounded upwards and underwent contraction on itself.

Neither is this the place for taking up that other controversy ; to wit, whether the blood alone serves for the nutrition of the body ? Aristotle in several places contends that the blood is the ultimate aliment of the body, and in this view he is supported by the whole body of physicians. But many things of difficult interpretation, and that hang but indifferently together, follow from this opinion of theirs. For when the medical writers speak of the blood in their physiological disquisitions, and teach that the above is its sole use and end, viz. : to supply nourishment to the body, they proceed to compose it of four humours, or juices, adducing arguments for such a view from the combinations of the four primary qualities ; and then they assert that the mass of the blood is made up of the two kinds of bile, the yellow and the black, of pituita, and the blood properly so called. And thus they arrive at their four humours, of which the pituita is held to be cold and moist ; the black bile cold and dry ; the yellow bile hot and dry ; and the blood hot and moist. Further, of each of these several kinds, they maintain that some are nutritious, and compose the whole of the body ; others, again, they say are excrementitious. Still further, they suppose that the blood proper is composed of the nutritious or heterogeneous portions ; but the constitution of the mass is such, that the pituita is a cruder matter, which the more powerful native heat can convert into perfect blood. They deny, however, that the bile can by any means be thus transformed into blood; although the blood, they say, is readily changed into bile, an event which they conceive takes place in melancholic diseases, through an excess of the concocting heat.

Now, if all this were true, and there be no retrogressive movement, viz. from black bile to bile, from bile to blood, they would be brought to the dilemma of having to admit that all the juices were present for the production of black bile, and that this was a principal and most highly concocted nutriment. It would further be imperative on them to recognize a kind of twofold blood, viz. one consisting of the entire mass of fluid contained in the veins, and composed of the four humours aforesaid; and another consisting of the purer, more fluid and spirituous portion, the fluid, which in the stricter sense they call blood, which some of them contend is contained in the arteries apart from the rest, and which they then depute upon sundry special offices. On their own showing, therefore, the pure blood is no aliment for the body, but a certain mixed fluid, or rather black bile, to which the rest of the humours tend.

Aristotle,[1] too, although he thought that the blood existed as a means of nourishing the body, still believed that it was composed as it were of several portions, viz. of a thicker and black portion which subsides to the bottom of the basin when the blood coagulates, and this portion he held to be of an inferior nature; [2] "for the blood," he says, "if it be entire, is of a red colour and sweet taste; but if vitiated either by nature or disease, it is blacker." He also will have it fibrous in part or partly composed of fibres, which being removed, he continues,[3] the blood neither sets nor becomes any thicker. He farther admitted a sanies in the blood: "Sanies is unconcocted blood, or blood not yet completely concocted, or which is as yet dilute like serum." And this part, he says, is of a colder nature. The fibrous he believed to be the earthy portion of the blood.

According to the view of the Stagirite, therefore, the blood

---

[1] De Part. Anim. lib. ii, cap. 3. [2] De Hist. Anim. lib. iii, cap. 19. [3] Ibid.

of different animals differs in several ways; in one it is more serous and thinner, a kind of ichor or sanies, as in insects, and the colder and less perfect animals; in another it is thicker, more fibrous, and earthy, as in the wild boar, bull, ass, &c. In some where the constitution is distempered, the blood is of a blacker hue; in others it is bright, pure, and florid, as in birds, and the human subject especially.

Whence, it appears, that in the opinion of the physicians, as well as of Aristotle, the blood consists of several parts, in some sort of the same description, according to the views of each. Medical men, indeed, only pay attention to human blood, taken in phlebotomy and contained in cups and coagulated. But Aristotle took a view of the blood of animals generally, or of the fluid which is analogous to it. And I, omitting all points of controversy, and passing by any discussion of the inconveniences that wait upon the opinions of writers in general, shall here touch lightly upon the points that all are agreed in, that can be apprehended by the senses, and that pertain more especially to our subject; intending, however, to treat of everything at length elsewhere.

Although the blood be, as I have said, a portion of the body,—the primogenial and principal part, indeed,—still, if it be considered in its mass, and as it presents itself in the veins, there is nothing to hinder us from believing that it contains and concocts nourishment within itself, which it applies to all the other parts of the body. With the matter so considered, we can understand how it should both nourish and be nourished, and how it should be both the matter and the efficient cause of the body, and have the natural constitution which Aristotle held necessary in a primogenial part, viz. that it should be partly of similar, partly of dissimilar constitution; for he says, " As it was requisite for the sake of sensation that there should be similar members in animal bodies, and as the faculty of perceiving, the faculty of moving, and the faculty of nourishing, are all contained in the same member (viz. the primogenate particle), it follows necessarily that this member, which originally contains inherent principles of the above kind, be extant both simply, that it may be capable of sensation of every description, and dissimilarly, that it may move and act. Wherefore, in the tribes that have blood, the heart is held to be such a member; in the bloodless tribes, however, it is proportional to their state."

Now, if Aristotle understands by the heart that which first appears in the embryo of the chick in ovo, the blood, to wit, with its containing parts — the pulsating vesicles and veins, as one and the same organ, I conceive that he has expressed himself most accurately; for the blood, as it is seen in the egg and the vesicles, is partly similar and partly dissimilar. But if he understands the matter otherwise, what is seen in the egg sufficiently refutes him, inasmuch as the substance of the heart, considered independently of the blood—the ventricular cone—is engendered long afterwards, and continues white without any infusion of blood, until the heart has been fashioned into that form of organ by which the blood is distributed through the whole body. Nor indeed does the heart even then present itself with the structure of a similar and simple part, such as might become a primogenial part, but is seen to be fibrous, fleshy, or muscular, and indeed is obviously what Hippocrates styled it,—a muscle or instrument of motion. But the blood, as it is first perceived, and as it pulsates, included within its vesicle, has as manifestly the constitution which Aristotle held necessary in a principal part. For the blood, whilst it is naturally in the body, has everywhere apparently the same constitution; when extravasated, however, and deprived of its native heat, immediately, like any dissimilar compound, it separates into several parts.

Were the blood destined by nature, however, for the nourishment of the body only, it would have a more *similar* constitution, like the chyle or the albumen of the egg; or at all events it would be truly one and a single body composed of the parts or juices indicated, like the other humours, such as bile of either kind, and pituita or phlegm, which retain the same form and character without the body, which they showed within their appropriate receptacles;—they undergo no such sudden change as the blood.

Wherefore, the qualities which Aristotle ascribed to a principal part are found associated in the blood; which as a natural body, existing heterogeneously or *dissimilarly*, is composed of these juices or parts; but as it lives and is a very principal animal part, consisting of these juices mingled together, it is

an animated *similar* part, composed of a body and a vital principle.   When this living principle of the blood escapes, however, in consequence of the extinction of the native heat, the
primary substance is forthwith corrupted and resolved into the
parts of which it was formerly composed; first into cruor, afterwards with red and white parts, those of the red parts that
are uppermost being more florid, those that are lowest being
black.   Of these parts, moreover, some are fibrous and tough,
(and these are the uniting medium of the rest,) others ichorous and serous, in which the mass of coagulum is wont to
swim.   Into such a serum does the blood almost wholly
resolve itself at last.   But these parts have no existence
severally in living blood; it is in that only which has become corrupted and is resolved by death that they are encountered.

Besides the constituents of the blood now indicated, there is
yet another which is seen in the blood of the hotter and stronger
animals, such as horses, oxen, and men also of ardent constitution.   This is seen in blood drawn from the body as it coagulates, in the upper part of the red mass, and bears a perfect
resemblance to hartshorn-jelly, or mucilage, or thick white of
egg.   The vulgar believe this matter to be the pituita; Aristotle
designated it the crude and unconcocted portion of the blood.

I have observed that this part of the blood differs both from
the others and from the mere serous portion in which the coagulated clot is wont to swim in the basin, and also from the
urine which percolates through the kidneys from the blood.
Neither is it to be regarded as any more crude or colder portion of the blood, but rather, as I conceive, as a more spiritual
part; a conclusion to which I am moved by two motives: first,
because it swims above the bright and florid portion—commonly
thought to be the arterial blood—as if it were hotter and more
highly charged with spirits, and takes possession of the highest
place in the disintegration of the blood.

Secondly, in venesection, blood of this kind, which is mostly
met with among men of warm temperament, strong and muscular, escapes in a longer stream and with greater force, as if
pushed from a syringe, in the same way as we say that the
spermatic fluid which is ejected vigorously and to a distance
is both more fruitful and full of spirits.

That this mucaginous matter differs greatly from the ichorous or watery part of the blood, which, as if colder than the rest, subsides to the bottom of the basin, appears on two distinct grounds : for the watery and sanious portion is too crude and unconcocted ever to pass into purer and more perfect blood ; and the thicker and more fibrous mucus swimming above the clot of the blood itself appears more concoct and better elaborated than this ; and so in the resolution or separation of the blood it comes that the mucus occupies the upper place, the sanies the lower ; the clot and red parts, however,—both those of a brighter and those of a darker colour,—occupy the middle space.

For it is certain that not only this part, but the whole blood, and indeed the flesh itself—as may be seen in criminals hung in chains—may be reduced to an ichorous sanies ; that is to say, become resolved into the matters of which they were composed, like salt into the lixivium from which it had been obtained. In like manner, the blood taken away in any cachexy abounds in serum, and this to such an extent that occasionally scarce any clot is seen—the whole mass of blood forms one sanies. This is observed in leucophlegmatia, and is natural in bloodless animals.

Further, if you take away some blood shortly after a meal, before the second digestion has been completed and the serum has had time to descend by the kidneys, or at the commencement of an attack of intermittent fever, you will find it sanious, inconcoct, and abounding in serum. On the contrary, if you open a vein after fasting, or a copious discharge of urine or sweat, you will find the blood thick, as if without serum, and almost wholly condensed into clot.

And in the same way as in coagulating blood you find a little of the afore-mentioned supernatant mucus, so if you expose the sanies in question, separated from the clot, to a gentle heat over the fire, you will find it to be speedily changed into the mucus ; an obvious indication that the water or sanies which separates from the blood in the basin, is perchance a certain element in the urine, but not the urine itself, although in colour and consistence it seems so in fact. The urine is not coagulated or condensed into a fibrous mucus, but rather into a lixivium ; the watery or sanious portion of the urine, however, when lightly boiled, does occasionally run into a mucus that swims through the fluid; in the same way, as the mucus in question rendered recrudescent by corruption, liquefies and returns to the state of sanies.

So far at this time have I thought fit to produce these my own observations on this constituent of the blood, intending to speak more fully of it as well as of the other constituents cognizable by the senses, and admitted by Aristotle and the medical writers.

That I may not seem to wander too widely from my purpose, I would here have it understood that with Aristotle I receive the blood as a part of the living animal body, and not as it is commonly regarded in the light of mere gore. The Stagirite says:[1] "The blood is warm, in the sense in which we should understand warm water, did we designate that fluid by a simple name, not viewing it as heated. For heat belongs to its nature; just as whiteness is in the nature of a white man. But when the blood becomes hot through any affection or passion, it is not then hot of itself. The same thing must be said in regard to the qualities of dryness and moistness. Wherefore, in the nature of such things they are partly hot and partly moist; but separated, they congeal and become cold; and such is the blood."

The blood consequently, as it is a living element of the body, is of a doubtful nature, and falls to be considered under two points of view. Materially and *per se* it is called nourishment; but formally and in so far as it is endowed with heat and spirits, the immediate instruments of the vital principle, and even with vitality (anima), it is to be regarded as the familiar divinity and preserver of the body, as the generative first engendered and very principal part. And as the prolific egg contains within it the matter, instrument, and framer of the future pullet, and all physicians admit a mixture of the seminal fluids of the two sexes in the uterus during or immediately after intercourse as constituting the mixed cause, both material and efficient, of the fœtus; so might one with more propriety maintain that the blood was both the matter and preserver of the body, though not the sole aliment; because it is observed that in animals which die of hunger, and in men who perish of

---

[1] De Part. Anim. lib. ii, cap. 3.

marasmus, a considerable quantity of blood is still found after death in the veins. And farther, in youthful subjects still growing, and in aged individuals declining and falling away, the relative quantity of blood continues the same, and is in the ratio of the flesh that is present, as if the blood were a part of the body, but not destined solely for its nourishment; for if it were so, no one would die of hunger so long as he had any blood left in his veins, just as the lamp is not extinguished whilst there is a drop of inflammable oil left in the cruise.

Now when I maintain that the living principle resides primarily and principally in the blood, I would not have it inferred from thence that I hold all bloodletting in discredit, as dangerous and injurious; or that I believe with the vulgar that in the same measure as blood is lost, is life abridged, because the sacred writings tell us that the life is in the blood; for daily experience satisfies us that bloodletting has a most salutary effect in many diseases, and is indeed the foremost among all the general remedial means : vitiated states and plethora of the blood, are causes of a whole host of diseases; and the timely evacuation of a certain quantity of the fluid frequently delivers patients from very dangerous diseases, and even from imminent death. In the same measure as blood is detracted, therefore, under certain circumstances, it may be said that life and health are added.

This indeed nature teaches, and physicians at all events propose to themselves to imitate nature ; for copious critical discharges of blood from the nostrils, from hemorrhoids, and in the shape of the menstrual flux, often deliver us from very serious diseases. Young persons, therefore, who live fully and lead indolent lives, unless between their eighteenth and twentieth year they have a spontaneous hemorrhage from the nose or lower parts of the body, or have a vein opened, by which they are relieved of the load of blood that oppresses them, are apt to be seized with fever or smallpox, or they suffer from headache and other morbid symptoms of various degrees of severity and danger. Veterinary surgeons are in the habit of beginning the treatment of almost all the diseases of cattle with bloodletting.

Of the inferences deducible from the course of the umbilical vessels in the egg.

We find the blood formed in the egg and embryo before any other part; and almost at the same moment appear its receptacles, the veins and the vesicula pulsans. Wherefore, if we regard the punctum saliens as the heart, and this along with the blood and the veins as constituting one and the same organ, conspicuous in the very commencement of the embryo, although we should admit that the proper substance of the heart was deposited subsequently, still we should be ready to admit with Aristotle that the heart (an organ made up of ventricles, auricles, vessels, and blood) was in truth the principal and primogenate part of the body, its own prime and essential element having been the blood, both in the order of nature and of genetic production.

The parts that in generation succeed the blood are the veins, for the blood is necessarily inclosed and contained in vessels; so that, as Aristotle observes, we find two meatus venales even from the very first, which canals, as we have shown in our history, afterwards constitute the umbilical vessels. It seems necessary, therefore, to say something here of the situation and course of these vessels.

In the first place, then, it is to be observed that all the arteries and veins have their origin from the heart, and are as it were appendices or parts added to the central organ. If therefore you carefully examine the embryo of the human subject, or one of the lower animals, and having divided the vena cava between the right auricle and the diaphragm, look into it upwards or towards the heart, you will perceive three foramina, the largest and most posterior of which tending to the spine is the vena cava; the anterior and lesser proceeds to the root and trunk of the umbilical vessels; the third and least of all enters the liver and is the origin and trunk of all the ramifications distributed to the convexity of that organ. Whence it clearly appears that the veins do by no means all proceed from the liver as their origin and commencement, but from the heart—unless indeed any one would be hardy enough to contend that a vessel proceeded from its branches, not the branches from the trunk of the vessel.

Moreover, as the vessels in question are distributed equally to the albumen and vitellus of the egg, not otherwise than as the roots of trees are connected with the ground, it is obvious that both of these substances must serve for the nutriment of the embryo, and that they are taken up and carried to it by these vessels. But this view is opposed to that of Aristotle, who everywhere maintains that the chick is formed from the albumen, and receives nourishment through the umbilicus alone. The albumen indeed is first consumed, and the yelk serves subsequently for food, supplying the place of the milk, which viviparous animals receive after their birth from their mothers. The food which nature provides for the young of viviparous tribes in the dug of the mother, she supplies in the yelk of the egg to the young of oviparous animals. Whence it happens, that when the albumen is almost wholly consumed, the vitellus still remains nearly entire in the egg, the chick being already perfect and complete; more than this, the yelk is still found in the abdomen of the chick long after its exclusion. Aristotle discovered some on the eighteenth day after the hatching; and I have myself seen a small quantity connected with the intestine at the end of six weeks from that epoch.

Nevertheless, from the yelk (which certainly does not decrease in the same ratio as the albumen whilst the chick is forming) that is taken into the abdomen of the chick, and from the distribution of vessels through its substance, the whole of these collecting into a single trunk which enters the porta of the liver, and doubtless carrying that portion of yelk they have absorbed for more perfect elaboration in that viscus—these and other arguments of the like kind force me to say that I cannot do otherwise than admit with Aristotle that the yelk supplies food to the chick, and is analogous to milk.

The whole of the yelk, indeed, does not remain after the foetus of the fowl is fully formed; for a certain portion of it has been liquefied on the very first appearance of the embryo, and receives branches of vessels no less than the albumen, by which, already prepared, it is carried as nourishment for the chick; still it is certain that the greater portion of the yelk remains after the disappearance of the albumen; that it is laid up in the abdomen of the chick when excluded, and, attracted or absorbed by the branches of the vena portæ, that it is finally carried to the liver.

It is manifest, therefore, that the chick when hatched, is nourished by the yelk in the first period of its independent existence. And as within the egg the embryo was nourished partly by the albumen, partly by the vitellus, but principally by the albumen, which is both present in larger quantity, and is more speedily consumed, so when the chick is hatched, and when all the nourishment that is taken must pass through the liver to undergo ulterior preparation, is it nourished partly by the vitellus and partly by chyle absorbed from the intestines, but principally by chyle, which the host of subdivisions of the mesenteric vessels seize upon, whilst there is but a single vessel from the porta distributed to the vitellus, and by and by but little of it remains. Nature, therefore, acts as does the nurse, who gradually habituates her infant to the food which is to take the place of her failing supply of milk. The pullet is thus gradually brought from food of more easy to food of more difficult digestion,—from yelk to chyle.

Wherefore there is every reason for what we perceive in connexion with the course of the veins in the egg. When the embryo first begins to be formed, they are distributed to the colliquament only, where the blood finds suitable nutriment and matter for the formation of the body; but by and by they extend into the thinner albumen, whence the chick, whilst it is yet in the state of gelatine or mucor, and resembles a maggot in form, derives its increase; the branches next extend into the thicker albumen, and then into the vitellus, that they may also contribute to the support of the fœtus, which, having at length arrived at maturity and been extruded, still preserves a portion of the yelk (or milk) within its abdomen, whereby it is maintained in part, in part by food selected and prepared for it by the mother, until it is able to look out for and to digest its own aliment. Thus does nature most wisely provide food through the whole round of generation, suited to the various strength of the digestive faculty in the future being. In the first period of the fœtal chick's existence a more delicate food is prepared for it; more advanced, firmer and firmer food is supplied; and this is the reason, I apprehend, wherefore, the perfect egg consists not only of two portions of different colours, but is even provided with two kinds of albumen.

Now all this that we discover from actual experience of the matter accords with the opinion of Aristotle, where he says :[1] "The part which is hot is best adapted to give form to the limbs; that which is more earthy rather conduces to the constitution of the body and is more remote. Wherefore in eggs of two colours, the animal begins to be engendered from the white (for the beginning of animal life is in the hot), and derives its nourishment from the yellow. In the warmer animals, consequently, these parts are kept distinct from one another, viz. that from which the beginning is derived, and that whence the nourishment is obtained, and the one is white, the other yellow."

From what has now been said it appears that the chick—and we shall show that it is not otherwise in all other animals—arises and is constituted as it were by a principle or soul inherent in the egg, and that in the same way the proper aliment is sought for and is supplied within the egg; whereby it comes that the chick is not dependent on its mother in the same way as plants are dependent on the ground; and it is not more correct to say that the chick is nourished by the blood of its mother, or that its heart beats, and that it lives through the spirits of its parent, than it would be to assert that it moved and felt through the organs, or grew and attained to adult age through the vital principle of its parent. It is manifest, on the contrary, and is allowed by all that the fœtal chick is nourished through its umbilical vessels; and that the vascular ramifications dispersed over the albumen and yelk imbibe nourishment from them and convey it to the fœtus. It is also admitted that the chick, when excluded from the shell, is supplied with nourishment, partly from yelk, partly from chyle, and that in either case the aliment passes by the same route, viz. by the vena portæ into the liver, the branches of this vessel effecting the transit.

It is therefore obvious, as I now say by the way, that the

---

[1] De Gen. Anim. lib. iii, cap. 1.

chyle by which all animals are nourished is brought by the mesenteric veins from the intestines; nor is there occasion to look for any new passage—by the lacteal vessels, to wit—or any route in adult animals other than that which we discover in the egg and chick. But we shall recur more fully in another place to the inconveniences of such an opinion as that referred to.

Lastly, from the structure of the umbilical vessels of the chick in ovo, some of which as stated in the history are veins, others arteries, it is legitimate to conclude that there is here a circular motion of the blood, such as we have already demonstrated in the animal body, in our book on the Motion of the Blood, and this for the sake of the nutrition and growth of the embryo, and because the umbilical veins are distributed to either fluid of the egg, that they may thence bring nutriment to the chick, and the arteries accompany the veins, that by their affluxive heat the alimentary matter may be duly concocted, liquefied, and made fit to answer the ends of nutrition.

And hence it happens that wherever veins—and here I would have it understood that both arteries and veins are intended—make their way into the albumen or vitellus, there these fluids look liquefied and different from the rest. For as soon as the branches of the veins shoot forth, the upper portion of the albumen in which they are implanted passing into colliquament, becomes transparent, whilst the lower portion, continuing thick and compact, is pushed into the inferior angle of the egg. In like manner a separation of the vitellus, as it seems into two portions, makes its appearance, the one being superior, and the other inferior, and these do not differ less from one another in character than melted differs from solid wax; now this division corresponds to the two parts which severally receive or do not receive blood-vessels.

Hence are we farther made more certain as to the commencement of animal generation and the prime inherent principle of the egg. For it is assuredly known that the cicatricula or spot on the yelk is the chief point in the egg, that to which all the rest are subordinate, and to which, if to any one thing more than another, is to be referred the cause, whatever it be, of fecundity in the egg:—certain it is that the generation of the embryo is begun within its precincts. Wherefore, as we have said, the first effect of incubation is to cause dilatation of the cicatricula, and the formation of the colliquament, in which the blood first flushes and veins are distributed, and where the effects of the native heat and the influence of the plastic power first show themselves. And then, the more widely the ramifications of these veins extend, in the same proportion do indications of the presence of the vital power and vegetative force appear. For every effect is a clear evidence of its efficient cause.

In a word I say,—from the cicatricula (in which the first trace of the native heat appears) proceeds the entire process of generation; from the heart the whole chick, and from the umbilical vessels the whole of the membranes called secundines that surround it. We therefore conclude that the parts of the embryo are severally subordinate, and that life is first derived from the heart.

EXERCISE THE FIFTY-FOURTH.

Of the order of the parts in Generation from an egg, according to Fabricius.

Having already determined what part is to be esteemed the first, the blood, to wit, with its receptacles, the heart, veins, and arteries, the next thing we have to do is to speak of the rest of the parts of the body and of the order and manner of their generation.

Fabricius, in whose footsteps we have resolved to tread, in speaking of the generation of the chick in ovo, passes in review the actions which take place in the egg, and by the effect of which the parts are produced, discussing them *seriatim*, as if a clearer view were thence to be obtained of the order or sequence of generation. "There are three primary actions," he says,[1] which present themselves in the egg of the bird: 1st, the generation of the embryo; 2d, its growth; 3d, its nourishment. The first, or generation, is the proper action of the egg; the second and third, viz. growth and nutrition, go on

---

[1] Op. supra cit. p. 41.

for the major part without the egg, though they are begun and also perfectly performed within it. Now these actions, as they flow from three faculties, the generative, the nutritive, and auctive, so do three operations follow them. From generation all the parts of the chick result; from increase and nutrition, the growth and maintenance of its body. From studying the formation of the chick, we perceive that, under the influence of the generative faculty, the parts of the creature which formerly had no existence are produced : the matter of the egg is changed into the organized body of a chicken. But whilst any part or substance undergoes transmutation into another, it must needs be that its proper essence undergoes change, otherwise would it still remain as it was and unaltered ; it must at the same time receive figure, position, and dimensions apt and convenient to its new nature ; and indeed it is into these two states or circumstances that procreation of matter resolves itself, viz. transformation and conformation. The transformative and the formative faculties would therefore be the cause of these functions ; and whilst one of them has produced every individual part of the chick, such as we see it, from the chalaza of the egg, the other has given it figure, articulations, and position, fitting it for its destined uses. The first, the transformative or alterative faculty, is entirely natural, and acts without all consciousness ; and taking the hot, the cold, the moist, and the dry, it alters all through the substance of the chalaza, and in altering this substance changes it into the component parts of the chick, that is to say, into flesh, bones, cartilages, ligaments, veins, arteries, nerves, and all the other similar and simple parts of the animal, and these, through the proper and innate heat and spirit of the semen of the cock, out of the substance of the egg, that is to say, its chalaza ; by altering and commuting, it engenders, creates, produces the proper substance of the chick, imparting at the same time to every substance its appropriate quality. The other, which is called the formative faculty, and which out of similar forms dissimilar parts,—namely, giving them elegance through figure, due dimensions, proper position, and congruous number—is much more noble than the former, is possessed of consummate sapience, and acts not naturally [or instinctively], but with election, and consciousness, and intelligence. For the formative faculty appears to have exact cognizance and foresight both of the future action and use of every part and organ. So much of the primary action of the egg, which is the generation of the chick, and to accomplish which both the semen of the cock as agent and fecundator, and the chalaza as matter are required. In the second place comes accretion or growth, which is accomplished by nutrition, whose faculties consist in attraction, retention, concoction, expulsion, and, finally, apposition, agglutination, and assimilation of food."

But for my part I neither regard such a distribution of actions as correct, or useful, or convenient in this place. It is incorrect, because those actions which he would make distinct in kind and in time—for instance, that parts are first produced similar by the alterative or transformative faculty, to be afterwards fashioned and organized by the formative faculty, and finally made to grow by the auctive faculty—are never apparent in the generation of the chick; for the several parts are produced and distinguished and increased simultaneously. For although in the generation of those animals which are formed by metamorphosis, where from matter previously existing, and already adequate in quantity and duly prepared, all the parts are made distinct and conformed by transformation, as when a butterfly is formed from a caterpillar, a silkworm from a grub, still in generation by epigenesis the thing is very different, nor do the same processes go on as in ordinary nutrition, which is effected by the various actions of different parts working together to a common end, the food being here first assumed and retained, then digested, next distributed, and finally agglutinated. Nor is the *similar constitution* the result of the transformative faculty, void of all foresight, as Fabricius imagined; but the organic comes from the formative faculty which proceeds with both consciousness and foresight. For generation and growth do not proceed without nutrition, nor nutrition or increase without generation; to nourish being in other terms to substitute for a certain quantity of matter lost as much matter of the same quality, flesh or nerve, in lieu of the matter, flesh or nerve, that has become effete. But what is this but to make or engender flesh or nerve? In like manner, growth cannot go on without generation, for all natural bodies are increased by the accession of new particles similar to those of which they formerly consisted, and this, taking place according to all their dimensions, they are distinguished as regards their parts, and are organized at the same time that they grow.

But to engender the chick is in truth nothing else than to fashion or make its several members and organs, which, although they are produced in a certain order, and some are postgenate to others,—the less important to the more principal organs— still, whilst the organs themselves are all distinguished, they are not engendered in such wise and order that the *similar* parts are first formed, and the *organic* parts afterwards compounded from them; or so that certain composing parts existed before other compounded parts which must be fashioned from them. For although the head of the chick and the rest of the body exist in the shape of a mucus or soft jelly, whence each of the parts is afterwards formed in sequence, and all are of *similar* constitution in the first instance, still are they simultaneously produced and augmented in virtue of the same processes directed by the same agent; and in the same proportion as the matter resembling jelly increases, in like measure are the parts distinguished; for they are engendered, transmuted, and formed simultaneously; similar and dissimilar parts exist together, and from a small similar organ a larger one is produced. The thing, in short, is not otherwise than it is among vegetables, where from the straw proceeds the ear, the awns, and the grain—distinctly, severally, and yet together; or as trees put forth buds, from which are produced leaves, flowers, fruit, and finally seed.

All this we learn from an attentive study of the parts and processes of the incubated egg, inasmuch, as from things done, actions or operations are apprehended; from operations, faculties or forces, and from these we then infer the artificer, generator, or cause. In the generation of the pullet, consequently, the actions or faculties of the engendering cause enumerated by Fabricius, namely, the metamorphic and formative, do not differ in kind, or even in the relation of sequence, as that one is first and the other second, but, as Aristotle is wont to say, are one and the same in reason; not as happens with reference to the actions of the nutritive faculty,—attraction, concoction, distribution and apposition, to wit,—which all come into play in several places at several times. Were this not so, the engen-

dering cause itself would be forced to make use of various instruments in order to accomplish its various operations.

Fabricius, therefore, asserts erroneously that the transmutative
force works with the properties of the elements,—hot, cold, moist
and dry—as its instruments; whilst the formative faculty acts
independently of these and by a more divine power, performing
its task with consciousness, as it seems, with foresight and election. But if he had looked more closely at the matter he
would have seen that the formative as well as the metamorphic
force made use of the hot and the cold, the moist and the dry, as
instruments; nor would he have been less struck with indications
of the Supreme Artificer's interference in the processes of nutrition and transformation than in that of formation itself. For
nature ordained each and all of these faculties to some definite
end, and everywhere labours with forethought and intelligence.
Whatever it is in the seeds of plants which renders them fertile
and exercises a plastic force in their interior; whatever it is
which in the egg performs the duty of a most skilful artificer,
producing and fashioning the parts of the pullet, warming,
cooling, moistening, drying, concocting, condensing, hardening,
softening and liquefying at once, impressing distinctive characters
on each of them by means of configuration, situation, constitution, temperament, number and order,—still is this something
at work, disposing and ordering all with no less of foresight,
intelligence, and choice in the business of transmuting, than in
the processes of nutrition, growth, and formation.

The concoctive and metamorphic, the nutritive and augmentive
faculties, which Fabricius would have it act through the qualities of hot, cold, moist and dry, without all consciousness, I
maintain, on the contrary, work no less to a definite end,
and with not less of artifice than the formative faculty, which
Fabricius declares has knowledge and foresight of the future
action and use of every particular part and organ. In the same
way as the arts of the physician, cook and baker, in which heat
and cold, moisture and dryness, and similar natural properties
are employed, require the use of reason no less than the mechanical arts in which either the hands or various instruments are
employed, as in the business of the blacksmith, statuary, potter,
&c.; in the same way, as in the greater world, we are told
that " All things are full of Jove,"—Jovis omnia plena—so

26

in the slender body of the pullet, and in every one of its actions, does the finger of God or nature no less obviously appear.

Wherefore, if from manifestations it be legitimate to judge of faculties, we might say that the vegetative acts appear rather to be performed with art, election, and foresight, than the acts of the rational soul and mind; and this even in the most perfect man, whose highest excellence in science and art, if we may take the God for our guide, is that he KNOW HIM-SELF.

A superior and more divine agent than man, therefore, appears to engender and preserve mankind, a higher power than the male bird to produce a young one from the egg. We acknowledge God, the supreme and omnipotent creator, to be present in the production of all animals, and to point, as it were, with a finger to his existence in his works, the parents being in every case but as instruments in his hands. In the generation of the pullet from the egg all things are indeed contrived and ordered with singular providence, divine wisdom, and most admirable and incomprehensible skill. And to none can these attributes be referred save to the Almighty, first cause of all things, by whatever name this has been designated,—the Divine Mind by Aristotle; the Soul of the Universe by Plato; the Natura Naturans by others; Saturn and Jove by the ancient Greeks and Romans; by ourselves, and as is seeming in these days, the Creator and Father of all that is in heaven and earth, on whom animals depend for their being, and at whose will and pleasure all things are and were engendered.

Moreover, as I have said, I neither hold this arrangement of the faculties of the vital principle, which Fabricius has placed at the head of his account of the organs of generation, as correct in itself, nor as useful or calculated to assist us in the matter we have in hand. For we do not attain to a knowledge of effects from a discussion of actions or faculties; the contrary is rather the case : from actions we ascend to a knowledge of faculties, inasmuch as manifestations are more cognizable to us than the powers whence they proceed, and the parts which we investigate already formed are more readily appreciated than the actions whence they proceed.

Neither is it well from the generation of a single chick from an egg, to venture upon general conclusions, which can in fact only be correctly arrived at after extensive observations on the mode of generation among animals at large. But of this matter I shall have more to say immediately.

Meantime, however, that we may come to the parts subservient to generation, as Fabricius says,[1] "let us consider and perpend in what order the organs subserving generation are produced—which are formed first, which last. In this investigation two bases are to be laid, one having reference to the corporeal, the other to the incorporeal; that is to say, to nature and the vital principle. The corporeal base," he continues, " I call that which depends on and proceeds from the nature of the body, and of which illustrations are readily supplied from things made by art; as for example, that every building requires a foundation upon which it may be established and reared; from whence walls are raised, by which both floors and ceilings are supported; then are all the supplementary parts added and ornaments appended :—and so, in fact, does nature strive in the construction of the animal body; for first she forms the bones as a foundation, in order that all the parts of the body may grow upon and be appended to and established around them. These are the parts, in other words, that are first formed and solidified; for as the bones derive their origin from a very soft and membranous substance, and by and by become extremely hard, much time is required to complete the formation of a bone, and it is therefore that they are first produced. Hence Galen did not compare the formation of the animal body to every kind of artificial structure, but particularly to a ship; for he says, as the commencement and foundation of a ship is the keel, from which the ribs, circularly curved, proceed on either side at moderate distances from each other, like the sticks of a hurdle, in order that the whole fabric of the vessel may afterwards be reared upon the keel as a suitable basis; so in the formation of the animal body does nature, by means of the outstretched spine and the ribs drawn around it, secure a keel and suitable foundation for the entire superstructure, which she then raises and perfects."

But experience teaches us that all this is very different in fact, and that the bones are rather among the last parts to be

---

[1] Op. supra cit. p. 43.

formed. The bones of the extremities and skull, and the teeth, do not arise any sooner than the brain, the muscles, and the other fleshy parts : in new-born fœtuses, perfect in other respects, the place of the bones is supplied by mere membranes or cartilages, which are only subsequently and in the lapse of time converted into bones; a circumstance which sufficiently appears in the crania of new-born infants, and in the state of their ribs and articulations.

And although it be true that the first rudiments of the body are seen in the guise of a recurved keel, still this is a soft mucous and jelly-like substance, which has no affinity in nature, structure, or office to bone; and although certain globules depend from thence, the destined rudiments of the head, still these contain no solid matter, but are mere vesicles full of limpid water, which are afterwards formed into the brain, cerebellum, and eyes, which are all subsequently surrounded by the skull, at a period, however, when the beak and nails have already acquired consistency and hardness.

This view of Fabricius is therefore both imperfect and incorrect; inasmuch as he does not think of what nature performs in fact in the work of generation, so much as of what in his opinion she ought to do, betrayed into this by his comparison with the edifice reared by art. As if nature had imitated art, and not rather art nature !—mindful of which he himself says afterwards :[1] " It were better to say that art learned of nature, and was an imitator of her doings ; for, as Galen everywhere reminds us, nature is both older and displays greater wisdom in her works than art."

And then when we admit that the bones are the foundation of the whole body, without which it could neither support itself nor perform any movement, it is still sufficient if they arise simultaneously with the parts that are attached to them. And indeed the things that are to be supported not yet existing, the supports would be established in vain. Nature, however, does nothing in vain ; nor does she form parts before there is a use for them. But animals receive their organs as soon as the offices of these are required. The first basis of Fabricius, therefore, is distinctly overthrown by his own observations on the egg, and the comparison drawn by Galen.

[1] Op. cit. p. 44.

He appears to have come nearer the truth where he says : [1] " The other basis of the parts to be formed first or last is obtained from nature, that is, from the vital principle by which the animal body is ruled and directed. If there be two grades of this principle, the vegetative and animal, the vegetative must be held prior in point of nature and time, inasmuch as it is common to plants and animals ; and assuredly the organs officiating in the vegetative office will be engendered and formed before those that belong to the sensitive and motive principle, especially to the chief organs which are in immediate relationship with the governing principle. Now these organs are two in especial—the liver and the heart : the liver as seat of concupiscence, of the vegetative or nutritive faculty; the heart, as the organ whose heat maintains and perfects the vegetative and every other faculty, and in this way has most intimate connexions and relations with the vegetative force. Whence, if after the third day you see the heart palpitating in the point where the chick is engendered, as Aristotle bears witness to the fact that you can, you will not be surprised but rather be disposed to admit that the heart belongs to the vegetative degree and exists for its sake. It is also consonant with reason that the liver should be engendered simultaneously with the heart, but should lie perdue or hidden, as it does not pulsate. And Aristotle himself admits that the heart and liver exist in the animal body for similar reasons ; so that where there is a heart there also is a liver discovered. If the heart and liver be the parts first produced, then, it is also fair to suppose that the other organs subserving these two should be engendered in the same manner,—the lungs which exist for the sake of the heart ; and, for the sake of the liver, almost all the viscera which present themselves in the abdomen."

Still is all this very different from the sequence we witness in the egg. Nor is it true that the liver is engendered simultaneously with the heart ; nor does the salve avail with which he would cover that infirmity where he says that the liver is concealed because it does not palpitate ; for the eyes and vena cava and carina are all conspicuous enough from the commencement, although none of them palpitate. How come the liver and lungs, if they be then extant, to be visible without any palpitation ? And then Fabricius himself has indicated a

[1] Op. cit. ut. sup.

minute point situated in the centre of his figure of the chick
of the fourth day, without stating, however, that it had any pulsation; and this he did not perceive to be the heart, but rather
believed it to be the rudiment of the body. It is certain, therefore, that Fabricius spoke only from conjecture and preconceived
ceived opinion of the origin of the liver; even in the same way
as others have done, Aldrovandus and Parisanus among the
number, who, lighting upon two points, and perceiving that
they did not pulsate simultaneously, straightway held that one
was the heart, the other the liver. As if the liver ever pulsated,
and these two points were aught but the two pulsating vesicles
replying to each other by alternate contractions, in the way
and manner we have indicated in our history!

Fabricius, therefore, is either deceived or deceives, when he
says, "In the first stage of the production of the chick, the
liver, heart, veins, arteries, lungs, and all the organs contained
in the cavity of the abdomen, are engendered together; and in
like manner are the carina, in other words, the head with the
eyes and entire vertebral column and thorax engendered." For
the heart, veins, and arteries are perfectly distinguished some
time before the carina; the carina, again, is seen before the
eyes; the eyes, beak, and sides before the organs contained in
the cavity of the abdomen; the stomach and intestines before
the liver or lungs; and there are still other particulars connected
with the order of production of the parts in generation, of which
we shall speak by and by.

He is also mistaken when he would have the vegetative portion of the vital principle prior in nature and time to the sensitive and motive element. For that which is prior in nature
is mostly posterior in the order of generation. In point of
time, indeed, the vegetative principle is prior; because without
it the sensitive principle cannot exist: an act—if the act of an
organic body—cannot take place without organs; and the
sensitive and motive organs are the work of the vegetative
principle; the sensitive soul before the existence of action, is
like a triangle within a quadrangle. But nature intended that
that which was primary and most noble should also be primary;
wherefore the vegetative force is by nature posterior in point of
order, as subordinate and ministrative to the sensitive and motive faculties.

Of the order of the parts according to Aristotle.

The following appear to be Aristotle's views of the order of generation : [1] "When conception takes place, the germ comports itself like a seed sown in the ground. For seeds likewise contain a first principle, which, existing in the beginning in potentia, by and by when it manifests itself, sends forth a stem and a root, by which aliment is taken up ; for increase is indispensable. And so in a conception, in which all the parts of the body inhere in potentia, and the first principle exists in a state of special activity."

This principle in the egg—the body analogous to the seed of a vegetable—we have called with Fabricius the spot or cicatricula, and have spoken of it as a very primary part of the egg, as that in which all the other parts inhere in potentia, and from whence each in its order afterwards arises. In this spot, in fact, is contained that—whatever it may be—by which the egg is made productive ; and here is the first action of the formative faculty, the first effect of the vegetative heat revealed.

This spot, as we have said, dilates from the very commencement of the incubation, and expands in circles, in the centre of which a minute white speck is displayed, like the shining point in the pupil of the eye ; and here anon is discovered the punctum saliens rubrum, with the ramifications of the sanguiferous vessels, and this as soon as the fluid, which we have called the colliquament, has been produced.

"Wherefore," adds Aristotle,[2] "the heart is the first part perceived in fact ; and this is in conformity not only with sense, but also with reason. For as that which is engendered is already disjunct and severed from both parents, and ought to rule and regulate itself like a son who comes of age and has his separate establishment, it must therefore possess a principle, an intrinsic principle, by which the order of the members may

De Gen. Anim. lib. ii. cap. 1   [2] Ibid.

be subsequently determined, and whatever is necessary to the
constitution of a perfect animal arranged. For if this principle
were at any time extrinsic, and entered into the body at a subsequent period, you would not only be in doubt as to the time
at which it entered, but as every part is distinct, you would
also see it as necessary that that should first exist from
which the other parts derive both increase and motion."   The
same writer elsewhere [1] asserts : " This principle is a portion of
the whole, and not anything added, or included apart.   For,"
he proceeds, "the generation of the animal completed, does
this principle perish, or does it continue ?   But nothing can be
shown existing intrinsically which is not a part of the whole
organized being, whether it be plant or animal; wherefore it
would be absurd to maintain that the principle in question
perished after the formation either of any one or of any number
of parts; for what should form those that were not yet produced?
Wherefore," he continues further, " they say not well who with
Democritus assert that the external parts of animals are those
first seen, and then the internal parts, as if they were rearing
an animal of wood and stone, for such a thing would include
no principle within itself.   But all animals have and hold a
principle in their interior.   Wherefore the heart is seen as the
first distinct part in animals that have blood ; for it is the origin
of all the parts, whether similar or dissimilar ; and the creature
that begins to feel the necessity of nourishment, must already
be possessed by the principle of an animal and a full-grown
fœtus."

From the above, it clearly appears that Aristotle recognizes
a certain order and commencement in animal generation,
namely, the heart, which he regards as the first produced and
first vivified part of the animal, and, like a son set free from
the tutelage of his parents, as self-sufficing and independent,
whence not only does the order of the parts proceed, but as that
by which the animal itself is maintained and preserved, receiving
from it at once life and sustenance, and everything needful to
the perfection of its being.   For as Seneca says : [2] " In the
semen is comprised the entire cause of the future man; and the
unborn babe has written within it the law of a beard and a

---

[1] De Gen. Anim. lib. ii, cap. 1.   [2] Nat. Quæst. lib. iii, cap. 29.

hoary head. For the whole body and the load of future years are already traced in delicate and obscure outlines in its constitution."

We have already determined whether the heart were this primigenial part or not; in other words, whether Aristotle's words refer to that part which, in the dissection of animals, is seen sooner than all the rest, the punctum saliens, to wit, with its vessels full of blood; and we have cordially assented to an answer in the affirmative. For I believe that the blood, together with its immediate instruments, the umbilical vessels, by which, as by roots, nutriment is attracted, and the pulsating vesicles, by which this nutriment is distributed, to maintain life and growth in every other part, are formed first and foremost of all. For as Aristotle[1] has said, it is the same matter by which a thing grows, and by which it is primarily constituted.

Many, however, err in supposing that different parts of the body require different kinds of matter for their nourishment. As if nutrition were nothing more than the selection and attraction of fit aliment; and in the several parts of the body to be nourished, no concoction, assimilation, apposition, and transmutation were required. This as we learn, was the opinion of Anaxagoras of old :

> Who held the principles of things to be
> Homœomeric :—bone to be produced
> Of small and slender bones ; the viscera
> Of small and slender viscera ; the blood
> Of numerous associate drops of blood.[2]

But Aristotle,[3] with the greatest propriety, observes : " Distinction of parts is not effected, as some think, by like being carried by its nature to like; for, besides innumerable difficulties belonging to this opinion in itself, it happens that each similar part is severally created ; for example, the bones by themselves, the nerves, the flesh, &c." But the nourishment of all parts is common and homogeneous, such as we see the albumen to be in the egg, not heterogeneous and composed of different parts. Wherefore all we have said of the matter from which parts are made, is to be stated of that by which they increase : all derive nourishment from that in which they exist in potentia, though

---

[1] De Gen. Anim. lib. ii, cap. 4.   [2] Lucret. lib. i.   [3] Loc. sup. cit.

26 §

not in act. Precisely as from the same rain plants of every kind increase and grow ; because the moisture which was a like power in reference to all, becomes actually like to each when it is changed into their substances severally : then does it acquire bitterness in rue, sharpness in mustard, sweetness in liquorice, and so on.

He explains, moreover, what parts are engendered before others, and assigns a reason which does not differ from the second basis of Fabricius. " The cause by which, and the cause of this cause, are different ; one is first in generation, the other in essence ;" by which we are to understand that the end is prior in nature and essence to that which happens for the sake of the end ; but that which happens for the sake of the end must be prior in generation. And on this ground Fabricius rightly infers that all those parts which minister to the vegetative principle, are engendered before those that serve the sensitive principle, inasmuch as the former is subordinate to the latter.

He subsequently adds the differences of those parts which are made for some special purpose : some parts, for example, are instituted for a purpose by nature, because this purpose ensues ; and others because they are instruments which the purpose employs. The former he designates genitalia, the latter instrumenta. For the end or purpose, he says, in some cases, is posterior, in others prior to that which is its cause. For both the generator and the instruments it uses must exist anteriorly to that which is engendered by or from them. The parts serving the vegetative principle, therefore, are prior to the parts which are the ministers of sense and motion. But the parts dedicated to motion and sensation are posterior to the motive and sensitive faculties, because they are the instruments which the motive and sensitive faculties employ. For it is a law of nature that no parts or instruments be produced before there be some use for them, and the faculty be extant which employs them. Thus there is neither any eye nor any motive organ engendered until the brain is produced, and the faculties preexist which are to see and to govern motion.

In like manner, as the pulsating vesicles serve as instruments for the motion of the blood, and the heart in its entire structure does the same, (as I have shown in the work on the Motion of the blood,) urging the blood in a ceaseless round through every part of the body, we see that the blood must exist before the heart, both in the order of generation and of nature and essence. For the blood uses the heart as an instrument, and moreover, when engendered it continues to nourish the organ by means of the coronary arteries, distributing heat, spirits, and life to it through their ramifications.

We shall have further occasion to show from an entire series of anatomical observations, how this rule of Aristotle in respect of the true priority of the parts is borne out. Meantime we shall see how he himself succeeds in duly inferring the causes of priority in conformity with his rule.

"After the prime part—viz. the heart—is engendered," he says, "the internal parts are produced before the external ones, the superior before the inferior; for the lower parts exist for the sake of the superior, and that they may serve as instruments, after the manner of the seeds of vegetables, which produce roots sooner than branches."

Nature, however, follows no such order in generation; nor is the instance quoted invariably applicable; for in beans, peas, and other leguminous seeds, in acorns, also, and in grain, it is easy to see that the stem shoots upwards and the root downwards from the same germ; and onions and other bulbous plants send off stalks before they strike root.

He then subjoins another cause of this order, viz.: "That as nature does nothing in vain or superfluously, it follows that she makes nothing either sooner or later than the use she has for it requires." That is to say, those parts are first engendered whose use or function is first required; and some are begun at an earlier period because a longer time is requisite to bring them to perfection; and that so they may be in the same state of forwardness at birth as those that are more rapidly produced. Just as the cook, having to dress certain articles for supper, which by reason of their hardness are done with difficulty, or require gentle boiling for a great length of time, these he puts on the first, and only turns subsequently to those that are prepared more quickly and with less expenditure of heat; and further, as he makes ready the articles that are to come on in the first course first of all, and those that are to be presented in the second course afterwards; so also does nature in the generation of animals only proceed at a later period to the construction of the soft and moist and fleshy parts, as requiring but a short time for their concoction and formation, whilst the hard parts, such as the bones, as requiring ample evaporation and abundant drying, and their matter long remaining inconcoct, she proceeds to fashion almost from the very beginning. "And the same thing obtains in the brain," he adds, "which, large in quantity and exceedingly moist at first, is by and by better concocted and condensed, so that the brain as well as the eye diminishes in size. The head is therefore very large at first, in comparison with the rest of the body, which it far surpasses because of the brain and the eyes, and the large quantity of moisture contained in them. These parts, nevertheless, are among the last to be perfected, for the brain acquires consistence with difficulty, and it is long before it is freed from cold and moisture in any animal, and especially in man. The sinciput, too, is consolidated the last, the bones here being quite soft when the infant sees the light."

He gives another reason, viz. because the parts are formed of different kinds of matter : " Every more excellent part, the sharer in the highest principle is, farther, engendered from the most highly concocted, the purest and first nutriment; the other needful parts, produced for the sake of the former, from the worse and excrementitious remainder. For nature, like the sage head of a family, is wont to throw away nothing that may be turned to any useful purpose. But he still regulates his household so that the best food shall be given to his children, the more indifferent to his menials, the worst to the animals. As then, man's growth being complete and mind having been superadded, (in other words, and, as I interpret the passage, adult man having acquired sense and prudence,) things are ordered in this way, so does nature at the period of production even compose the flesh and the other more sensitive parts of the purest matter. Of the excrementitious remainder she makes the bones, sinews, hair, nails, and other parts of the same constitution. And this is the reason why this is done last of all, when nature has an abundant supply of recrementitious material." Our author then goes on to speak of " a twofold order of aliment :" "one for nutrition, another for growth ;" "the nutritive is the one which supplies existence to the whole and to the parts; the augmentative, that which causes increase to the bulk."

This is in accordance with what we find in the egg, where the albumen supplies a kind of purer aliment adapted to the nutrition of the embryo in its earlier stages, and the yelk affords the material for the growth of the chick and pullet. The thinner albumen, moreover, as we have seen, is used in fashioning the first and more noble parts; the thicker albumen and the yelk, again, are employed in nourishing and making these to grow, and further in forming the less important parts of the body. For," he says, "the sinews, too, are produced in the same way as the bones, and from the same material, viz.: the seminal and nutritive excrementitious matter. But the nails, hair, horns, beak, and spurs of birds, and all other things of the same description, are engendered of the adventitious and nutritive aliment, which is obtained both from the mother and from without." And then he gives a reason why man, whilst other animals are endowed by nature with defensive and offensive arms, is born naked and defenceless, which is this: that whilst in the lower animals these parts are formed of remainders or excrements, man is compounded of a purer material, "which contains too small a quantity of inconcoct and earthy matter."

Thus far have we followed Aristotle on the subject of 'The Order in Generation,' the whole of which seems to be referrible to one principle, viz.: the perfection of nature, which in her works does nothing in vain and has no short-comings, but still does that in the best manner which was best to be done. Hence in generation no part would either precede or follow, did she prefer producing them altogether, viz.: in circumstances where she acts freely and by election; for sometimes she works under compulsion, as it were, and beside her purpose, as when through deficiency or superabundance of material, or through some defect in her instruments, or is hindered of her ends by external injuries. And thus it occasionally happens that the final parts are formed before the instrumental parts,—understanding by final parts, those that use others as instruments.

And as some of the parts are genital, nature making use of them in the generation of other parts, as the means of removing obstacles the presence of which would interfere with the due progress of the work of reproduction, and others exist for other special ends; it therefore happens that for the disposition of material, and other requisites, some parts are variously engendered before others, some of them being begun earlier but completed at a later period, some being both begun and perfected at an earlier period, and others being begun together but perfected at different times subsequently. And then the same order is not observed in the generation of all animals, but this is variously altered; and in some there is nothing like succession, but all the parts are begun and perfected simultaneously, by metamorphosis, to wit, as has been already stated. Hence it follows, in fine, that the primogenate part must be of such a nature as to contain both the beginning and the end, and be that for whose sake all the rest is made, namely, the living principle, or soul, and that which is the potential and genital cause of this, the heart, or in our view the blood, which we regard as the prime seat of the soul, as the source and perennial centre of life, as the generative heat, and indeed as the inherent heat; in a word, the heart is the first efficient of the whole of the instrumental parts that are produced for the ends of the soul, and used by it as instruments. The heart, according to Aristotle, I say, is that for which all the parts of animals are made, and it is at the same time that which is at once the origin and fashioner of them all.

Of the order of the parts in generation as it appears from observation.

That we may now propose our own views of the order of the parts in generation as we have gathered it from our observations, it appears that the whole business of generation in all animals may be divided into two periods, or connected with two structures: the ovum, i. e. the conception and seed, or that, whatever it be, which in spontaneous productions corresponds to the seed, whether with Fernelius it be called "the native celestial heat in the primogenial moisture," or with Aristotle, "the vital heat included in moisture." For the conception in viviparous animals, as we have said, is analogous to the seed and fruit of plants; in the same way as it is to the egg of oviparous creatures; to worms in spontaneously engendered animals, or to certain vesicles fruitful by the vital warmth of their included moisture. In each and all of these the same things inhere which might with propriety lead to their being called seeds; they are all bodies, to wit, from which and by which, as previously existing matter, artificer and organ, the whole of an animal body is primarily engendered and produced.

The other structure is the embryo produced from the seed or conception. For both the matter and the moving and efficient cause, and the instruments needful to the operation, must necessarily precede operation of any and every kind.

We have already examined the structure of the egg. Now the embryo to which it gives birth, in so far as this can be made out by observation and dissection, particularly among the more perfect animals with [red] blood, appears to be perfected by four principal degrees or processes, which we reduce to as many orders, in harmony with the various epochs in generation; and we shall demonstrate that what transpires in the egg also takes place in every conception or seed.

The first process is that of the primogenial and genital part, viz. the blood with its receptacles, in other words, the heart and its vessels.

And this part is first engendered for two principal reasons: 1st, because it is the principal part which uses all the rest as instruments, and for whose sake the other parts are formed; and, 2d, because it is the 'prime genital part, the origin and author of the rest. The part, in a word, in which inhere both the principle whence motion is derived, and the end of that motion, is obviously father and sovereign.

In the generation of this first part, which in the egg is accomplished in the course of the fourth day, although I have not been able to observe any order or sequence, inasmuch as the whole of its elements,—the blood, the vessels, and the pulsating vesicles—appear simultaneously, I have nevertheless imagined, as I have said, that the blood exists before the pulse, because, according to nature's laws, it must be antecedent to its receptacles. For the substance and structure of the heart, namely, the conical mass with its auricles and ventricles, as they are produced long

subsequently along with the other viscera, so must they be referred to the same class of parts as these, namely, the third.

In the production of the circulating system the veins are
sooner seen than the arteries; such at least is our conclusion.

The second process, which begins after the fourth day, is indicated by a certain concrescence, which I designate vermiculum
—worm or maggot; for it has the life and obscure motions of a
maggot; and as it concretes into a mucous matter, it divides
into two parts, the larger and superior of which is seen to be
conglobed, and divided, as it were, into thin vesicles,—the
brain, the cerebellum, and the two eyes; the less, again, constituting the carina, arises over the vena cava and extends in
the line of its direction.

In the genesis of the head, the eyes are first perceived; by
and by a white point makes its appearance in the situation of
the beak, and the slime drying around it, it becomes invested
with a membrane.

The outline of the rest of the body follows about the same
period. First, from the carina something like the sides of a
ship are seen to arise; the parts having an uniform consistence
in the beginning, but the ribs being afterwards prefigured by
means of extremely fine white lines. The instruments of locomotion next arise—the legs and wings; and the carina and the
extremities adnate to it are then distinguished into muscles,
bones, and articulations.

These two rudiments of the head and trunk appear simultaneously, but as they grow and advance to perfection subsequently, the trunk increases and acquires its shape much more
speedily than the head; so that this, which in the first instance
exceeded the whole trunk in size, is now relatively much smaller.
And the same thing occurs in regard to the human embryo.

The same disparity also takes place between the trunk and
the extremities. In the human embryo, from the time when
it is not longer than the nail of the little finger, till it is of the
size of a frog or mouse, the arms are so short that the extremities of the fingers could not extend across the breast, and the
legs are so short that were they reflected on the abdomen they
would not reach the umbilicus.

The proportion of the body to the extremities in children
after their birth continues excessive until they begin to stand

and run. Infants, therefore, resemble dwarfs in the beginning, and they creep about like quadrupeds, attempting progressive motion with the assistance of all their extremities; but they cannot stand erect until the length of the leg and thigh together exceeds the length of the rest of the body. And so it happens, that when they first attempt to walk, they move with the body prone, like the quadruped, and can scarcely rise so erect as the common dunghill fowl.

And so it happens that among adult men the long-legged—they who have longer legs, and especially longer thighs—are better walkers, runners, and leapers than square-built, compact men.

In this second process many actions of the formative faculty are observed following each other in regular order, (in the same way as we see one wheel moving another in automata, and other pieces of mechanism,) and all arising from the same mucaginous and similar matter. Not indeed in the manner that some natural philosophers would have it when they say, "that like is carried to its like." We are rather to maintain that parts are moved, not changing their places, but remaining and undergoing change in hardness, softness, colour, &c., whence the diversities between *similar* parts; those things appearing *in act* which were before *in power*.[1] The extremities, spine, and rest of the body, namely, are formed, grow, and acquire outline and complexion together; the extremities, comprising bones, muscles, tendons, and cartilages, all of which on their first appearance were similar and homogeneous, become distinguished in their progress, and, connected together, compose organs, by whose mutual continuity the whole body is constituted. In like manner, the membrane growing around the head, the brain is composed, and the lustrous eyes receive their polish out of a perfectly limpid fluid.

That is to say, nature sustains and augments the several parts by the same nourishment with which she fashioned them at first, and not, as many opine, with any diversity of aliment and particles similar to each particular structure. As she is increasing the mucaginous mass or maggot, like a potter she first divides her material, and then indicates the head and trunk

---

[1] De Gen. Anim. lib. ii, cap. 4.

and extremities; like a painter, she first sketches the parts in outline, and then fills them in with colours; or like the ship-builder, who first lays down his keel by way of foundation, and upon this raises the ribs and roof or deck: even as he builds his vessel does nature fashion the trunk of the body and add the extremities.   And in this work she orders all the variety of similar parts—the bones, cartilages, membranes, muscles, tendons, nerves, &c.—from the same primary jelly or mucus. For thick filaments are produced in the first instance, and these by and by are brought to resemble cords; then they are rendered cartilaginous and spinous; and, lastly, they are hardened and concocted into bones.   In the same way the thicker membrane which invests the brain is first cartilaginous and then bony, whilst the thinner membrane merely consolidates into the pericranium and integument.   In similar order flesh and nerve from soft mucus are confirmed into muscle, tendon, and ligament; the brain and cerebellum are condensed out of a perfectly limpid water into a firm coagulum; for the brain of infants, before the bones of the head have closed, is soft and diffluent, and has no greater consistence than the curd of milk.

The third process is that of the viscera, the formation of which in the chick takes place after the trunk is cast in outline, or about the sixth or seventh day,—the liver, lungs, kidneys, cone and ventricles of the heart, and intestines, all become visible nearly at the same moment; they appear to arise from the veins, and to be connected with them in the same way as fungi grow upon the bark of trees. They are, as I have already said, gelatinous, white, and bloodless, until they take on their proper functions.   The stomach and intestines are first discovered as white and tortuous filaments extending lengthwise through the abdomen; along with these the mouth appears, from which a continuous canal extends to the anus, and connects the superior with the inferior parts.   The organs of generation likewise appear about the same time.

Up to this period all the viscera, the intestines, and the heart itself inclusive, are excluded from the cavities of the body and hang pendulous without, attached as it were to the veins.   The trunk of the body presents itself, in fact, like a boat undecked or a house without a roof, the anterior walls of the thorax and abdomen not being yet extant to close these cavities.

But as soon as the sternum is fashioned the heart enters into the chest as into a dwelling which it had built and arranged for itself; and there, like the tutelary genius, it enters on the government of the surrounding mansion, which it inhabits with its ministering servants the lungs. The liver and stomach are by and by included within the hypochondria, and the intestines are finally surrounded by the abdominal parietes. And this is the reason wherefore without dissection the heart can no longer be seen pulsating in the hen's egg after the tenth day of incubation.

About this epoch the point of the beak and the nails appear of a fine white colour; a quantity of chylous matter presents itself in the stomach; a little excrement is also observed in the intestine, and the liver being now begun, some greenish bile is perceived; facts from which it clearly appears that there is another digestion and preparation of nutriment going on besides that which takes place by the branches of the umbilical veins; and it is reasonable matter of doubt how the bile, the excrementitious matter of the second digestion, can be separated by the instrumentality of the liver from the other humours, when we see it produced at the same time as this organ.

In the order now indicated are the internal organs generated universally; in all the animals which I have dissected, particularly the more perfect ones, and man himself, I have found them produced in the same manner: in these, in the course of the second, third, and fourth month, the heart, liver, lungs, kidneys, spleen, and intestines present themselves inchoate and increasing, and all alike of the same white colour which belongs to the body at large. Wherefore these early days are not improperly spoken of as the days when the embryo is *in the milk;* for with the exception of the veins, particularly those of the umbilicus, everything is as it were spermatic in appearance.

I am of opinion that the umbilical arteries arise after the veins of the same name, because the arteries are scarcely to be discovered in the course of the first month, and take their rise from the branches that descend to either lower extremity. I do not believe, therefore, that they exist until that part of the body whence they proceed is formed. The umbilical veins, on the contrary, are conspicuous long before any part of the body is begun.

What I have now said I have derived from numerous dissections of human embryos of almost every size; for I have had them for inspection from the time they were like tadpoles, till they were seven or eight fingers' breadth in length, and from thence onwards to the full time.   I have examined them more particularly, however, through the second, third, and fourth months, in the course of which the greatest number of changes take place, and the order of development is seen with greatest clearness.

In the human embryo, then, of the age of two months, what we have spoken of as taking place in the "second process," is observed to occur.   For I rather think that during the first month there is scarcely anything of the conception in the uterus—at all events, I have never been able to discover anything. But the first month past, I have repeatedly seen conceptions thrown off, and similar to the one which Hippocrates mentions as having been voided by the female pipe-player, of the size of a pheasant's or pigeon's egg.   Such conceptions resemble an egg without its shell ; they are, namely, of an oval figure; the thicker membrane or chorion with which they are surrounded, however, is seen to be covered with a white mucor externally, particularly towards the larger end ; internally it is smooth and shining, and is filled with limpid and sluggish water—it contains nothing else.

In the course of the second month I have frequently seen an ovum of this description, or somewhat larger, thrown off with the symptoms of abortion, viz. ichorous lochia ; the ovum being sometimes entire, at other times burst, and covered with bloody coagula.   Within it was smooth and slippery ; it was covered with adhering blood without.   Its form was that which I have just described.   In some of these aborted ova, I have discovered embryos, in others I could find none.   The embryo, when present, was of the length of the little finger-nail, and in shape like a little frog, save that the head was exceedingly large and the extremities very short, like a tadpole in the month of June, when it gets its extremities, loses its tail, and assumes the form of a frog.   The whole substance was white, and so soft and mucilaginous, that unless immersed in clear water, it was impossible to handle it.   The face was the same as that of the embryo of one of the lower animals—the dog or cat, for instance, without lips, the mouth gaping, and extending from ear to ear.

Many women, whose conceptions, like the wind-eggs of fowls, are barren and without an embryo, miscarry in the third month.

I have occasionally examined aborted ova of this age, of the size of a goose's egg, which contained embryos distinct in all their parts, but misshapen. The head, eyes, and extremities were distinct, but the muscles were indistinct; there were no bones, but certain white lines in their situations, and as it seemed, soft cartilages. The substance of the heart was extremely white, and consisted of two ventricles of like size and thickness of walls, forming a cone with a double apex, which might be compared to a small twin-kernel nut. The liver was very small and of the general white colour. Through the whole of this time, i. e. during the first three months, there is scarcely any appearance of a placenta or uterine cake.

In every conception of this description I have seen, I have always found a surrounding membrane containing a large quantity of watery fluid, between which and the body of the embryo, suspended by its middle by means of a long and twisted umbilical cord, there is such disproportion, that it is impossible to regard this liquid as either sweat or urine; it seems far more probable that like the colliquament in the hen's egg, it is a fluid destined by nature for the nourishment of the fœtus. Nor was there any indication to be discovered of these conceptions or ova having been connected with the uterus; there was only on the external surface of their larger extremity a greater appearance of thickening and wrinkling, as if the rudiments of the future placenta had existed there.

These conceptions, therefore, appear to me in the light of ova, which are merely cherished within the uterus, and, like the egg in the uterus of the fowl, grow by their own inherent powers.

In the fourth month, however, it is wonderful to find what rapid strides the fœtus has made : from the length of the thumb it has now grown to be a span long. All the members, too, are distinct and are tinged with blood; the bones and muscles can be distinguished; there are vestiges of the nails, and the fœtus now begins to move lustily. The head, however, is excessively large; the face without lips, cheeks, and nose; the gape of the mouth is enormous, and the tongue lies in its middle; the eyes are small, without lids to cover them; the middle integument of the regions of the forehead and sinciput is not yet cartilaginous, far less bony; but the occiput is somewhat firm and in some sort cartilaginous, indicating that the skull already begins to acquire solidity.

The organs of generation have now made their appearance, but the testes are contained within the abdomen, in the situation of the female uterus, the scrotum still remaining empty. The female organs are yet imperfect, and the uterus with its tubes resembles the two-horned uterus of the lamb.

The placenta, of larger size, and now attached to the uterus, comprises nearly one half of the entire conception, and presented itself to my eye as a fleshy or fungous excrescence of the womb, so firmly was its gibbous portion connected all around with the uterine walls, which had now grown to greater thickness. The branches of the umbilical vessels struck into the placenta like the roots of a tree into the ground, and by their means was the conception now, for the first time, connected with the uterus.

The brain presented itself as a large and soft coagulum, full of ample vessels. The ventricles of the heart were of equal capacity, and their walls of the same thickness. In the thorax, and covered by the ribs, three cavities, nearly of the same dimensions, were perceived; of these the lowest was occupied by the lungs, which are full of blood, and of the same colour as the liver and kidneys; the middle cavity was filled by the heart and pericardium; the superior cavity, again, was possessed by the gland called the thymus, which is now of very ample size.

In the stomach there was some chyle discovered, not very different in character from the fluid in which the embryo swam. It also contained some white curdled matter, not unlike the mucous sordes which the nurse washes particularly from between the folds of the skin of new-born infants. In the upper part of the intestines there was a small quantity of excrementitious or chylous matter; the lower bowels contained meconium. In the urinary bladder there was urine, and in the gall bladder bile. The intestinum cœcum, that appendix of the colon, was empty as in the adult, and apparently superfluous, not as in the lower animals—the hog, horse, hare, constituting as it were another stomach. The omentum, or apron, floated over the intestines at large like a thin and transparent veil or cloud.

The kidneys at this epoch are not yet formed into a smooth and continuous rounded mass, as in the adult, but are compacted of numerous smaller masses, as we see them in the calf and sturgeon, as if there were a renal globule or nipple placed at the extremity of each division of the ureter, from the orifice of which the urine distilled. Over the kidneys two bodies, first observed by Eustachius, are discovered, very abundantly supplied with blood, so that their veins, which anatomists designate as venæ adiposæ, are not much smaller than the emulgents themselves. The liver and spleen, according to their several proportions, are equally full of blood.

I may here observe, by the way, that in every strong and healthy human fœtus we everywhere discover milk ; it is particularly abundant in the thymus gland, though it is also found in the pancreas, through the whole of the mesentery, and in certain lacteal veins and glands, as it seems, situated between the divisions of the mesenteric vessels. Moreover, it can be pressed and indeed sometimes flows spontaneously from the breasts of newly-born infants, and nurses imagine that this is beneficial to the infant.

And it clearly appears that this fluid, which abounds in the ovum, is no excrementitious matter thrown off by the embryo, nothing like urine or sweat, because its relative quantity is diminished as the period of parturition approaches, when the fœtus is of course larger, and, as it consumes a greater quantity of nutriment, accumulates excrementitious matter more abundantly than it did in the first months of pregnancy. Let it be added, that the bladder is at this time distended with urine. For my own part I have never been able to discover that conduit for the urine, from the bladder to the umbilicus, which anatomists describe under the name of urachus ; I have, on the contrary, frequently seen urine escaping by the penis, but never by any urachus, when the bladder was pressed upon with the hand.

So much for what I have observed with reference to the order of the parts in the development of the human fœtus.

In the fourth and last process the parts of the lowest state and order are produced, those, namely, that do not exist as needful to the being or to the maintenance of the individual, but only as defences against external injury, as ornaments, or as weapons of offence.

The outermost part of all, the skin, with its several append-ages,—cuticle, hair, wool, feathers, scales, shells, claws, hooves, and other items of the same description, may be regarded as the principal means of defence or protection. And it is well devised by nature, who, indeed, never does aught amiss, that these parts are the last to be engendered, inasmuch as they could never be of use or avail as defences until the animal was born. The common domestic pullet is therefore born covered with down only, not with feathers, like certain other birds which have to be speedily prepared for flight, because it has to seek its food on foot, not on the wing, and by active running about hither and thither. In like manner the young of ducks and geese, which feed swimming, have their feathers and wings perfected at a later period than their feet and legs. It is otherwise with swallows, however, which have to fly sooner than to walk, be-cause they feed on the wing.

The down of the pullet begins to appear after the fourteenth day, the foetus being already perfect in all its parts. When the feathers first show themselves, they are in the guise of points within the skin, but by and by the feathers project, like plants from the ground, increase in length, become unfolded, invest the whole body, and protect it against the inclemencies of the atmosphere.

Feathers differ from quills in form, use, place of growth, and order of production. The pullet is feathered before it has any quills, for the quill-feathers only grow in the wings and tail, and also spring more deeply, from the very lowest part of the integument, or even from the periosteum, and serve essentially as instruments of motion; the feathers again arise superficially from the skin, and are everywhere present as means of protection.

"Nails, hair, horn, and the like," says Aristotle,[1] "are en-gendered from the skin; whence it happens that they change colour with the skin; for the white and black and particoloured are so in consequence of the colour of the skin whence they

---

[1] De Gener. Anim. lib. ii, cap. 4.

arise." In the bird, however, this is not so; for whatever the colour of the feathers, the skin is still never otherwise than of one tint, viz., white. And then the same feather or quill is frequently seen of different and often brilliant colours in different parts for the ornament of the creature.

In the human fœtus the skin and all the parts connected with it are in like manner perfected the last of all. In the earlier periods, consequently, we find neither lips, cheeks, external ears, eyelids, nor nose; and the last part to grow together is the upper lip in the course of the middle line of the body.

Man comes into the world naked and unarmed, as if nature had destined him for a social creature, and ordained him to live under equitable laws and in peace; as if she had desired that he should be guided by reason rather than be driven by force; therefore did she endow him with understanding, and furnish him with hands, that he might himself contrive what was necessary to his clothing and protection. To those animals to which nature has given vast strength, she has also presented weapons in harmony with their powers; to those that are not thus vigorous, she has given ingenuity, cunning, and singular dexterity in avoiding injury.

Ornaments of all kinds, such as tufts, crests, combs, wattles, brilliant plumage, and the like, of which some vain creatures seem not a little proud, to say nothing of such offensive weapons as teeth, horns, spurs, and other implements employed in combat, are more frequently and remarkably conferred upon the male than the female. And it is not uninteresting to remark, that many of these ornaments or weapons are most conspicuous in the male at that epoch when the females come into season, and burn with desire of engendering. And whilst in the young they are still absent, in the aged they also fail as being no longer wanted.

Our common cock, whose pugnacious qualities are well known, so soon as he comes to his strength and is possessed of the faculty of engendering, is distinguished by his spurs, and ornamented with his comb and beautiful feathers, by which he charms his mates to the rites of Venus, and is furnished for the combat with other males, the subject of dispute being no empty or vainglorious matter, but the perpetuation of the stock in this line or in that; as if nature had intended that he who could best defend himself and his, should be preferred to others for the continuance of the kind. And indeed all animals which are better furnished with weapons of offence, and more warlike than others, fall out and fight, either in defence of their young, of their nests or dens, or of their prey; but more than all for the possession of their females. Once vanquished, they yield up possession of these, lay aside their strut and haughty demeanour, and, crest-fallen and submissive, they seem to consume with grief; the victor, on the contrary, who has gained possession of the females by his prowess, exults and boastfully proclaims the glory of his conquest.

Nor is this ornamenting anything adventitious and for a season only; it is a lasting and special gift of nature, who has not been studious to deck out animals, and especially birds only, but has also thrown an infinite variety of beautiful dyes over the lowly and insensate herbs and flowers.

EXERCISE THE FIFTY-SEVENTH.

Of certain paradoxes and problems to be considered in connexion with this subject.

Thus far have we spoken of the order of generation, whereby the differences between those creatures that are engendered by metamorphosis and those that are developed by epigenesis, as well as between those that are said to proceed from a worm and those that arise from an egg, have been made to appear. The latter are partly incorporated from a prepared matter, and are nourished and increased from a certain remaining matter; the former are incorporated from the whole of the matter present; the latter grow and are formed simultaneously, and after their birth continue to wax in size and finally attain maturity; the former increase at once, and from a grub or caterpillar grow into an aurelia, and are then produced, consummately formed, as butterflies, moths, and the like. Wherefore Aristotle, as Fabricius[1] observes: " As he assigns a sort

---

[1] Fabricius, Op. cit. p. 46.

of twofold nature to the egg, and a twofold egg in this kind, so does he assert a twofold action and a twofold animal engendered. For," he proceeds, "from the first eggs, which are the primordia of generation, a worm is constantly produced; viz. : from the eggs of flies, ants, bees, silkworms, &c., in which some fluid is contained, and from the whole of which fluid the worm is engendered; but from the second eggs, formed by the worms themselves, butterflies are engendered and disclosed, viz. : flying animals contained in a shell, or follicle, or egg, which shell giving way the winged creature escapes; precisely as Aristotle[1] has it where he speaks of the egg of the locust." Finally, whilst the higher animals produced from eggs are perfected by a succession of parts, the lower creatures that arise in this way, or that are formed by metamorphosis, are produced at one effort, as it were, and entire. And in the same way are engendered both those creatures that are said to arise spontaneously, by chance or accident, and derive their first matter or take their origin from putrefaction, filth, excrement, dew, or the parts of plants and animals, as well as those that arise congenerately from the semen of animals. Because this is common to all living creatures, viz. : that they derive their origin either from semen or eggs, whether this semen have proceeded from others of the same kind, or have come by chance or something else. For what sometimes happens in art occasionally occurs in nature also; those things, namely, take place by chance or accident which otherwise are brought about by art. Of this Aristotle[2] quotes health as an illustration. And the thing is not different as respects the generation, in so far as it is from seed, of certain animals : their semina are either present by accident, or they proceed from an univocal agent of the same kind. For even in fortuitous semina there is an inherent motive principle of generation, which procreates from itself and of itself; and this is the same as that which is found in the semina of congenerative animals,—a power, to wit, of forming a living creature. But of this matter we shall have more to say shortly.

From what has just been said, however, several paradoxes present themselves for consideration. For when we see the cicatricula enlarging in the egg, the colliquament concocted

---

Hist. Anim. lib. v, cap. 28.   [2] Metaph. lib. vii, cap. 9.

and prepared, and a variety of other particulars all tending, not without foresight, to the development of the embryo, before the first rudiment or the merest particle of this is conspicuous, what should hinder us from believing that the calidum innatum and the vegetative soul of the chick are in existence before the chick itself? For what is competent to produce the effects and acts of life, except their efficient cause and principle, heat, namely, and the faculty of the vegetative soul? Therefore it would seem that the soul was not the act of the organic body possessing life in potentia; for we regard the chick with its appropriate form as the consequence of such an act. But where can we suppose the form and vital principle of the chick to inhere save in the chick itself? unless indeed we admitted a separation of forms and conceded a certain metamorphosis.

Now this appears most obviously where the same animal lives, as Aristotle has it, by or under a succession of forms, for example, a caterpillar, a chrysalis, a butterfly. For it is of necessity the same efficient, nutrient, and conservative principle that possesses each of these, although under different forms; unless we allow that there is one vital principle in the youth, another in the man, a third in the aged individual, or maintain that the forms of the grub and caterpillar are the same as those of the silkworm and butterfly. Aristotle has entered very fully into this subject, and we shall ourselves have more to say on it immediately.

It appears further paradoxical to maintain that the blood is produced, and moves to and fro, and is imbued with vital spirits, before any sanguiferous or locomotive organs are in existence. Neither is it less new and unheard-of to assert, that sensation and motion belong to the foetus before the brain is formed; for the foetus moves, contracting and unfolding itself, when there is nothing more than a little limpid water in the place of the brain.

Moreover, the body is nourished and increases before the organs appropriated to digestion, viz. the stomach and abdominal viscera, are formed. Sanguification, too, which is entitled the second digestion, is perfect before the first, or chylification, which takes place in the stomach, is begun. The excrementitious products of the first and second digestions, namely, excrement in the intestines, urine and bile in the urinary and gall bladder, are contemporaneous with the existence of the concocting organs themselves. Lastly, not only is there a soul or vital principle present in the vegetative part, but even before this there is inherent mind, foresight, and understanding, which from the very commencement to the being and perfect formation of the chick, dispose and order and take up all things requisite, moulding them in the new being, with consummate art, into the form and likeness of its parents.

In reference to this subject of family likeness, we may be permitted to inquire as to the reason why the offspring should at one time bear a stronger resemblance to the father, at another to the mother, and, at a third, to progenitors, both maternal and paternal, further removed? particularly in cases where at one bout, and at the same moment, several ova are fecundated. And this too is a remarkable fact, that virtues and vices, marks and moles, and even particular dispositions to disease are transmitted by parents to their offspring; and that while some inherit in this way, all do not. Among our poultry some are courageous, and pugnaciously inclined, and will sooner die than yield and flee from an adversary; their descendants, once or twice removed, however, unless they have come of equally well-bred parents, gradually lose this quality; according to the adage, "the brave are begotten by the brave." In various other species of animals, and particularly in the human family, a certain nobility of race is observed; numerous qualities, in fact, both of mind and body, are derived by hereditary descent.

I have frequently wondered how it should happen that the offspring, mixed in so many particulars of its structure or constitution, with the stamp of both parents so obviously upon it, in so many parts, should still escape all mixture in the organs of generation; that it should so uniformly prove either male or female, so very rarely an hermaphrodite.

Lastly, many things are present before they appear, and some are begun among the very first which are completed among the very last, such as the eyes, the organs of generation, and the beak.

Several doubts and difficulties have thence arisen as to the principality and relative dignity of the several members, in which they who are fond of such things have displayed their ingenuity. Among the number: whether the heart gives life and virtue to the blood; or, rather, the blood to the heart. Whether the blood be extant for the sake of the body as matter, nourishment, and instrument; or, on the contrary, the body and its parts are the cause of the blood, and constituted for the sake of the vital principle which especially inheres in it. In like manner, whether the auricles or the ventricles of the heart are the chief, the auricles being the first to live and pulsate, the last to die. Further, whether the left ventricle, which in man is of greater length, and is also surrounded with thicker and more fleshy walls, and is regarded as the source of the spirits, be hotter, more spirituous, excitable, and excellent, than the right, which contains a larger quantity of blood, and is the last to become unstrung by death; in which the blood of the dying accumulates, congeals, and is deprived of life and spirit; to which, moreover, as to a fountain head, the first umbilical veins bring their blood, and from which they themselves derive their origin.

So much appears from careful observation of the order observed in the production of the parts, and certain other points that follow as deductions from these, and do not a little militate against the commonly received physiological doctrines, viz.: since it is manifest that sensation and motion exist before the brain, all sensation and motion do not proceed from the brain; from our history it is clearly ascertained that sense and movement inhere in the very first drop of blood produced in the egg, before there is a vestige of the body. The first scaffolding or rudiment of the body, too, which we have said is merely mucilaginous, before any of the extremities are visible, and when the brain is nothing more than a limpid fluid, if lightly pricked, will move obscurely, will contract and twist itself like a worm or caterpillar, so that it is very evidently possessed of sensation.

There are yet other arguments deduced from sense and motion whence we should infer that the brain was not so much the first principle of the body, in the way the medical writers maintain, as the heart, agreeably to Aristotle's view.

The motions and actions which physicians style *natural*, because they take place involuntarily, and we can neither prevent nor moderate, accelerate nor retard them by our will, and they therefore do not depend on the brain, still do not occur entirely without causing sensation, but proclaim themselves subject to sense, inasmuch as they are aroused, called forth, and changed thereby. When the heart, for example, is affected with palpitation, tremor, lipothymia, syncope, and with great variety in the extent, rapidity, and order or rhythm of its pulsations, we do not hesitate to ascribe these to morbific causes implicating, deranging its sensation. For whatever by its divers movements strives against irritations and troubles must necessarily be endowed with sensation.

The stomach and bowels, disturbed by the presence of vitiated humours, are affected with ructus, flatus, vomiting, and diarrhœa; and as it lies not in our power either to provoke or to restrain their motions, neither are we aware of any sensation dependent on the brain which should arouse the parts in question to motions of the kind.

It is truly wonderful to observe the effect of taking a solution of antimony, which we neither distinguish by the taste, nor find any inconvenience from, whether in the swallowing or the rejection. Nevertheless there is a certain discriminating sense in the stomach which distinguishes what is hurtful from what is useful, and by which vomiting is induced.

Nay, the flesh itself readily distinguishes a poisoned wound from one that is not poisoned, and on receipt of the former contracts and condenses itself, whereby phlegmonous tumours are produced, as we find in connexion with the stings of bees, gnats, and spiders.

I have myself, for experiment's sake, occasionally pricked my hand with a clean needle, and then having rubbed the same needle on the teeth of a spider, I have pricked my hand in another place. I could not by my simple sensation perceive any difference between the two punctures; nevertheless there was a capacity in the skin to distinguish the one from the other; for the part pricked with the envenomed needle immediately contracted into a tubercle, and by and by became red, and hot, and inflamed, as if it collected and girded itself up for a contest with the poison for its overthrow.

The sensations which accompany affections of the uterus, such as twisting, decubitus, prolapse, ascent, suffocation, &c., and other inconveniences and irritations, do not depend on

the brain or on common sensation; yet neither are these to
be presumed as happening without all consciousness. For
that which is wholly without sense is not seen to be irritated by any means, neither can it be stimulated to motion or
action of any kind. Nor have we any other means of distinguishing between an animate and sentient thing and one that
is dead and senseless than the motion excited by some other
irritating cause or thing, which as it incessantly follows, so
does it also argue sensation.

But we shall have an opportunity of speaking farther of this
matter when we discuss the actions and uses of the brain.
Respect for our predecessors and for antiquity at large inclines
us to defend their conclusions to the extent that love of truth
will allow. Nor do I think it becoming in us to neglect and
make little of their labours and conclusions who bore the
torch that has lighted us to the shrine of philosophy. I am,
therefore, of opinion that we should conclude in this way : we
have consciousness in ourselves of five principal senses, by
which we judge of external objects; but we do not feel with
the same sense by means of which we are conscious that we
feel—seeing with our eyes, we still do not know by them that
we see, but by another sense or sensitive organ, namely, the
internal common sensation or common sensorium, by which
we examine those things that reach us through each of the
external sensoria, and distinguish that which is white from
that which is sweet or hard. Now this sensorium commune
to which the species or impressions of all the external instruments of sensation are referred, is obviously the brain, which
along with its nerves and the external organs annexed, is held
and esteemed to be the adequate instrument of sensation.
And this brain is like a sensitive root to which a variety of
fibres tend, one of which sees, another hears, a third touches,
and a fourth and a fifth smell and taste.

But as there are some actions and motions the government
or direction of which is not dependent on the brain, and which
are therefore called *natural*, so also is it to be concluded that
there is a certain sense or form of touch which is not referred
to the common sensorium, nor in any way communicated
to the brain, so that we do not perceive by this sense that we
feel; but, as happens to those who are deranged in mind, or

who are agitated to such a degree by violent passion that they feel no pain, and pay no regard to the impressions made on their senses, so must we believe it to be with this sense, which we therefore distinguish from the proper animal sense. Now such a sense do we observe in zoophytes or plant-animals, in sponges, the sensitive plant, &c.

Wherefore, as many animals are endowed with both sense and motion without having a common sensorium or brain, such as earthworms, caterpillars of various kinds, chrysalides, &c., so also do certain natural actions take place in the embryo and even in ourselves without the agency of the brain, and a certain sensation takes place without consciousness. And as medical writers teach that the natural differ from the animal actions, so by parity of reason does the natural sense of touch differ from the animal sense of touch,—it constitutes, in a word, another species of touch; and whilst the one is communicated to the common sensorium, the other is not so communicated.

Further, it is one thing for a muscle to be contracted and moved, and another for it by regulated contractions and relaxations to perform any movement, such as progression or prehension. The muscles or organs of motion, when affected with spasms or convulsions from an irritating cause, are assuredly moved no otherwise than the decapitated cock or hen, which is agitated with many convulsive movements of its legs and wings, but all confused and without a purpose, because the controlling power of the brain has been taken away:—common sensation has disappeared, under the controlling influence of which these motions were formerly coordinated to progression by walking or to flight.

We therefore conceive the fact to be that all the natural motions proceed from the power of the heart, and depend on it; the spontaneous motions, however, and those that complete any motion which physicians entitle an animal motion, cannot be performed without the controlling influence of the brain and common sensation. For inasmuch as by this common sensation we are conscious of our perceptions, so also are we conscious that we move, and this whether the motion be regular or otherwise.

We have an excellent example of both of these kinds of motion in respiration. For the lungs, like the heart, are con-

tinually carried upwards and downwards by a natural movement, and are excited by any irritation to coughing and more
frequent action; but they cannot form and regulate the voice,
nor can singing be executed, without the assistance, and in
some sort the command, of the sensorium commune.

But these matters will be more fully handled when we come
to speak of the actions and uses of the brain, and to consider
the vital principle or soul. So much we have thought fit to
say by the way, that we might show the respect in which we
hold our illustrious teachers, and our anxiety to carry them
along with us in our labours.

EXERCISE THE FIFTY-EIGHTH.

Of the nutrition of the chick in ovo.

That the authority of the ancients is not to be rashly thrown
off appears in this: it was formerly current doctrine, though
many at the present day, Fabricius[1] among the number, reject
it as a delusion and a foolish idea, that the embryo sucked in
its mother's womb. This idea nevertheless had Democritus,
Epicurus, and Hippocrates for its supporters; and the father
of physic contends for it on two principal grounds: " Unless
the foetus sucked," he says,[2] "how should excrements be
formed? or how should it know how to suck immediately after
it is born?"

Now, whilst in other instances it is customary to swear by
the bare statement of this ancient and most distinguished
writer, his *ipse dixit* (αὐτὸς ἔφη) sufficing, because he here
makes an assertion contrary to the commonly received
opinion, Fabricius not only denies the statement, but spurns
the arguments in support of his conclusion. We, however,
leave it to the judgment of skilful anatomists and learned
physicians to say whether our observations on the generation of
animals do not proclaim this opinion of Hippocrates to be not
merely probable, but even necessary.

All admit that the foetus in utero swims in the midst of an

[1] De Form. Foetu, pp. 19 et 134.   [2] Lib. de Carn. et de Nat. Pueri.

abundance of a watery fluid, which in our history of the egg we have spoken of as the colliquament, this fluid modern authorities regard as the sweat and excrement of the fœtus, and ascribe as its principal use the protection of the uterus against injury from the fœtus during any violent motion of the mother in running or leaping; and, on the other hand, the defence of the fœtus from injury through contact with neighbouring bones, or an external cause, particularly during the period when its limbs are still delicate and weak.

Fabricius[1] ascribes additional uses to this fluid, viz. " that it may moisten and lubricate all the parts around, and dispose the neck of the uterus to facile and speedy dilatation to the utmost extent; and all this is not less assisted by that thick, white, excrementitious matter of the third digestion, neglected by the ancients, which is unctuous and oily, and farther prevents the sweat, which may occasionally be secreted sharp and salt in quality, from excoriating the tender body of the fœtus."

I readily acknowledge all the uses indicated, viz. that the tender fœtus may be secure against all sudden and violent movements of the mother, that he may ride safe in the " bat's wings," as they are called, and, surrounded with an abundance of water, that he may escape coming into contact with his mother's sides, being restrained by the retinacular fluid on either hand : this circumambient fluid must certainly protect the body which floats in its middle from all external injury. But, as in many other instances, my observations compel me here to be of a different opinion from Fabricius. In the first place, I am by no means satisfied that this fluid is the sweat of the fœtus. And then I do not believe that the fluid serves those important purposes in parturition which he indicates; and much less that it is ever so sharp and saline that an unctuous covering was requisite to protect the fœtus from its erosive effects, particularly in those cases where there is already a thick covering of wool, or hair, or feathers. The fluid, in fact, has a pleasant taste, like that of watery milk, so that almost all viviparous animals lap it up, and cleanse their new-born progeny by licking them with their tongues, greedily

---

[1] Op. cit. p. 137.

swallowing the fluid, though none of them was ever seen to touch any of the excrements of their young.

Fabricius spoke of this fluid as saline and acrimonious, because he believed it to be sweat. But what inconvenience, I beseech you, were sweat to the chick, already covered with its feathers?—if indeed any one ever saw a chicken sweat. Nor do I think he could have said that the use of this fluid in the egg was, by its moistening and lubrifying qualities, to facilitate the birth of the chick; for the drier and older the shell of the egg, the more friable and fragile it becomes. Finally, were it the sweat of the embryo, or fœtus, it ought to be most abundant nearest the period of parturition : the larger the fœtus and the more food it consumes, the more sweat must it necessarily secrete. But shortly before the exclusion of the chick from the egg, namely, about the nineteenth or twentieth day, there is none of the fluid to be seen, because as the chick grows it is gradually taken up; so that if the thing be rightly viewed, the fluid in question ought rather to be regarded as nutriment than as excrement, particularly as he has said that the chick in the egg breathes, and lets its chirping be heard, which it certainly would not do were it surrounded with water.

But all experienced obstetricians know that the watery fluid of the secundines is of no great use either in lubricating the parts or in facilitating the progress of parturition in the way Fabricius would have it. For the parts surrounding the vulva are relaxed of themselves, and by a kind of proper maturity at the full time, without any assistance from the uterine waters; and particularly those that offer the greatest obstacles to the advance of the fœtus, namely, the ossa pubis and the os coccygis, to which the attention of the midwife is especially directed in assisting the woman in labour. For midwives are much less studious to anoint the soft parts with any emollient salves, lest they tear, than careful to pull the os coccygis outwards, a business in which, if the fingers do not suffice, they have recourse to the uterine speculum, applied by the hand of the experienced surgeon, an instrument having three sides or branches, one of which bearing on the os coccygis, the other two on the ossa pubis, the business of distension is effected by force. For the head of the child that is about

to be born, when it makes the turn, and is forced downwards, relaxes and opens the os uteri; but coming down
he will stick fast, and scarcely be brought forth if he chance
to abut upon the point of the os coccygis, and immediately the
case is one not without danger both to the child and mother. But
nature's intention was obviously to relax and soften all the parts
concerned; and the attendant knows that when the uterine
orifice is discovered in a soft and lax condition, by the finger
introduced, it is an infallible sign that the delivery is at hand
even though the waters have not broken. Indeed—and I do
not speak without experience—if anything remains in the
uterus for expulsion, either after delivery or at any other time,
and the uterus make efforts to get rid of it, the orifice both
descends lower and is found soft and relaxed. If the uterine
orifice recedes, and is found somewhat hard after delivery, it is
a sign of the woman's restoration to health.

Taught by like experience, I assert that the ossa pubis frequently become loosened during labour, their cartilaginous
connexion being softened, and the whole hypogastric region
enlarged in the most miraculous manner, not, however, by any
pouring out of watery fluids, but spontaneously, as ripe fruit
gapes that the included seed may find an exit. The degree in
which the coccyx may impede delivery, however, is apparent
among quadrupeds having tails, which can neither bring forth,
nor even discharge the excrement from their bowels, unless the
tail be raised; if you but depress the tail with your hand, you
prevent the exit of the dung.

Moreover, the most natural labour of all is held to be that
in which the fœtus and afterbirth, the waters inclusive, or the
ovum, is expelled entire. Now if the membranes have not
given way, and the waters have not escaped, it comes to pass
that the surrounding parts are more than usually distended
and dilated by the labour pains, in consequence, to wit, of the
entire and tense state of the membranes, by which it happens
that the fœtus is produced more speedily, and with a less
amount of effort, although with more suffering to the mother.
In cases of this kind we have known women who were suffering
much in their travail in consequence of the too great distension, immensely relieved by the rupture of the membranes
and the sudden escape of the waters, the laceration being

effected either with the nails of the midwife or the use of a pair of forceps.

Experienced midwives are farther aware that if the waters come away before the orifice of the uterus is duly dilated, the woman is apt to have a lingering time and a more difficult delivery, contrary to Fabricius's notion of the waters having such paramount influence in softening and lubricating the parts.

Moreover, that the fluid which we have called colliquament is not the sweat of the fœtus is made obvious, both from the history of the egg and of the uterogestation of other animals : it is present before the fœtus is formed in any way, before there is a trace of it to be seen ; and whilst it is still extremely small and entirely gelatinous, the quantity of water present is very great, so that it seems plainly impossible that so small a body should produce such a mass of excrementitious fluid.

It happens besides that the ramifications of the umbilical veins are distributed over and terminate upon the membrane which incloses this fluid, precisely as on the membranes of the albumen and yelk of the egg, a circumstance from which, and the thing being viewed as it is in fact, it appears to be clearly proclaimed that this fluid is rather to be regarded as food than as excrement.

To me, therefore, the opinion of Hippocrates appears more probable than that of Fabricius and other anatomists, who look on this liquid as sweat, and believe that it must prove detrimental to the fœtus. I am disposed, I say, to believe that the fluid with which the fœtus is surrounded may serve it for nourishment; that the thinner and purer portions of it, taken up by the umbilical veins, may serve for the constitution and increase of the first formed parts of the embryo; and that from the remainder or the milk, taken into the mouth by suction, passed on to the stomach by the act of deglutition, and there digested or chylified, and finally absorbed by the mesenteric veins, the new being continues to grow and be nourished. I am the more disposed to take this view from certain not impertinent arguments, which I shall proceed to state.

As soon as the embryo acquires a certain degree of perfection it moves its extremities, and begins to prove the actions of the organs destined to locomotion. Now I have seen the chick in ovo, surrounded with liquid, opening its mouth, and any fluid that thus gained access to the fauces must needs have been swallowed; for it is certain that whatever passes the root of the tongue and gains the top of the œsophagus, cannot be rejected by any animal with a less effort than that of vomiting. This fact is acted upon every day by veterinary practitioners, who in administering medicated drinks and pills or boluses to cattle, seize the tongue, and having put the article upon its root beyond the protuberant part, the animal cannot do otherwise than swallow it. And if we make the experiment ourselves, we find that a pill carried between the finger and thumb as far as the root of the tongue and there dropped, immediately the action of deglutition is excited, and unless vomiting be produced the pill is taken down. If the embryo swimming in the fluid in question, then, do but open his mouth, it is absolutely necessary that the fluid must reach the fauces; and if the creature then move other muscles, wherefore should we not believe that he also uses his throat in its appropriate office and swallows the fluid?

It is further quite certain that in the crop of the chick,—and the same thing occurs in reference to the stomach of other embryos—there is a certain matter having a colour, taste, and consistence, very similar to that of the liquid mentioned, and some of it in the stomach digested to a certain extent, like coagulated milk; and further, whilst we discover a kind of chyle in the upper intestines, we find the lower bowels full of stercoraceous excrements. In like manner we perceive the large intestines of the fœtuses of viviparous animals to contain excrements of the same description as those that distend them when they feed on milk. In the sheep and other bisulcated animals we even find scybala.

Towards the seventeenth day we find dung very obviously near the anus of the chick; and shortly before the extrusion I have seen the same matter expelled and contained within the membranes. Volcher Coiter, a careful and experienced dissector, states that he has observed the same thing.

Wherefore should we doubt, then, that the fœtus in utero sucks, and that chylopoiesis goes on in its stomach, when we find present both the principles and the recrementitious products of digestion?

And then, when we find the bladder both of the bile and the

urine full of those excrements of the second digestion, wherefore should we not conclude that the first digestion, or chylopoiesis, has preceded ?

The embryo, therefore seeks for and sucks in nourishment by the mouth ; and you will readily believe that he does so if you rip him from his mother's womb and instantly put a finger in his mouth; which Hippocrates thinks he would not seize had he not previously sucked whilst in the womb. For we are accustomed to see young infants trying various motions, making experiments, as it were, approaching everything, moving their limbs, attempting to walk, and uttering sounds, acts all of which when taught by repeated experience, they afterwards come to execute with readiness and precision. But the fœtus so soon as it is born, aye, before it is born, will suck; doubtless as it had done in the uterus long before. For I have found by experience that the child delayed in the birth, and before it has cried or breathed, will seize and suck a finger put into its mouth. A new-born infant, indeed, is more expert at sucking than an adult, or than he is himself if he have but lost the habit for a few days. For the infant does not suck by squeezing the nipple with his lips as we should, and by suction in the common acceptation ; he rather seems as if he would swallow the nipple, drawing it wholly into his throat, and with the aid of his tongue and palate, and chewing, as it were, he milks his mother with more art and dexterity than an adult could practise. He therefore appears to have learned that by long custom, and before he saw the light, which we know full well he unlearns by a very brief discontinuance.

These and other observations of the same kind make it extremely probable that the chick in ovo is nourished in a twofold manner, namely, by the umbilical and by the mesenteric veins. By the former he imbibes a nourishment that is well nigh perfectly prepared, whence the first-formed parts are engendered and augmented ; by the latter he receives chyle for the structure and growth of the other remaining parts.

But the reason is perhaps obscure why the same agent should perform the work of nutrition by means of the same matter in a variety of ways, since nature does nothing in vain. We shall therefore endeavour to explain this.

What is taken up by the umbilical veins is the purer and

more limpid part; and the rest of the colliquament in which the fœtus swims is like crude milk, or milk deprived of its purer portion. The purer part does not require any of that ulterior concoction of which the remainder stands in need; and to undergo which it is taken into the stomach, where it is transmuted into chyle. Similar to this is the crude and watery milk which is found in the breasts immediately after parturition. The liquefied albumen of the egg, and the crude or watery milk of the mammæ seem to have in all respects the same colour, taste, and consistence. For the first flow of milk is serous and watery, and women are wont to express water from their breasts before the milk comes white, concocted, and perfect.

Just as the colliquament found in the crop of the chick is a kind of crude milk, whilst the same fluid discovered in the stomach is concocted, white, and curdled; so in viviparous animals, before the milk is concocted in the mammæ, a kind of dew and colliquament makes its appearance there, and the colliquament only puts on the semblance of milk after it has undergone concoction in the stomach. And so it happens, in Aristotle's opinion, that the first and most essential parts are formed out of the purer and thinner portion of the colliquament, and are increased by the remaining more indifferent portion after it has undergone elaboration by a new digestion in the stomach. In the same way are the other less important parts developed and maintained. Thus has nature, like a fond and indulgent mother, been sedulous rather to provide superfluity, than to suffer any scarcity of things necessary. Or it might be said to be in conformity with reason to suppose that the fœtus, now grown more perfect, should also be nourished in a more perfect manner, by the mouth, to wit, and by a more perfect kind of aliment, rendered purer by having undergone the two antecedent digestions and been thereby freed from the two kinds of excrementitious matter. In the beginning and early stages, nourished by the ramifications of the umbilical veins, it leads in some sort the life of a plant; the body is then crude, white, and imperfect; like plants, too, it is motionless and impassive. As soon, however, as it begins by the mouth to partake of the same aliment farther elaborated, as if feeling a diviner influence, boasting a higher grade of vegetative existence, the gelatinous mass of the body is changed into flesh, the organs of motion are distinguished, the spirits are perfected, and motion begins; nor is it any longer nourished like a vegetable, by the roots, but, living the life of an animal, it is supported by the mouth.

Of the uses of the entire egg.

Having now gone through the several changes and processes which must take place in the hen's egg, in order that it may produce a chick, Fabricius proceeds to consider the uses of the egg at large, and of its various parts; nor does he restrict himself to the hen's egg, but condescends upon eggs in general. Among other things he inquires: wherefore some eggs are heterogeneous and composed of different elements; and others are homogeneous and similar? such as the eggs of insects, and those creatures that are engendered from the whole egg, viz. by metamorphosis, and are not engendered from one part of the egg, and nourished by another part.

I have no purpose myself of entering on a general consideration of eggs of all kinds and descriptions; I have not yet given the history of all, but only of the hen's egg; so that I shall here limit myself to a survey of the uses of the common hen's egg, keeping in view the end of all its actions, which is nothing less than the production and completion of a new being, as Fabricius has well and truly said.[1]

Among the points having reference to the whole egg, Fabricius speaks of the form, dimensions, and number of eggs. "The figure of the egg is round," he says,[2] "in order that the mass of the chick may be stowed in the smallest possible space; for the same cause that God made the world round, namely, that it might embrace all things; and it is from this, as Galen conceives, that this figure is always felt to be most agreeable and consonant to nature. Further, as it has no angles exposed to injury from without, it is, therefore, the safest figure, and the

---

[1] Loc. cit. p. 50.   [2] Lib. x, de usu part.

one best adapted to effect the exclusion of the chick." It had been well after such a preface to have assigned satisfactory causes why hen's eggs are not spherical, like the eggs of fishes, worms and frogs, but oblong and pointed; to have shown what there is in them which hinders the presumed perfection of figure. Now to me the form of the egg has never appeared to have aught to do with the engenderment of the chick, but to be a mere accident; and to this conclusion I come the rather when I see such diversities in the shape of the eggs of different hens. They vary, in short, in conformity with the variety that obtains among the uteri of different fowls, in which, as in moulds, they receive their form.

Aristotle,[1] indeed, says that the longer-shaped eggs produce females, the rounder males. I have not made any experiments upon this point myself. But Pliny[2] asserts, in opposition to Aristotle, that the rounder eggs produce females, the others males. Now were there any certainty in such statements, either in one way or the other, some hens would always produce males, others always females, inasmuch as the eggs of the same hen are in many instances always of one figure, namely, either much rounded or acutely pointed. Horace[3] thought that the oblong eggs, as being the more perfect and better corcocted, and therefore the better flavoured, produced males.

I willingly pass by the reasons alleged by Fabricius for the form of eggs, as being all irrelevant.

The size of an egg appears to bear a proportion to the size of the fœtus produced from it; large hens, too, certainly lay large eggs. The crocodile, however, lays eggs the size of those of the goose; nor does any animal attain to larger dimensions from a smaller beginning. It would seem, too, that the size of the egg and the quantity of matter it contained had some connexion with its fecundity, inasmuch as the very small eggs called centenines are all barren.

The number of eggs serves the same end as abundance of conceptions among viviparous animals—they secure the perpetuity of the species. Nature appears to have been particularly careful in providing a numerous offspring to those animals which, by reason of their pusillanimity or bodily weakness, hardly

---

[1] Hist. Anim. lib. vi, cap. 2.   [2] Lib. x, cap. 52.   [3] Plin. ibid.

defend themselves against the attacks of others ; she has coun-
terbalanced the shortness of their own lives by the number of
their progeny. " Nature," says Pliny,[1] " has made the timid
tribes among birds more fruitful than the bold ones." All
generation as it is instituted by nature for the sake of perpetuating species, so does it occur more frequently among those
that are shorter-lived and more obnoxious to external injury
lest their race should fail. Birds that are of stronger make,
that prey upon other creatures, and therefore live more securely
and for longer terms scarcely lay more than two eggs once a
year. Pigeons, turtle and ring-doves, that lay but a couple of
eggs, make up for the smallness of the number by the frequency of laying, for they will produce young as often as ten
times in the course of a year. They therefore engender greatly
although they do not produce many at a time.

Of the uses of the yelk and albumen.

" An egg," says Fabricius,[2] " properly so called, is composed
of many parts, because it is the organ of the engenderer, and
Galen everywhere insists on the constitution of an organ as im-
plying multiplicity of parts." But this view leads us to ask
whether every egg must not be heterogeneous, seeing that every
egg is organic? And every egg, indeed, even that of the fish
and insect, appears to be composed of several different parts,—
membranes, coverings, defences ; nor is the included matter by
any means without diversity of constitution in different parts.

Fabricius agrees farther, and correctly, with Galen, when he
says :[3] Some parts of the egg are the chief instruments of the
actions that take place in it, others may be styled necessary,—
without them no actions could take place ; others exist that the
action which takes place may be better performed ; others, in
fine, are destined for the safety and preservation of all of these."
But he is mistaken when he says : " If we speak of the prime

---

[1] Lib. x, cap. 52.   [2] Op. supra, id. p. 47.   [3] Ib. p. 48.

action, which is the generation of the chick, the chief cause of this is the semen and the chalazæ, these two being the prime cause of the generation of the chick, the semen being the efficient cause, the chalaza the matter only." Now according to the opinion of Aristotle, it must be allowed that that which generates is included in the egg; but Fabricius denies that the semen of the cock is contained in the egg.

Nor does he wander less wide of the mark when he speaks of the chalazæ as the matter from which, by the influence of the semen galli, the chick is incorporated. For the chick is not produced either from one or the other, nor yet from both of the chalazæ, as we have shown in our history. Neither is the generation of the chick effected by metamorphosis, nor by any new form assumed and division effected in the chalazæ, but by epigenesis, in the manner already explained. Nor are the chalazæ especially fecundated by the semen of the male bird, but the cicatricula rather, or the part which we have called the eye of the egg, from which, when it enlarges, the colliquament is produced, in and from which, subsequently, the blood, the veins, and the pulsating vesicles proceed, after which the whole body is gradually formed. Moreover, on his own admission, the semen of the cock never enters the uterus of the hen, and yet it fecundates not only the eggs that are already formed, but others that are yet to be produced.

Fabricius refers the albumen and vitellus to the second action of the egg, which is the nutrition and growth of the chick. " The vitellus and albumen," he says,[1] " are in quantity commensurate with the perfect performance of this action, and with the due development and growth of the chick. The shell and membranes are therefore the safety of the whole of the egg as well as the security of its action. But the veins and arteries which carry nourishment are organs without which the action of the egg, in other words, the growth and nutrition of the chick, would not take place." It is uncertain, however, whether the umbilical vessels of the embryo or the veins and arteries of the mother, whence the egg is increased, are here to be understood. For a like reason the uterus and incubation ought to be referred to this last class of actions.

[1] Op. cit. p. 48.

We have to do, then, with the two fluids of the egg, the albumen and the vitellus; for these, before all the other parts, are formed for the use of the embryo, and in them is the second action of the egg especially conspicuous.

The egg of the common hen is of two colours internally, and consists of two fluids, severally distinct, separated by membranes, and in all probability of different natures, and therefore having different ends to serve, inasmuch as they are distinguished by different extensions of the umbilical veins, one of them proceeding to the white, another to the yelk. " The yelk and white of the egg are of opposite natures," says Aristotle,[1] " not only in colour, but also in power. For the yelk is congealed by cold; the white is not congealed, but is rather liquefied; on the contrary, the white is coagulated by heat, the yelk is not coagulated, but remains soft, unless it be overdone, and is more condensed and dried by boiling than by roasting." The vitellus getting heated during incubation, is rendered more moist; for it becomes like melted wax or tallow, whereby it also takes up more room. For as the embryo grows, the albumen is gradually taken up and becomes inspissated; but the yelk, even when the fœtus has attained perfection, appears scarcely to have diminished in size; it is only more diffluent and moist, even when the fœtus begins to have its abdomen closed in.

Aristotle[2] gives the following reason for the diversity: " Since the bird cannot perfect her offspring within herself, she produces it along with the aliment needful to its growth in the egg. Viviparous animals again prepare the food (milk) in another part of their body, namely, the breasts. Now nature has done the same thing in the egg; but otherwise than as is generally presumed, and as Alcmæon Crotoniates states it, for it is not the albumen but the vitellus which is the milk of the egg."

For as the fœtus of a viviparous animal draws its nourishment from the uterus whilst it is connected with its mother, like a plant by its roots from the earth; but after birth, and when it has escaped from the womb, sucks milk from the breast, and thereby continues to wax in size and strength, the

---

[1] Hist. Anim. lib. vii, cap. 2.   [2] De Gen. Anim. lib. iii, cap. 2.

chick finds the analogue of both kinds of food in the egg. So that whilst in viviparous animals the uterus exists within the parent, in oviparous the parent may rather be said to exist within the uterus (the egg). For the egg is a kind of exposed and detached uterus, and in it are included in some sort vicarious mammæ. The chick in the egg, I say, is first nourished by albumen, but afterwards, when this is consumed, by the yelk or by milk. The umbilical vascular connexion with the albumen, therefore, when this fluid is used up, withers and is interrupted when the abdomen comes to be closed, and before the period of exclusion arrives, so that it leaves no trace of its existence behind it: in viviparous animals, on the contrary, the umbilical cord is permanent in all its parts up to the moment of birth. The other canal that extends to the vitellus, however, is taken up along with this matter into the abdomen, where being stored, it serves for the support of the delicate fœtus until its beak has acquired firmness enough to seize and bruise its food, and its stomach strength sufficient to comminute and digest it; just as the young of the viviparous animal lives upon milk from the mammæ of its mother, until it is provided with teeth by which it can masticate harder food. For the vitellus is as milk to the chick, as has been already said; and the bird's egg, as it stands in lieu both of uterus and mammæ, is furnished with two fluids of different colours, the white and the yelk.

All admit this distinction of fluids. But I, as I have already said, distinguish two albumens in the egg, kept separate by an interposed membrane, the more external of which embraces the other within it, in the same way as the yelk is surrounded by the albumen in general. I have also insisted on the diverse nature of these albumens; distinguished both by situation and their surrounding membranes, they seem in like manner calculated for different uses. Both, however, are there for ends of nutrition, the outermost, as that to which the branches of the umbilical veins are earliest distributed, being first consumed, and then the inner and thicker portion; last of all the vitellus is attacked, and by it is the chick nourished, not only till it escapes from the shell but for some time afterwards.

But upon this point we shall have more to say below, when we come to speak of the manner in which the fœtuses of viviparous animals are developed, and at the same time demonstrate that these all derive their origin from eggs, and live by a twofold albuminous food in the womb. One of these is thinner, and contained within the ovum or conception; the other is obtained by the umbilical vessels from the placenta and uterine cotyledons. The fluid of the ovum resembles a dilute albumen in colour and consistence; it is a sluggish, pellucid liquid, in all respects similar to that which we have called the colliquament of the egg, in which the embryo swims, and on which it feeds by the mouth. The fluid which the fœtus obtains from the uterine placenta by the aid of the umbilical vessels is more dense and mucaginous, like the inspissated albumen. Whence it clearly appears that the fœtus in utero is no more nourished by its parent's blood than is the suckling afterwards, or the chick in ovo; but that it is nourished by an albuminous matter concocted in the placenta, and not unlike white of egg.

Nor is the contemplation of the Divine Providence less useful than delightful when we see nature, in her work of evolving the fœtus, furnishing it with sustenance adapted to its varying ages and powers, now more easy, by and by more difficult of digestion. For as the fœtus acquires greater powers of digesting, so is it supplied with food that is successively thicker and harder. And the same thing may be observed in the milk of animals generally: when the young creature first sees the light the milk is thinner and more easy of concoction; but in the course of time, and with increased strength in the suckling, it becomes thicker, and is more abundantly stored with caseous matter. Those flabby and delicate women, therefore, who do not nurse their own children, but give them up to the breast of another, consult their health indifferently; for mercenary nurses being for the major part of more robust and hardy frames, and their milk consequently thicker, more caseous, and difficult of digestion, it frequently happens that milk of this kind given to the infants of such parents, particularly during the time of teething, is not well borne, but gives rise to crudities and diarrhœas, to griping, vomiting, fever, epilepsy, and other formidable diseases of the like nature.

What Fabricius says,[1] and strives to bolster up by certain

[1] Op. cit. p. 34.

reasonings, of the chalazæ standing for the matter of the chick, we have already thrown out in our history, and at the same time have made it manifest that the substance of the chick and its first rudiments were produced whilst the chalazæ were still entire and unchanged, and in a totally different situation.

Neither is it true, as he states,[1] "that the chalazæ, rendered fruitful by the semen of the cock, stand in the place of seed, and that from them the chick is produced." Nor are the chalazæ, as he will have it,[2] "in colour, substance, and bodily properties so like seed, or bear so strong a resemblance to the embryo in a boiled egg, that we may rightly conceive all the parts designated spermatic to be thence engendered." I am rather of opinion that the fluid which we have called colliquament, or the thinner portion of the albumen liquefied and concocted, is to be regarded as of the nature of seed, and, if the testimony of our eyes is to be credited, as a substitute for it.

The observation of this venerable old man is therefore unnecessary when he says,[3] "As the whole animal body is made up of two substances very different from one another, and even of opposite natures, viz. hot and cold—among the hot parts being included all those that are full of blood and of a red colour; among the cold all those that are exsanguine and white—these two orders of parts doubtless require a different and yet a like nourishment, if it be true that we are nourished by the same things of which we are made. The spermatic, white, and cold parts, therefore, require white and cold nourishment; the sanguineous, red, and hot parts, again, demand nourishment that is red and hot. And so is the cold white of the egg properly held to nourish the cold and white parts of the chick, and the hot and sanguine yelk regarded as a substitute for the hot and purple blood. In this way do all the animal parts obtain nourishment suitable and convenient for them." Now we by no means admit that the two fluids or matters of the egg are there as appropriate means of nourishment for different orders of parts. For we have already said that the heart, lungs, kidneys, liver, spleen, muscles, bones, ligaments, &c., &c., were all alike and indiscriminately white and bloodless on their first formation.

[1] Op. cit. p. 54.   [2] Ib. p. 57.   [3] Ib. p. 55.

29

Further, on the preceding view of Fabricius it would follow that the heart, lungs, liver, spleen, &c., were not spermatic parts, did not originate from the seed (which he, however, will by no means allow), inasmuch as they too are by and by nourished by the blood and grow out of it; for every part is both formed and nourished by the same means, and nutrition is nothing more than the substitution of a like matter in the room of that which is lost.

Nor would he find less difficulty in answering the question how it happens that when the albumen in the egg is all consumed, the cold and white parts, such as the bones, ligaments, brain, spinal marrow, &c., continue to be nourished and to grow by means of the vitellus? which to these must be nourishment as inappropriate as albumen to the hot, red, and sanguine parts.

Adopting the views commented on, indeed, we should be compelled to admit that the hot and sanguineous parts were the last to be produced: the flesh after the bones; the liver, spleen, and lungs after the ligaments and intestinal canal; and further, that the cold parts of the chick must come together and attain maturity, the white being all the while consumed, and the hot parts be engendered subsequently, when the vitellus fails and ceases from nourishing them; and then it would be certain that all the parts could not take their rise in and be constituted out of the same clear liquid. All such conclusions, however, are refuted by simple ocular inspection.

I add another argument to those already supplied: the eggs of cartilaginous fishes—skates, the dog-fish, &c.,—are of two colours—their yelks are of a good deep colour; nevertheless all the parts of these fishes are white, bloodless, and cold, not even excepting the substance of their liver. On the contrary, I have seen a certain breed of fowls of large size, their feathers black, their flesh well supplied with blood, their liver red; yet were the yelks of the eggs of these fowls—fruitful eggs— of the palest shade of yellow, not deeper than the tint of ripe barley straw.

Fabricius, however, seems in these words[1] to retract all he has but just said: "There is one thing to be particularly

---

[1] Op. cit. p. 55.

wondered at both in the yelk and the white, viz. that neither of them being blood, they are still so near to the nature of blood that they in fact differ but very slightly from it—there is but little wanting to constitute either of them blood; so that little labour and a very slight concoction suffice to effect the change. The veins and arteries distributed to the membranes of both the white and yelk are consequently seen replete with blood at all times; the white and yelk nevertheless continuing possessed of their own proper nature, though either, so soon as it is imbibed by the vessels, is changed into blood, so closely do they approach in constitution to this fluid."

But if it be matter of certainty that blood exists no less in the vessels distributed to the albumen than in those sent to the vitellus, and that both of these fluids are so closely allied to blood in their nature, and turn into blood so readily; who, I beseech you, will doubt that the blood, and all the parts which are styled sanguineous, are nourished and increased through the albumen as well as the vitellus?

Our author, however, soon contrives a subterfuge from this conclusion: "Although all this be true," he says,[1] "still must we conceive that the matter which is imbibed by the veins from the yelk and white is only blood in the same sense as the chyle in the mesenteric veins, in which nothing but blood is ever seen; now chyle is but the shadow of blood, and is first perfected in the liver; and in like manner the matter taken up by the veins from the white and yellow is only the shadow of blood," &c. Be it so; but hiding under this shadow, he does not answer the question, wherefore the blood and blood-like parts should not, for the reasons cited, be equally well nourished by the albumen as by the vitellus?

Had our author, in like manner, asserted that the hotter parts are rather nourished by that blood which is derived from the vitellus than by that attracted from the albumen, and the colder parts, on the other hand, by that which is derived from the albumen, I should not myself have been much disposed to gainsay him.

There is one consideration in the whole question, however, which is sorely against him; it is this—how is the blood

---

[1] Op. cit. p. 55.

formed in the egg? by what agent is either white or yelk turned into blood whilst the liver is not yet in existence? For in the egg, at all events, he could not say that the blood was transfused from the mother. He says, indeed, "This blood is produced and concocted in the veins rather than in the liver; but it becomes bone, cartilage, flesh, &c. in the parts themselves, where it undergoes exact concoction and assimilation." In this he adds nothing; he neither tells us how or by what means perfect blood is concocted and elaborated in the minute veins both of the albumen and vitellus, the liver, as I have said, not having yet come into existence,— not a particle of any part of the body, in fact, having yet been produced by which either concoction or elaboration might be effected. And then, forgetful of what he has previously said, viz. that the hot and hæmatous parts are nourished by the vitellus and the cold and anæmic parts by the albumen, he is plainly in contradiction with himself when he admits that the same blood is turned into bone, cartilage, flesh, and all other parts.

More than this, Fabricius has slipped the greatest difficulty of all, the source of not a little doubt and debate to the medical mind, viz. how the liver should be the source and artificer of the blood, seeing that this fluid not only exists in the egg before any viscus is formed, but that all medical writers teach that the parenchymata of the viscera are but effusions of blood? Is the work the author of its workman? If the parenchyma of the liver come from the blood, how can it be the cause of the blood?

What follows is of the same likelihood: "There is another reason wherefore the albumen should be separated from the yelk, namely, that the fœtus may swim in it, and be thus supported, lest tending downwards by its own weight, it should incline to one particular part, and dragging, should break the vessels, in preventing which the viscidity and purity of the albumen contribute effectually. For did the fœtus grow amid the yelk, it might readily sink to the bottom, and so cause laceration of that body." Sufficiently jejune! For what, I entreat, can the *purity* of the albumen contribute to the support of the embryo? Or how should the thinner albumen sustain it better than the thicker and more earthy yelk? Or where the danger, I ask, of its sinking down, when we see that the egg in incubation is always laid on its side, and there is nothing to fear either for the ascent or the descent of the embryo? It is indubitable, indeed, that not only does the embryo of the chick float in the egg, but that the embryo of every animal during its formation floats in the uterus; this however takes place amidst the fluid which we have called colliquament, and neither in the albumen nor vitellus, and we have elsewhere given the reason wherefore this is so.

"Aristotle informs us," says Fabricius, "that the vitellus rises to the blunt end of the egg when the chick is conceived; and this because the animal is incorporated from the chalaza, which adheres to the vitellus; whence the vitellus which was in the middle is drawn towards the upper wider part of the egg, that the chick may be produced where the natural cavity exists, which is so indispensable to its well-being." The chalaza, however, is certainly connected still more intimately with the albumen than with the yelk.

My mode of interpreting the ascent in question is this: the spot or cicatricula conspicuous on the membrana vitelli, expands under the influence of the spirituous colliquament engendered within it, and requiring a larger space, it tends towards the blunt end of the egg. The liquefied portion of the vitellus and albumen, diluted in like manner, and concocted and made more spirituous, swims above the remaining crude parts, just as the inferior particles of water in a vessel, when heated, rise from the bottom to the top, a fact which every medical man must have observed when he had chanced to put a measure of thick and turbid urine into a bath of boiling water, in which case the upper part first becomes clear and transparent. Another example will make this matter still more plain. There is an instrument familiar to almost everybody, made rather for amusement than any useful purpose, nearly full of water, on the surface of which float a number of hollow glass beads which by their lightness and swimming together support a variety of figures, Cupids with bows and quivers, chariots of the sun, centaurs armed, and the like, which would else all sink to the bottom. So also does the eye of the egg, as I have called it, or first colliquament, dilated by the heat of the incubating fowl

and genital virtue inherent in the egg, expand, and thereby
rendered lighter, rise to the top, when the vitellus, with which
it is connected follows.   It is because the cicatricula, formerly
situated on the side of the vitellus, now tends to rise directly
upwards that the thicker albumen is made to give place, and
the chalazæ are carried to the sides of the egg.

Of the uses of the other parts of the egg.

The shell is hard and thick that it may serve as a defence
against external injury to the fluids and the chick it includes.
It is brittle, nevertheless, particularly towards the blunt end,
and as the time of the chick's exclusion draws near, doubtless
that the birth may suffer no delay.   The shell is porous also;
for when an egg, particularly a very recent one, is dressed
before the fire, it sweats through its pores.   Now these pores
are useful for ventilation; they permit the heat of the incubating hen to penetrate more readily, and the chick to have
supplies of fresh air; for that it both breathes and chirps in the
egg before its exclusion is most certain.

The membranes serve to include the fluids, and therefore
are they present in the same number as these, and therefore
is the colliquament also invested, as soon as it is produced, with
a tunica propria, which Aristotle[1] refers to in these words: " A
membrane covered with ramifications of blood-vessels already
surrounds the clear liquid," &c.   But the exit of the chick
being at hand, and the albumen and colliquament being entirely
consumed, all the membranes, except that which surrounds the
vitellus, are dried up and disappear; the membrana vitelli, on
the contrary, along with the yelk, is retracted into the peritoneum of the chick and included in the abdomen.   Of the
membranes two are common to the whole egg, which they surround immediately under the shell; the rest belong, one to the
albumen, one to the yelk, one to the colliquament; but all still
conduce to the preservation and separation of the parts they

---

[1] Hist. Anim. lib. vi, cap. 3.

surround. The outer of the two common membranes which adheres to the shell is the firmer, that it may take no injury from the shell; the inner one again is smooth and soft, that it may not hurt the fluids; in the same way, therefore, as the meninges of the brain protect it from the roughness of the superincumbent skull. The internal membranes, as I have said, include and keep separate their peculiar fluids, whence they are extremely thin, pellucid, and easily torn.

Fabricius ascribes great eminence and dignity to the chalazæ, regarding them as the parts whence the chick is formed; he, however, leaves the spot or cicatricula connected with the membrana vitelli without any office whatsoever, looking on it merely as the remains of the peduncle whence the vitellus was detached from the vitellarium in the superior uterus of the hen. In his view the vitellus formerly obtained its nourishment either by this peduncle or the vessels passing through it; but when detached, and no longer nourished by the hen, a simple trace of the former connexion and important function alone remains.

I however am of opinion that the uses of the chalazæ are no other than those I have assigned them, namely, that they serve as poles to the microcosm of the egg, and are the association of all the membranes convoluted and twisted together, by which not only are the several fluids kept in their places, but also in their distinct relative positions. But I have absolute assurance that the spot or cicatricula in question is of the very highest importance; it is the part in which the calor insitus nestles; where the first spark of the vital principle is kindled; for the sake of which, in a word, the whole of the rest of the fluids and all the membranes of the egg are contrived. But this has been already insisted on above.

Formerly, indeed, I did think with Fabricius that this cicatricula was the remains or trace of the detached peduncle; but I afterwards learned by more accurate observation that this was not the case; that the peduncle, by which the vitellus hangs, was infixed in no such limited space as we find it in apples and plums, and in such a way as would have given rise to a scar on its separation. This peduncle, in short, expands like a tube from the ovary on towards the vitellus, the horizon of which it embraces in a bipartite semicircle, not otherwise than the tunica conjunctiva embraces the eye; and this in suchwise that the superior part of the vitellus, or the hemisphere which regards the ovary, is almost free from any contact or cohesion with the peduncle, in the superior part of the cup or hollow of which nevertheless, but somewhat to the side, the spot or cicatricula in question is placed. The peduncles becoming detached from the vitelli can therefore in no way be said to leave any trace of their attachments behind them. Of the great importance of this spot in generation I have already spoken in the historical portion of my work.

But I have still, always following my old teacher Fabricius as my guide on the way, to treat of the uses of the cavity in the blunt end of the egg.

Fabricius enumerates various conveniences arising from this cavity, according to its dimensions. I shall be brief on the subject: it contains air, and is therefore useful in the ventilation of the egg, assisting the perspiration, refrigeration, and respiration, and finally the chirping of the chick. Whence this cavity, small at first, is larger by and by, and at last becomes of great size, as the several offices mentioned come into play.

Thus far have we spoken of the generation of the egg and chick, and of the uses of the several parts of the egg; and to the type exhibited we have referred the mode of generation of oviparous animals in general. We have still to speak of the generation of viviparous animals, in doing which we shall as before refer all to a single familiarly known species.

EXERCISE THE SIXTY-SECOND.

An egg is the common origin of all animals.

" Animals," says Aristotle,[1] " have this in common with vegetables, that some of them arise from seed, others arise spontaneously; for as plants either proceed from the seed of other plants, or spring up spontaneously, having met with some primary condition fit for their evolution, some of them deriving their nourishment from the ground, others arising from and living on other plants; so are some animals engendered from cognate forms, and others arise spontaneously, no kind of cognate

[1] Hist. Anim. lib. 5, cap. 1.

seed having preceded their birth; and whilst some of them are generated from the earth, or putrefying vegetable matter, like so many insects, others are produced in animals themselves and from the excrementitious matters of their parts." Now the whole of these, whether they arise spontaneously, or from others, or in others, or from the parts or excrements of these, have this in common, that they are engendered from some principle adequate to this effect, and from an efficient cause inherent in the same principle. In this way, therefore, the primordium from which and by which they arise is inherent in every animal. Let us entitle this the primordium vegetale or vegetative incipience, understanding by this a certain corporeal something having life in potentia; or a certain something existing *per se*, which is capable of changing into a vegetative form under the agency of an internal principle. Such primordia are the eggs of animals and the seeds of plants; such also are the conceptions of viviparous animals, and the worm, as Aristotle calls it, whence insects proceed: the primordia of different living things consequently differ from one another; and according to their diversities are the modes of generation of animals, which nevertheless all agree in this one respect, that they proceed from the vegetal primordium as from matter endowed with the virtue of an efficient cause, though they differ in respect of the primordium which either bursts forth, as it were, spontaneously and by chance, or shows itself as fruit or seed from something else preceding it. Whence some animals are spoken of as spontaneously produced, others as engendered by parents. And these last are again distinguished by their mode of birth, for some are oviparous, others viviparous, to which Aristotle[1] adds a vermiparous class. But if we take the thing as simple sense proclaims it, there are only two kinds of birth, inasmuch as all animals engender others either in actu—virtually, or in potentia—potentially. Animals which bring forth in fact and virtually are called viviparous, those that bring forth potentially are oviparous. For every primordium that lives potentially, we, with Fabricius, think ought to be called an egg, and we make no distinction between the worm of Aristotle and an egg, both because to the eye there is no difference,

---

[1] Hist. Anim. lib. i, cap. 5.

and because the identity is in conformity with reason. For
the vegetal primordium which lives potentially is also an animal potentially. Nor can the distinction which Aristotle[1]
made between the egg and the worm be admitted: for he defines an egg to be that "from part of which an animal is produced; whilst that," he says elsewhere,[2] "which is totally
changed, and which does not produce an animal from a part
only, is a worm." These bodies, however, agree in this, that
they are both inanimate births, and only animals potentially;
both consequently are eggs.

And then Aristotle himself, whilst he speaks of worms in
one place, designates them by the name of eggs in another.[3]
Treating of the locust, he says,[4] "its eggs become spoiled in
autumn when the season is wet;" and again, speaking of the
grasshopper, he has these words, "when the little worm
has grown in the earth it becomes a matrix of grasshoppers
(tettigometra);" and immediately afterwards, "the females are
sweeter after coitus, for then they are full of white eggs."

In this very place, indeed, where he distinguishes between
an egg and a worm, he adds:[5] "but the whole of this tribe
of worms, when they have come to their full size, are changed
in some sort into eggs; for their shell or covering hardens,
and they become motionless for a season, a circumstance that
is plainly to be seen in the vermiculi of bees and wasps, and
also in caterpillars." Every one indeed may observe that the
primordia of spiders, silkworms, and the like, are not less to
be accounted eggs than those of the crustacea and mollusca,
and almost all fishes, which are not actually animals, but are
potentially possessed of the faculty of producing them. Since,
then, those creatures that produce actually are called viviparous, and those that produce potentially either pass without
any general distinguishing title or are called oviparous and particularly as such productions are vegetal primordia, analogous to
the seeds of plants, which true eggs must needs be held to be,
the conclusion is, that all animals are either viviparous or
oviparous.

But as there are many species of oviparous animals, so must

---

[1] De Gen. Anim. lib. iii, cap. 9.   [4] Hist. Anim. lib. v, cap. 30.
[2] Hist. Anim. lib. i, cap. 5.   [5] De Gen. Anim. lib. iii, cap. 9.
[3] Ib. lib. v, cap. 29.

there also be several species of eggs; for every primordium is not alike fit to receive or assume every variety of animal form indifferently. Though we admit, therefore, that eggs in a general sense do not differ, yet when we find that one is perfect, another imperfect, it is obvious that they differ essentially from one another. Perfect eggs are such as are completed in the uterus, where they obtain their due dimensions before being extruded; of this kind are the eggs of birds. Imperfect eggs, again, are such as are prematurely excluded before they are of the full size, but increase after they are laid; of this description are the eggs of fishes, crustacea and mollusca; the primordia of insects, which Aristotle entitles worms, are farther to be referred to this class, as well as the primordia of those animals that arise spontaneously.

Moreover, although perfect eggs are of two colours, in other words, are composed of albumen and vitellus, some are still only of one hue, and consist of albumen alone. In like manner, of imperfect eggs, some from which a perfect animal proceeds are properly so called; such are the eggs of fishes; others are improperly so styled, they engendering an imperfect animal, namely, a worm, grub, or caterpillar, a kind of mean between a perfect and an imperfect egg, which, in respect of the egg or the primordium itself, is an animal endowed with sense and motion, and nourishing itself; but in respect of a fly, moth or butterfly, whose primordium it is potentially, it is as a creeping egg, and to be reputed as adequate to its own growth; of this description is the caterpillar, which having at length completed its growth is changed into a chrysalis or perfect egg, and ceasing from motion, it is like an egg, an animal potentially.

In the same way, although there are some eggs from the whole of which a perfect animal is produced by metamorphosis, without being nourished by any remains of the substance of the egg, but forthwith finds food for itself abroad, there are others from one part of which the embryo is produced, and from the remainder of which it is nourished:—although, I repeat, there are such differences among eggs, still, if we be permitted to conclude on the grounds of sense and analogy, there is no good reason wherefore those that Aristotle calls worms should not be spoken of as eggs; inasmuch as all vegetal principles are not indeed animals actually, but are so potentially, are true animal seeds, analogous to the seeds of vegetables, as we have already demonstrated in the particular instance of the hen's egg. All animals are, therefore, either viviparous or oviparous, inasmuch as they all either produce a living animal in fact, or an egg, rudiment, or primordium, which is an animal potentially.

The generation of all oviparous animals may therefore be referred to that of the hen's egg as a type, or at all events deduced from thence without difficulty, the same things and incidents that have been enumerated in connexion with the common fowl being also encountered in all other oviparous animals whatsoever. The various particulars in which they differ one from another, or in which they agree, either generally, or specifically, or analogically, will be subsequently treated of when we come to speak of the generation of insects and the animals that arise equivocally. For as every generation is a kind of way leading to the attainment of an animal form, as one race of animal is more or less like or unlike another, their constituent parts either agreeing or disagreeing, so does it happen in respect of their mode of generation. For perfect nature, always harmonious with herself in her works, has instituted similar parts for similar ends and actions : to arrive at the same results, to attain the same forms, she has followed the same path, and has established one and the same method in the business of generation universally.

Wherefore as we still find the same parts in the perfect or two-coloured egg of every bird, so do we also observe the same order and method pursued in the generation and development of their embryos as we have seen in the egg of the common fowl. And so also are the same things to be noted in the eggs of serpents and of reptiles, or oviparous quadrupeds, such as tortoises, frogs, and lizards, from all the perfect two-coloured eggs of which embryos are produced and perfected in the same manner. Nor is the case very different in regard to fishes. But of the manner in which spiders and the crustacea, such as shrimps and crabs, and the mollusca, such as the cuttlefish and calamary, arise from their eggs; of the conditions also upon which worms and grubs first proceed from the eggs of insects, which afterwards change into chrysalides or aurelias, as if they reverted anew to the state of eggs, from which at length emerge flies or butterflies—of the several respects in which these differ in their mode of generation from an egg, from what we have found in the hen's egg, will be matter for remark in the proper place.

Although all eggs consisting of yelk and white are not produced and fecundated in the same manner, but some are made prolific through the intercourse of male and female, and others in some other way (as of fishes); and although there is some difference even in the mode in which eggs grow, some attaining maturity within the body of the parent, others continuing to be nourished and to grow when extruded, there is still no reason why an embryo should not be developed in the same precise manner in every egg—always understood as perfect—as it is in the egg of the hen. Wherefore the history which has been given of the evolution of the chick from the hen's egg may be regarded as applicable to the generation of all other oviparous animals whatsoever, as well as to the inferences or conclusions which may be deduced from thence.

Of the generation of viviparous animals.

Thus far have we treated mainly of the generation of oviparous animals; we have still to speak particularly of the other species of generation, the viviparous, to wit, in which many things identical with those we have noticed in oviparous generation will come to be observed. These we have reduced into order, and here at length present for consideration. Even the parts that appear paradoxical and in contradiction with the current views of generation will, I believe, be found entirely in conformity with truth.

Among viviparous animals, man, the most perfect of all creatures, occupies the foremost place; after him come our ordinary domestic animals, of which some are soliped, such as the horse and ass; others bisulcate, as the ox, goat, sheep, deer, and hog; others digitate, such as the dog, cat, rabbit, mouse, and others of the same description; from the modes of whose generation a judgment may be formed of that of all other viviparous animals. Wherefore I shall propose a single genus, by way of general example or type, as we did in the case of the oviparous class; this made familiar to us, will serve as a light or standard, by means of which all the others may be judged of by analogy.

The reasons that led me to select the hen's egg as the measure of eggs in general have been already given: eggs are of little price, and are everywhere to be obtained, conditions that permit repeated study, and enable us cheaply and readily to test the truth of statements made by others.

We have not the same facilities in studying the generation of viviparous animals: we have rarely, if ever, an opportunity of dissecting the human uterus; and then to enter on the subject experimentally in the horse, ox, sheep, goat, and other cattle, would be attended with immense labour and no small expense; dogs, cats rabbits, and the like, however, will supply those with subjects who are desirous of putting to the test of experiment the matters that are to be delivered by us in this place.

Fabricius of Aquapendente, as if every conception of a viviparous animal were in a certain sense an egg, begins his treatise with the egg as the universal example of generation; and among other reasons for his conclusions assigns this in particular:[1] "Because the study of the egg has the most extensive application, the greater number of animals being engendered from eggs." Now we, at the very outset of our observations, asserted that ALL animals were in some sort produced from eggs. For even on the same grounds, and in the same manner and order in which a chick is engendered and developed from an egg, is the embryo of viviparous animals engendered from a pre-existing conception. Generation in both is one and identical in kind: the origin of either is from an egg, or at least from something that by analogy is held to be so. An egg is, as already said, a conception exposed beyond the body of the parent, whence the embryo is produced; a conception is an egg remaining within the body of the parent until the foetus has acquired the requisite perfec-

---

[1] De Form. Ovi et Pulli, cap. 1.

tion; in everything else they agree; they are both alike primordially vegetables, potentially they are animals. Wherefore, the same theorems and conclusions, though they may appear paradoxical, which we drew from the history of the egg, turn out to be equally true with regard to the generation of animals generally. For it is an admitted fact that all embryos, even those of man, are procreated from some conception or primordium. Let us, therefore, say that that which is called primordium among things arising spontaneously, and seed among plants, is an egg among oviparous animals, i. e. a certain corporeal substance, from which, through the motions and efficacy of an internal principle, a plant or an animal of one description or another is produced; but the prime conception in viviparous animals is of the same precise nature, a fact which we have found approved both by sense and reason.

What we have already affirmed of the egg, viz. that it was the sperma or seed of animals and analogous to the seeds of plants, we now affirm of the conception, which is indeed the seed of an animal, and therefore also properly called ovum or egg. Because "a true seed," according to Aristotle,[1] "is that which derives its origin from the intercourse of male and female, and possesses the virtues of both; such as is the seed of all vegetables, and of some animals, in which the sexes are not distinct, and is, as that which is first mingled from male and female, a kind of promiscuous conception or animal; for it has those things already that are recognised of both;" i. e. matter adapted to nourish the fœtus, and a plastic or formative and effective virtue. And so in like manner is a conception the fruit of the intercourse of male and female, and the seed of the future embryo; it therefore does not differ from an egg.

" But that which proceeds from the generant is the cause which first obtains the principle of generation, (i. e. it is the efficient cause,) and ought to be called the geniture,"[2] not the seed, as is commonly done both by the vulgar and philosophers at the present time; because it has not that which is required of both the concurring agents, neither is it analogous to the seeds of plants. But whatever possesses this, and corresponds to the seeds of vegetables, that too is rightly entitled egg and conception.

[1] De Gen. Anim. lib. 1, cap. 18.   [2] Ibid.

Further, the definition of an egg, as given by Aristotle,[1] is perfectly applicable to a conception :—" An egg," he says, " is that the principal part of which goes to constitute an animal, the remainder to nourish the animal so constituted." Now the same thing is common to a conception, as shall be made to appear visibly from the dissection of viviparous animals.

Moreover, as the chick is excluded from the egg under the influence of warmth derived from the incubating hen or obtained in any other way, even so is the fœtus produced from the conception in the uterus under the genial warmth of the mother's body. In few words, I say, that what oviparous animals supply by their breast and incubation, viviparous animals afford by their uterus and internal embrace. For the rest, in all that respects the development, the embryo is produced from the conception in the same manner and order as the chick from the egg, with this single difference, that whatever is required for the formation and growth of the chick is present in the egg, whilst the conception, after the formation of the embryo, derives from the uterus of the mother whatever more is requisite to its increase, by which it continues to grow in common with the fœtus. The egg, on the contrary, becomes more and more empty as the chick increases; the nutriment that was laid up in it is diminished; nor does the chick receive aught in the shape of new aliment from the mother; whilst the fœtus of viviparous animals has a continued supply, and when born, moreover, continues to live upon its mother's milk. The eggs of fishes, however, increase through nourishment obtained from without; and insects and crustaceous and molluscous animals have eggs that enlarge after their extrusion. Yet are not these called eggs the less on this account, nor, indeed, are they therefore any the less eggs. In like manner the conception is appropriately designated by the name of ovum or egg, although it requires and procures from without the variety of aliment that is needful to its growth.

Fabricius gives this reason for some animals being oviparous, for all not producing living offspring : " It is," he says, " that eggs detained in the uterus till they had produced their chicks would interfere with the flight of birds, and weigh them

---

[1] Hist. Anim. lib. i, cap. v.

down by their weight. Serpents would also be hindered in their alternate zig-zag movements by a multitude of eggs in the abdomen. In the body of tortoises, with their hard and girding shell, there is no room for any store or increase of eggs; nor would the abdomen of fishes suffice for the multitude of eggs they must spawn were these to grow to any size. It was, therefore, matter of necessity that those creatures should lay their eggs imperfect. It seems most natural that an animal should retain and cherish its conception in its interior until the fœtus it produces has come to maturity; but nature sees herself compelled, as it were, occasionally to permit the premature birth of various eggs, and to provide them, without the body of the parent, with the nourishment they require for their complete development. As to everything that refers to the evolution of the fœtus, all animals are engendered from an oviform primordium; I say oviform, not as meaning that it has the precise configuration of an egg, but the nature and constitution of one; this being common in generation, that the vegetal primordium whence the fœtus is produced, including the nature of an egg, corresponding in its proportions to the seed of a plant, pre-exists. In all vegetal primordia, consequently, whether eggs, or having the form of eggs, there are inherent the nature and conditions of an egg, properties which the seeds of plants have in common with the eggs òf animals. The primordium of any animal, whatsoever, is therefore called seed and fruit; and in like manner the seed of every plant is spoken of as a kind of conception or egg.

And this is the reason why Aristotle says:[1] "Animals that engender internally have something formed in the fashion of an egg after their first conception: there is a fluid contained within a delicate membrane, like en egg without the shell. And this is the cause why the disorders of the conception, which are apt to occur in the early period, are called discharges." Such a discharge is particularly observed among women when they miscarry in the course of the first or second month. I have repeatedly seen such ova aborted at this time; and such was the one which Hippocrates has described as having been thrown off by the female pipe-player in consequence of a fall.

---

[1] De Gen. Anim. lib. iii, cap. 9.

30

In the uterus of all animals there is consequently present a prime conception or primordium, which, on Aristotle's testimony,[1] "is like an egg surrounded with a membrane from which the shell had been removed." This fact will appear still more plainly from what is about to be said. Meantime let us conclude with the philosopher, "that all living creatures, whether they swim, or walk, or fly, and whether they come into the world with the form of an animal or of an egg, are engendered in the same manner."

EXERCISE THE SIXTY-FOURTH.

The generation of viviparous animals in general is illustrated from the history of that of the hind and doe, and the reason of this selection.

It was customary with his Serene Majesty, King Charles, after he had come to man's estate, to take the diversion of hunting almost every week, both for the sake of finding relaxation from graver cares, and for his health; the chase was principally the buck and doe, and no prince in the world had greater herds of deer, either wandering in freedom through the wilds and forests, or kept in parks and chases for this purpose. The game during the three summer months was the buck, then fat and in season; and in the autumn and winter, for the same length of time, the doe. This gave me an opportunity of dissecting numbers of these animals almost every day during the whole of the season when they were rutting, taking the male, and falling with young; I had occasion, so often as I desired it, to examine and study all the parts, particularly those dedicated to the offices of generation.

I shall therefore consider the generation of viviparous animals in general, from the particular history of the hind and doe, as the instance most convenient to me; and as I have done above, in speaking of oviparous generation, where I have referred everything to the common fowl, so shall I here, in dis-

[2] Hist. Anim. lib. vii, cap. 7.

cussing viviparous generation, refer all to the fallow deer and roe. In taking this course, I am not moved by the same reasons as I was in reference to the hen's egg; but because the great prince, whose physician I was, besides taking much pleasure in such inquiries, and not disdaining to bear witness to my discoveries, was pleased in his kindness and munificence to order me an abundant supply of these animals and repeated opportunities of examining their bodies.

I therefore propose to give the history of generation in the hind and doe as I have observed it during a long series of years, and as most familiar to me, believing that from thence something certain in reference to the generation of other viviparous animals may be concluded. In giving a faithful narrative of this history, I shall not abstain in its course from introducing particulars worthy of note that have either been observed accidentally and by the way, or that are the result of particular dissections instituted for the purpose of arriving at conclusions, the subjects of these having been other bisulcated, hoofed, or multungulated animals, or, finally, man himself. We shall give a simple narrative of the series of formations of the fœtus, following the footsteps of nature in the process.

EXERCISE THE SIXTY-FIFTH.

Of the uterus of the hind and doe.

About to treat of the generation of the hind and doe, our first business will be to speak of the place where it proceeds, or of the uterus, as we have done above, in giving the history of the common fowl, by which all that follows will be more easily and readily understood. And history has this great pre-eminence over fable, that it narrates the events which transpired in certain places at certain times, and therefore leads us to knowledge by a safe and assured way.

Now that we may have a clearer idea of the uterus of the hind, I shall describe both its external and internal structure, following the uterus of the human female as my guide. For man is the most consummate of creatures, and has therefore the genital as well as all other parts in higher perfection than any other animal. The parts of the female uterus consequently present themselves with great distinctness, and by reason of the industry of anatomists in this direction are believed to be particularly well known to us.

We meet with many things in the uterus of deer which we encounter in the uterus of the human female; and we also observe several that differ. In the vulva or os externum we find neither labia, nor clitoris, nor nymphæ, but only two openings, one for the urine, adjacent to the pecten, or os pubis, the other the vagina, lying between the meatus urinarius and the anus. A cuticular or membranous fold, such as we have noted in the hen, stretching downwards from the anus, acts as a velabrum, supplies the place of nymphæ and labia pudendi, and guards against injury from without. This velabrum must be somewhat retracted by the female when she copulates, or at all events must be raised by the penis of the male as it enters the vulva.

The symphysis pubis being divided in deer, and the legs widely separated, the urinary bladder, the vagina which is entered by the penis of the buck, and the cervix uteri, are all seen in their relative situations, not otherwise than they are in women; the ligamenta suspensoria, with the veins, arteries, and testicles, as they are called, also come into sight; the cornua of the uterus in these creatures are also more remarkable than any other part of this organ.

As for the vessels called vasa præparantia and vasa deferentia seu ejaculantia, you will discover nothing of the kind here, nor indeed in any other female animal that I am aware of. The anatomists who believe that women emit a seminal fluid sub coitu have been too eager in their search after such vessels; for in some they are not met with at all, and where they do occur they never present themselves with anything of uniformity of character. Wherefore it seems most likely that women do not emit any semen sub coitu, which is in conformity as I have said with what the greater number of women state. And although some of warmer temperament shed a fluid in the sexual embrace, still that this is fruitful semen, or is a necessary requisite to conception, I do not believe; for many women conceive without having any emission of the kind, and some even without any kind of pleasurable sensation whatsoever. But of these things more in another place.

The vulva, or vagina uteri, which extends from the os externum to the inner orifice of the uterus, is situated in the hind, as well as in the human female, between the urinary bladder and the intestinum rectum, and corresponds in length, width, and general dimensions, with the penis of the male. When this part is laid open it is found occupied lengthwise by rugæ and furrows, admitting of ready distension, and lubricated with a sluggish fluid. At its bottom we observe a very narrow and small orifice, the commencement of the cervix uteri, by which whatever is propelled outwards from the cavity of the uterus must pass. This is the corresponding orifice to that which medical men assert is so firmly closed and sealed up in the pregnant woman and virgin, that it will not even admit the point of a probe or fine needle.

The os uteri is followed by the cervix or process, which is much longer and rounder than in woman, and also more fibrous, thicker, and nervous; it extends from the bottom of the vagina to the body of the uterus. If this cervix uteri be divided longitudinally, you perceive not only its external orifice at the bottom of the vagina, its surface in close contact, and so firmly agglutinated that not even air blown into the vagina will penetrate the cavity of the uterus, but five other similar constrictions placed in regular order, firmly contracted against the entrance of any foreign body and sealed with gelatinous mucus; just as we find the narrow orifice of the woman's uterus plugged with a yellowish glutinous mass. A like constriction of parts, all firmly closed, and precluding all possibility of entrance, Fabricius has found in the uterine neck of the sheep, sow, and goat. In the deer there are very distinctly five of these constrictions, or so many orifices of the uterus constricted and conglutinated, which may all justly be looked upon as so many barriers against the entrance of anything from without. Such particular care has nature taken, that if the first barrier were forced by any cause or violence, the second should still stand good, and so the third, and the fourth, and the fifth, determined apparently that nothing should enter. A probe pushed from within outwards, however, from the cavity of the uterus towards the vagina, passes through readily. A way had to be

left open for the escape of flatus, menstrual blood, and other
excreted fluids; but even the smallest and most subtile things,
air, for instance, and the seminal fluid are precluded all access
from without.

In all animals this uterine orifice is found obstructed or
plugged up in the same way as it is wont to be in women,
among whom we have sometimes known the outlet so much constricted that the menses, lochia, and other humours were retained
in the womb, and became the exciting cause of most severe
hysterical symptoms.   In such cases it became necessary to
contrive a suitable instrument with which the os uteri being
opened, the matters that stagnated within were discharged,
when all the accidents disappeared.   By this contrivance injections could also be thrown into the cavity of the uterus, and
by means of these I have cured internal ulcers of the womb,
and have occasionally even found a remedy for barrenness.

The cavity of the uterus in the deer is extremely small, and
the thickness of its walls not great; the body of the womb in
these animals is, in fact, but a kind of vestibule, or ante-room,
in the cavity of which a passage opens to the right and left
into either cornu.

For the parts are different in almost all animals from what they
are in woman, in whom the principal part of the uterus is its body,
and the cervix and cornua are mere appendices, that scarcely
attract attention.   The neck is short; the cornua are slender
round processes extending from the fundus uteri like a couple of
tubes, which anatomists indeed commonly speak of as the vasa
ejaculatoria.   In the deer, however, as in all other quadrupeds,
except the ape and the solipeds, the chief organ of generation
is not the body but the horns of the uterus.   In the human
female and the solipedia, the uterus is the 'place' of conception,
in all the rest the conception is perfected in the cornua; and
this is the reason why writers so commonly speak of the cornua
uteri in the lower animals under the simple name of the uterus,
saying that the uterus in certain animals is bipartite, whilst in
others it is not, understanding by the word uterus the place in
which conception takes place, this in the majority of viviparous and especially of multiparous animals being the cornua, to
which moreover all the arteries and veins distributed to the
organs of generation are sent.   We shall therefore, in treating

of the history of generation in the deer employ the words uterus and horns of the uterus promiscuously.

In the human female, as I have said, the two tubes that arise near the cervix uteri and there perforate its cavity have no analogy to the parts generally called cornua, but, on the contrary, in the mind of some anatomists, to the vasa spermatica. By others again they are called the spiramenta uteri—the breathing tubes of the uterus; and by others still they are called the vasa deferentia seu reservantia, as if they were of the same nature as the canals so designated in the male; whilst they in fact correspond to the cornua of the uterus in other animals, as most clearly appears from their situation, connexion, length, perforation, general resemblance, and also office. For as many of the lower animals regularly conceive in the cornua uteri, so do women occasionally carry their conceptions in the cornu, or this tube, as the learned Riolanus[1] has shown from the observations of others, and as we ourselves have found it with our own eyes.

These cornua terminate in a common cavity which, as stated, forms a kind of porch or vestibule to the uterus, and corresponds in the deer to the neck of the womb in women; in the same way as the tubes in question in the human female correspond to the cornua uteri in the deer. Now this name of cornua has been derived from the resemblance of the parts to the horns of an animal; and in the same way as the horns of a goat or ram are ample at the base, arched and protuberant in front, and bent-in behind, so are these horns of the uterus in the hind and doe capacious inferiorly, and taper gradually off superiorly, as they are reflected towards the spine. Further, as the horns of the animal are unequally tuberculated and uneven in front, but smooth behind, so are the horns of the uterus tuberculated, as it were, and uneven, through the presence of cells, something like those of the colon, inferiorly and anteriorly; but superiorly, and on the aspect towards the spine, they are continuous and smooth, and present themselves secured and bound down by a ligamentous band; they at the same time gradually decrease in size like horns. Did one take a piece of empty intestine, such as is used for making sausages, and draw-

---

[1] Anthropologia, lib. ii, cap. 34.

ing a tape through it, tied this on one side, he would have it puckered and constricted on that side, and thrown into cells similar to those of the colon on the opposite side. Such is the structure of the cornua of the uterus in the hind and doe. In other animals it is different; for there the cells are either much larger, or they are entirely wanting. The cells of the cornua uteri of the hind and doe, however, are not all of the same size; the first that is met with is much larger than any of the others; and here it is that the conception is generally lodged.

As the uterus, tubes, or cornua, and other parts appertaining in the human female are connected with the pubes, spine, and surrounding structures by the medium of broad and fleshy membranes, by suspensory bands, as it were, which anatomists have designated by the name of bats' wings, because they have found that the uterus suspended in this way resembled a bat with its wings expanded, so also are the cornua uteri, together with the testes [ovaries], on either side, and all the uterine vessels, connected with the neighbouring parts, particularly with the spine, by means of a firm membrane, within the folds of which are suspended all the parts that have been mentioned, and which serves the same office with reference to these uterine structures as the mesentery does to the intestines, and the mesometrium to the uterus of the fowl. In the same way, too, as the mesenteric arteries and veins are distributed to the intestines through the mesentery, are the uterine vessels distributed to the uterus through the membrane in question; in which also certain vessels and glands are perceived on either side, which by anatomists are generally designated the testicles [the ovaries.]

The substance of the horns of the uterus in the hind and doe is skinny or fleshy, like the coats of the intestines, and has a few very minute veins ramified over it. This substance you may in anatomical fashion divide into several layers, and note different courses of its component fibres, fitting them to perform the several motions and actions required, retention, namely, and expulsion. I have myself frequently seen these cornua moving like earthworms, or in the manner in which the intestines may at any time be observed, twisting themselves with an undulatory motion, on laying open the abdomen of a recently slaughtered animal, by which they move on the chyle and excrements to inferior portions of the gut, as if they were surrounded and compressed with a ring forced over them, or were stripped between the fingers.

The uterine veins, as in woman, all arise from the vena cava, near the emulgents; the arteries (and this also is common to the deer and the human subject) arise from the crural branches of the descending aorta. And as in the pregnant woman the uterine vessels are relatively larger and more numerous than in any other part of the body, this is likewise the case in the pregnant hind and doe. The arteries, however, contrary to the arrangement in other parts of the body, are much more numerous than the veins; and air blown into them makes its way into the neighbouring veins, although the arteries cannot be inflated in their turn by blowing into the veins. This fact I also find mentioned by Master Riolanus; and it is a cogent argument for the circulation of the blood discovered by me; for he clearly proves that whilst there is a passage from the arteries into the veins, there is none backwards from the veins into the arteries. The arteries are more numerous than the veins, because a large supply of nourishment being required for the fœtus, it is only what is left unused that has to be returned by the latter channels.

In the deer as well as in the sheep, goat, and bisulcate animals generally, we find testicles; but these are mere little glands, which rather correspond in their proportions to the prostate or mesenteric glands, the use of which is to establish divarications for the veins, and to store up a fluid for lubricating the parts, than for secreting semen, concocting it into fecundity, and shedding it at the time of intercourse. I am myself especially moved to adopt this opinion, as well by numerous reasons which will be adduced elsewhere, as by the fact that in the rutting season, when the testes of the buck and hart enlarge and are replete with semen, and the cornua of the uterus of the hind and doe are greatly changed, the female testicles, as they are called, whether they be examined before or after intercourse, neither swell nor vary from their usual condition; they show no trace of being of the slightest use either in the business of intercourse or in that of generation.

It is surprising what a quantity of seminal fluid is found in the vesiculæ seminales and testicles of moles and the larger kinds of mice at the season of intercourse; this circumstance corresponds with what we have already noticed in the cock, and the great change perceptible in the organs of generation of both sexes; nevertheless, the glands, which are regarded as the female testes, continue all the while unchanged and without departure from their pristine appearance.

All that has now been said of the uterus and its horns in hinds and does applies in major part to viviparous animals in general, but not to the human female, inasmuch as she conceives in the body of the uterus, but all these, with the exception of the horse and ass, in the horns of the organ; and even the horse and ass, although they appear to carry their fruit in the uterus, still is the *place* of the conception in them rather of the nature of an uterine horn than the uterine body.   For the *place* here is not bipartite indeed, but it is oblong, and different from the human uterus both in its situation, connexions, structure, and substance; it bears a greater affinity to the superior uterus or uterine process of the fowl, where the egg grows and becomes surrounded with the albumen, than to the uterus of the woman.

EXERCISE THE SIXTY-SIXTH.

Of the intercourse of the hind and doe.

So much for the account of the uterus of the female deer, where we have spoken briefly upon all that seemed necessary to the history of generation, viz. the 'place' of conception, and the parts instituted for its sake.   We have still to speak of the action and office of this 'place,' in other words, of intercourse and conception.

The hind and doe admit the male at one and only one particular season of the year, namely, in the middle of September, after the Feast of the Holy Cross; and they bring forth after the middle of June, about the Feast of St. John the Baptist (24th June).   They, therefore, go with young about nine months, not eight, as Pliny says;[1] with us, at all events,

---

[1] Lib. viii, cap. 32.

they produce in the ninth month after they have taken the buck.

At the rutting season the bucks herd with the does; at other times they keep severally apart, the males, particularly the older ones, associating together, and the females and younger males trooping and feeding in company. The rutting season lasts for a whole month, and it begins later if the weather have been dry, earlier if it have been wet. In Spain, as I am informed, the deer are hardly in rut before the beginning of October, wet weather not usually setting in there until this time; but with us the rutting season rarely continues beyond the middle of October.

At this time deer are rendered savage by desire, so that they will attack both dogs and men, although at other seasons they are so timid and peaceable, and immediately betake themselves to flight on the barking of even the smallest dog.

Every male knows all his own females, nor will he suffer any one of them to wander from his herd : with a run he speedily drives back any straggler; he walks jealously from time to time among his wives; looks circumspectly about him, and the careful guardian of his own, he shows himself the watchful sentinel. If a strange doe commit any offence, he does not pursue her very eagerly, but rather suffers her to get away; but if another buck approach he instantly runs to meet him, and gives him battle with his antlers.

The hind and doe are held among the number of the chaster animals; they suffer the addresses of the male reluctantly, who, like the bull, mounts with violence, and unless forced or tired out, they resist him; which disinclination of the females appears also to be the reason of their herding together, and confining themselves to their own males, who are always the older and better armed; for when any strange male approaches them they immediately take to flight, and seek refuge in their own herd, and protection to their chastity, as it seems, from their proper husband.

If a younger male finds a female straying alone, he immediately pursues her, and when she is worn out and unable to fly farther he mounts and forces her to his pleasure.

The males all provide themselves what are called rutting places; that is to say, they dig a trench, or they take their stand upon an acclivity, whither they compel their females to come in turn. The female that is to be leapt stands with her hind feet in the trench prepared for the purpose, stooping or lowering her haunches somewhat, if need be; by which the male is enabled, pressing forward upon her in the same way as a bull, to strike her, in technical language, and finish the business of copulation at one assault.

Old and sturdy bucks have a considerable number of does in their herds, as many as ten, and even fifteen; younger and weaker males have fewer. Keepers say that the doe is sated with two, or at most with three leaps; once she has conceived she admits the male no more.

The lust of the male cools when he has served his females; he becomes shyer, and much leaner; he deserts his herd and roams alone, and feeds greedily to repair his wasted strength, nor does he afterwards approach a female for a whole year.

When the male is capable of intercourse the hair on his throat and neck grows black, and the extremity of the prepuce becomes of the same colour, and stinks abominably. The females take the male but rarely, and only in the night or in dusky places, which are, therefore, always chosen by the males for their connubial pleasures. When two stags engage in battle, as frequently happens, the vanquished yields possession of his females to the victor.

EXERCISE THE SIXTY-SEVENTH.

Of the constitution or change that takes place in the uterus of the deer in the course of the month of September.

We now come to the changes that take place in the genital parts of the female after intercourse, and to the conception itself. In the month of September, then, when the female deer first comes in season, her cornua uteri, uterus, or place of conception, grows somewhat more fleshy and thick, softer also, and more tender. In the interior of either cornu, at that part, namely, which looks drawn together by a band, and is turned towards the spine, we observe, protruding in regular succession, five caruncles, soft warts, or papillæ. The first of these is larger than any of the others, and each in succession is smaller than the one before it, just as the cornua themselves become smaller and smaller towards their termination. Some of the caruncles grow to the thickness of the largest finger, and look like proud flesh; some are white, others of a deeper red.

From the 26th to the 28th of September, and also subsequently, in the month of October, the uterus becomes thicker, and the carunculæ mentioned come to resemble the nipples of the woman's breast: you might fancy them ready to pour out milk. Having removed their apex that I might examine their internal structure, I found them made up of innumerable white points compacted together, like so many bristles erect, and connected by means of a certain mucous viscidity; compressed between the fore finger and thumb, from the base upwards, a minute drop of blood oozed out from each point, a fact which led me, after farther investigation, to conclude that they were entirely made up of the capillary branches of arteries.

During the season of intercourse, therefore, the uterine vessels, particularly the arteries, are observed to be more numerous and of larger size; although the parts called the female testes, as I have said above, are neither larger nor more highly gorged with blood than before, and do not appear to be altered in any way from their former state.

The inner aspect of the uterus or cornua uteri, where it is puckered into cells, is as smooth and soft as the ventricles of the brain, or the glans penis within the prepuce. Nothing, however, can be discovered there—neither the semen of the male, nor aught else having reference to the conception—during the whole of the months of September and October, although I have instituted repeated dissections with a view of examining the conception at this period. The males have been doing their duty all the while; nevertheless, reiterated dissection shows nothing. This is the conclusion to which I have come, after many years of observation. I have only occasionally found the five caruncles so close together that they formed a kind of continuous protuberance into the interior of the uterus. But when, after repeated inspections, I still found nothing more in the uterus, I began to doubt, and to ask

myself whether the semen of the male could by any possibility
make its way—by attraction or injection—to the seat of the
conception?   And repeated examination led me to the conclusion that none of the semen whatsoever reached this seat.

Of what takes place in the month of October.

Repeated dissections performed in the course of the month
of October, both before the rutting season was over and after
it had passed, never enabled me to discover any blood or
semen, or a trace of anything else, either in the body of the
uterus or in its cornua.   The uterus was only a little larger,
and somewhat thicker; and the caruncles were more tumid
and florid, and, when strongly pressed with the finger, discharged small drops of blood, much in the manner in which a
little watery milk can be squeezed from the nipples of a
woman in the fourth month of her pregnancy.   In one or two
does, indeed, I found a green and ichorous matter, like an
abscess, filling the cavity of the uterus, which was preternaturally extenuated; in other respects these animals were healthy,
and in as good condition as others which I examined at the
same time.

Towards the end of October and beginning of November,
the rutting season being now ended, and the females separat-
ing themselves from the males, the uterus begins (in some
sooner, in others later) to shrink in size, and the walls of its
internal cavity, inflated in appearance, to bulge out; for where
the cells existed formerly there are now certain globular masses
projecting internally, which nearly fill the whole cavity, by
which the sides are brought into mutual contact, and almost
agglutinated, as it seems, so that there is no interval between
them.   Even as we have seen the lips of boys who, in robbing a
hive, had been stung in the mouth, swollen and enlarged, so
that the oral aperture was much contracted, even so does the internal surface of the uterus in the doe enlarge, and become filled
with a soft and pulpy substance, like the matter of the brain,

that fills its cavity and involves the caruncles, which, though not larger than before, look whiter, and as if they had been steeped in hot water, much as the nurse's nipple appears immediately after the infant has quitted it. And now I have not found it possible by any compression to force blood out of the caruncles as before.

Nothing can be softer, smoother, more delicate, than the inner aspect of the uterus thus raised into tubers. It rivals the ventricles of the brain in softness, so that without the information of the eye we should scarcely perceive by the finger that we were touching anything. When the abdomen is laid open immediately after the death of the animal, I have frequently seen the uterus affected with a wavy and creeping motion, such as is perceived in the lower part of a slug or snail whilst it is moving, as if the uterus were an animal within an animal, and possessed a proper and independent motion. I have frequently observed a movement of the same kind as that just described in the intestines, whilst engaged in vivisections; and indeed such a motion can both be seen and felt in the bodies of dogs and rabbits whilst they are alive and uninjured. I have also observed a corresponding motion in the testes and scrotum of men; and I have even known women upon whom, in their eagerness for offspring, such palpitations have imposed. But whether the uterus in hysterical females, by ascending, descending, and twisting, experiences any such motion or not, I cannot take upon me to declare; and whether the brain, in its actions and conceptions, moves in anything of a similar manner or not, though a point difficult of investigation, I am inclined to look upon as one by no means unworthy of being attempted.

Shortly afterwards, the tubercular elevations of the inner surface of the uterus that have been mentioned begin to shrink; it is as if, losing a quantity of moisture, they became less plump. In some instances, indeed, though rarely, I have observed something like purulent matter adhering to them, such as is usually seen on the surface of wounds and ulcers when they are digested, as it is said, they pour out smooth and homogeneous pus. When I first saw this matter, I doubted whether it was the semen of the male or not, or a substance concocted from its purer portion. But as it was only in exceedingly rare instances that I met with such matter, and as twenty days had then passed since the doe had had any intercourse with the buck, and farther, as the matter was not viscid and tenacious, or spumous, such as the seminal fluid presents itself to us, but rather friable, purulent looking, and inclining to yellow, I came to the conclusion that it was the effect of accident, a sweat or exudation in consequence of violent exercise previous to death; just as in a catarrh the thinner defluxion of the nose is by and by changed into a thicker mucus.

Having frequently shown this alteration in the uterus to his majesty the king as the first indication of pregnancy, and satisfied him at the same time that there was nothing in the shape of semen or conception to be found in the cavity of the organ, and he had spoken of this as an extraordinary fact to several about him, a discussion at length arose : the keepers and huntsmen asserted at first that it was but an argument of a tardy conception occasioned by the want of rain. But by and by, when they saw the rutting season pass away, I still continuing to maintain that things were in the same state, they began to say that I was both deceived myself and had misled the king, and that there must of necessity be something of the conception to be found in the uterus. These men, however, when I got them to bring their own eyes to the inquiry, soon gave up the point. The physicians, nevertheless, held it among their αδύνατα—their impossibilities—that any conception should ever be formed without the presence of the semen masculinum, or some trace remaining of a fertile intercourse within the cavity of the womb.

That this important question might be the more satisfactorily settled in all time to come, his highness the king ordered about a dozen does to be separated from the bucks towards the beginning of October, and secluded in the inclosure, which is called the course, at Hampton Court, because the animal placed there has no means of escape from the dogs let loose upon it. Now that no one might say the animals thus secluded retained any of the semen received from the last connexions with the male, I dissected several of them before the rutting season had passed, and ascertained that no seminal fluid remained in the uterus, although the others were found to be

pregnant in consequence of the preceding intercourse—impregnated by a kind of contagion as it appears—and duly produced
their fawns at the proper time.

In the dog, rabbit, and several other animals, I have found
nothing in the uterus for several days after intercourse. I
therefore regard it as demonstrated that after fertile intercourse
among viviparous as well as oviparous animals, there are no remains in the uterus either of the semen of the male or female
emitted in the act, nothing produced by any mixture of these
two fluids, as medical writers maintain, nothing of the menstrual
blood present as 'matter' in the way Aristotle will have it; in
a word, that there is not necessarily even a trace of the conception to be seen immediately after a fruitful union of the
sexes. It is not true, consequently, that in a prolific connexion
there must be any prepared matter in the uterus which the
semen masculinum, acting as a coagulating agent, should congeal, concoct, and fashion, or bring into a positive generative
act, or, by drying its outer surface, include in membranes.
Nothing certainly is to be seen within the uterus of the doe
for a great number of days, namely, from the middle of September up to the 12th of November.

It appears moreover that all females do not shed seminal
fluid into the uterus during intercourse; that there is no trace
either of seminal fluid or menstrual blood in the uterus of the
hind or doe, and many other viviparous animals. But as to
what it is which is shed by women of warmer temperament no
less than by men during intercourse, accompanied with failure
of the powers and voluptuous sensations; whether it be necessary to fecundation, whether it come from the testes femi-
ninæ, and whether it be semen and prolific, is discussed by us
elsewhere.

And whilst I speak of these matters, let gentle minds forgive
me, if, recalling the irreparable injuries I have suffered, I here
give vent to a sigh. This is the cause of my sorrow:—whilst
in attendance on his majesty the king during our late troubles
and more than civil wars, not only with the permission but by
command of the Parliament, certain rapacious hands stripped
not only my house of all its furniture, but what is subject of
far greater regret with me, my enemies abstracted from my
museum the fruits of many years of toil. Whence it has come

31

to pass that many observations, particularly on the generation of insects, have perished, with detriment, I venture to say, to the republic of letters.

Of what takes place in the uterus of the doe during the month of November.

Taught by the experience of many years I can state truly that it is from the 12th to the 14th of November that I first discover anything which belongs to the future offspring in the uterus of the hind.

I remember, indeed, that in the year of grace 1633, the signs of conception, or the commencements of the embryos, made their appearance somewhat earlier; because the weather was then cloudy and wet. In does, too, which have rutted six or seven days sooner than hinds, I have always discovered something of the future fœtus about the 8th or 9th of November. What this is and how it is begun I shall proceed to state.

A little before anything is perceptible, the substance of the uterus or its horns appears less than it was before the animals began to rut, the white caruncles are more flaccid, as I have said, and the protuberances of the internal coat subside somewhat, and are corrugated and look moist. For about the date above mentioned certain mucous filaments like spiders' webs are observed drawn from the extremities, or superior angles of the cornua through the middle of either, and also through the body of the uterus. These filaments becoming conjoined present themselves as a membranous and gelatinous tunic or empty sac. Even as the plexus choroides is extended through the ventricles of the brain, is this oblong sac produced through the whole of either horn and the intervening cavity of the uterus, insinuating itself between the wrinkles of the flabby internal tunic, and sending delicate fibres among the aforementioned rounded protuberances, being nearly in the same manner as the pia mater dips between the convolutions of the brain.

Within a day or two this sac becomes filled with a clear,

watery, sluggish albuminous matter, and now presents itself as a long-shaped pudding full of fluid. It adheres by its external glutinous matter to the containing walls of the uterus, but so that it is still easily separated from these; for if it be taken hold of cautiously in the strait of the uterus, where it is constricted in its course, it can be drawn entire out of either horn.

The conception arrived at this stage removed entire, presents itself with the figure of a wallet or double pudding; externally, it is covered with a purulent-looking matter; internally, it is smooth, and contains in its cavity a viscid fluid not unlike the thinner white of egg.

This is the conception of the hind and doe in its first stage. And since it has now the nature and state of an egg, and the definition given by Aristotle of an egg is applicable to it, namely: " A body from one part of which an animal is produced, the remainder serving as nourishment to that which is engendered;" and farther, as it is the primordium of the future fœtus, it is therefore called the ovum, or egg of the animal, in conformity with that passage of the philosopher where he says :[2] " Those animals which engender internally, have a certain oviform body produced after the first conception. For a humour is included within a delicate membrane, such as that which you find under the shell in the egg of the hen; wherefore the blightings of conceptions that are apt to take place about this period are called fluxes." This conception, therefore, as we have already said of the egg, is the true sperma or seed, comprising the virtue of both sexes in itself, and is analogous to the seed of the vegetable. So that Aristotle, describing the first conception of women, says,[3] that it is " covered with a membrane like an egg from which the shell has been removed;" such as Hippocrates describes as having been passed by the female pipe-player. And I have myself frequently seen such ova, of the size of pigeons' eggs, and containing no fœtus, discharged by women about the second month after conception; when the ovum was of the size of a pheasant's or hen's egg, the embryo could be made out, the size of the little finger nail, floating within it. But the membrane surrounding the conception has not yet acquired any annexed placenta; neither is

[1] Hist. Anim. lib. i, cap. 5 ; et De Gen. Anim. lib. ii, cap. 9.
[2] De Gen. Anim. lib. iii, cap. 9.　　　　[3] Hist. Anim. lib. vii. cap. 7.

it connected with the uterus; there is only at its upper and blunter part a kind of delicate mossy or woolly covering which stands for the rudiments of the future placenta. The inner aspect is smooth and polished, and covered with numerous ramifications of the umbilical vessels. In the third month this ovum exceeds a goose's egg in size, and includes a perfect embryo of the length of two fingers' breadths. In the fourth month it is larger than an ostrich's egg. All these things I have noted in the numerous careful dissections of aborted ova which I have made.

In the way above indicated do the hind and doe, affected by a kind of contagion, finally conceive and produce primordia, of the nature of eggs, or the seeds of plants, or the fruit of trees, although for a whole month and more they had exhibited nothing in the uterus, the conception being perfected about the 18th, at furthest, the 21st of November, and having its seat now in the right, now in the left horn, occasionally in both at once. The ovum at this time is full of a colliquate matter, transparent, crystalline, similar to that fluid which in the hen's egg we have called the colliquament or eye, of far greater purity than that fluid in which the embryo by and by floats, and contained within a proper tunic of extreme tenuity, and orbicular in form. In the middle of the ovum, vascular ramifications and the punctum saliens—the first or rudimentary particle of the fœtus—and nothing else, are clearly to be perceived. This is the first genital part, which, once constituted, is not only already possessed by the vegetative, but also by the motive soul; and from this are all the other parts of the fœtus, each in its order, generated, fashioned, disposed, and endowed with life, almost in the same manner as we have described the chick to be produced from the colliquament of the egg.

Both of the humours mentioned are present in the conceptions of all viviparous animals, and are regarded by many as the excrements of the fœtus,—one the urine, the other the sweat, although neither of them has any unpleasant taste, and they are always and at all periods present in conceptions, even before a particle of the fœtus has been produced.

Of the membranes investing the two fluids, of which there are only two, the outer is called the chorion, the inner the amnion. The chorion includes the whole conception, and ex-

tends into either cornu; the amnion swimming in the midst
of the liquid of the former, is found in one of the horns only,
except in the cases where there is a twin conception, when there
is an amnion present in each of them; just as in a twin-fraught
egg there are two colliquaments.   Where there are two fœtuses
consequently, both are contained in one common conception,
in one egg, as it were, with its two separate collections of crystalline fluid included.   If you incise the external membrane
at any point, the more turbid fluid which it contains immediately escapes from either horn of the uterus; but the crystalline liquid in the interior of the amnion does not escape at
the same time unless the membrane have been simultaneously
implicated.

The vein which is first discerned in the crystalline fluid within
the amnion takes its rise from the punctum saliens, and assumes
the nature and duty of an umbilical vessel; increasing by degrees it expands into various ramifications distributed through
the colliquament, so that it seems certain that the nourishment
is in the first instance derived from the colliquament alone in
which the fœtus swims.

I have exhibited this point to his serene highness the king,
still palpitating in the uterus laid open; it was extremely minute
indeed, and without the advantage of the sun's light falling
upon it from the side, its tremulous motions were not to be
perceived.

When the ovum with the colliquament entire was placed in
a silver or pewter basin filled with tepid water, the punctum
saliens became beautifully distinct to the spectators.   In the
course of the next ensuing days, a mucilage or jelly, like a tiny
worm, and having the shape of a maggot, is found to be added;
this is the rudiment of the future body.   It is divided into two
parts, one of which is the head, the other the trunk, precisely
in the same way as we have already seen it in the generation of
the chick in ovo.   The spine, like a keel, is somewhat bent;
the head is indifferently made up of three small vesicles or
globules, and swimming in transparent water grows amain, and
by degrees assumes its proper shape.   There is only this to be
observed, that the eye in embryos of oviparous animals is much
larger and more conspicuous than that of viviparous animals.

After the 26th of November the fœtus is seen with its body

nearly perfect, in one case in the right in another in the left horn of the uterus; in twin cases in both horns.

At this time, too, the male embryo is readily distinguishable from the female by means of the organs of generation. These parts are also very conspicuous in the human embryo, and make their appearance at the same time as the trachea.

Males and females are met with indifferently in the right and left horn of the uterus. I have, however, more frequently found females in the right, males in the left horn; and I have made the same observation in does that carried twins, as well as in the sheep. It is certain, therefore, that the right or left side has no appropriate virtue in conferring sex; neither is the uterus, nor yet the mother herself, the fashioner or framer of the fœtus, any more than the hen is of the pullet in the egg which she incubates. In the same way as the pullet is formed and fashioned in the egg by an internal and inherent agent, is the fœtal form produced from the uterine ovum of the hind and doe.

It is indeed matter of astonishment to find a fœtus formed and perfected within the amnion in so short a space of time after the first appearance of the blood and punctum saliens. On or about the 19th or 20th day of November this punctum first becomes visible; on the 21st the shapeless vermiculus or maggot that is to form the body of the future animal is perceived; and in the course of from six to seven days afterwards a fœtus so perfect in all its parts is seen, that a male can be distinguished from a female by the organs of generation, and the feet are formed, the hooves being cleft, the whole having a mucous consistency and a pale yellowish colour.

The substance of the uterus begins to be extenuated immediately after the appearance of the embryo; contrary to what takes place in the human female, whose uterus grows every day thicker and fleshier with the advancing growth of the fœtus. In the hind and doe, on the other hand, the more the embryo augments the more do the cornua of the uterus assimilate themselves to the intestines; that horn in particular in which the fœtus is contained looks like a bag or pouch, and exceeds the opposite one in dimensions.

The ovum or conception, thus far advanced, and with its included fœtus perfectly distinct, has still contracted no adhesions to its mother's sides: the whole can most readily be withdrawn from the uterus, as I have ascertained with an ovum which contained a fœtus nearly the length of the thumb. It is manifest, therefore, that the fœtus up to this period has been nourished by the albumen alone that is contained within the conception; in the same way as we have ascertained the process to go on within the hen's egg. The mouths of the umbilical veins are lost and obliterated between the albumen and neighbouring humours of the conception and their containing membranes; but nowhere is there as yet any connexion with the uterus, although by these veins alone is nourishment supplied to the embryo. And as in the egg the ramifications of the veins are first sent to the colliquament, (in the same way as the roots of trees penetrate the ground,) and afterwards take their course to the external tunic called the chorion, whereon, for the sake of the nourishment, they are dispersed in an infinity of ramifications through the albuminous fluid contained within the outer membrane, so have I observed veins in the chorion of a human abortion; and Aristotle[1] also states "that membrane to be crowded with veins."

If the fœtus be single its umbilical vessels are distributed to both horns, and a few twigs are also sent to the intervening body of the uterus; but if the conception be double, one in either horn, each sends its umbilical vessels to its own horn alone; the embryo in the right horn deriving nourishment from the right part of the conception, that in the left from the left portion of the same. In other respects the twin-conception here is precisely similar to the twin-conception of the egg.

Towards the end of November, then, all the parts are clearly and distinctly to be distinguished, and the fœtus is now of the size of a large bean or nutmeg; its occiput is prominent, as in the chick, but its eyes are smaller; the mouth extends from ear to ear, the cheeks and lips, as consisting of membranous parts, being perfected at a very late period. In the fœtuses of all animals, indeed, that of man inclusive, the oral aperture without lips or cheeks is seen stretching from ear to ear; and this is the reason, unless I much mistake, why so many are born with the upper lip divided as it is in the hare and camel, whence

[1] Hist. Anim. lib. vii, cap. 7.

the common name of *hare-lip* for the deformity. In the development of the human fœtus the upper lip only coalesces in
the middle line at a very late period.

I have frequently put a fœtus the size of a large bean, swimming in its extremely pure nutritive fluid within the transparent
amnion, into a silver basin filled with the clearest water, and
have noted these particulars as most worthy of observation :—
The brain of somewhat greater consistency than white of egg,
like milk moderately coagulated, and of an irregular shape, and
without any covering of skull, is contained within a general investing membrane. The cerebellum projects in a peak, as in
the chick. The conical mass of the heart is of a white colour,
and all the other viscera, the liver inclusive, are white and
spermatic-looking. The trunk of the umbilical veins arises
from the heart, and passing the convexity of the liver, perfo-
rates the trunk of the vena portæ, whence, advancing a little
and subdividing into a great number of branches, it is distributed to the colliquament and tunica choroidea in innumerable
fine filaments. The sides of the body ascend on either hand
from the spine, so that the thorax presents itself in the guise of
a boat or small vessel, up to the period at which the heart and
lungs are included within its area, precisely and in all respects
as we have seen it in the development of the chick. The heart,
intestines, and other viscera, are very conspicuous, and present
themselves as appendages of the body, until the thorax and abdomen being drawn around them, and the roof, as it were, put
on the building, they are concealed within the compages of these
cavities. At this time the sides both of the thorax and abdomen are white, gelatinous, and apparently identical in structure,
save that a number of slender white lines are perceived in the
walls of the thorax, as indications of the future ribs, whereby a
distinction is here made between the bony and fleshy compages of the cavity.

I have also occasionally observed in conceptions of the sheep,
which were sometimes twin, sometimes single, of corresponding
age and about a finger's breadth in length, that the form of
the embryo resembled a small lizard of the size of a wasp or
caterpillar; the spine being curved into a circle, and the head
almost in contact with the tail. In the double conceptions
both were of the same size, as if produced at once and simul-

taneously; each floated distinctly within the fluid of its own amnion; but although one lay in the right, the other in the left horn of the uterus, they were still both included in the same double sac or wallet, both belonged to the same ovum, and were surrounded by the same common external fluid. The mouth was large, but the eyes were mere points, so that they could scarcely be seen, very different, therefore, from what occurs among birds. The viscera in these embryos were also pendulous without the body,—not yet inclosed within the appropriate cavities. The outer membrane or chorion adhered in no way to the uterus, so that the entire conception was readily removed. Within the substance of the chorion innumerable branches of the umbilical vessels were conspicuous, but having no connexion whatsoever with the walls of the uterus; a circumstance to which allusion has already been made in the case of the deer; the distribution was in fact very much as we have found it on the external tunic of the hen's egg. There were but two humours, and the same number of containing tunics, of which the chorion extending through both cornua, and full of a more turbid fluid, gave general configuration to the ovum or conception. The tunica amnios again is almost invisible, like the tunica arachnoides of the eye, and embraces the crystalline humour in which the embryo floats.

The fluid of the amnion was, in proportion, but a hundredth, or shall I say a thousandth, to that of the chorion; although the crystalline humour of the amnion was still in such quantity that no one could reasonably imagine it to be the sweat of the very small embryo that floated within it. It was, further, extremely limpid, and seemed to be without anything like bad taste or smell. It was, as we have already observed of the deer, in all respects like watery milk, and had none of the obnoxious qualities of an excrement. I add, that if this fluid were of an excrementitious nature it ought to increase in quantity with the growth of the fœtus. But I have found precisely the opposite of this to obtain in the conception of the ewe, so that shortly before she lambs there is scarce a drop of the fluid in question remaining. I am, therefore, rather inclined to regard it as aliment than as excrement.

The internal tunic of the uterus of the ewe is covered with caruncles innumerable, as the heavens are with stars. These are not unlike crabs' eyes, and I have called them by this name; but they are smaller, like pendulous warts, glandular and white, sticking within the coats of the uterus, and somewhat excavated towards the conception; otherwise than in the deer, consequently, in which the caruncles corresponding to these rather project towards the embryo. These caruncles are gorged with blood, and their inner surface, where they regard the conception, is perceived to be beset with black sanguineous points. The umbilical vessels of the embryo were not yet connected with these caruncles, nor did the conception itself adhere to the uterus.

I find nothing of an allantois, of which something has been said as a tunic distinct from the chorion, in the conception of the ewe. At a later period, indeed, when the embryo is larger, when the ovum or conception has contracted adhesions with the uterus, and the umbilical vessels have penetrated the caruncles, the chorion extends further, and at its extremities on either side, and as it were in a couple of appendices, there is a certain fluid of a yellow colour, which you might call excrementitious, kept separate and distinct.

The human conception scarcely differs in any respect from an egg during the first months of pregnancy. I have observed a clear fluid, like the more liquid white of an egg, to be included within an extremely delicate membrane. At this time the placenta had not yet appeared, and the entire conception was of the size of a pigeon's, or perhaps a pheasant's egg. The embryo itself, of the length of the little finger nail, and having the form of a small frog, was conspicuous enough. The body was broad, the oral aperture widely cleft, the legs and arms like the stalks of flowers just risen above the ground, the occiput prominent, or rather forming a vesicle appended to the rest of the head, such as we have described the rudiments of the future cerebellum in the chick.

In another human conception of about the fiftieth day, the ovum was as large as a hen's or a turkey's egg. The embryo was as long as a large bean, the head of very large relative dimensions, and dominated by the cerebellum as by a kind of crest. The brain itself was of the consistence of curdled milk. Instead of a cranium there was a coriaceous membrane, in some places cartilaginous, and divided down the forehead to the roots of the nostrils; the face looked like the muzzle of a dog. There were no external ears, nor any nose, yet could the rudiments of the trachea passing down to the lungs, and those of the penis, be detected. The two auricles of the heart presented themselves like eyes, of a black colour.

In the body of a woman who died of fever I found an hermaphrodite embryo nearly of the same size. The pudendum was like that of the rabbit, the labia standing for prepuce, the nymphæ for glans. In the upper part the root of the penis was also apparent, and on either side for the testicle there was the lax skin of the scrotum. The uterus was extremely diminutive, and in figure like that of the ewe or mole, with two horns. And as the prostate glands are situated near the penis of the boy, so were the testicles (ovaries) of visible dimensions, seen adjacent to these cornua. Externally considered, the sex seemed that of the male; internally, however, it was rather that of the female. The uterus of the mother was of great size, having the urinary bladder connected with it as an appendage. In the embryo, on the contrary, the bladder was large with the uterus of very small dimensions attached to it.

All the human ova that have been described above were, like those of the ewe, shaggy externally, and besmeared with a kind of gelatine, or glutinous matter. At this epoch, too, there was neither any placenta apparent, nor any visible connexion with the uterus; neither was there any implantation into the substance of the uterus of the umbilical vessels scattered over the surface of the conception itself.

As in the deer, so in the sheep, goat, and other bisulcated animals, do we find more than one fœtus in the same conception, just as in twin-fraught eggs we find two chicks surrounded by the same albumen. But in the dog, rabbit, hog, and other viviparous animals that produce a considerable number at a litter, the thing is otherwise. In these each fœtus has two humours, these being severally surrounded with their proper membranes.

In the bitch there are a number of knots or constrictions along the whole course of either cornu of the uterus, between each of which the appropriate humours and a single embryo are contained. In the hare and rabbit we observe a number of balls, like the eggs of serpents, so that the horns of the uterus look like a pair of bracelets composed of so many amber beads strung upon a thread. The conception of the hare bears a strong resemblance to an acorn, the placenta embracing the embryo like a cup, and the humours inclosed in their membranes depending like the gland or nut.

Of the conception of the deer in the course of the month of December.

In the beginning of December the fœtus is seen larger, every way more perfect, and the length of the finger. The heart and other viscera which formerly hung externally are now concealed within the cavities of the body, so that they can no longer be seen without dissection.

The conception, or ovum, by the medium of the five caruncles which we have already spoken of as present in either cornu, is now in connexion with the uterus at an equal number of points; still the union is not so strong but that a very slight rather than a great effort suffices to break it. When the conception is detached, we perceive points or depressions on the surface of the chorion at the places where the adhesions to the uterus had existed, these spots being further covered with a certain viscid and wrinkled matter, as if this had been the bond of union between the mother and the ovum. Thus have we the nature and use of these caruncles made known to us : seen in the first instance as fungi or excrescences growing from the sides of the uterus, they are now recognized in connexion with the conception, as standing instead of the placenta or uterine cake in the human subject, and performing the same office. These caruncles are in fact but as so many nipples, whence the embryo by means of its umbilical vessels receives the nourishment that is supplied by the mother, as shall be clearly shown by what is to follow.

The size and capacity of the uterus, by which name we understand the cornua, or place occupied by the conception, is increased in proportion to the growth of the embryo; in suchwise, however, that the horn in which the fœtus is lodged is larger than the other.

The conception or ovum is single, whether one or several embryos are evolved from it; and it extends, as already said, into both of the horns, so that it presents itself with the shape of a double pudding, or rather of a single pudding having a constriction in its middle. Proceeding rounded and slender from the upper extremity of one of the horns, the conception gradually enlarges, and is produced into that common cavity which in the human female is called the uterus or matrix; (because, by conceiving and cherishing her offspring in this place the woman is made a mother;) the conception of the deer, passing through a kind of isthmus in the body of the uterus, is narrowed; but by and by, escaping into the other cornu, it there expands at first, but anon contracts again, and finally ends as it began in a tapering extremity. The whole conception, therefore, taken out entire, resembles a wallet filled with water on either side; and hence the chorion is also called allantois, because the conception in the lower animals, such as the deer, looks like an intestine inflated, or stuffed and tied in the middle.

In the embryo anatomized at this period every internal part is seen distinct and perfect; particularly the stomach, intestines, heart, kidneys, and lungs, which, divided into lobes, but having the proper form of the organs, look bloody. The colour of the lungs is deeper than it is in those fœtuses that have breathed, because the lungs, dilated by the act of respiration, assume a whiter tint. And by this indication is it known whether a mother has brought forth a living or dead child; in the former case the colour of the lungs is changed, and the change remains though the infant have died immediately afterwards.

In the female fœtus the testes—improperly so called—are seen situated near the kidneys at the extremities of the cornua uteri on either side; they are relatively of larger size than in the adult, and, like the caruncles of the uterus, look white.

In the stomach of the fœtus there is a watery fluid contained, not unlike that in which it swims, but somewhat more turbid or less transparent. It resembles the milk that begins to be secreted in the breasts of pregnant women about the fourth or

fifth month of pregnancy, and may be pressed out of the
nipples, or it is like the drink which we call white posset.

In the small intestines there is an abundance of chyle concocted from the same matter; in the colon greenish fæces and
scybala begin to appear.

I do not find the urachus perforate; neither do I perceive
any difference between the tunica allantoides or allantois, which
is said to contain urine, and the chorion. Neither do I detect
any urine in the secundines, but only in the bladder, where
indeed it is present in large quantity. The bladder, of an oblong form, is situated between the umbilical arteries as they
proceed from the bifurcation of the descending aorta.

The liver is rudely sketched and almost shapeless, as if it
were a mere accidental part; it looks like a red coloured mass
of extravasated blood. The brain, with some pretensions to
regularity of outline, is contained within the dura mater. The
eyes are concealed under the eyelids, which are as firmly glued
together as we find them in puppies for some short time after
birth, so that I found it scarcely possible to separate them and
open the eyes. The breast-bones and ribs have a certain degree of firmness, and the colour of the muscles changes from
white to blood red.

By the great number of dissections which I performed in the
course of this month, I was every day confirmed in my opinion
that the carunculæ of the uterus perform the office of the placenta; they are at this time found of a reddish colour, turgid,
and of the size of walnuts. The conception, which had previously adhered to the caruncles by the medium of mucor or
glutinous matter only, now sends the branches of its umbilical vessels into them, as plants send their roots into the
ground, by which it is fastened and may be said to grow to the
uterus.

About the end of December the fœtus is a span long, and I
have seen it moving lustily and kicking; opening and shutting
its mouth; the heart, inclosed in the pericardium, when exposed, was found pulsating strongly and visibly; its ventricles,
however, were still uniform, of equal amplitude of cavity and
thickness of parietes; and each ending in a separate apex,
they form together a double-pointed cone. Occasionally I have
seen the fluid contained in the auricles of the heart, which at

this time present themselves as ample sacs filled with blood, continuing to pulsate for some short time after the ventricles themselves had left off contracting.

The internal organs, all of which had lately become perfect, were now larger and more conspicuous. The skull was partly cartilaginous, partly osseous. The hooves were yellowish, flexible, and soft, resembling those of the adult animal softened in hot water. The uterine caruncles, of great magnitude and like immense fungi, extended over the whole cavity of the uterus, and plainly performed the office of placentæ, for numerous and ample branches of the umbilical vessels penetrated their substance there to imbibe nutritive matter for the growth of the embryo. As in the fœtus after birth, the chyle is now carried by the mesenteric veins to the porta of the liver.

Where there is a single fœtus the umbilical vessels are distributed to the whole of the carunculæ, both those of the horn where the fœtus is lodged and those of the opposite horn; where there is a pair of embryos formed, the umbilical vessels of each only extend to the caruncles of the horn appropriated to it.

The smaller umbilical veins in tending towards the fœtus, form larger and larger trunks by coalescing, until at length two great canals are formed, which in conjunction pour their blood into the vena cava and vena portæ. But the umbilical arteries, which arise from the division of the descending aorta, form two trunks of small size, not remarkable save for their pulse: proceeding to the boundary of the conception, in other words, to the conjunction of the placenta or carunculæ with the ramifications of the umbilical veins, they first divide into numerous capillary twigs, and then are lost in others that are invisible.

As the extremities of the umbilical veins within the uterus terminate in the caruncles, so the uterine vessels on the outside, which are large and numerous, and bring the blood from the mother towards the uterus, by means of the vessels of the suspensory ligaments, terminate externally on the caruncles. It is to be noted, also, that the internal vessels are almost all veins ; the external vessels, again, are in many instances branches of arteries. In the placenta of the woman, if it be carefully examined immediately after delivery, a much larger number of arteries than of veins, and these of larger size, will be found dispersed on every side in innumerable subdivisions to the very edge of the mass.   In the same kind of spongy parenchyma of the spleen, the number of the arteries is also greater than that of the veins.

The exterior uterine vessels run to the uterus, as I have said, not to the ovaries (testiculi) situated in the suspensory ligament, as some suppose.

I have remarked an admirable instance of the skill of nature, in the bulge or convexity of the caruncles turned towards the conception : a quantity of white and mucilaginous matter is discovered in a number of cavities, cotyledons, or little cups ; these are all as full of this matter as we ever see waxen cells full of honey ; now this matter, in colour, consistency, and taste, is extremely like white of egg.   On tearing the conception away from the caruncles, you will perceive numbers of suckers or capillary branches of the umbilical veins, looking like lengthened filaments, extracted at the same time from every one of the cotyledons and pits, and from amidst their mucilaginous contents ; very much as we see the delicate filaments of the roots of herbs following the stem when it is pulled out of the ground.

It is clearly ascertained from this that the extremities of the umbilical vessels are not conjoined by any anastomosis with the extremities of the uterine vessels ; that they do not imbibe any blood from them, but that they end and are obliterated in that mucilaginous matter, and from it take up their nourishment, nearly in the same way as at an earlier period they had sought for aliment from the albuminous humour contained within the membranes of the conception.   In the same manner, consequently, as the chick in ovo is nourished by the white of the egg through its umbilical vessels, is the fœtus of the hind and doe nourished by a similar albuminous matter laid up in these cells, and not directly from the blood of the mother.

These carunculæ might therefore with propriety be called the uterine liver, or the uterine mammæ, seeing that they are organs adapted for the preparation and concoction of that albuminous aliment, and fitting it for absorption by the veins.   In those viviparous animals consequently that have neither caruncles nor placentæ, as the horse and the hog, the fœtus is nourished up to the moment of its birth by fluids contained within the conception or ovum; nor has the ovum in these animals at any time a connexion with the uterus.

From all of what precedes it is manifest that in both the classes of viviparous animals alluded to, those, namely, that are provided with carunculæ or cotyledons, and those that want them, and perhaps in viviparous animals generally, the fœtus in utero is not nourished otherwise than the chick in ovo; the nutritive matter, the albumen, being of the same identical kind in all. As in the egg the terminations of the umbilical vessels are in the white and yelk, so in the hind and doe, and other animals furnished with uterine cotyledons like them, the final distributions of the umbilical vessels are sent to the humours that are included within the conception or ovum, and to the albumen that is stored in the cotyledons, or cup-like cavities of the carunculæ, where they open and end. And this is further obvious from the fact of the extremities of the umbilical vessels, when they are drawn out of the afore-mentioned mucor, looking completely white; a certain proof that they absorb this mucilage liquefied only, and not blood. The same arrangement may very readily be observed to obtain in the egg.

The human placenta is rendered uneven on its convex surface, and where it adheres to the uterus, by a number of tuberous projections, and it seems indeed to adhere to the uterus by means of these; it is not consequently attached at every point, but at those places only where the vessels pierce it in search of nourishment, and at those where, in consequence of this arrangement, an appearance as if of vessels broken short off is perceived. But whether the extremities of these vessels suck up blood from the uterus, or rather a certain concocted matter of the nature of albumen, as I have described the thing in the hind and doe, I have not yet ascertained.

Finally, that the truth just announced may be still more fully confirmed, it is found that by compressing the uterine caruncles between the fingers, about a spoonful of the nutritive fluid in question may be obtained from each of them, as from a nipple, unmixed with blood, which is not obtained even with forcible pressure. Moreover, the caruncle thus milked and emptied, like a compressed sponge, contracts and becomes flaccid, and is seen to be pierced with a great number of holes. From everything, therefore, it appears that these caruncles are uterine mammæ, or fountains and receptacles of nutritive albumen.

The month of December at an end, the caruncles adhere less firmly to the uterus than before, and a small matter suffices to detach them. The larger the fœtus grows, indeed, the nearer it is to its term, the more readily are the caruncles detached from the uterus, so that, like ripe fruit from the tree, they slip at length from the uterus of themselves, and as if they had formed an original element in the conception.

Separated from the uterus you may perceive in the prints which they leave points pouring out blood; these are the arteries that entered them. But if you now detach the conception from the caruncles, no blood is effused; none escapes, save from the ends of the vessels proceeding from the conception, although it does seem more consonant with reason to suppose that blood should be shed from the caruncles than from the conception when they are forcibly separated. For, as the caruncles or cotyledons have an abundance of uterine branches distributed to them, and they are generally believed to receive blood for the nourishment of the fœtus, we should expect that they would appear replete with blood. Nevertheless, as I have said, they yield no blood either under milking or compression, and the reason of this is that they contain albumen rather than blood, and rather store up than prepare this matter. It seems manifest, therefore, that the fœtus in utero is not nourished by its mother's blood, but by this albuminous fluid duly elaborated. It may even be perhaps that the adult animal is not nourished immediately by the blood, but rather by something mixed with the blood, which serves as the ultimate aliment; as may perhaps be more particularly shown in our PHYSIOLOGY and particular treatise on the Blood.

The truth of that passage of Hippocrates[1] where it said that " those whose acetabula or cotyledons are full of mucor, abort," has always been suspected by me; for this is no excrementitious matter or cause of miscarriage, but nourishment and a source of life. But Hippocrates, by the word acetabula, perhaps, understood something else than the parts so called in the uterus of the lower animals, for they are wanting in women;

---

[1] Lib. de Nat. Mul., de morb. vulg. et s. v, Aph. 45.

nor does the placenta in the human subject contain any collections of albuminous matter in distinct cavities.

Modern medical writers, following the Arabians, speak of three nutritious humours—dew, gluten, and cambium; these Fernelius designates nutritious juices; as if he had wished to imply that the parts of our bodies were not immediately nourished by the blood as ultimate nutriment, but by these secondary juices. The first of them, like dew, bathes all the minutest particles of the body on every side : this fluid, become thicker by an ulterior concoction, and adhering to the parts, is called gluten; finally, altered and assimilated by the proper virtue of the part, it is called cambium.

He who espoused such views might designate the matter which is contained in the cotyledonous cavities of the deer as gluten or nutritious albumen, and maintain that as the ultimate nourishment destined for each of the particular parts of the fœtus it was analogous to the albumen or vitellus of the egg. For as we but lately stated, with Aristotle, that the yelk of the egg was analogous to milk, so do we think it not unreasonable to assert, that the matter lodged in the cotyledons, or acetabula of the uterine placenta, stands instead of milk to the fœtus so long as it remains in the uterus; in this way the caruncles approve themselves a kind of internal mammæ, the nutritive matter of which, transferred at the period of parturition to the proper mammæ, there assumes the nature of milk, an arrangement by which the fœtus is seen to be nourished with the same food after it has begun its independent existence, as it was whilst it lodged in the uterus. Between the two-coloured eggs of oviparous animals, consequently, or the eggs that consist of a white and a yelk, and the ova or conceptions of viviparous animals, there is only this difference, that in the former the vitellus (which is a secondary nutritive matter) is prepared within the egg, and at the period of birth, being stored within the abdomen of the young creature, serves it as food; whilst in the latter, the nutritive juice is laid up within acetabula, and after birth is transferred to the mammæ; so that the chick is nourished with milk inclosed in its interior, whilst the fœtus of the viviparous animal draws its nourishment from the breasts of its mother.

In the months of January, February, &c., as nothing new or

worthy of note occurs which has not been already mentioned, (more than the growth of the hair, teeth, horns, &c.) but the parts only grow larger without reference to the process of generation, it seems unnecessary to say more upon such points at present.

I have frequently examined the conceptions of sheep during the same intervals. These I find, as in the deer, extending into both horns of the uterus, and presenting the figure of a wallet or double sausage. In several of them I found two fœtuses; in others only one: they were without a trace of wool on the surface, and the eyelids were so closely glued together that they could not be opened; the hooves, however, were present. Where there were two embryos they were contained in the opposite horns of the uterus, and without any regard to sex with reference to the right or left horn, the male being sometimes in the right, sometimes in the left, and the female the same; both, however, were, in every instance, included within one and the same common external membrane or chorion. The extreme ends of this membrane were stained on either hand with a yellow or bilious excrement, and appeared to contain something turbid or excrementitious in their interior.

Many caruncles, or miniature placentas of different sizes, were discovered, and otherwise disposed than in the hind and doe. In the sheep they look like rounded fungi with the foot-stalks broken off, and are contained in the coats of the uterus; their rounded or convex aspects are turned to the uterus, (a circumstance, by the way, common to the cow and sheep,) their concave aspects, which are the smooth ones, being turned towards the fœtus. The larger branches of the vessels are also distributed to the concave portion, as in the human placenta. The branches in extension of the umbilical vessels connected with the caruncles, grow pretty firmly into them, so that when I attempted to separate them the rounded portion was rather torn from the interior of the uterus than from the ovum or conception; different, consequently, from what we observed in the deer, where the chorion was readily detached from the cotyledons of the caruncules, and where the convexity of the caruncule, connected with the conception, is separable, whilst the concavity, or rather the pedicle or root, is firmly adherent to the uterus. In other respects the function

seems to be the same in both cases ; in both the same acetabula are discovered, and the same viscid and albuminous mucus
can be pressed out in both, as it can also in the cow.

In the conception that contains a single fœtus, the umbilical vessels are distributed to the whole of the caruncules of
either horn ; but the one in which the fœtus itself is contained,
swimming in its crystalline fluid within the amnion, is larger
than the other. In the cases where there are two fœtuses
present, each has its own separate or appropriate caruncles, and
does not send its umbilical vessels in quest of nourishment beyond the cornu in which it is lodged.

In male fœtuses, the testes contained in the scrotum, of
large size for the age, hang externally. Female fœtuses, again,
have their dugs in the same situation, furnished with nipples
like the breasts of women.

In the compound stomach of the fœtus, namely the omasus
and abomasus, a clear fluid is discovered, similar to that in
which it floats ; the two liquids agreeing obviously in smell,
taste, and consistency. There is also a quantity of chyle in
the upper part of the intestinal tube ; in the inferior portion a
greenish-coloured excrement and scybala, such as we find when
the animal is feeding on grass. The liver is discovered of considerable size, the gall-bladder of an oblong shape, and in some
cases empty.

In so far as the order in which the several parts are produced is concerned, we have still found the same rule to be
observed in the hind and doe as in the egg, and we believe
that the same law obtains among viviparous animals generally.

EXERCISE THE SEVENTY-FIRST.

Of the innate heat.

As frequent mention is made in the preceding pages of the
calidum innatum, or innate heat, I have determined to say a
few words here, by way of dessert, both on that subject and on
the *humidum primigenium*, or radical moisture, to which I am
all the more inclined because I observe that many pride them-

selves upon the use of these terms without, as I apprehend,
rightly understanding their meaning.   There is, in fact, no
occasion for searching after spirits foreign to, or distinct from,
the blood; to evoke heat from another source; to bring
gods upon the scene, and to encumber philosophy with any
fanciful conceits; what we are wont to derive from the stars is
in truth produced at home: the blood is the only calidum innatum, or first engendered animal heat; a fact which so clearly
appears from our observations on animal reproduction, particularly of the chick from the egg, that it seems superfluous to
multiply illustrations.

There is, indeed, nothing in the animal body older or more
excellent than the blood; nor are the spirits which are distinguished from the blood at any time found distinct from it;
for the blood without heat or spirit is no longer blood, but
cruor or gore.   " The blood," says Aristotle,[1] " is hot in a
certain manner, in that, namely, in virtue of which it exists as
blood,—just as we speak of hot-water under a single term; as
subject, however, and in itself finally, blood is blood, it is not
hot : so that as blood is in a certain way hot *per se,* so is it
also in a certain way not hot *per se :* heat is in its essence or
nature, in the same way as whiteness is in the essence of a
white man; but where blood is by affection or passion, it is
not hot *per se.*"

We physicians at this time designate that as spirit which
Hippocrates called *impetum faciens,* or moving power; im-
plying by this whatever attempts aught by its own proper
effort, and causes motion with rapidity and force, or induces
action of any kind; in this sense we are accustomed to speak
of spirit of wine, spirit of vitriol, &c.   And therefore it is that
physicians admit as many spirits as there are principal parts or
operations of the body, viz. animal, vital, natural, visual, auditory, concoctive, generative, implanted, influent, &c. &c.   But
the blood is the first produced and most principal part of the
body, endowed with each and all of these virtues, possessed of
powers of action beyond all the rest, and therefore, κατ᾽ ἐξο-
χήν—in virtue of its pre-eminence, meriting the title of spirit.

Scaliger, Fernelius, and others, giving less regard to the

---

[1] De Part. Anim. lib. ii, cap. 3.

admirable qualities of the blood, have imagined other spirits of an aerial or ethereal nature, or composed of an ethereal or elementary matter, a something more excellent and divine than the innate heat, the immediate instrument of the soul, fitted for all the highest duties. Now their principal motive for this was the consideration that the blood, as composed of elements, could have no power of action beyond these elements or the bodies compounded of them. They have, therefore, feigned or imagined a spirit, different from the ingenerate heat, of celestial origin and nature; a body of perfect simplicity, most subtile, attenuated, mobile, rapid, lucid, ethereal, participant in the qualities of the quintessence. They have not, however, anywhere demonstrated the actual existence of such a spirit, or that it was superior to the elements in its powers of action, or indeed that it could accomplish more than the blood by itself. We, for our own parts, who use our simple senses in studying natural things, have been unable anywhere to find anything of the sort. Neither are there any cavities for the production and preservation of such spirits, either in fact or presumed by their authors. Fernelius, indeed, has these words:[1] "He who has not yet completely mastered the matter and state of the ingenerate heat, let him cast an eye upon the structure of the body, and turn to the arteries, and contemplate the sinuses of the heart and the ventricles of the brain. When he observes them empty, containing next to no fluid, and yet feels that he must own such parts not made in vain, or without a design, he will soon, I conceive, be brought to conclude that an extremely subtile aura or vapour fills them during the life of the animal, and which, as being of extreme lightness, vanished insensibly when the creature died. It is for the sake of cherishing this aura that by inspiration we take in air, which not only serves for the refrigeration of the body, by a business that might be otherwise accomplished, but further supplies a kind of nourishment."

But we maintain that so long as an animal lives, the cavities of the heart and the arteries are filled with blood. We further believe the ventricles of the brain to be indifferently fitted for any so excellent office, and that they are rather formed for secreting some excrementitious matter. What shall we say,

---

[1] Physiologia, lib. iv, cap. 2.

too, when we find the brain of many animals unfurnished with ventricles? And supposing it were true that any kind of air or vapour was found there, seeing that all nature abhors a vacuum, still it does not seem over probable that it should be of heavenly origin and possessed of such superlative virtues. But what we admire most of all is that a spirit, the native of the skies, and endowed with such admirable qualities, should be nourished by our common and elementary air; especially when we see it maintained that the elements can do nothing that is beyond their natural powers.

It is admitted, moreover, that the spirits are in a perpetual state of flux, and most readily dissipated and corrupted; nor indeed can they endure for an instant unless renovated by due supplies of their appropriate nutriment,—they as much require incessant nourishing as the primum vivens, or first animate atom of the body. What occasion is there, then, I ask, for this extraneous inmate, for this ethereal heat? when the blood is competent to perform all the offices ascribed to it, and the spirits cannot separate from the blood even by a hair's breadth without destruction; without the blood, indeed, the spirits can neither move nor penetrate anywhere as distinct and independent matters. And whether they are engendered and are fed and increased, as some suppose, from the thinner part of the blood, or from the primigenial moisture, as others imagine, all still confess that they are nowhere to be found apart from the blood, but are inseparably connected with it as the aliment that sustains them, even as the flame of a lamp or candle is inseparably connected with the oil or tallow that feeds it. The tenuity, subtilty, mobility, &c. of the spirits, therefore, bring no kind of advantage more than the blood, which it seems they constantly accompany, already possesses. The blood consequently suffices, and is adequate to be the immediate instrument of the soul, inasmuch as it is everywhere present, and moves hither and thither with the greatest rapidity. Nor can it be admitted that there are any other bodies or qualities of a spiritual and incorporeal nature, or any more divine kinds of heat, such as light, as Cæsar Cremoninus,[1] a great adept in the Aristotelian philosophy, strenuously contends against Albertus that there are.

[1] Dictato vii.

If it be said that these spirits reside in the primigenial moisture as in their ultimate aliment, and flow from thence through the whole body to nourish its several parts, they propound a simple impossibility, viz. that the ingenerate heat, that primigenial element of the body, nourished itself, yet serves for the nourishment of the body at large. Upon such grounds the thing nourished and the thing that nourishes would be one and the same, and itself would both nourish and be nourished; which could in no way be effected; inasmuch as it is by no means probable that the nourishment should ever be mixed with the thing nourished, for things mixed must have equal powers and mutually act on one another; and, according to Aristotle's dictum, "where there is nutrition, there there is no mixture." But as nutrition takes place everywhere, the nutriment is one thing, and that which is nourished by it is another, and it is altogether indispensable that the one pass into the other.

But as it is thought that the spirits, and the ultimate or primigenial aliment, or something else, is contained in animals which acts in a greater degree than the blood above the forces of the elements, we are not sufficiently informed what is understood by the expression, " acting above the forces of the elements ;" neither are Aristotle's words rightly interpreted where he says,[1] " every virtue or faculty of the soul appears to partake of another body more divine than those which are called elements. . . . . For there is in every seed a certain something which causes it to be fruitful, viz. what is called heat, and that not fire or any faculty of the kind, but a spirit such as is contained in semen and frothy bodies ; and the nature inherent in that spirit is responsive in its proportions to the element of the stars. Wherefore fire engenders no animal; neither is anything seen to be constituted of the dense, or moist, or dry. But the heat of the sun and of animals, and not only that which is stored up in semen, but even that of any excrementitious matter, although diverse in nature, still contains a vital principle. For the rest, it is obvious from this that the heat contained in animals is not fire, neither does it derive its origin from fire." Now I maintain the same things of the innate heat and

---

[1] De Gen. Anim. lib. ii, cap. 3.

the blood; I say that they are not fire, and neither do they derive their origin from fire. They rather share the nature of some other, and that a more divine body or substance. They act by no faculty or property of the elements; but as there is a something inherent in the semen which makes it prolific, and as, in producing an animal, it surpasses the power of the elements, —as it is a spirit, namely, and the inherent nature of that spirit corresponds to the essence of the stars,—so is there a spirit, or certain force, inherent in the blood, acting superiorly to the powers of the elements, very conspicuously displayed in the nutrition and preservation of the several parts of the animal body; and the nature, yea, the soul in this spirit and blood, is identical with the essence of the stars. That the heat of the blood of animals during their lifetime, therefore, is neither fire, nor derived from fire, is manifest, and indeed is clearly demonstrated by our observations.

But that this may be made still more certain let me be permitted to digress a little from my subject, and, in a few words, to show what is meant by the word "spirit," and what by the phrases "superior in action to the forces of the elements," "to have the properties of another body, and that more divine than those bodies which are called elements," and "the nature inherent in this spirit which answers to the essence of the stars."

We have already had occasion to say something both of the nature of "spirit" and "the vital principle," and we shall here enter into the subject at greater length. There are three bodies—simple bodies—which seem especially entitled to receive the name, at all events, to perform the office of "spirit," viz. fire, air, and water, each of which, by reason of its ceaseless flux and motion, expressed by the words flame, wind, and flood, appears to have the properties of life, or of some other body. Flame is the flow of fire, wind the flow of air, stream or flood the flow of water. Flame, like an animal, is self-motive, self-nutrient, self-augmentative, and is the symbol of our life. It is therefore that it is so universally brought into requisition in religious ceremonies: it was guarded by priestesses and virgins in the temples of Apollo and Vesta as a sacred thing, and from the remotest antiquity has been held worthy of divine worship by the Persians and other ancient nations; as if God were most conspicuous in flame, and spoke to us from fire as he did to

Moses of old. Air is also appropriately spoken of as " spirit,"
having received the title from the act of respiration. Aristotle [1]
himself admits, "that there is a kind of life, and birth, and
death of the winds." Finally, we speak of a running stream
as " living water."

These three, therefore, inasmuch as they have a kind of life,
appear to act superiorly to the forces of the element, and to
share in a more divine nature ; they were, therefore, placed
among the number of the divinities by the heathen. When
any excellent work or process appeared, surpassing the powers
of the naked elements, it was held as proceeding from some more
divine agent. "To act with power superior to the powers of
the elements," therefore, and, on that account, "to share in the
properties of some more divine thing, which does not derive its
origin from the elements," appear to have the same signification.

The blood, in like manner, " acts with powers superior to the
powers of the elements" in the fact of its existence, in the forms
of primordial and innate heat, in semen and spirit, and its producing all the other parts of the body in succession ; proceeding at all times with such foresight and understanding, and
with definite ends in view, as if it employed reasoning in its acts.
Now this it does not, in so far as it is elementary, and as deriving its origin from fire, but in so far as it is possessed of
plastic powers and endowed with the gift of the vegetative soul,
as it is the primordial and innate heat, and the immediate and
competent instrument of life. Αἷμα, τὸ ζωτικὸν τοῦ ἀνθρώπου :
The blood is the living principle of man, says Suidas ; and the
same thing is true of all animals ; an opinion which Virgil
seems to have wished to express when he says :

> " Una eademque via sanguisque animusque sequuntur."
> And by one path the blood and life flowed out.

The blood, therefore, by reason of its admirable properties
and powers, is " spirit." It is also celestial; for nature, the soul,
that which answers to the essence of the stars, is the inmate of
the spirit, in other words, it is something analogous to heaven,
the instrument of heaven, vicarious of heaven.

In this way all natural bodies fall to be considered under a

---

[1] De Gen. Anim. lib. iv, cap. ultimum.

twofold point of view, viz. either as they are specially regarded, and are comprehended within the limits of their own
proper nature, or are viewed as the instruments of some more
noble agent and superior power.   For as regards their peculiar
powers, there is, perhaps, no doubt but that all things subject
to generation by birth, and to death and decay, derive their
origin from the elements, and perform their offices agreeably to
their proper standard ; but in so far as they are the instruments
of a more excellent agent, and are governed by that, not acting
of their own proper nature, but by the regimen of another;
therefore is it, therein is it, that they seem to participate with
another and more divine body, and to surpass the powers of
the ordinary elements.

In the same way, too, is the blood the animal heat, in so
far, namely, as it is governed in its actions by the soul; for it
is celestial as subservient to heaven ; and divine, because it is
the instrument of God the great and good.   But this we have
already spoken of above, where we have shown that male and
female were the instruments of the sun, heaven, and Supreme
Preserver, when they served for the generation of the more
perfect animals.

The inferior world, according to Aristotle, is so continuous
and connected with the superior orbits, that all its motions and
changes appear to take their rise and to receive direction from
thence.   In that world, indeed, which the Greeks called Κόσμος
from its order and beauty, inferior and corruptible things wait
upon superior and incorruptible things ; but all are still subservient to the will of the supreme, omnipotent, and eternal
Creator.

They, therefore, who think that nothing composed of the
elements can show powers of action superior to the forces exer-
cised by these, unless they at the same time partake of some
other and more divine body, and on this ground conceive the
spirits they evoke as constituted partly of the elements, partly
of a certain ethereal and celestial substance—these persons, I
say, appear to me to reason indifferently.   In the first place
you will scarcely find any elementary body which in acting
does not exceed its proper powers : air and water, the winds
and the ocean, when they waft navies to either India and round
this globe, and often by opposite courses, when they grind,

bake, dig, pump, saw timber, sustain fire, support some things, overwhelm others, and suffice for an infinite variety of other and most admirable offices—who shall say that they do not surpass the powers of the elements? In like manner what does not fire accomplish? in the kitchen, in the furnace, in the laboratory, [in the steam-engine], softening, hardening, melting, subliming, changing, [and setting in motion], in an infinite variety of ways! What shall we say of it when we see iron itself produced by its agency?—iron "that breaks the stubborn soil, and shakes the earth with war!"—iron that in the magnet (to which Thales therefore ascribed a soul) attracts other iron, "subdues all other things, and seeks besides I know not what inane," as Pliny[1] says; for the steel needle only rubbed with the loadstone still steadily points to the great cardinal points; and when our clocks constantly indicate the hours of the day and night,—shall we not admit that all of these partake of something else, and that of a more divine nature, than the elements? And if in the domain and rule of nature so many excellent operations are daily effected surpassing the powers of the things themselves, what shall we not think possible within the pale and regimen of nature, of which all art is but imitation? And if, as ministers of man, they effect such admirable ends, what, I ask, may we not expect of them, when they are instruments in the hand of God?

We must, therefore, make the distinction and say, that whilst no primary agent or prime efficient produces effects beyond its powers, every instrumental agent may exceed its own proper powers in action; for it acts not merely by its own virtue, but by the virtue of a superior efficient.

They, consequently, who refuse such remarkable faculties to the blood, and go to heaven to fetch down I know not what spirits, to which they ascribe these divine virtues, cannot know, or at all events, cannot consider that the process of generation, and even of nutrition, which indeed is a kind of generation, for the sake of which they are so lavish of admirable properties, surpasses the powers of those very spirits themselves, nor of the spirits only, but of the vegetative, aye, even the sensitive, and I will venture to add, the rational soul. Powers, did

---

[1] Lib. xxxvi, cap. 16.

I say? It far exceeds even any estimate we can form of the rational soul; for the nature of generation, and the order that prevails in it, are truly admirable and divine, beyond all that thought can conceive or understanding comprehend.

That it may, however, more clearly appear that the remarkable virtues which the learned attribute to the spirits and the innate heat belong to the blood alone, besides what has already been spoken of as conspicuous in the egg before any trace of the embryo appears, as well as in the perfect and adult fœtus, the few following observations are made by way of further illustration, and for the sake of the diligent inquirer. The blood considered absolutely and by itself, without the veins, in so far as it is an elementary fluid, and composed of several parts—of thin and serous particles, and of thick and concrete particles called cruor—possesses but few, and these not very obvious virtues. Contained within the veins, however, inasmuch as it is an integral part of the body, and is animated, regenerative, and the immediate instrument and principal seat of the soul, inasmuch, moreover, as it seems to partake of the nature of another more divine body, and is transfused by divine animal heat, it obtains remarkable and most excellent powers, and is analogous to the essence of the stars. In so far as it is spirit, it is the hearth, the Vesta, the household divinity, the innate heat, the sun of the microcosm, the fire of Plato; not because like common fire it lightens, burns, and destroys, but because by a vague and incessant motion it preserves, nourishes, and aggrandizes itself. It farther deserves the name of spirit, inasmuch as it is radical moisture, at once the ultimate and the proximate and the primary aliment, more abundant than all the other parts; preparing for and administering to these the same nutriment with which itself is fed, ceaselessly permeating the whole body, cherishing and keeping alive the parts which it has fashioned and added to itself, not otherwise assuredly than the superior stars, the sun and moon especially, in maintaining their own proper orbits, continually vivify the stars that are beneath them.

Since the blood acts, then, with forces superior to the forces of the elements, and exerts its influence through these forces or virtues, and is the instrument of the Great Workman, no one can ever sufficiently extol its admirable, its divine faculties.

In the first place, and especially, it is possessed by a soul which is not only vegetative, but sensitive and motive also; it penetrates everywhere and is ubiquitous; abstracted, the soul or the life too is gone, so that the blood does not seem to differ in any respect from the soul or the life itself (anima); at all events, it is to be regarded as the substance whose act is the soul or the life. Such, I say, is the soul, which is neither wholly corporeal nor yet wholly incorporeal; which is derived in part from abroad, and is partly produced at home; which in one way is part of the body, but in another way is the beginning and cause of all that is contained in the animal body, viz. nutrition, sense, and motion, and consequently of life and of death alike; for whatever is nourished, is itself vivified, and *vice versa*. In like manner, that which is abundantly nourished increases; what is not sufficiently supplied shrinks; what is perfectly nourished preserves its health; what is not perfectly nourished falls into disease. The blood, therefore, even as the soul, is to be regarded as the cause and author of youth and old age, of sleep and waking, and also of respiration; all the more and especially as the first instrument in natural things contains the internal moving cause within itself. It therefore comes to the same thing, whether we say that the soul and the blood, or the blood with the soul, or the soul with the blood, performs all the acts in the animal organism.

We are too much in the habit, neglecting things, of worshipping specious names. The word blood, signifying a substance, which we have before our eyes, and can touch, has nothing of grandiloquence about it; but before such titles as spirits, and calidum innatum or innate heat, we stand agape. But the mask removed, as the error disappears, so does the idle admiration. The celebrated stone, so much vaunted for its virtues by Pipinus to Migaldus, seems to have filled not only him but also Thuanus, an excellent historian, with wonder and admiration. Let me be allowed to append the riddle: " Lately," says he, " there was brought from the East Indies to our king a stone, which we have seen, wonderfully radiant with light and effulgence, the whole of which, as if burning and in flames, was resplendent with an incredible brilliancy of light. Tossed hither and thither, it filled the ambient air with beams that were scarcely bearable by any eyes. It was also extremely impatient of the earth; if you essayed to cover it, it forthwith and of itself burst forth with violence, and mounted on high.   No man could by any art contain or inclose it in any confined place; on the contrary, it appears to delight in free and spacious places. It is of the highest purity, of the greatest brightness, and is without stain or blemish. It has no certain shape, but a shape uncertain and changing every moment.   Of the most consummate beauty, it suffers no one to touch it; and if you persist too long or obstinately, it will do you injury, as I have observed it repeatedly to do in no trifling measure.   If anything be by chance taken from it by persevering efforts, it is (strange to say) made nothing less thereby.   Its custodier adds farther, that its virtues and powers are useful in a great variety of ways, and even—especially to kings—indispensably necessary; but these he declines to reveal without being first paid a large reward." The author might have added of this *stone* that it was neither hard nor soft, and exhibited a variety of forms and colours, and had a singular trick of trembling and palpitating, and like an animal—although itself inanimate—consumed a large quantity of food every day for its nutrition or sustenance.   Farther, that he had heard from men worthy of credit, that this stone had formerly fallen from heaven to earth; that it was the frequent cause of thunder and lightning, and was still occasionally engendered from the solar beams refracted through water.

Who would not admire so remarkable a stone, or believe that it acted with a force superior to the forces of the elements, that it participated in the nature of another body, and possessed an ethereal spirit? especially when he found that it responded in its proportions to the essence of the sun. But with Fernelius[1] for Œdipus, we find the whole enigma resolving itself into "Flame."

In the same way, did I paint the blood under the garb of a fable, and gave it the title of the philosopher's stone, and propose all its wonderful faculties and operations in enigmatical language, many would doubtless think a great deal of it; they would readily believe that it could act with powers superior to those of the elements, and they would not unwillingly allow it to be possessed of another and more divine body.

---

[1] De Abdit. rer. caus. lib. ii, cap. 27.

Of the primigenial moisture.

We have now dignified the blood with the title of the innate heat; with like propriety, we believe, that the fluid which we have called the crystalline colliquament, from which the fœtus and its parts primarily and immediately arise, may be designated the radical and primigenial moisture. There is certainly nothing in the generation of animals to which this title can with better right be given.

We call this the radical moisture, because from it arises the first particle of the embryo, the blood, to wit; and all the other posthumous parts arise from it as from a root; and they are procreated and nourished, and grow and are preserved by the same matter.

We also call it primigenial, because it is first engendered in every animal organism, and is, as it were, the foundation of the rest; as may be seen in the egg, in which it presents itself after a brief period of incubation, as the first work of the inherent fecundity and reproductive power.

This fluid is also the most simple, pure, and unadulterated body, in which all the parts of the pullet are present potentially, though none of them are there actually. It appears that nature has conceded to it the same qualities which are usually ascribed to first matter common to all things, viz. that potentially it be capable of assuming all forms, but have itself no form in fact. So the crystalline humour of the eye, in order that it might be susceptible of all colours, is itself colourless; and in like manner are the media or organs of each of the senses destitute of all the other qualities of sensible things: the organs of smelling and hearing, and the air which ministers to them, are without smell and sound; the saliva of the tongue and mouth is also tasteless.

And it is upon this argument that they mainly rely who maintain the possibility of an incorporeal intellect, viz. because it is susceptible of all forms without matter; and as the hand is called the " instrument of instruments," so is the intellect

33

called " the form of forms," being itself immaterial and wholly without form; it is, therefore, said to be possible or potential, but not passible.

This fluid, or one analogous to it, appears also to be the ultimate aliment from which Aristotle taught that the semen, or geniture, as he calls it, is produced.[1] I say the ultimate aliment, called dew by the Arabians, with which all the parts of the body are bathed and moistened. For in the same way as this dew, by ulterior condensation and adhesion, becomes alible gluten and cambium, whence the parts of the body are constituted, so, mutatis mutandis, in the commencement of generation and nutrition, from gluten liquefied and rendered thinner is formed the nutritious dew: from the white of the egg is produced the colliquament under discussion, the radical moisture and primigenial dew. The thing indeed is identical in either instance, if any credit be accorded to our observations; and in fact neither philosophers nor physicians deny that an animal is nourished by the same matter out of which it is formed, and is increased by that from which it was engendered. The nutritious dew, therefore, differs from the colliquament or primigenial moisture only in the relation of prior and posterior; the one is concocted and prepared by the parents, the other by the embryo itself, both juices, however, being the proximate and immediate aliment of animals; not indeed "first and second," according to that dictum, " contraria ex contrariis," but ultimate, as I have said, and as Aristotle himself admonishes us, according to that other dictum, " similia ex similibus augeri," " like is necessarily increased by its like." There is in either fluid a proximate force, in virtue of which, no obstacles intervening, it will pass spontaneously, or by the law of nature, into every part of the animal body.

Such being the state of the question, it is obvious that all controversy about the matter of animals and their nourishment may be settled without difficulty. For as some believe that the semen or matter emitted in intercourse is taken up from every part of the body, so do they derive from this the resemblance of the offspring to the parents. Aristotle has these words: " Against the opinion of the ancients, it may

---

[1] De Gen. Anim. lib. i, cap. 18, et lib. iv, cap. 1.

be said that as they avow the semen to be a derivative from all parts else, we believe the semen to be disposed of itself to form every part; and whilst they call it a colliquament, we are rather inclined to regard it as an excrement" (he had, however, said shortly before that he entitled excrement the remains of the nourishment, and colliquament that which is secreted from the growth by a preternatural resolution); "for that which arrives last, and is the excrement of what is final, is in all probability of the same nature; in the same way as painters have very commonly some remains of colours, which are identical with those they have applied upon their canvass; but anything that is consuming and melting away is corrupt and degenerate. Another argument that the seminal fluid is not a colliquament, but an excrement, is this: that animals of larger growth are less prolific, smaller creatures more fruitful. Now there must be a larger quantity of colliquament in larger than in smaller animals, but less excrement; for as there must be a large consumption of nourishment in a large body, so must there be a small production of excrement. Farther, there is no place provided by nature for receiving and storing colliquament; it flows off by the way that is most open to it; but there are receptacles for all the natural excrements—the bowels for the dry excrements, the bladder for the moist; the stomach for matters useful; the genital organs, the uterus, the mammæ for seminal matter—in which several places they collect and run together." After this he goes on by a variety of arguments to prove that the seminal matter from which the fœtus is formed is the same as that which is prepared for the nutrition of the parts at large. As if, should one require some pigment from a painter, he certainly would not go to scrape off what he had already laid on his canvass, but would supply the demand from his store, or from what he had over from his work, which was still of the same nature as that which he might have taken away from his picture. So and in like manner the excrement of the ultimate nutriment, or the remainder of the gluten and dew, is carried to the genital organs and there deposited; and this view is most accordant with the production of eggs by the hen.

The medical writers, too, who hold all the parts to be originally formed from the spermatic fluid, and consequently speak of these under the name of spermatic parts, say that the semen is formed from the ultimate nourishment, which with Aristotle they believe to be the blood, being produced by the virtue of the genital organs, and constituting the "matter" of the foetus. Now it is obvious enough that the egg is produced by the mother and her ultimate nutriment, the nutritious dew, to wit. That clear part of the egg, therefore, that primigenial, or rather antegenial colliquament, is more truly to be reputed the semen of the cock, although it is not projected in the act of intercourse, but is prepared before intercourse, or is gathered together after this, as happens in many animals, and as will perhaps be stated more at length by and by, because the geniture of the male, according to Aristotle, coagulates.

When I see, therefore, all the parts formed and increasing from this one moisture, as "matter," and from a primitive root, and the reasons already given combine in persuading us that this ought to be so, I can scarcely refrain from taunting and pushing to extremity the followers of Empedocles and Hippocrates, who believed all similar bodies to be engendered as mixtures by association of the four contrary elements, and to become corrupted by their disjunction; nor should I less spare Democritus and the Epicurean school that succeeded him, who compose all things of congregations of atoms of diverse figure. Because it was an error of theirs in former times, as it is a vulgar error at the present day, to believe that all similar bodies are engendered from diverse or heterogeneous matters. For on this footing, nothing even to the lynx's eye would be similar, one, the same, and continuous; the unity would be apparent only, a kind of congeries or heap—a congregation or collection of extremely small bodies; nor would generation differ in any respect from a [mechanical] aggregation and arrangement of particles.

But neither in the production of animals, nor in the generation of any other "similar" body (whether it were of animal parts, or of plants, stones, minerals, &c.), have I ever been able to observe any congregation of such a kind, or any divers miscibles pre-existing for union in the work of reproduction. For neither, in so far at least as I have had power to perceive, or as reason will carry me, have I ever been able to trace any "similar" parts, such as membranes, flesh, fibres, cartilage, bone, &c.,

produced in such order, or as coexistent, that from these, as the elements of animal bodies, conjoined organs or limbs, and finally, the entire animal, should be compounded. But, as has been already said, the first rudiment of the body is a mere homogeneous and pulpy jelly, not unlike a concrete mass of spermatic fluid; and from this, under the law of generation, altered, and at the same time split or multifariously divided, as by a divine fiat, from an inorganic an organic mass results; this is made bone, this muscle or nerve, this a receptacle for excrementitious matter, &c.; from a similar a dissimilar is produced; out of one thing of the same nature several of diverse and contrary natures; and all this by no transposition or local movement, as a congregation of similar particles, or a separation of heterogeneous particles is effected under the influence of heat, but rather by the segregation of homogeneous than the union of heterogeneous particles.

And I believe that the same thing takes place in all generation, so that similar bodies have no mixed elements prior to themselves, but rather exist before their elements (these, according to Empedocles and Aristotle, being fire, air, earth, and water; according to chemists, salt, sulphur, and mercury; according to Democritus, certain atoms), as being naturally more perfect than these. There are, I say, both mixed and compound bodies prior to any of the so called elements, into which they are resolved, or in which they end. They are resolved, namely, into these elements according to reason rather than in fact. The so-called elements, therefore, are not prior to those things that are engendered, or that originate, but are posterior rather—they are relics or remainders rather than principles. Neither Aristotle himself nor any one else has ever demonstrated the separate existence of the elements in the nature of things, or that they were the principles of " similar" bodies.

The philosopher,[1] indeed, when he proceeds to prove that there are elements, still seems uncertain whether the conclusion ought to be that they exist *in esse*, or only *in posse;* he is of opinion that in natural things they are present in power rather than in action; and therefore does he assert, from the division, separation, and solution of things, that there

---

[1] Lib. iii, de Cœlo, cap. 31.

are elements. It is, however, an argument of no great cogency to say that natural bodies are primarily produced or composed of those things into which they are ultimately resolved; for upon this principle some things would come out composed of glass, ashes, and smoke, into which we see them finally reduced by fire; and as artificial distillation clearly shows that a great variety of vapours and waters of different species can be drawn from so many different bodies, the number of elements would have to be increased to infinity. Nor has any one among the philosophers said that the bodies which, dissolved by art, are held pure and indivisible in their species, are elements of greater simplicity than the air, water, and earth, which we perceive by our senses, which we are familiar with through our eyes.

Nor, to conclude, do we see aught in the shape of miscible matter naturally engendered from fire; and it is perhaps impossible that it should be so, since fire, like that which is alive, is in a perpetual state of fluxion, and seeks for food by which it may be nourished and kept in being; in conformity with the words of Aristotle,[1] that "Fire is only nourished, and is especially remarkable in this." But what is nourished cannot itself be mingled with its nutriment. Whence it follows that it is impossible fire should be miscible. For mixture, according to Aristotle, is the union of altered miscibles, in which one thing is not transformed into another, but two things, severally active and passive, into a third thing. Generation, however, especially generation by metamorphosis, is the distribution of one similar thing having undergone change into several others. Nor are mixed similar bodies said to be generated from the elements, but to be constituted by them in some certain way, solvent forces residing in them at the same time.

These considerations, however, properly belong to the section of Physiology, which treats of the elements and temperaments, where it will be our business to speak of them more at large.

---

[1] De Gen. et Corrup. lib. ii, cap. 50.

ON PARTURITION.

ON PARTURITION.

ON generation follows parturition, that process, viz. by which the fœtus comes into the world and breathes the external air. I have, therefore, thought it well worth while, and within the scope of my design, to treat briefly of this subject. With Fabricius, then, I shall consider the causes, the manner, and the seasons of this process, as well as the circumstances which both precede and follow it. The circumstances which occur immediately previous to birth, and which, in women especially, indicate that the act of parturition is not far distant, are, on the one hand, such a preparation and arrangement on the part of the mother as may enable her to get rid of her offspring; and on the other, such a disposition of the fœtus as may best facilitate its expulsion.

With respect to the latter, viz. the position of the fœtus, Fabricius says,[1] "that it is disposed in a globular form and bent upon itself, in order that its extremities and prominent points generally may not injure the uterus and the containing membranes; another reason being that it may be packed in as small a space as possible." For my own part, I cannot think that these are the reasons why the limbs of the fœtus are always kept in the same position. Swimming and moving about, as it does, in water, it extends itself in every direction, and so turns and twists itself that occasionally it becomes entangled in a marvellous manner in its own navel-string. The truth is, that all animals, whilst they are at rest or asleep,

---

[1] De Form. Fœt. cap. ix, p. 40.

fold up their limbs in such a way as to form an oval or globular figure : so in like manner embryos, passing as they do the greater part of their time in sleep, dispose their limbs in the position in which they are formed, as being most natural and best adapted for their state of rest. So too the infant in utero is generally found disposed after this manner : the knees are drawn up towards the abdomen, the legs flexed, the feet crossed, and the hands directed to the head, one of them usually resting on the temples or ears, the other on the chin, in which situation white spots are discernible on the skin as the result of friction; the spine, moreover, is curved into a circle, and the neck being bowed, the head falls upon the knees. In such a position is the embryo usually found, as that which we naturally take in sleep; the head being situated superiorly, and the face usually turned towards the back of the mother. A short time, however, before birth the head is bent downwards towards the orifice of the uterus, and the fœtus, as it were, in search of an outlet, dives to the bottom. Thus Aristotle:[1] "All animals naturally come forth with the head foremost; but cross and foot presentations are unnatural." This, however, does not hold universally; but as the position in utero varies, so too does the mode of exit; this may be observed in the case of dogs, swine, and other multiparous animals. The human fœtus even has not always the same position; and this is well known to pregnant women, who feel its movements in very different parts of the uterus, sometimes in the upper part, sometimes in the lower, or on either side.

In like manner the uterus, when the term of gestation is completed, descends lower (in the pelvis), the whole organ becomes softer, and its orifice patent. The "waters" also, as they are vulgarly called, "gather;" that is, a portion of the chorion, in which the watery matter is contained, gets in front of the fœtus, and falls from the uterus into the vagina; at the same time the neighbouring parts become relaxed and dilatable; in addition to which the cartilaginous attachments of the pelvic bones so lose their rigidity that the bones themselves yield readily to the passage of the fœtus, and thus greatly in-

---

[1] Hist. Anim. lib. vii, cap. 7.

crease the area of the hypogastric region. When all these circumstances concur, it is quite clear that delivery is not far distant. Nature, in her provident care, contrives this dilatation of the parts in order that the fœtus may come into the world like the ripe fruit of a tree; just as she fills the breasts of the mother with milk that the being who is soon to enjoy an independent existence may have whereon to subsist. These, then, are the circumstances which immediately precede birth; and thus it happens that the presence of milk has especially been regarded as a sign of approaching delivery—milk, I mean, of a character suitable for the sustenance of the offspring; and this, according to Aristotle,[1] is only visible at the period of birth; it is therefore never observed before the seventh month of pregnancy.

Fabricius[2] maintains that on the subject of parturition there were two special heads of inquiry, viz. the time at which and the manner in which the process took place. Under the first of these heads he considers the term of utero-gestation; under the second, the way in which the fœtus comes into the world.

Aristotle[3] thought that the term of utero-gestation varied much. " There is," he says, " a certain definite term to each animal, determined in the majority of cases by the animal's duration of life; for it follows of necessity that a longer period is required for the production of the longer-lived animals." He attributes, however, the chief cause to the size of the animal; " for it is scarcely possible," he continues, " that the vast frames of animals or of aught else can be brought to perfection in a short period of time. Hence it is that in the case of mares and animals of cognate species, though their duration of life is small, their term of utero-gestation is considerable; and thus the elephant carries its young-for the space of two years, the reason being its enormous size, for each animal has a definite magnitude, beyond which it cannot pass." I would add, that the material of which each is formed has also its fixed limit in point of quantity. He says, moreover, " There is good reason why animals should have the periods of gestation, generation, and duration of life in certain cycles—I mean by cycle, a day, night, month, and year, and

---

[1] De Gen. Anim. lib. iv, cap. 8, et lib. vii, cap. 5.　　[2] Page 141.
[3] De Gen. Anim. lib. iv, cap. 4 et ult.

the time which is described by these; also the motions of the
moon—for these are the common origin of generation to all.
For it is in accordance with reason that the cycles of inferior
things should follow those of the higher." Nature, then, has
decreed that the birth and death of animals should have their
period and limit after this manner.

Just as the birth of animals depends on the course of the
sun and moon, so have they various seasons for copulation and
different terms of utero-gestation, these last being longer or
shorter according to circumstances. "In the human species
alone," says the philosopher in the same part of his works,
"is the period of utero-gestation subject to great irregularity.
In other animals there is one fixed time, but in man several;
for the human fœtus is expelled both in the seventh and tenth
months, and at any period of pregnancy between these; moreover, when the birth takes place in the eighth month, it is possible for the infant to live." In the majority of animals there
is a distinct season for bringing forth their young; this is
generally found to be in the spring, when the sun returns, but
in many species it is in the summer, and in some in the
autumn, as is the case with the cartilaginous fishes. Hence it
is that animals, as the time of labour approaches, seek their
accustomed haunts, and provide a safe and comfortable shelter
where they may bring forth and rear their young. Hence, too,
the title "bird-winds," applied to those gales which prevail toward
the beginning of spring, the word owing its origin to the fact
of certain birds at that period of the year availing themselves
of these winds to accomplish their migrations. In like manner stated seasons are observed by those fishes which congregate in myriads in certain places for the purpose of rearing
their young. Moreover, in the spring, as soon as caterpillars
fall under our notice (their ova, as may be observed by the
way, like to invisible atoms, being for the most part carried by
the winds, and not owing their origin, as commonly supposed,
to spontaneous generation, or to be looked upon as the result
of putrefaction), straightway the trees put forth their buds,
soon to be devoured by these creatures; and these in their
turn fall victims to birds innumerable, and are carried to the
nest as food for the young brood. So constantly does this
hold, that whenever strange species of caterpillars fall under

notice, at the same time we are sure to see some rare and foreign birds, as if the latter had chased the former from some remote corner of the earth. Now in both of these classes of creatures the time for bringing forth their young is the same. Physicians, too, when these phenomena occur, are enabled to predict the approach of sundry strange diseases. Bees bring forth in the month of May, when honey abounds; wasps in the summer, when the fruit is ripe; and this is analogous to what takes place in viviparous animals, who produce their young at the period when their milk is best adapted for their offspring. But other animals of the non-migratory classes, in the same way, at stated seasons seek a place to deposit their young as they do a store of food. And thus it results that the countryman is able to decide what are the proper seasons for ploughing, sowing, and getting in his harvest, forming his opinion chiefly from the approach of flocks of birds, and especially of the seminivora. There are, however, some animals in whom there is no fixed time for production, and this is chiefly the case with those which are called domestic, and live with the human species. These both copulate and produce their young at uncertain seasons, and the reason probably is to be sought for in the larger quantity of food they consume, and the consequent inordinate salacity. But in these, as in the human species, the process of parturition is often difficult and dangerous.

There are other animals also on whom the course of the moon has influence, and which consequently copulate and bring forth their young at certain periods of the year—rabbits, mice, and the human female may be instanced. "For the moon," observes Plutarch,[1] "when half full, is represented as greatly efficacious in shortening the pains of labour, and this she effects by moderating and relaxing the humours—hence, I think, those surnames of Diana are derived, Locheia, i. e. the tutelar deity of childbirth, and Eilytheia, otherwise Lucina; for Diana and the moon are synonymous."

"In all other animals," says Pliny,[2] "there are stated seasons and periods for production and utero-gestation; in man alone are they undetermined." And this is, to a great extent, true;

---

[1] Sympos. lib. iii. qu. 10.　　　　[2] Lib. vii, cap. 5.

for in his case, although nature has laid down for the most part certain boundaries, yet there is sometimes a vast difference in individuals, and instances are recorded of women bringing forth viable children, some in the seventh, and others in the fourteenth month. Further, although Aristotle[1] asserts "that the majority of eight months' children in Greece die," he still admits "that they survive in Egypt and in some other countries, where the women have easy labours;" and although he says "that children born before the seventh month can under no circumstances survive, and that the seventh month is the first in which anything like maturity exists, and that the feebleness of children born even then is such as to make it necessary to wrap them in wool," he still allows "that these are viable." Franciscus Valesius tells us of a girl in his time, who, although a five months' child, had arrived at the age of twelve years. Adrianus Spigelius[2] also records the case of a certain courier, " who proved to the satisfaction of all, on the public testimony of the city of Middleburgh, that he was born at the commencement of the sixth month, and that his frame was so slight and fragile that his mother found it necessary to wrap him up in cotton until such times as he was able to bear the ordinary dress of infants." Avicenna[3] also states that a sixth months' child is very capable of surviving. In like manner it is proved, both by ancient and modern authorities, that children may live who are born after the completion of the eleventh month. "We are told," says Pliny,[4] "by Massurius, that when his inheritance was claimed by the next heir, Lucius Papyrius the prætor gave the decision against the claimant, although, by his mother's account, Massurius was a thirteen months' child—the ground of the judgment being that the term of utero-gestation had not been as yet accurately determined. There was indeed, not so long since, a woman in our own country who carried her child more than sixteen months, during ten of which she distinctly felt the movements of the fœtus, as indeed did others, and at last brought forth a living infant. These are rare contingencies, I will allow; and therefore it is hardly fair of Spigelius to blame Ulpianus the lawyer because he regarded as legitimate no child born after the completion of the

---

[1] Hist. Anim. lib. vii. cap. 4.

[2] In Epist. de incerto tempore partus.

[3] Lib. ix, De Nat. Anim. c. ult.

[4] Loco procitato.

tenth month. Both laws and precepts of art, we must remember, have reference to the general rules of vital processes. Besides, it is impossible to deny that many women, either for purposes of gain or from fear of punishment, have simulated pregnancy, and not hesitated to swear to the truth of their assertion :—others again have frequently been deceived, and fancied themselves pregnant, whilst the uterus has contained no product of conception. On this point Aristotle's[1] words may be quoted : "The exact period at which conception takes place in the case of those born after the eleventh month can scarcely be ascertained. Women themselves do not know the time at which they conceive ; for the uterus is often affected by flatulent disorders, and if under these circumstances conception takes place, women imagine this flatulency to mark the period of conception, because they have recognized certain symptoms which accompany actual conception."

In the case of other women in whom the fœtus has died in the third or fourth month, then putrefied, and come away in the form of fetid lochial discharges, we have known superfœtation to take place ; and yet these same women have persisted that they have brought forth their children after the completion of the fourteenth month. "It happens sometimes," says Aristotle,[2] "that an abortion takes place, and ten or twelve products of superfœtation come away. But if the (second) conception takes place soon after (the first), the woman goes to the full time with the second, and brings forth both as twins. This was said to have been the case in the fable of Iphicles and Hercules. And it is a subject which admits of proof ; for it is known of a woman that she brought forth one child resembling her husband, and another like a man with whom she had had adulterous intercourse. Another woman became pregnant of twins, and conceived another by superfœtation. Her labour came on, and she brought forth the twins well formed and at their proper time, whilst the third child was at the fifth month, and so died immediately."

A certain maid-servant being gotten with child by her master, to conceal her disgrace, fled to London in the month of September; here she was delivered, and returned home with her

---

[1] Hist. Anim. lib. vii, cap. 4. [2] Ibid.

health restored. In December, however, the birth of another child, conceived by superfœtation, proclaimed to the world the fault she had committed. "It happened to another woman," adds the philosopher, "to be delivered of a seven months' child, and afterwards of twins at the full term, the single child dying, the twins surviving. Other women also, having become pregnant of twins, have miscarried of one, and borne the other to the full term." It is very easy to understand how, if the earlier or later product of superfœtation come away after three or four months have elapsed, that mistakes may be made in calculating the subsequent months, especially by credulous and ignorant women. We have sometimes observed, both in women and other animals, the product of conception perish, and come away gradually in the form of a thin fluid, somewhat resembling fluor albus. Not long since a woman in London, after an abortion of this kind, conceived anew, and brought forth a child at the proper period. Subsequently, however, after a lapse of some months, as she was engaged in her ordinary duties, without any pain or uneasiness, there came away piecemeal some dark bones belonging to the fœtus of which she had formerly miscarried. I was able to recognize in some of the fragments portions of the spine, femur, and other bones.

I am acquainted with a young woman, the daughter of a physician with whom I am very intimate, who experienced in her own person all the usual symptoms of pregnancy; after the fourteenth week, being healthy and sprightly, she felt the movements of the child within the uterus, calculated the time at which she expected her delivery, and when she thought, from further indications, that this was at hand, prepared the bed, cradle, and all other matters ready for the event. But all was in vain. Lucina refused to answer her prayers; the motions of the fœtus ceased; and by degrees, without inconvenience, as the abdomen had increased so it diminished; she remained, however, barren ever after. I am acquainted also with a noble lady who had borne more than ten children, and in whom the catamenia never disappeared except as the result of impregnation. Afterwards, however, being married to a second husband, she considered herself pregnant, forming her judgment not only from the symptoms on which she usually relied, but also from the movements of the child, which were frequently felt both by herself and her sister, who occupied the same bed with her. No arguments of mine could divest her of this belief. The symptoms depended on flatulence and fat. Hence the best ascertained signs of pregnancy have sometimes deceived not only ignorant women, but experienced midwives, and even skilful and accurate physicians—so that as mistakes are liable to arise, not only from deception on the part of the women themselves, but also from the erroneous tokens of pregnancy, I should say that no rule is to be rashly laid down with respect to births taking place before the seventh or after the fourteenth month.

Unquestionably the ordinary term of utero-gestation is that which we believe was kept in the womb of his mother by our Saviour Christ, of men the most perfect; counting, viz. from the festival of the Annunciation, in the month of March, to the day of the blessed Nativity, which we celebrate in December. Prudent matrons, calculating after this rule, as long as they note the day of the month in which the catamenia usually appear, are rarely out of their reckoning; but after ten lunar months have elapsed, fall in labour, and reap the fruit of their womb the very day on which the catamenia would have appeared, had impregnation not taken place.

As regards the causes of labour, Fabricius, besides that of Galen[1] (who held " that the fœtus was retained in utero until it was sufficiently grown and nourished to take food by the mouth," according to which theory weakly children ought to remain in utero longer than others, which they do not), gives another and a better reason, viz. " the necessity the fœtus feels for more perfectly cooling itself by respiration, since the child breathes immediately on birth, but does not take food by the mouth. This is not only the case," he continues, " in man and quadrupeds, but has been particularly observed in birds : these, small as they are, and furnished as yet with but tender bills, peck through the egg-shell at the point where they have need of respiration; and they do this rather through want of breath than of food, since the instant they quit the shell the function of respiration begins, whilst they remain without eating for two days, or longer." This point, however, whether

---

[1] De Non Part. lib. xv, cap. 7.

the object of respiration be really to "cool" the animal, shall be discussed elsewhere at greater length.

In the mean time I would propose this question to the learned—How does it happen that the foetus continues in its mother's womb after the seventh month? seeing that when expelled after this epoch, not only does it breathe, but without respiration cannot survive one little hour; whilst, as I before stated, if it remain in utero, it lives in health and vigour more than two months longer without the aid of respiration at all. To state my meaning more plainly—how is it that if the foetus is expelled with the membranes unbroken, it can survive some hours without risk of suffocation; whilst the same foetus, removed from its membranes, if air has once entered the lungs, cannot afterwards live a moment without it, but dies instantly? Surely this cannot be from want of "cooling," for in difficult labours it often happens that the foetus is retained in the passages many hours without the possibility of breathing, yet is found to be alive; when, however, it is once born and has breathed, if you deprive it of air it dies at once. In like manner children have been removed alive from the uterus by the Cæsarean section many hours after the death of the mother; buried as they are within the membranes, they have no need of air; but as soon as they have once breathed, although they be returned immediately within the membranes, they perish if deprived of it. If any one will carefully attend to these circumstances, and consider a little more closely the nature of air, he will, I think, allow that air is given neither for the "cooling" nor the nutrition of animals; for it is an established fact, that if the foetus has once respired, it may be more quickly suffocated than if it had been entirely excluded from the air: it is as if heat were rather enkindled within the foetus than repressed by the influence of the air.

Thus much, by the way, on the subject of respiration; hereafter, perhaps, I may treat of it at greater length. As the arguments on either side are very equally balanced, it is a question of the greatest difficulty.

To return to parturition. Besides the reasons alluded to above, viz. "the necessity for respiration and the want of nourishment," Fabricius gives another; he says, "that the weight of the foetus becomes so great as to exert considerable pressure, and the bulk such that the uterus is unable to retain it, added to which the quantity of excrementitious matter is so much increased that it cannot be contained by the membranes." [1]

Now it has been shown above that the uterine humours are not excrementitious. Nor do the weight and bulk of the fœtus help us to a more probable explanation; for the fœtus suspended in water weighs but slightly on the placenta or uterus; besides which some nine months' children are very small, much less in fact than many fœtuses of eight months, nevertheless they do not abide longer in the womb. And as to weight, any twins of eight months are far heavier than a single nine months' child; yet they are not expelled before nine months are completed. Nor do we find a better reason in "want of nutriment;" twins, and even more children, are abundantly supplied with support up to the full term; and the milk which after delivery is sufficient for the nourishment of the child, could equally well, if transferred to the uterus, nourish the fœtus there.

I should rather attribute the birth of the child to the following reason—that the juices within the amnion, hitherto admirably adapted for nutriment, at that particular period either fail or become contaminated by excrementitious matter. I have touched on this subject before. The variation in the term of utero-gestation, occurring as it does chiefly in the human species, I believe to depend on the habits of life, feebleness of body, and on the various affections of the mind. And thus in the case of domesticated animals, owing to their indolence and overfeeding, the seasons both of copulation and production are less fixed and certain than in the wilder tribes. So women in robust health usually experience easy and rapid labours; the contrary holding good in those whose constitutions are shattered by disease. For the same thing befalls them that happens to plants, the seeds and fruits of which come later and less frequently to perfection in cold climates than in those where the soil is good and the sun powerful. Thus oranges in this country usually remain on the tree two years before they arrive at maturity; and figs, which in Italy ripen two or three times annually, scarcely come to perfection in our climate:—the

[1] P. 142.

same thing happens to the fruit of the womb; it depends on the abundance or deficiency of nutriment, on the strength or weakness of body, and on the right or wrong ordering of life with reference to what physicians call the "non-naturals," whether the child arrives sooner or later at maturity, i. e. is born.

Fabricius describes the manner of parturition as follows: "The uterus having been so enlarged by the bulk of the fœtus that it will admit of no further distension without risk, and thus excited to expulsion, is drawn into itself by the action of the transverse fibres, and diminishes its cavity. Thus whilst previously neither the excrementitious matters from their quantity, nor the fœtus from its bulk, could be contained within it, the uterus, contracted and compressed as it is now, becomes still less able to retain them. Wherefore, first of all, the membranes, as being the weaker parts, and suffering most pressure, are ruptured, and give exit to the waters, which are of a very fluid consistence, for the purpose of lubricating the passages. Then follows the fœtus, which tends towards, and, as it were, assaults the uterine aperture, not only by the force of its own gravity as no longer floating in water, but compressed and propelled by the action of the uterus: the abdominal muscles and the diaphragm also assist mightily in the entire process."

Now in these words Fabricius rather describes the process of defæcation or an abortion than a genuine and natural birth. For although in women, as a general rule, the membranes are ruptured before the escape of the fœtus, it is not universally so; nor does it hold in the case of other animals which bring forth their young enveloped in their membranes. This can be observed in the bitch, ewe, mare, and others, and more particularly in the viper, which conceives an ovum of an uniform colour and soft shell (resembling in fact the product of conception in the woman); this is retained until the fœtus is completely formed; it is then expelled entire, and, according to Aristotle,[1] is broken through by the young animal on the third day. It sometimes happens, however, that kittens, whilst yet in utero, gnaw through the membranes, and so come into the world uninvolved.

[1] Hist. Anim. lib. v, cap. 34.

And so also, according to the observation of experienced midwives, women have occasionally expelled the child with the membranes unbroken. And this kind of birth, in which the fœtus is born enveloped in its coverings, appears to me by far the most natural; it is like the ripe fruit which drops from the tree without scattering its seed before the appointed time. But where it is otherwise, and the placenta, subsequently to birth, adheres to the uterus, there is great difficulty in detaching it, grave symptoms arise, fetid discharges, and sometimes gangrene occur, and the mother is brought into imminent peril.

Since then the process of parturition, as described by Fabricius, does not apply to all animals, but to women alone, and this not universally, but only where the labour is premature, and, as it were, forced, we must regard it not so much as a description of a natural as of a preternatural and hurried delivery, in fact, of an abortion.

In natural and genuine labour two things are required, which mutually bear upon and assist each other: these are, the mother which produces, and the child to be produced; and unless both are ready to play their part, the labour will hardly terminate favorably, requiring as it does the proper maturity of both. For if, on the one hand, the fœtus, from restlessness and over-desire to make its way out, does violence to the uterus, and thus anticipates the mother; or if, on the contrary, the mother, owing to feebleness of the uterus, or any other circumstance necessitating expulsion, is beforehand with the fœtus, this is to be looked upon rather as the result of disease than as a natural and critical birth. The same may be said of those cases where parts only of the product of conception escape, whilst others remain; for instance, if the fœtus itself is disposed to come away when the placenta is not yet separated from the uterus, or, on the other hand, if the placenta is separated when the fœtus is not rightly placed, or the uterus is not sufficiently relaxed to allow of its passage. Hence it is that midwives are so much to blame, especially the younger and more meddlesome ones, who make a marvellous pother when they hear the woman cry out with her pains and implore assistance, daubing their hands with oil, and distending the passages, so as not to appear ignorant in their art—giving besides medicines to excite the expulsive powers, and when they would hurry the labour, retarding it and making it unnatural, by leaving behind portions of the membranes, or even of the placenta itself, besides exposing the wretched woman to the air, wearying her out on the labour-stool, and making her, in fact, run great risks of her life. In truth, it is far better with the poor, and those who become pregnant by mischance, and are secretly delivered without the aid of a midwife; for the longer the birth is retarded the more safely and easily is the process completed.

Of unnatural labours, therefore, there are chiefly two kinds: either the fœtus is born before the proper time (and this constitutes an abortion), or else subsequently to it, when a difficult or tedious labour is the result, either from the due time and order not being preserved, or from the presence of dangerous symptoms; these arise either from failure of the expelling powers on the part of the mother, or from sluggishness on the part of the fœtus in making its way out; it is when both perform their proper parts that a safe and genuine labour results.

Fabricius ascribes the business of expelling the offspring to the uterus; and he adds, "the abdominal muscles and the diaphragm assist in the business." It seems to me, however, on deep investigation, that the throes of childbirth, just as sneezing, proceed from the motion and agitation of the whole body. I am acquainted with a young woman who during labour fell into so profound a state of coma that no remedies had power to rouse her, nor was she in fact able to swallow. When called to her, finding that injections and other ordinary remedies had been employed in vain, I dipped a feather in a powerful sternutatory, and passed it up the nostrils. Although the stupor was so profound that she could not sneeze, or be roused in any way, the effect was to excite convulsions throughout the body, beginning at the shoulders, and gradually descending to the lower extremities. As often as I employed the stimulus the labour advanced, until at last a strong and healthy child was born, without the consciousness of the mother, who still remained in a state of coma.

We can observe the manner of labour-pains in other animals, as the bitch, sheep, and larger cattle, and ascertain that they do not depend on the action of the uterus and abdomen only, but on the efforts of the whole body.

The degree in which the offspring contributes to accelerate and

facilitate birth is made clear from observations on oviparous animals; in these it is ascertained that the shell is broken through by
the fœtus and not by the mother.   Hence it is probable that in
viviparous animals also the greater part of delivery is due to
the fœtus—to its efforts, I mean, not to its gravity, as Fabricius
would have it.   For what can gravity do in the case of quadrupeds standing or sitting, or in the woman when lying down?
Nor are the efforts of the fœtus to get out, the result, as he
believes, of its own bulk or of that of the waters; the waters, it
is true, when the fœtus is dead and decomposed, by their putrid
and acrimonious nature, stimulate the uterus to expel its contents; but it is the fœtus itself which, with its head downwards, attacks the portals of the womb, opens them by its own
energies, and thus struggles into day.   Wherefore a birth of
this kind is held the more speedy and fortunate; " it is contrary to nature," says Pliny,[1] " for a child to be born with the
feet foremost; hence those so born were called Agrippæ, i. e.
born with difficulty"—(ægre parti), for in such the labour is
tedious and painful.   Notwithstanding this, in cases of abortion, or where the fœtus is dead, or, in fact, when any difficulty
arises in the delivery so as to require manual aid, it is better
that the feet should come first; they act as a wedge on the
narrow uterine passages.   Hence, when we chiefly depend upon
the fœtus, as being lively and active, to accomplish delivery, we
must do our best that the head escape first; but if the business
is to be done by the uterus, it is advisable that the feet come
foremost.

    We are able to observe in how great a degree the fœtus con-
tributes to delivery, not only in birds, which, as I have said
above, break through the shell by their own powers, but also
in many other animals.   All kinds of flies and butterflies pierce
the little membrane in which they lie concealed as " aureliæ ;"
the silkworm also, at its appointed time, softens by moistening,
and then eats through the silken bag which it had spun round
itself for protection, and makes its way out without any foreign
aid.   In the same manner wasps, hornets, all insects in fact,
and fishes of every kind, are born by their own will and powers.
This can be best seen in the skate, fork-fish, lamprey, and the

<hr />

[1] Lib. vii, cap. 8.

cartilaginous fishes generally. These conceive a perfect two-coloured egg, made up, that is, of albumen and yelk, and contained in a strong quadrangular shell; from this, still retained within the uterus, the young fish is formed : it then breaks through the shell, and makes its way out. In an exactly similar manner the young viper eats through the egg-shell, sometimes whilst it remains in utero, sometimes when within the passages, at others two or three days after birth. Hence arose the fable of the young viper eating through the womb of its mother, and so avenging its father's death; it does, in fact, nothing but what the young of every animal does, breaking though the membranes which envelope it, either in the delivery itself, or a short time subsequently to that event.

We learn moreover from positive observations how much the fœtus contributes to its own birth. A woman in my own neighbourhood, and I speak as having knowledge of the circumstance, died one evening, and the body was left by itself in a room ; the next morning an infant was found between the thighs of the mother, having evidently forced its way out by its own efforts. Gregorius Nymmanus has collected several instances of a similar kind from trustworthy authors.

I am further acquainted with a woman who had the whole length of the vagina so torn and injured in a difficult labour, that subsequently, after she had again become pregnant, not only did the parts in the neighbourhood of the nymphæ, but the whole cavity of the vagina as far as the orifice of the uterus, become adherent; this went to such an extent that coition became impossible, nor could a probe be passed up, nor was there any passage left for the ordinary discharges. When her labour came on her sufferings were so dreadful that all hope of delivery was abandoned. She therefore gave up the keys to her husband, arranged her affairs, and took leave of her friends who were present. On a sudden, however, by the violent efforts of the fœtus the whole space was burst through, and a vigorous infant born; thus was the fœtus the salvation both of itself and its mother, besides opening the way for subsequent children. By the exhibition of proper remedies the mother recovered her former good state of health.

The following instance is even more remarkable. A white mare of great beauty had been presented to her Serene High-

ness the Queen, and in order that its symmetry and usefulness might not be impaired by foal-bearing, the grooms, as is
the custom, had infibulated the animal with iron rings. This
mare (by what chance I know not, nor could the grooms inform me) was got with foal; and at length, when no one suspected anything of the kind, she foaled in the night, and a
living foal was found the next morning by the mother's side.
When I heard of the circumstance I went immediately to the
place, and found the sides of the vulva still fastened together
by the rings, but the whole pudendum on the left side so
thrust and torn away from the pelvis by the almost incredible
efforts of the fœtus, that a gap sufficiently wide was made to
admit of its escape. Such is the force and vigour of a full-
grown and healthy fœtus.

But, on the contrary, if the fœtus is diseased or feeble, or is
born before the full term, it must be considered more an abortion than a regular birth, the fœtus being expelled rather than
born; and thus for some days after birth it neither properly
takes the breast nor gets rid of its excretions.

And yet the following example will show that the uterus
also contributes towards delivery. A poor washerwoman had
long suffered from procidentia uteri to such an extent that a
tumour hung between the thighs as large as the fist. As no
remedies had been applied, the prolapsed part became so rough
and wrinkled as to take on the appeararance of the scrotum,
and in this state she suffered less than at the commencement
of her illness. When consulted on her case, I ordered her to
keep her bed for several days, to employ fomentations and oint-
ments, and after the uterus was returned, to keep it in its
place by means of pessaries and bandages, until by the use of
strengthening applications it should be fixed firmly in its place.
This plan was followed by some success; but she soon suffered
a relapse, when compelled by her circumstances to follow her
usual occupations, and continue long in the erect position. She
bore, however, her inconvenience with patience, the uterus at
times protruding, at others not doing so. At night she could
usually reduce it, and it remained for some time in its proper
place. After the lapse of a few days she returned, and complained that the uterus was so swelled from the use, as she
thought, of the remedies, and especially of the fomentations, that

it could not any longer be retained. By using some applications she was enabled to accomplish the reduction; but the cure was only temporary, for as soon as she stood up, and followed her ordinary occupations, the uterus immediately gave her much inconvenience by its weight, and at length entirely prolapsed. And now it hung down to the middle of the thigh, like the scrotum of a bull, to such an extent that I suspected not only the vagina but also the uterus to be inverted, or that there was some kind of uterine hernia. At length the tumour exceeded in magnitude a man's head, acquired a resisting character, and hung down as low as the knees; it also gave her much pain, and prevented her walking except in the prone position; added to which it discharged a sanious fluid from its inferior part, as if some portion had ulcerated. On ocular inspection (for I did not employ the touch) I feared that cancer or carcinoma might result, and so thought of the ligature or excision; in the mean time I advised the employment of soothing fomentations to ease the pain. The following night, however, a fœtus of a span long, perfectly formed, but dead, was expelled from the tumour, and was brought to me the next day. I took out the intestines, and kept it in cold water without decomposition for many months, showing it to my friends as an extraordinary object of curiosity. The proper skin in this fœtus was not yet formed, but in its place there was a pellicle, which could be stripped off entire, like that on a baked apple; underneath all the muscles of the body could be distinctly seen, the fœtus being very lean. I shall describe at another opportunity what I discovered in this fœtus on dissection. I have mentioned the case on this occasion to show that it was the uterus alone which excited the abortion, and expelled the fœtus by its own efforts.

Fabricius[1] suggests two circumstances as especially worthy of admiration in and after birth: first, the dilatation of the uterus at the time of birth; secondly, the way in which after birth it is restored to its usual small size. He wonders how the uterus can be so distended as to allow the fœtus to escape, and afterwards in so short a period return to its pristine state. He says, "that with Galen[2] we can only wonder, but not understand," how the neck of the uterus, a part so thick, hard,

---

[1] De Form. Fœt. p. 142.   [2] De Usu Part. lib. xv, cap. 7.

and closely sealed, as not to admit a probe, can suffer such distension at the time of delivery. He gives,[1] however, the following reason: "that the unimpregnated uterus is of a thick and hard consistence, and so is its orifice, but when impregnated is yielding and soft, and in proportion as the term of delivery approaches, both the body of the uterus and its orifice become more and more yielding." He believes this to arise " from the distension which the uterus undergoes, and that when this distension takes place, the compact and plaited, so to speak, body of the uterus is expanded and unfolded; thus what was before thick and hard becomes soft and yielding, and ready to admit of the passage of the fœtus." He adds subsequently, " Some one may ask—if all this is correct, how is it that in pregnant animals the uterine aperture is so closed that it will not admit a probe? I answer, that this is so because the uterus, whilst it is being distended and undone, like a closely-folded piece of linen, begins to undergo these changes at its superior part; the lower portions then gradually widen, until the power of distension arrives at the aperture; this generally takes place at the period of birth. With reason then is the uterine orifice closely shut in the first months of pregnancy, whilst it is still hard and thick, but inclined to dilate in the latter ones. Thus much may be said about the unknown cause of Galen. Other circumstances may be mentioned as conducing to the dilatation of the orifice; for instance, the excretions of the fœtus, such as the sweat and urine; for although these are contained in their proper receptacles and membranes, yet some degree of moisture may be communicated to the uterine aperture, especially as it lies low, and always in the immediate neighbourhod of these humours; added to which, mucous and slimy matters are always found about the orifice." But in my opinion this great man is wrong; for the neck of the uterus is not hard from being folded on itself, but in consequence of its own proper substance and cartilaginous nature; and the accidental causes which he gives can have but little weight towards furthering the dilatation. This, doubtless, like every other contrivance in the human body, is owing to the divine providence of Nature, which directs her workmanship to

[1] P. 143.

certain ends, actions, and uses.   The structure, then, of the
uterus is such, that immediately on conception it shuts up
closely its cartilaginous aperture, for the purpose of retaining
the seed; this part subsequently, at birth, and that the fœtus
may escape, like fruit on the tree, comes to maturity and softens, and this not by any unfolding of its tissue, but by a change
in its natural character.   For a loosening and softening takes
place even in the commissural attachments of bones, as in those
between the haunches and the sacrum, the pubes, and the pieces
of the coccyx.   It is a truly wonderful thing that the little
point of a sprouting germ, say of the almond or another
fruit, should break the shell which a hammer can scarcely
crush; or that the tender fibres of the ivy-root should penetrate the narrow chinks of the stone, and at length cause rents
in mighty walls.   But it does not appear so marvellous that
the parts of the woman, when distended by labour, should recover their natural firmness, if we consider the state of the male
organ in coition, and how soon it subsequently becomes soft
and flaccid.   A greater matter for wonder is it, and surpassing
all these " foldings," that the substance of the uterus, as the
fœtus increases, not only is day by day enlarged and distended
or unfolded, as it were, to take Fabricius's notion, but that it
should become more thick, fleshy, and strong.   We may even,
with Fabricius, marvel still more at the means by which the
mass of the uterus, by the intervention of the ordinary lochial
discharges, returns to its original size in so few days; for this
is not the case with other tumours or abscesses; these require
a longer period for dispersion, being made up of unnatural
matters, and such as require digestion, a process opposed to
the power of expulsion.   Yet this is not more worthy of admiration than the other works of nature, for " all things are full
of God," and the Deity of nature is ever visibly present..
     In the last place, it is object of great wonder to Fabricius
how those vessels of the fœtus (meaning the oval opening
out of the vena cava into the pulmonary vein, and the duct
from the pulmonary artery into the aorta, on which subjects I
have entered fully in my Essay on the Circulation of the
Blood) immediately after birth begin to shrivel up and become obliterated.   He is driven to that reason given by

Aristotle,[1] and already cited by me, which is, that all parts are made for a certain function, and if the function ceases to be required that they themselves disappear. The eye sees, the ear hears, the brain perceives, the stomach digests, not because such characters and structures (naturally) belong to these organs; but they are endowed with such characters and structures to accomplish the functions appointed them by nature.

On grounds like these it would appear that the uterus holds the first place among the organs destined for generation; for the testicles are made to produce semen, the semen is for the purposes of intercourse, and coition itself, or the emission of the semen, is instituted by nature that the uterus may be fecundated and generation result.

I have said before that an egg is, as it were, the fruit of an animal, and a kind of external uterus. Now, on the other hand, we may regard the uterus as an egg remaining within. For as trees are gay with leaves, flowers, and fruit at stated periods, and oviparous animals at one time conceive and produce eggs, at another become effete, so that neither the "place" or the part that contained them can be found, so have viviparous animals their spring and autumn allotted them. At the season of fecundation the genital organs, especially in the female, undergo great changes, so much so that in birds, the ovary, which at other times is scarcely visible, now becomes turgid; and the belly of the fish, near about the time of spawning, far exceeds in bulk the rest of the body, owing to the enormous number of ova and the quantity of semen contained within it. In very many viviparous animals the genital organs, that is, the uterus and spermatic vessels, are not always found presenting the same mode and course of action and structure; but as they are capable or not of conception, so changes take place, and to such an extent that the organs can hardly be recognized as the same. In nature, just as there is nothing lacking, so is there nothing superfluous; and thus it happens that the organs of generation wither away and are lost when there is no longer any use for them.

At the period of coitus in the hare and mole, the testicles

---

[1] De Gen. Anim. lib. i, cap. 5.

of the male become visible, and in the female the horns of the uterus appear. In truth, it is most marvellous to see what an enormous quantity of semen is contained in full-grown moles and mice at those times, whilst at others no semen can be seen, and the testicles are shrunk and retracted. So also when the reproductive faculty ceases in the female, the uterus is found with difficulty, and it is scarcely possible to distinguish the sexes.

The uterus, especially in the woman, varies extraordinarily as it is fecundated or not, both in constitution and in the results of that constitution—I mean in position, size, form, colour, thickness, hardness, and density. In the girl, before the age of puberty, the breasts are no larger than those of the boy, and the uterus is a small, white, membranous organ, destitute of vessels, and not larger than the top of the thumb, or a large bean. In like manner in old women, as the breasts are collapsed, so is the uterus shrunken, flaccid, withered, pale, and void of vessels and blood. I attribute the suppression of the catamenia in elderly women to this cause; in them the menstruous fluid either escapes as hemorrhoidal flux, or is prematurely stopped, to the injury of the health. For when the uterus becomes cold and almost lifeless, and all its vessels are obliterated, the superfluous blood boils up, and either falls back and stagnates, or else is diverted into the neighbouring veins. On the contrary, in those pale virgins who labour under chronic maladies, and in whom the uterus is small and the catamenia stagnate, " by coition," says Aristotle,[1] " the excrementitious menstrual fluid is drawn downwards, for the heated uterus attracts the humours, and the passages are opened." In this way their maladies are greatly lessened, seeing that want of action on the part of the uterus exposes the body to various ills. For the uterus is a most important organ, and brings the whole body to sympathize with it. No one of the least experience can be ignorant what grievous symptoms arise when the uterus either rises up or falls down, or is in any way put out of place, or is seized with spasm—how dreadful, then, are the mental aberrations, the delirium, the melancholy, the paroxysms of frenzy, as if the affected person were under the dominion of spells, and all arising from unnatural states of the uterus. How

---

[1] De Gen. Anim. lib. iii, cap. 1.

many incurable diseases also are brought on by unhealthy menstrual discharges, or from over-abstinence from sexual intercourse where the passions are strong!

Nor are the changes which take place in the virgin less observable when the uterus first begins to enlarge and receive warmth; the complexion is improved, the breasts enlarge, the countenance glows with beauty, the eyes lighten, the voice becomes harmonious; the gait, gestures, discourse, all are graceful. Serious maladies, too, are cured either at this period or never.

I am acquainted with a noble lady who for more than ten years laboured under furor uterinus and melancholy. After all remedies had been employed without success, she became affected with prolapsus uteri. Contrary to the opinion of others, I predicted that this last accident would prove salutary, and I recommended her not to replace the uterus until its over-heat had been moderated by the contact of the external air. Circumstances turned out as I anticipated, and in a short time she became quite well; the uterus was returned to its proper situation, and she lives in good health to the present day.

I also saw another woman who suffered long with hysterical symptoms, which would yield to no remedies. After many years her health was restored on the uterus becoming prolapsed. In both cases, when the violence of the symptoms was abated, I returned the uterus, and the event proved favorable. For the uterus, when stimulated by any acrid matter, not only falls down, but like the rectum irritated by a tenesmus, thrusts itself outwards.

Various, then, is the constitution of the uterus, and not only in its diseased, but also in its natural state, that is, at the periods of fecundity and barrenness. In young girls, as I said, and in women past childbearing, it is without blood, and about the size of a bean. In the marriageable virgin it has the magnitude and form of a pear. In women who have borne children, and are still fruitful, it equals in bulk a small gourd or a goose's egg; at the same time, together with the breasts, it swells and softens, becomes more fleshy, and its heat is increased; whilst, to use Virgil's expression with reference to the fields,

> " Superat tener omnibus humor,
> Et genitalia semina poscunt."

Wherefore women are most prone to conceive either just before or just subsequent to the menstrual flux, for at these
periods there is a greater degree of heat and moisture, two
conditions necessary to generation. In the same manner when
other animals are in heat, the genital organs are moist and
turgid.

Such is the state of the uterus as I have found it before
birth. In pregnant women, as I have before stated, the uterus
increases in proportion to the fœtus, and attains a great size.
Immediately after birth, I have seen it as large as a man's head,
more than a thumb's breadth in thickness, and loaded with
vessels full of blood. It is, indeed, most wonderful, and, as
Fabricius remarks, quite beyond human reason, how such a
mass can diminish to so vast an extent in the space of fifteen
or twenty days. It happens as follows : immediately on the
expulsion of the fœtus and its membranes, the uterus gradually
contracts, narrows its neck, and shrinks inwardly into itself;
partly by a process of diaphoresis, partly by means of the lochia,
its bulk insensibly lessens ; and the neighbouring parts, bones,
abdomen, and all the hypogastric region, at the same time diminish and recover their firmness. The lochial discharge at first
resembles pure blood; it then becomes of a sanious character, like
the washings of flesh, and is otherwise pale and serous. At this
last stage, when no longer tinged with blood, the women call
it "the coming of the milk," for the reason probably that at
that time the breasts are loaded with milk, and the lochia sensibly diminish ; as if the nutritive matter was then transferred
to the breasts from the uterus.

In other animals the process is shorter and simpler ; in them
the parts concerned recover their ordinary bulk and consistence
in one or two days. In fact, some, as the hare and rabbit,
admit the buck, and again become fecundated, an hour after
kindling. In like manner, I have stated that the hen admits
the cock immediately on laying. Women, as they alone have
a menstruous, so have they alone a lochial discharge ; added to
which they are exposed to disorders and perils immediately
after birth, either from the uterus, through feebleness, contracting too soon, or from the lochia becoming vitiated or sup-
pressed. For it often happens, especially in delicate women,
that foul and putrid lochia set up fevers and other violent

symptoms. Because the uterus, torn and injured by the separation of the placenta, especially if any violence has been used, resembles a vast internal ulcer, and is cleansed and purified by the free discharge of the lochia. Therefore do we conclude as to the favorable or unfavorable state of the puerperal woman from the character of these excretions. For if any part of the placenta adhere to the uterus, the lochial discharges become fetid, green, and putrid; and sometimes the powers of the uterus are so reduced that gangrene is the result, and the woman is destroyed.

If clots of blood, or any other foreign matter, remain in the uterine cavity after delivery, the uterus does not retract nor close its orifice; but the cervix is found soft and open. This I ascertained in a woman, who, when laboring under a malignant fever, with great prostration of strength, miscarried of a fœtus exhibiting no marks of decomposition, and who afterwards lay in an apparently dying state, with a pulse scarcely to be counted, and cold sweats. Finding the uterine orifice soft and open, and the lochia very offensive, I suspected that something was undergoing decomposition within; whereupon I introduced the fingers and brought away a "mole" of the size of a goose's egg, of a hard, fleshy, and almost cartilaginous consistence, and pierced with holes, which discharged a thick and fetid matter. The woman was immediately freed from her symptoms, and in a short time recovered.

When the neck of the uterus contracts in a moderate degree after birth, and certain pains, called by the midwives "after pains," ensue, in consequence of the difficulty with which the clots are expelled, the case is considered a favorable one, and is so in fact; for it indicates vigour on the part of the uterus, and that it is inclined readily to contract to its usual bulk; the result of which is that the lochia are duly expelled, and health restored to the woman.

But I have observed in some women the uterine orifice so closed immediately after parturition, that the blood has been retained in the uterus, and then, becoming putrid, has induced the most dangerous symptoms; and when art did not avail to promote its exit, the woman has presently died.

A noble lady in childbed being attacked with fever for want of the ordinary lochial discharge, had the pudenda swollen and hot; finding the uterine orifice hard and firmly closed, I forcibly dilated the part by means of an iron instrument sufficiently to admit of my introducing a syringe and throwing up an injection; the effect of which was that grumous and fetid blood, to the amount of several pounds, flowed away, with present relief of the symptoms.

The wife of a doctor of divinity was brought to me; a lady of a very tolerable constitution, but who was barren, and having an extreme desire for progeny, had tried all kinds of prescriptions in vain. In her the catamenia appeared at their proper period; but at times, especially after horse exercise, a bloody and purulent discharge came from the uterus, and then, in a short time, ceased suddenly. Some considered the case as one of leucorrhœa; others, led chiefly by the fact that the discharge was not continually present, and in small quantities, but appeared by intervals and in abundance, suspected a fistulous ulcer; whereupon they examined the whole vagina by means of a speculum uteri, and appied various remedies, but in vain; when I was at length called to her. I opened the uterine orifice, and immediately two spoonfuls of pus came away of a sanious character and tinged with streaks of blood. On seeing this I said that there was a hidden ulcer in the uterine cavity, and by applying suitable remedies I restored her to her former state of health. But during the time when I was engaged in her cure, when the ordinary remedies did not appear to be doing much good, I applied stronger ones, suspecting as I did that the ulcer was of long standing, and perhaps covered by exuberant granulations. I therefore added a little Roman vitriol to the injection employed previously, the effect of which was to make the uterus contract suddenly and become as hard as a stone; at the same time various hysterical symptoms showed themselves, such, I mean, as are generally supposed by physicians to arise from constriction of the uterus, and the rising of " foul vapours" therefrom. The symptoms continued some time, until by the application of soothing and anodyne remedies the uterus relaxed its orifice; upon which the acrid injection, together with a putrid sanies, was expelled, and in a short time the patient recovered.

I have introduced this account from my " medical observations" for the purpose of showing how acutely sensible the uterus is, and how readily it closes on the approach of danger, especially when urgent symptoms accompany the puerperal state. Women are peculiarly subject to these accidents, especially those among them who lead a luxurious life, or whose health is naturally weak, and who easily fall into disorders. Country women, and those accustomed to a life of labour, do not become dangerously ill on such small grounds. Some of them may be found pregnant a month after delivery; whilst two months frequently elapse before others are able to set about the ordinary occupations of life.

It is laid down by Hippocrates,[1] that as many days are required for the "after-purgings" as there are for the formation of the fœtus; therefore there are more for a female than a male child. "But this," says Scaliger,[2] "is false; for in none of our women do "the cleansings" last more than a month; in very many they cease on the fifteenth day; in some even on the seventh day: and I have seen a case where they lasted only until the third day, although the woman had borne twins." Galen has many observations on this subject in his work περὶ κυουμένων, (On the Formation of the Fœtus.) In the New World, it is said that the woman keeps apart the day only on which she is delivered, and then returns to her ordinary occupations.

I will add, in conclusion, an extraordinary instance told me by the noble Lord George Carew, Earl of Totness, and long Lord-Lieutenant of Munster in Ireland—he who wrote the history of these times. A woman, great with child, was following her husband, who served as a soldier, and it happened that the army, when on the march, was compelled to halt for the space of an hour near a small river which impeded their passage; whereupon the woman, who felt her labour at hand, retired to a neighbouring thicket, and there, without the aid of a midwife or any other preparation, gave birth to twins; after she had washed both herself and them in the running stream, she wrapped the infants in a coarse covering, tied them on her back, and the same day marched barefoot twelve miles with the army, without the slightest harm ensuing. The following day the Viceroy, Earl Mountjoy, who at that time was leading an

---

[1] Lib. de Fœtu. [2] Com. in Arist. Hist. Anim. lib. vii, cap. 3.

army against Kinsale, then occupied by the Spaniards, and the Earl of Totness, were so affected by the strange incident, that they appeared at the font, and had the infants called by their own names.

ON

THE UTERINE MEMBRANES AND HUMOURS.

UTERINE MEMBRANES AND HUMOURS.

"FOUR kinds of bodies" are enumerated by Hieronymus Fabricius[1] "as existing externally to the fœtus; these are the umbilical vessels, the membranes, the humours, and a fleshy substance." On these subjects, guided by my observations, I shall briefly state wherein I differ from him; first, however, giving his statement in his own words.

"There are," he says, "three membranes, two of which envelope the whole fœtus, but the third does not do so. Of those which envelope the whole fœtus, the innermost, immediately investing one, is called ἄμνιον, i. e. the mantle. That which fol·lows next is entitled by the Greeks χόριον; the Latins, however, have not given it a name, although some interpreters have thought proper erroneously to call it " secundæ" or " secundina," the secundines; this also envelopes the entire fœtus. The third is called ἀλλαντοειδὴς, i. e. gut-like, from its resemblance to a stuffed intestine; it does not entirely encompass the fœtus, but is applied upon the thorax and part of the abdomen, and extends to either horn of the uterus." He allows that this last membrane is only found in the fœtus of the sheep and cow; he asserts also that it is continuous with the urachus, and by means of this receives the urine from the bladder. Hence, he goes on, " horned animals, in whom this allantois is found, have the urachus so wide and straight, that it resembles a small intestine; it gradually decreases in size until it reaches the fundus of the bladder; whence it would appear to owe its

[1] Lib. de Form. Fœt. cap. 1.

origin rather to the intestine than to the bladder itself. But in man and other animals furnished with incisors in both jaws, and in whom the allantois is wanting, the size of the urachus is so diminished, that although it rises from the fundus of the bladder as a single tube, it afterwards splits into innumerable fibres, which pass beyond the umbilicus together with the vessels, and carry the urine into the chorion, although the exact mode in which it does so cannot be demonstrated." On this ground he accuses Arantius of a double error—first, his denial of the existence of the urachus in man; and, secondly, his assertion that the fœtus passes its urine through the genital organs.

For my own part, I must confess I am a willing party to the errors of Arantius, if errors they are to be called. For I am quite sure, if pressure be made on the bladder of a full-grown fœtus, whether of man or of any other animal, that urine will flow by the genitals. But I have never seen an urachus, nor observed that the urine is propelled into the membranes by making pressure on the bladder. I have indeed seen in the sheep and deer what appeared to be a process of bladder between the umbilical arteries, and which contained urine; but it in no way resembled the urachus as described by Fabricius. Not that I would obstinately deny the existence of an allantois; for the minor membranes are so delicate and transparent (those, for example, which we have described as existing between the two "whites" of the egg) that they may easily escape observation. Moreover, in the hen's egg a white excrementitious matter, and even fæces are found between the colliquament and albumen, i. e. between the amnion and chorion; this I have mentioned before, and Coiterus has also observed it. Added to which, the membrane of the colliquament itself, in which the fœtus swims, although it is so exceedingly transparent and delicate that Fabricius himself allows nothing can be imagined more so, nevertheless (for according to him all membranes, however thin, are double) may nature sometimes find herself compelled to deposit urine or some other matter between its duplicatures. An allantois of this kind I am ready to allow Fabricius; but that other intestine-like body produced into either horn of the uterus, I do not discover among the membranes in cloven-footed animals, nor aught else, in fact, except the conception itself. I can only find, as I before said, a process of the bladder, situated between the umbilical arteries, which contains an excrementitious matter, and varies in length in different animals. Wherefore, in my opinion, the tunic which Fabricius calls the allantois is, in fact, the chorion; and the ancients applied the name of allantois to it on account of its resemblance to a double intestine. For that external membrane, constricted in the middle, and resembling a saddle-bag in form, which is stretched upwards to each horn of the uterus, and in its passage is pinched in by that part of the uterus which connects the horns, is in truth the chorion; and in the sheep, goat, roe, fallow-deer, and other cloven-footed animals, it can be raised by the hand in the middle of its course, and easily extracted whole; this is the same as what is called the "conception" or ovum. Like an egg, it contains within itself two fluids, and the foetus with its appendages; it is possessed besides of those characters which Aristotle attributes to the egg; these are, that out of part of it the embryo is originally formed, and that the remainder constitutes the sustenance of the new animal, as has been frequently explained. I believe, then, the tunic which Fabricius called the allantois to be either the chorion or else some unnatural structure formed out of the reduplication of the membranes. It is accordingly only found to exist in some animals, and not always in these; it cannot be traced from the commencement of conception, and in some animals it is more apparent than in others: whilst in others nothing can be seen except a mere process of the bladder. Besides, Fabricius himself allows that its purpose is not to envelope the foetus, but to contain its urine. In truth, I must think that he has described it rather to defend the doctrine of the ancients, than because he really believed he had discovered such a membrane, or that it served any good purpose. For he allows, with the ancients, and every medical school, that the chorion contains urine, when he says [1] that there are two humours encircling the foetus, one, viz. in the amnion, consisting of sweat; the other in the chorion, consisting of urine. It is, therefore, clear that the ancients under the two names understood one and the same membrane; and that in

---

[1] Cap. i.

the cloven-footed animals they called it " allantois," on account
of its form; but in others " chorion," because they thought
its object was to receive the urine. Wherefore they allow that
this tunic is neither found in man nor any of the other animals.
For what need can there be of another tunic to retain the urine,
when they themselves admit that the office of doing so belongs
especially to the chorion? There can be no probable reason assigned why this tunic should exist in the sheep, goat, and the
other cloven-footed animals, and not also in the dog, cat, mouse,
and others. For in truth, if the object of this membrane were to
contain the urine, the fœtus of the sheep and cow must secrete
a much larger quantity than those of animals furnished with incisors in both jaws; there must then either be three different
humours, or at least two receptacles for the urine. For myself,
I am sure that the chorion from the first is full of water. I
will not, however, enter into controversies; I would rather
record what I have found by my own observations.

To do as Fabricius has done, and give the structure of the
full-grown and perfect embryo, is one thing, but it is another to
enter fully on the subject of its generation and first formation :
just as they are very different things to describe the ripe fruit
of an apple or any other tree, and to explain the manner in
which it is produced from the germ. I will, therefore, briefly go
through the stages by which the " conception" is brought to
maturity, in which way the true doctrines in the matter of the
membranes and other fœtal appendages will be better ascertained.

In the production of all living creatures, as I have before
said, this invariably holds, that they derive their origin from a
certain primary something or primordium which contains within
itself both the " matter" and the "efficient cause;" and so is, in
fact, the matter out of which, and that by which, whatsoever is
produced is made. Such a primary something in animals (whether they spring from parents, or arise spontaneously, or from
putrefaction) is a moisture inclosed in some membrane or shell;
a similar body, in fact, having life within itself either actually or
potentially; and this, if it is generated within an animal and
remain there, until it produce an " univocal" (not equivocal)
animal, is commonly called a " conception;" but if it is exposed to the air by birth, or assumes its beginning under other

circumstances, (than within an animal), it is then denominated an "egg," or "worm." I think, however, that in either case the word "primordium" should be used to express that from whence the animal is formed; just as plants owe their origin to seeds: all these "primordia" have one common property—that of vitality.

I find a "primordium" of this kind in the uterus of all viviparous animals before any trace of a fœtus appears: there is a clear, thick, white fluid (like the albumen of the egg) inclosed in a membrane, and this I call the ovum. In the roe, fallow-deer, sheep, and other cloven-footed animals, it fills the whole uterus and both its horns.

In process of time an extremely limpid and pure watery fluid (similar to that which in the hen's egg I have called the colliquament) is secreted by this "primordium" or "ovum;" in clearness and brilliancy far exceeding the remaining fluid of the ovum in which it is contained. It is of a circular form, and inclosed in a very delicate and transparent membrane of its own called the "amnion." The other fluid, of a denser and thicker character, is contained in the outer envelope, or chorion, which is in immediate contact with the concave surface of the uterus, and which also encompasses the entire ovum: the shape of this second membrane varies according to that of the uterus: in some animals it is oval, in others oblong, but in those with cloven feet it resembles a saddle-bag. After a short time a red pulsating point shows itself within the transparent substance, and from this point exceedingly fine twigs, or rather rays of vessels, start forth. By and by the first aggregated portion of the body makes its appearance, folded upon itself orbicularly, and somewhat resembling a grub: the remaining parts follow in the order described in our history. For I have ascertained that the production of the fœtus from their ova or "conceptions" in viviparous animals, takes place exactly in the same way as the growth of the chick within the egg.

As I before observed, "conceptions" in viviparous animals vary in form, number, and in their modes of attachment to the uterus. At first, especially in the cloven-footed animals, the "conception" does not adhere to the uterus, but is only in contact with, and fills and distends the organ, and can be easily extracted entire. In cloven-footed animals, which conceive within the horns of the uterus, and also in the solidungula, one ovum only of this kind is found, and that stretching up into either horn of the uterus: and although these animals sometimes produce one, sometimes two young at a birth, and so sometimes one, sometimes two colliquaments are found, one in the right, the other in the left horn of the uterus, yet the two are always contained in one and the same ovum.

In other animals, however, the number of ova answers to the number of foetuses, and within them are as many colliquaments: this is the case in the dog, cat, mouse, and other animals of this kind with teeth in either jaw. In cloven-footed animals the ovum is shaped like a saddle-bag: the form, in fact, under which Fabricius represented the allantois. In the mare, the figure of the uterus internally resembles an oblong bag; in the woman it is of a globular form.

In animals in whom the "conception" adheres to the uterus, (and in very many it does not do so until the foetus is fully formed), this takes place in various modes. In some it is adherent in one place by the intervention of a fleshy substance, which in the woman is called the "placenta," from its resemblance to a round cake (placenta): in others it is attached at many points by certain fleshy bodies, or "carunculæ:" these are five in number in the hind and doe; more numerous, but of smaller size, in the cow; and in the sheep they are in great numbers and of various sizes. In dogs and cats these fleshy bodies entirely surround each ovum like a girdle. A similar substance, in the hare and mole, grows to the side of the uterus: like the human placenta, which embraces about half the "conception," (just as the cup does the acorn at the commencement of its growth), it is attached by its convex aspect to the uterus, and by its concave surface to the chorion.

With these observations premised, I shall now state my opinions on the humours, membranes, fleshy substance of the uterus, and the distribution of the umbilical vessels, in the order described by Fabricius.

The words δεύτερα and ὕστερα are correctly understood by Fabricius[1] to answer to "secundæ" and "secundina" (the

---

[1] Cap. v.

secundines) : and by these are implied not only the membranes, but everything which comes away from the uterus at the last stage of parturition, or at least not long after it, viz. the humours, membranes, fleshy substance, and umbilical vessels.

Of the Humours.

The doctrines inculcated on the subject of the humours, and which, as being entertained by the ancients, Fabricius regards as certain truths requiring no further proof, are altogether inconsistent and false; the doctrines, I mean, that the fluid within the amnion, wherein the fœtus swims, consists of sweat; and that within the chorion of urine. For both these humours are found in the "conception" before any trace of the fœtus is visible; added to which, the fluid they call urine can be seen before that which they regard as sweat. In truth, these humours, especially the outer one, may be observed in unfruitful conceptions where nothing like a fœtus is discoverable.

Women sometimes expel conceptions of this kind, analogous to the subventaneous or wind egg. Aristotle[1] says they are called "fluxes;" among ourselves they are termed "false conceptions," or "slips." An ovum of this kind was aborted in the case of Hippocrates's pipe-player. "In all creatures," we are informed on the authority of Aristotle,[2] "which breed another within themselves, immediately on conception an egg-like body is formed; that is to say, a body in which a fluid is contained within a delicate membrane just like an egg with the shell removed." The humour in the chorion, which Fabricius and other physicians consider to be urine, Aristotle seems to have regarded as the seminal fluid (spermatis sive genituræ liquor). He says,[3] "when the semen is received into the uterus, after a certain time it becomes surrounded by a membrane, and if expulsion takes place before the fœtus is formed, it has the appearance of an egg with the shell removed and covered by its membrane : this mem-

---

[1] De Gen. Anim. lib. iii, cap. 9.   [2] Ibid.
[3] Hist. Anim. lib. vii, cap. 7.

brane, moreover, is loaded with vessels." It is, in fact, the chorion; so called from the conflux or multitude of veins. I have often observed ova of this kind escape in the second and third month; they are frequently decomposed internally, and come away gradually in the form of a leucorrhœal discharge, and thus the hopes of the parent are lost.

Another reason why these humours cannot be sweat and urine, is, that they exist in such abundance at the very beginning;—for the purpose, no doubt, of preventing the body of the fœtus from coming in contact with the adjacent parts when the mother runs, jumps, or uses violent exertion of any kind.

Added to which, many animals never sweat at all, (and we must remember what is said by Aristotle,[1] " that all creatures which swim, walk, or fly," I will add serpents and insects, whether viviparous or oviparous, or generated spontaneously, "are produced after the same manner,") as is the case with birds, serpents, and fishes, which neither sweat nor pass urine. The dog and cat also never sweat; neither in fact does any animal in which the urinary secretion is very abundant. Besides, it is impossible that urine can be passed before the kidneys and bladder are formed.

Moreover, and this is the strongest argument that can be brought forward, those humours can never be excrementitious into which so many branches of the umbilical vessels are distributed by means of the chorion; these vessels, in fact, in this manner taking up nourishment, (as it were from a large reservoir,) and then conducting it to the fœtus.

Besides what need is there of an allantois, if the fluid within the chorion is urine? And if that in the amnion is sweat, why does Nature, who contrives all things well, ordain that the fœtus should float about in its own excrement? And why, too, should the mother (as is the case with some animals) immediately after birth, so greedily devour the excretions of its own offspring, together with the containing membranes? Some have even observed that if the animal fails to eat up these matters it does not give its milk freely.

Notwithstanding these arguments, it may possibly be ima-

---

[1] Hist. Anim. lib. vii, cap. 7.

gined by some that the humours which I believe serve for the nutrition of the fœtus are excrementitious, led chiefly by the fact that they increase as the fœtus grows larger, and in some animals are observed to exist in immense quantities at the period of birth (at which time it might be supposed that all alimentary matters would have been absorbed), and serve besides other uses hardly compatible with their supposed function of nutrition. I nevertheless most confidently assert my belief that these humours are at the commencement destined for the nourishment of the fœtus, just as the colliquament and albumen are in the case of the chick; but that, in course of time, when the thinner and purer portions are absorbed, the remainder takes on the character of excrementitious matter, but still has its uses, and in some animals especially conduces to the safety of the fœtus, and also greatly facilitates birth. For just as wine becomes poor and tasteless when the spirit has evaporated; and as all excreted matters owe their origin for the most part to what has been previously food; so, after all the nutrient portions of the fluid contained in the chorion have been taken up by the fœtus, the remainder become excrementitious, and is applied to the above-mentioned uses. But all the fluid of the amnion is usually consumed by the time of birth; so that it is probable the fœtus seeks its exit on account of deficiency of nutriment.

Lastly, if any other fluid is ever contained within the allantois, and this is sometimes the case, I believe it to be unnatural. For sometimes we see women at their delivery have an enormous flow of water, sometimes a distinctly double flow; and this the midwives call the " by-waters." And so some women are seen with the abdomen immensely distended, and yet they bring forth a little shrivelled fœtus accompanied by a vast flow of water. Some imagine that a larger quantity of water is found with weakly and female children, whilst stronger and male fœtuses have a smaller share. I have often seen the waters come away in the middle of pregnancy, and abortion not take place, the child remaining strong and vigorous until birth. Since, then, there are naturally two collections of fluid, one in the chorion, the other in the amnion, so it sometimes happens that unnatural accumulations take place either in membranes of their own, or between the duplicatures of the chorion.

Of the Membranes.

With respect to the membranes or tunics of the uterus; as their special office is to contain the " waters," and as these waters are two only, it is pretty certain that the membranes themselves do not necessarily or usually exceed that number.

Those who enumerate three tunics are, I believe, in error, owing to the ancients having described the same membrane at one time under the title of " chorion," from the concourse of veins, at another under the name of " allantois" from its form.

Unquestionably, every " conception" is inclosed in two en-velopes, just as the brain is surrounded by its two membranes; every tree and fruit, moreover, has it double bark ; and lastly, seeds and fruits are protected by a double covering, the outer-most of which is harder and stronger than the inner one.

Of the above-mentioned membranes, the innermost (that which contains the colliquament or purer fluid,) is exceed-ingly delicate ; it is called the " amnion," i. e. the mantle, from the way in which it is disposed round the foetus. The outer tunic, however, is much thicker and stronger, and has received the name of " chorion," " because," says Fabricius, " a multitude of arteries and veins are aggregated together and arranged in it, as it were, after the manner of a chorus. Hence one of the tunics of the eye has been denominated χοροειδἠς (choroid) from its vessels having a similar arrangement to those in the chorion; the plexus of arteries and veins in the ven-tricles of the brain has also gained its name from the same circumstance."

The chorion fills the whole uterus, and contains a viscid and rather turbid fluid; whilst the placenta, or carunculæ, adhere to its outer surface, and thus attach the " conception" to the uterus.

In the woman it is usually adherent to the amnion at its lower portion; nor can it be separated there without diffi-culty. In cloven-footed animals the chorion is of very large size, and contains a hundred times more fluid than the amnion: this last membrane at first is scarcely as large as a nutmeg, or broad bean, and is generally found in one or other horn of the uterus ; that, namely, in which the embryo lies.

In the woman, more particularly, the chorion is externally rough and viscous, but internally it is smooth, slippery, and interwoven with abundance of vessels. In the woman, also, the upper part is thick and soft, but the lower is thinner and more membranous in character.

The placenta in the woman grows to the upper part of this membrane. In the sheep, numerous carunculæ adhere to it at various points. In the fallow and red deer the ovum is united to the uterus in five places only ; whilst in the mare it is in contact with the inner surface of the uterus by an almost infinite number of points of attachment. Hence Fabricius[1] states that in almost all viviparous animals there is a soft, loose, porous, and thick fleshy body of a dark colour, in intimate union with the terminations of the umbilical vessels ; he compares it to a sponge, or to the loose parenchyma of the liver or spleen ; hence, too, it was called by Galen[2] " glandular flesh ;" and it is now commonly known by the name of the uterine liver, in which the extremities of the umbilical vessels ramify to bring nutriment from the uterus to the fœtus.

But this fleshy substance is not found in all animals, nor at all periods of utero-gestation ; but in those alone in which the conception adheres to the uterus; and then only when it becomes attached for the purpose of taking up nutriment. At the commencement the " conception" (like an egg placed within the uterus) is found in contact with every part of the uterus, yet at no point is it adherent ; but produces and nourishes the embryo out of the humours contained within it, as I have explained in the instance of the hen's egg. This adhesion, or growing together, first takes place, and the fleshy mass (constituting the bond of union between the " conception" and the uterus) is first produced, when the fœtus becomes perfectly formed, and, through want either of different or more abundant nourishment, dispatches the extremities of the umbilical vessels to the uterus, that from hence, (as plants do from the earth by their radicles) it may absorb the nutrient juices. For in the beginning, as I have said, when the " punctum saliens" and the blood can alone be seen, the ramifications of the umbilical vessels are only visible in the colliquament and amnion. When,

---

[1] Cap. iii.   [2] 5 Aphor. xlv.

however, the fabric of the body is completely formed, the ramifications extend further, and are distributed in vast numbers
throughout the chorion, that from the albuminous fluid which
there exists, they may obtain nourishment for the fœtus.

Hence it is manifest that the young of viviparous animals
are at the beginning nourished in exactly the same manner as
the chick in the egg; and that they are detained within the
uterus in order that (when they can no longer supply themselves with nutriment from their own stores) they may form
adhesions to it by means of this fleshy substance, and receiving
more abundant supplies of food from the mother, may be nourished and made to grow.

Wherefore Fabricius has rightly observed, that in some
animals the "conception" is scarcely attached to the uterus at
all. Thus the sow and the mare have no such fleshy mode of
union,—but in them the ovum or "conception," as in the beginning it is formed out of the humours of the uterus, so it is
nourished subsequently by the same means; just as the ovum
of the hen is supplied with aliment at the expense of the albuminous matter without any connexion whatever with the uterus:
and thus the fœtus is furnished with aliment by the "conception" in which it is contained, and is nourished as the chick is
from the fluids of the egg. This is a strong argument that the
fœtus of viviparous animals is no more nourished by the blood
of the mother than the chick in the egg; and moreover, that
the fluid within the chorion is neither urine nor any other excrementitious matter; but serves for the support of the fœtus.
Although, as I have before remarked, it is possible when all the
nutrient portions have been taken up, the remainder may degenerate into excrementitious matter resembling urine. This
is also clear from what I formerly observed of the cotyledons
in the deer, viz., that in these animals the fleshy mass was of
a spongy character, and constituted, like a honeycomb, of innumerable shallow pits filled with a muco-albuminous fluid, (a
circumstance already observed by Galen[1]); and that from this
source the ramifications of the umbilical vessels absorbed the
nutriment and carried it to the fœtus: just as, in animals
after their birth, the extremities of the mesenteric vessels are
spread over the coats of the intestines and thence take up chyle.

[1] Lib. de Dissect. Uteri, cap. ult.

Of the Placenta.

In my opinion, then, the placenta and carunculæ have an office analogous to that of the liver and mamma. The liver elaborates for the nourishment of the body, the chyle previously taken up from the intestines : the placenta, in like manner, prepares for the fœtus alimentary matters which have come from the mother. The mammæ also, which are of a glandular structure, swell with milk, and although in some animals they are not even visible at other times, they become full and tumid at the period of pregnancy; so, too, the placenta, a loose and fungus-like body, abounds in an albuminous fluid, and is only to be found at the period of pregnancy. The liver, I say, then, is the nutrient organ of the body in which it is found ; the mamma is the same of the infant, and the placenta of the embryo. And just as the mother forms more milk from her food than is requisite to sustain her own flesh and blood, which milk is digested and elaborated in the mamma ; so do those animals, furnished with a placenta, supply to the fœtus nourishment which is purified in that organ. Hence it happens that the embryo is furnished with good or bad nutriment just as the mother takes wholesome or unwholesome food, and in proportion as it is elaborately prepared or not in these uterine structures. For some embryos have a more perfect structure provided for them, such as that fleshy substance mentioned above, which in some is altogether wanting. In some, also, the placenta is observed to be thicker, larger, and more loaded with blood ; whilst in others it is more spongy and white, like the thymus or pancreas. But there is not more variety found in the placenta than in the mamma or viscera generally : for instance, the liver in some animals is red and filled with blood, in others, as is the case with fishes and some cachectic persons in the human species, it is of much paler hue. The mare feeds on crude grass, and does not ruminate ; the sow gorges itself with any unclean food ; and in both the placenta, or organ for perfecting the aliment, is wanting.

Rightly then is it observed by Fabricius,[1] that " this fleshy

---

[1] Cap. iii.

structure, differs much in shape, size, position, and number in different kinds of animals. The human female has one placenta only; as is the case with the mouse, rabbit, guinea-pig, dog, and cat :" so also with many animals which have the toes distinct, and incisor teeth in both jaws. " All those which have the hoof cloven and incisors in one jaw only, have several placentæ, whether they be domesticated animals, like the sheep, cow, and goat, or wild, as the red-deer, roe, fallow-deer, and others of the same kind. Again, where there is only one of these fleshy structures it either resembles a cake, (whence its name placenta), as in the human female, rabbit, hare, mole, mouse, and guinea-pig ; or else it is like a girdle or bandage encircling the trunk of the body, as in the dog, cat, ferret, and the like." In some it resembles the cup or chalice of the acorn, and surrounds the greater part of the " conception," as in the hare and rabbit, its convex part adhering to the uterus, the concave looking towards the fœtus. " Again, in animals which have this structure in the form of a cake, although the shape is similar, the situation in which it is found is very different. In the human female it adheres to the fundus of the uterus, and is as far removed from the fœtus as possible, their connexion being effected by means of long vessels. In the mouse, guinea-pig, and rabbit, it is attached partly in the region of the loins, partly at the sides of the thorax. Those animals which have numerous placentæ are all furnished with incisors in one jaw only, as the sheep, cow, goat, red-deer, roe, and the like. Yet in these some variety is observable."

For in the sheep the carunculæ are many in number, and of different magnitudes, the largest being of the size of a nutmeg, the smallest of that of a pea or vetch : they are also of a rounded form and reddish hue, with their convex portion turned towards the uterus, something in the semblance of soft warts or nipples. " In the cow they are larger, wider, and whiter, more like a spongy or fungoid body," and they appear to take their origin from the chorion. In the red or fallow-deer they are five only in number; these spring from the walls of the uterus, and thrust themselves inwards, exhibiting their depressions or acetabula on the side of the fœtus. But in all animals it is observed that the carunculæ adhere firmly to the uterus, and cannot be separated from it without considerable difficulty, except at the period of birth; at which time they become loosened from their attachments and fall like ripe fruit. If they are forcibly torn from the uterus, I have observed the greater part of the blood that escapes to flow, not from the "conception," but from the uterus itself.

Fabricius,[1] when discussing the mode of union between the "fleshy substance" and the uterus, uses many arguments, but in my opinion weak ones, to prove that the umbilical vessels anastomose with those of the uterus: yet he seems chiefly to have done so to countenance the old opinion once held almost by all; for he confesses that he can make no positive assertion on the subject, "because the fleshy mass itself stands in the way of any accurate investigation." Yet neither reason nor observation would lead us to believe that more anastomoses exist in the uterus, than in the liver between the branches of the vena portæ and the cava; or in the mamma, between the vessels which transmit blood and those which carry milk. There may be, indeed, at places a juxtaposition of vessels, and sometimes the insertion of one into the coats of another; but the perfect coalition and union, described by Fabricius, never exist. Were it so, the veins and arteries ought to be continuous; for the vessels which bring the blood from the mother into the uterus and carunculæ are arteries, whilst those which pass from the uterus to the fœtus are veins, as is readily apparent; for they carry blood from the placenta into the vena cava.

Hence the opinion of Arantius seems to me to be the true one, viz. that the orifices of the umbilical veins are in no way continuous with the uterine vessels. For there is a smaller number of vessels carrying blood to the uterus than there is of veins returning it to the fœtus; and the greater part of the roots of those terminate in the chorion. Yet Fabricius, either from respect to the ancients, or through an envious feeling towards Arantius, most pertinaciously holds to the old opinion.

[1] De Form. Fœt. p. 122.

Of the Acetabula.

Fabricius[1] has ascertained nothing on the subject of the " cotyledons" or " acetabula ;" he gives only the various opinions of the ancients. In the former part of my work, however, in the history of the fœtus in the deer, I have mentioned the animals in which acetabula are found; at the same time I described them as constituting numerous cells of a small size scattered throughout the carunculæ, or " fleshy substance," and filled with an albuminous or mucilaginous fluid, like a honeycomb full of honey.

In the deer they greatly resemble in shape the cavity of the haunch-bone which receives the head of the thigh; hence their name in Greek, κοτυλήδονες (little measures); and in Latin, acetabula, because they resemble the little cups formerly brought to table filled with vinegar for sauce.

These cavities do not exceed in size the holes in a large sponge, and a delicate ramification of the umbilical vessels penetrates deeply into each of them; for in them aliment is laid up for the fœtus, not indeed constituted of blood, as Fabricius would have it, but matter of a mucous character, and greatly resembling the thicker part of the albumen in the egg. Hence it is clear, as I have before observed, that the fœtus in cloven-footed animals (as indeed in all others) is not nourished by the blood of the mother.

Aristotle's[2] statement, " that the acetabula gradually diminish with the growth of the fœtus, and at last disappear," is not borne out by experiment; for as the fœtus increases so do the carunculæ; the acetabula at the same time become more capacious and numerous, and more full of the albuminous matter.

If the carunculæ are pressed no blood escapes, but just as water or honey can be squeezed from a sponge or honeycomb, so if pressure is made a whitish fluid oozes from out of the acetabula, which then become shrunk, white, and flaccid, and at last come to resemble a nipple, or a large flabby wart.

Cap iv   [2] Hist. Anim. lib. vii. cap. 8.

Aristotle asserts, with truth, that acetabula are not found in all animals ; for they do not exist in the woman, nor (as far as I know) in any animal which possesses a single fleshy substance or placenta. As to the uses of the carunculæ, I believe that, like the mamma, they elaborate not blood but a fluid resembling albumen, and that this serves for the nourishment of the fœtus.

Of the Umbilical Cord.

Fabricius gives an elegant description, as well as most beautiful figures, of the umbilical vessels. " The veins," he says,[1] " which pass from the uterus in the direction of the fœtus are always closely united and become larger and larger as they proceed ; nor does this mutual interlacement cease until all end in two large trunks ; these penetrate the fœtus at the umbilicus, and become one vein of great size, which is inserted into the liver of the fœtus, and has a communication both with the vena cava and vena portæ. In like manner the arteries which accompany the veins, being many in number and exceedingly minute, pass from the uterus towards the fœtus, and, gradually uniting and increasing in size, terminate in two large trunks ; these, after penetrating the umbilicus, separate from the veins, and attaching themselves to the lateral surface of the bladder by the intervention of a membrane, proceed downwards on either side and become continuous with the branches of the aorta descending to the thigh." It must be observed, however, that this description of Fabricius applies only to the umbilical vessels of the human fœtus, and not to the young of every animal. Nor even does it hold in the case of the human fœtus except when it is full grown ; for at the beginning the arteries make little show, and are so small as to require the eyes of a lynx to see them ; nor afterwards indeed are they distinguishable except by their pulsation : in other particulars they resemble veins. Since then, as I have elsewhere shown, the very small branches of arteries do not pulsate, in so far as the eye is concerned, there can be no difference between them and veins. The arteries, I say, at this time are so fine and

[1] Op. cit. cap. 2.

minute, that they are woven, as it were, like the most delicate threads, into the tissues of the veins, or rather in some obscure manner insinuate themselves into them; hence they almost entirely elude the sight. But all the veins, by a retrograde movement, unite their twigs and terminate in one trunk like the branches of a tree, in the same manner as the mesenteric veins, all of which terminate in the vena portæ.

Near the embryo [the umbilical veins] are divided into two trunks, but when entered within it they constitute one umbilical vein, which ends in the vena cava, near the right auricle of the heart, and passes through the liver, entering the vena portæ; giving off no branches besides until it leaves the convex portion of the liver by a very large orifice. So that if the vena cava is opened from the right auricle downwards and emptied of blood, three apertures may be seen close to each other; one is the entrance of the vena cava descendens, the second that of the hepatic vein, which ramifies throughout the convex portion of the liver, and the third is the origin of the umbilical vein. Hence it is quite clear that the origin of the veins is by no means to be looked for in the liver; inasmuch as the orifice of the vena cava descendens is much larger than the hepatic branch, which is indeed equalled in size by the umbilical vein. For the branches are not said to be the origin of their trunk; but where the trunk is greatest there the origin of the veins is to be looked for, and this is the case at the entrance of the right ventricle: here, then, the origin of all veins, and the storehouse of the blood must be placed.

To return to the umbilical vessels, which are not subdivided in the same way in all animals; for in some two or more branches of veins are found within the body of the fœtus,—some of which pass through the liver, whilst others join the portal and mesenteric veins. In the human fœtus, at a distance of three or four fingers' breadth from the umbilicus, the trunks of the arteries and veins are involved together in a complicated manner, (as if one were to twist several waxen tapers in the form of a stick,) and are besides covered and held together by a thick gelatinous membrane. This cord passes on towards the chorion, and when arrived at the concave portion of the placenta and the inner surface of the chorion, splits into innumerable branches; these divide again, and constitute the means by which the nutrient matter is taken up, as by rootlets, and distributed to the fœtus. The veins of the cord are marked at various places by knots or varices, resembling vesicles filled with blood; this is a contrivance of nature to prevent the blood rushing too violently to the fœtus. From the number of these knots superstitious midwives are accustomed to predict the number of the future offspring; and if none can be seen at all they pronounce that the woman will be ever after barren : they also absurdly prophesy by the distance between the knots about the interval to take place between the birth of each child, and also of its sex from their colour.

A like arrangement of the umbilical vessels is found in almost all fœtuses furnished with a single placenta, as in the dog, mouse, and others; but in these the cord is shorter and less convoluted. In the ox, sheep, red-deer, fallow-deer, hog, and others, in which the nutrient material is not supplied from one fleshy mass or placenta, but from several, the umbilical vessels are distributed in a different manner. The branches and extremities of these vessels are not only disseminated through the fleshy substance, but still more and chiefly through the membrane of the chorion itself by means of the most delicate fibres; exactly in the same way as the vessels are distributed in the human fœtus, without the aid of the cord, before the " conception" adheres to the uterus. Hence it is plain that the embryo does not derive all its nourishment from the placenta, but receives a considerable portion of it from the fluid contained in the chorion.

As to the uses of the umbilical vessels, I cannot agree with Fabricius, for he imagines that all the blood is supplied to the fœtus from the uterus by means of the veins, and that the vital spirits are transmitted from the mother by the arteries. He also asserts that no part of the fœtus performs any common function, but that each individual portion looks only to itself, how it may be nourished, grow, and be preserved. In like manner, because he has found no nerve in the umbilical cord, he refuses to allow sensation or voluntary motion to the fœtus. Just as if the uterus or placenta of the mother were the heart or first source whence these functions are derived to the fœtus, and whence heat flows in and is distributed through all its parts. All these are manifest errors. For the human fœtus, even before the completion of the fourth month, (in some animals sooner,) in no obscure manner moves, rolls about, and kicks, especially if it suffer from cold, heat, or any external source of inconvenience. Moreover, the "punctum saliens" (whilst yet the heart is not) moves to and fro, with an evident pulsation, and distributes blood and spirits; and this part, as I have before stated, if languid and nearly extinct through cold, will, if warmth be applied, again be restored and live. In the Cæsarean section, also, it is quite clear that the life of the embryo does not immediately depend upon the mother, and that the spirits do not proceed from her; for I have often seen the fœtus extracted alive from the uterus when the mother has been dead some hours. I have also known the rabbit and hare survive when extracted from the uterus of the dead mother. Besides, in a tedious labour we learn whether the infant is alive or not by the pulsation of the umbilical arteries; and it is certain that these arteries receive their impulse from the heart of the fœtus and not of the mother, for the rhythm of the two differs: this can be easily ascertained if one hand is applied to the wrist of the mother and the other to the umbilical cord. Nay, in the Cæsarean section, when the embryo is still enveloped in the chorion, I have often found the umbilical arteries pulsating, and the fœtus lively, even when the mother was dead and her limbs stiffened. It is not, therefore, true that the "spirits" pass from the mother to the fœtus through the arteries; nor is it more so that the umbilical or fœtal vessels anastomose with those of the uterus. The fœtus has a proper life of its own, and possesses pulsating arteries filled with blood and "spirits," long before the "conception," in which it is formed and dwells, is attached to the uterus; just as it is with the chick in the egg.

In my treatise on the Circulation of the Blood I have shown the uses of the arteries, both in the fœtus and in the adult, to be very different from what is generally supposed, and my views receive confirmation from the subject now under consideration.

In truth, the "secundines" are part of the "conception," and depend upon it, borrowing thence their life and faculty of growth. For, just as in the mesentery, the blood is propelled to the intestines by the branches of the cœliac and mesenteric arteries, and returns thence by means of the veins to the liver and heart, together with the chyle, so in like manner do the umbilical arteries carry the blood to the secundines; which blood, together with the nutrient fluid, is brought back by the veins to the fœtus. Hence it is that these arteries do not proceed immediately from the heart, as if they were the principal vessels, but take their origin from the arteries of the lower limbs, as being of inferior rank, use, and magnitude.

Adrian Spigelius lately published a book entitled ' On the Formation of the Fœtus ' (de Formato Fœtu); in which he treats of the uses of the umbilical arteries, and proves, by powerful arguments, that the fœtus does not receive vital " spirits" from the mother through the arteries; he also answers fully the arguments on the other side. He could also have shown by the same arguments that neither is the blood transferred to the fœtus from the vessels of the mother by means of the branches of the umbilical veins; this is especially clear from the case of the hen's egg, and also of the Cæsarean section. In truth, if heat and life flow to the blood from the mother, should she die the child must straightway be destroyed also, for the same fatality must attach to both; nay, the child must be the first to perish; for as dissolution approaches, the subordinate parts languish and grow chill before the principal ones, and so the heart fails last of all. The blood, I mean of the fœtus, would be the first to lose its heat and become unfit to perform its functions were it derived from the uterus, since the uterus would be deprived of all vital heat before the heart.

ON CONCEPTION.

ON CONCEPTION.

FABRICIUS has indeed recounted many wonderful things on the subject of parturition; for my own part, I think there is more to admire and marvel at in conception. It is a matter, in truth, full of obscurity; yet will I venture to put forth a few things— rather though as questions proposed for solution—that I may not appear to subvert other men's opinions only, without bringing forward anything of my own. Yet what I shall state I wish not to be taken as if I thought it a voice from an oracle, or desired to gain the assent of others by violence; I claim, however, that liberty which I willingly yield to others, the permission, viz. in subjects of difficulty to put forward as true such things as appear to be probable until proved to be manifestly false.

It is to the uterus that the business of conception is chiefly intrusted: without this structure and its functions conception would be looked for in vain. But since it is certain that the semen of the male does not so much as reach the cavity of the uterus, much less continue long there, and that it carries with it a fecundating power by a kind of contagious property, (not because it is then and there in actual contact, or operates, but because it previously has been in contact); the woman, after contact with the spermatic fluid in coitu, seems to receive influence, and to become fecundated without the co-operation of any sensible corporeal agent, in the same way as iron touched by the magnet is endowed with its powers and can attract other iron to itself. When this virtue is once received the woman exercises a plastic power of generation, and produces a being after her own image; not otherwise than the plant, which we see endowed with the forces of both sexes.

Yet it is a matter of wonder where this faculty abides after intercourse is completed, and before the formation of the ovum or "conception." To what is this active power of the male committed? is it to the uterus solely, or to the whole woman? or is it to the uterus primarily and to the woman secondarily? or, lastly, does the woman conceive in the womb, as we see by the eye and think by the brain?

For although the woman conceiving after intercourse sometimes produces no fœtus, yet we know that phenomena occur which clearly indicate that conception has really taken place, although without result. Over-fed bitches, which admit the dog without fecundation following, are nevertheless observed to be sluggish about the time they should have whelped, and to bark as they do when their time is at hand, also to steal away the whelps from another bitch, to tend and lick them, and also to fight fiercely for them. Others have milk or colostrum, as it is called, in their teats, and are, moreover, subject to the diseases of those which have actually whelped; the same thing is seen in hens which cluck at certain times, although they have no eggs on which to sit. Some birds also, as pigeons, if they have admitted the male, although they lay no eggs at all, or only barren ones, are found equally sedulous in building their nests.

The virtue which proceeds from the male in coitu has such prodigious power of fecundation, that the whole woman, both in mind and body, undergoes a change. And although it is the uterus made ready for this, on which the first influences are impressed, and from which virtue and strength are diffused throughout the body, the question still remains, how it is that the power thus communicated remains attached to the uterus? is it to the whole uterus or only to a part of it? nothing is to be found within it after coitus, for the semen in a short time either falls out or evaporates, and the blood, its circle completed, returns from the uterus by the vessels.

Again, what is this preparation or maturity of the uterus which eagerly demands the fecundating seed? whence does it proceed? Certain it is, unless the uterus be ready for coition every attempt at fecundation is vain; nay, in some animals, at no other time is the male admitted. It happens occasionally, I allow, that this maturity arrives earlier in some from the solicitations of the male animal; it is itself, however, a purely natural result, just as is the ripening of the fruit in trees. What these changes are I will now recount, as I have found them by observation.

The uterus first appears more thick and fleshy; then its inner surface, the future residence, that is, of the "conception," becomes softer, and resembles in smoothness and delicacy the ventricles of the brain; this I have already described in the deer and other cloven-footed tribes. But in the dog, cat, and other multiparous and digitated animals, the horns of the uterus—clearly corresponding to the round tubes of the woman [Fallopian tubes], the appendices of the intestines in birds, or the ureters in man—exhibit little protuberances at certain intervals, which swell up and become extremely soft; these, after intercourse, appear to open themselves, (as I have observed in deer;) from them the first white fluid transudes into the uterus, and out of this the "conception," or ovum, is formed. In this way the uterus, by means of the male, (like fruit by the summer's heat,) is brought to the highest pitch of maturity, and becomes impregnated.

But since there are no manifest signs of conception before the uterus begins to relax, and the white fluid or slender threads (like the spider's web) constituting the "primordium" of the future "conception," or ovum, shows itself; and since the substance of the uterus, when ready to conceive, is very like the structure of the brain, why should we not suppose that the function of both is similar, and that there is excited by coitus within the uterus a something identical with, or at least analogous to, an "imagination" (phantasma) or a "desire" (appetitus) in the brain, whence comes the generation or procreation of the ovum? For the functions of both are termed "conceptions," and both, although the primary sources of every action throughout the body, are immaterial, the one of natural or organic, the other of animal actions; the one (viz. the uterus) the first cause and beginning of every action which conduces to the generation of the animal, the other (viz. the brain) of every action done for its preservation. And just as a "desire" arises from a conception of the brain, and this conception springs from some external object of desire, so also from the male, as being the more perfect animal, and, as it were, the most

37

natural object of desire, does the natural (organic) conception arise in the uterus, even as the animal conception does in the brain.

From this desire, or conception, it results that the female produces an offspring like the father. For just as we, from the conception of the "form" or "idea" in the brain, fashion in our works a form resembling it, so, in like manner, the "idea," or "form," of the father existing in the uterus generates an offspring like himself with the help of the formative faculty, impressing, however, on its work its own immaterial "form." In the same way art, which in the brain is the εἶδος or "form" of the future work, produces, when in operation, its like, and begets it out of "matter." So too the painter, by means of conception, pictures to himself a face, and by imitating this internal conception of the brain carries it out into act; so also the builder constructs his house according to previous conception. The same thing takes place in every other action and artificial production. Thus, what education effects in the brain, viz. art, with its analogue does the coitus of the male endow the uterus, viz. the plastic art; hence many similar or dissimilar fœtuses are produced at the same coitus. For if the productions and first conceptions of art (the mere imitations of nature) are in this way formed in the brain, how much more probable is it that copies (exemplaria) of animal generation and conception should in like manner be produced in the uterus?

And since Nature, all of whose works are wonderful and divine, has devised an organ of this kind, viz. the brain, by the virtue and sensitive faculty of which the conceptions of the rational soul exist, such as the desires and the arts, the first principles and causes of so many and such various works, of which man, by means of the impulsive faculty of the brain, is by imitation the author; why should we not suppose that the same Nature, who in the uterus has constructed an organ no less wonderful, and adapted it by means of a similar structure to perform all that appertains to conception, has destined it for a similar or at least an analogous function, and intended an organ altogether similar for a similar use? For as the skilful artificer accomplishes his works by ingeniously adapting his instruments to each, so that from the substance and shape of these instruments it is easy to judge of their use and application, with no less certainty than we have been taught by Aristotle [1] to recognize the nature of animals from the structure and arrangement of their bodily organs; and as physiognomy instructs us to judge of a man's disposition and character from the shape of his face and features, what should prevent us from supposing that where the same structure exists there is the same function implanted?

But it is so unfairly ordered that, when customary and familiar matters come to be debated, this very familiarity lessens their importance and our wonder; whilst things of much less moment, because they are novel and rare, appear to us far greater objects of marvel. Whoever has pondered with himself how the brain of the artist, or rather the artist by means of his brain, pictures to the life things which are not present to him, but which he has once seen; also in what manner birds immured in cages recall to mind the spring, and chant exactly the songs they had learned the preceding summer, although meanwhile they had never practised them; again, and this is more strange, how the bird artistically builds its nest, the copy of which it had never seen, and this not from memory or habit, but by means of an imaginative faculty (phantasia), and how the spider weaves its web, without either copy or brain, solely by the help of this imaginative power; whosoever, I say, ponders these things, will not, I think, regard it as absurd or monstrous, that the woman should be impregnated by the conception of a general immaterial "idea," and become the artificer of generation.

I know well that some censorious persons will laugh at this, —men who believe nothing true but what they think so themselves. Yet this that I do is the practice of philosophers, who, when they cannot clearly comprehend how a thing really is brought to pass, devise some mode for it in accordance with the other works of nature, and as near as possible to what is true. And indeed all those opinions which we now regard as of the greatest weight, were at the beginning mere figments and imaginations, until confirmed by experiments addressed to the senses, and made credible by a knowledge of their positive causes. Aris-

---

[1] Analyt. lib. ii, cap. 35.

totle[1] says "that philosophers are in some sort lovers of fables, seeing that fable is made up of marvels." And indeed men were first led to cultivate philosophy from wondering at what they saw. For my own part, then, when I see nothing left in the uterus after intercourse to which I can ascribe the principle of generation, any more than there is in the brain anything discoverable after sensation and experience, which are the prime sources of art, and when I find the structure of both alike, I have devised this fable. Let learned and ingenious men consider of it, let the supercilious reject it, and those who are peevish and scoffing laugh if they please.

Since, then, nothing can be apprehended by the senses in the uterus after coition, and since it is necessary that there be something to render the female fruitful, and as this is probably not material, it remains for us to take refuge in the notion of a mere conception and of " species without matter" (species sine materiâ), and imagine that the same thing happens here as every one allows takes place in the brain, unless indeed there be some one " whom the gods have moulded of better clay," and made fit to discover some other efficient cause besides any of those enumerated.

Some philosophers of our time have returned to the old opinion about atoms, and so imagine that this generative contagion, as indeed all others, proceeds from the subtile emanations of the semen of the male, which rise like odorous particles, and gain an entrance into the uterus at the period of intercourse. Others invoke to their aid incorporeal spirits, such as demiurgi, angels, and demons. Others regard it as a process of fermentation. Others devise other theories. I pray, therefore, a place for this conjecture of mine until something certain is established in the matter.

Many observations have been made by me which would easily overthrow the opinions I have mentioned, so easy is it to say what a thing is not rather than what it is; this is not, however, the place to introduce them, although elsewhere it is my intention to do so. On the present occasion I shall only observe, if that which is called by the common name of " contagion," as arising from the contact of the spermatic fluid in

---

[1] Metaphys. lib. i, cap. 2.

intercourse, and which remains in the woman (without the actual presence of the semen) as the efficient of the future offspring— if, I say, this contagion (whether it be atoms, odorous particles, fermentation, or anything else) is not of the nature of any corporeal substance, it follows of necessity that it is incorporeal. And if on further inquiry it should appear that it is neither spirit nor demon, nor soul, nor any part of the soul, nor anything having a soul, as I believe can be proved by various arguments and experiments, what remains, since I am unable myself to conjecture anything besides, nor has any one imagined aught else even in his dreams, but to confess myself at a stand-still? "For whoever," says Aristotle,[1] "doubts and wonders, confesses his ignorance; therefore if to escape the imputation of ignorance, ingenious men have turned to philosophy, it is clear they follow their pursuit for the sake of knowledge, and not from any other motive."

It must not, then, be imputed to me for blame, if, eager for knowledge, and approaching untrodden ground, I have presented aught which at first sight may appear made up or fabulous. For as everything is not to be received at once with an unthinking credulity, so that which has been long and painfully considered must not be straightway rejected, even although it fail to catch the eye of the quick-sighted. Aristotle himself wrote a book, 'De Mirabilibus auditis,' on hearsay wonders; and elsewhere he says,[2] "We must not only thank those in whose opinions we acquiesce, but those also who have said aught (to the purpose) although superficially. For these bring in something to the common stock, in this, that they exercise and train our habits. For if Timotheus had not existed, we should have lost much music. Yet if Phrynis had not been we should have had no Timotheus. So is it with those who have laid down any truth. For we have received some opinions from certain philosophers, yet were there others to whom these owed their existence."

Influenced, then, by the example and authority of so great a man, and not to appear resolute only to subvert the doctrines of others, I have preferred proposing a fanciful opinion rather than none at all, playing in this the part of Phrynis to

---

[1] Metaphys. lib. i, cap. 2.　　　[2] Ibid. lib. ii, cap. 1.

Timotheus, my object being to shake off the sloth of the age we live in, to rouse the intellects of the studious, and, rather than that the diligent investigator of nature should accuse me of indolence, to bid him laugh at my ill-formed and crude notions.

In truth, there is no proposition more magnificent to investigate or more useful to ascertain than this: How are all things formed by an "univocal" agent? How does the like ever generate the like ? And this not only in productions of art (for so house builds house, face designs face, and image forms image), but also in things relating to the mind, for mind begets mind, opinion is the source of opinion. Democritus with his atoms, and Eudoxus with his chief good which he placed in pleasure, impregnated Epicurus ; the four elements of Empedocles, Aristotle; the doctrines of the ancient Thebans, Pythagoras and Plato; geometry, Euclid. By this same law the son is born like his parents, and virtues which ennoble and vices which degrade a race are sometimes passed on to descendants through a long series of years. Some diseases propagate their kind, as lepra, gout, syphilis, and others. But why do I speak of diseases, when the moles, warts, and cicatrices of the progenitor are sometimes repeated in the descendant after many generations?[1] " Every fourth birth," says Pliny,[2] " the mark of the origin of the Dacian family is repeated on the arm." Why may not the thoughts, opinions, and manners now prevalent, many years hence return again, after an intermediate period of neglect ? For the divine mind of the Eternal Creator, which is impressed on all things, creates the image of itself in human conceptions.

Having, therefore, overcome some difficulties relating to the subject, I feel a greater desire to enter into it a little more closely, and this with two objects in view—first, that what I have hitherto treated cursorily may seem to carry with it a greater weight of probability ; and secondly, to stir up the intellects of the studious to search more deeply into so obscure a subject.

To illustrate the matter, let A stand for the fecundated egg (the " matter" that is of the future chick), which is alterable or

---

[1] Arist. Hist. Animal. lib. vii, cap. 6 ; et De Gen. Anim. lib. i, cap. 17.

[2] Lib. vii, cap. 11.

convertible into the chick, and is in fact the chicken in posse. Let B be that which fecundates the egg, and thus distinguishes it from an unfruitful egg, i. e. the " efficient cause" of the chick, or that which puts the egg in motion, and converts it into a chick. And let C be the chick, or " final cause," for the sake of which both the egg and that which fecundates the egg exist, the actual chick, namely, or " reason" why the chick is.

Now we take for granted, as demonstrated by Aristotle,[1] that every prime mover is " combined with" that which is moved by it. And these things are more particularly said by him to be " together" which are generated or produced at the same moment of time : thus that which moves and that which is moved are actually together, and where one is there the other is also ; for it is evident that when the effect is present the cause must be so too.

Whenever, then, A (i. e. the fecundated egg) is actually in being, B (i. e. the internal moving and "efficient" or fecundating cause) is also actually in being. But when B is actually in being, C also (i. e. the immaterial " form" of the chick) must, at least in some sort, be existing too. For B is the internal efficient cause of the chick, that, namely, which alters A (the egg) into C (the " reason" why the chick is). Since, then, everything which moves coexists with that which is moved by it, and every cause with its effect, it follows that C coexists with B ; for the " final cause," both in nature and art, is primary to all other causes, since it moves, and is not itself moved; but the " efficient" moves, because it is impelled by the " final cause." There inheres, in some way or other, in every " efficient cause" a ratio finis (a final cause), and by this the efficient, co-operating with Providence, is moved.

The authority of Aristotle is clearly on my side : " That," he says,[2] " appears to hold the chief place among natural causes which we signify under this expression, ' cujus gratiâ'—for whose sake. For this is the ' reason ;' but the ' reason' is the chief thing, as well in artificial as in natural subjects. For when a physician explains what health is, either by definition or description, or a workman a house, he is accustomed to give

---

[1] Physiologia, lib. vii, cap. 3. [2] De Part. Anim. lib. i, cap. 1.

the reasons and causes of what he does, and adds why he does it; although that cause, ' cujus gratiâ,' and the reason ' for the sake of the good and fair,' are joined rather to the works of nature than to those of art."

" The end," he elsewhere says,[1] " is this ' cujus gratiâ' (for whose sake), as health is the thing for the sake of which we walk. For why does a man walk? We answer, for the sake of his health; and when we have thus said, we think we have given a ' cause;' and whatever else is further interposed, by means of another agent, is done for the sake of this end, as dieting, or purging, or drugs, or instruments, are all for the sake of health; for all these are for the sake of the end." Again, " It is our business always to seek the primary cause of everything, For instance, a man builds a house because he is a builder, but he is a builder by reason of the art of building; this then (the art) is a prior cause; and so in all things." Hence it is that he asserts[2] " that the cause which first moves, and in which the ' reason' and ' form' lie, is greater and more divine than the ' material cause.' "

In all natural generation, therefore, both the " matter" out of which and the " efficient cause" by which (namely, A, the thing which is moved, and B, the thing moving) are alike for the sake of the animal begotten or to be begotten; for that which moves and is not itself moved, viz. C, is in (inest) both. For both those (viz. A and B) are at the same time capable of motion, and are moreover moved, viz. the thing fecundating, B, (which both moves and is moved) and the thing fecundated, A, the " matter," viz. or ovum, which is moved and changed only. Wherefore if no moveable thing is actually moved, unless the thing which moves is present, so neither will " matter" be moved, nor the " efficient" effect anything, unless the first moving cause be in some way present; and this is the " form" or " species" which is without matter, and is the prime cause. " For the efficient and generating," according to Aristotle,[3] " in so far as they are so, belong to that which is effected and generated." The following syllogism, therefore, may be framed out of these first and necessary predicates:

[1] Physiologia, lib. ii, tract. 3.   [2] De Gen. Anim. lib. ii, cap. 1.
[3] Ibid. cap. 4.

Whenever B is actually in existence, C also is actually in existence (i. e. moving in some way).

Whenever A is actually in existence, B is also in actual existence.

Therefore whenever A is in actual existence, C is also in actual existence.

Natural and artificial generation take place after the same manner.[1] Both are instituted for the sake of something further, and by a kind of providence both direct themselves to a proposed end;—both too are first moved by some "form" conceived without matter, and are the products of this conception. The brain is the organ of one kind of conception (for in the soul, the organ of which is the brain, art, without the intervention of matter, is the "reason" or first cause of the work), the uterus or ovum of the other.

The "conception," therefore, of the uterus or the ovum resembles, at least in some sort, the conception of the brain itself, and in a similar way does the "end" inhere in both. For the "species" or "form" of the chick is in the uterus or ovum without the intervention of matter, just as the "reason" of his work is in the artist, e. g. the "reason" of the house in the brain of the builder.

But since the phrase "to be in" is perhaps equivocal, and things are said to be coexistent in various senses, I affirm, further, and say, that the "species" and immaterial "form" of the future chick are, in some sort, the cause of the impregnation or fecundation of the uterus, because after intercourse no corporeal substance can be found within that organ.

But how this immaterial cause, this first principle, exists alike in the uterus and brain, or how the conceptions of the brain and uterus, answering to art and nature, resemble or differ from each other, and in what way the thing which fecundates (viz. the internal efficient cause whereby the animal is generated) exists alike in the male and his semen and in the woman and her uterus—in the egg also, the mixed work of both sexes—and wherein their differences consist, I shall subsequently attempt to explain when I treat generally of the generation of animals (as well of those creatures which are produced by metamor-

---

[1] Arist. de Part. Anim. lib. i, cap. 1.

phosis, viz. insects, as of spontaneously generated beings, in whose ova or " primordia," as in all other seeds, the " species" or immaterial " form" plainly dwells, the moving principle, as it were, of those things which are to be generated), and when I speak of the soul and its affections, and how art, memory, and experience are to be regarded as the conceptions of the brain alone.

THE ANATOMICAL EXAMINATION

OF THE BODY OF

THOMAS PARR,

WHO DIED AT THE AGE OF ONE HUNDRED AND FIFTY-TWO YEARS;

MADE BY

WILLIAM HARVEY,

OTHERS OF THE KING'S PHYSICIANS BEING PRESENT,

ON THE 16TH OF NOVEMBER, THE ANNIVERSARY OF THE BIRTHDAY

OF HER SERENE HIGHNESS

HENRIETTA MARIA, QUEEN OF GREAT BRITAIN, FRANCE AND IRELAND.

[This account first appeared in the work of Dr. Bett, entitled: " De Ortu et Natura Sanguinis," 8vo. London, 1669, the MS. having been presented to Bett by Mr. Michael Harvey, nephew of the author, with whom Bett informs us he was on terms of intimacy.—Ed.]

ANATOMICAL EXAMINATION OF THE BODY
OF THOMAS PARR.

THOMAS PARR, a poor countryman, born near Winnington, in the county of Salop, died on the 14th of November, in the year of grace 1635, after having lived one hundred and fifty-two years and nine months, and survived nine princes. This poor man, having been visited by the illustrious Earl of Arundel when he chanced to have business in these parts, (his lordship being moved to the visit by the fame of a thing so incredible,) was brought by him from the country to London; and, having been most kindly treated by the earl both on the journey and during a residence in his own house, was presented as a remarkable sight to his Majesty the King.

Having made an examination of the body of this aged individual, by command of his Majesty, several of whose principal physicians were present, the following particulars were noted :

The body was muscular, the chest hairy, and the hair on the fore-arms still black; the legs, however, were without hair, and smooth.

The organs of generation were healthy, the penis neither retracted nor extenuated, nor the scrotum filled with any serous infiltration, as happens so commonly among the decrepid; the testes, too, were sound and large; so that it seemed not improbable that the common report was true, viz. that he did public penance under a conviction for incontinence, after he had passed his hundredth year; and his wife, whom he had married as a widow in his hundred-and-twentieth year, did not deny that he had intercourse with her after the manner of other husbands with their wives, nor until about twelve years back had he ceased to embrace her frequently.

The chest was broad and ample; the lungs, nowise fungous, adhered, especially on the right side, by fibrous bands to the ribs. They were much loaded with blood, as we find them in cases of peripneumony, so that until the blood was squeezed out they looked rather blackish. Shortly before his death I had observed that the face was livid, and he suffered from difficult breathing and orthopnœa. This was the reason why the axillæ and chest continued to retain their heat long after his death: this and other signs that present themselves in cases of death from suffocation were observed in the body.

We judged, indeed, that he had died suffocated, through inability to breathe, and this view was confirmed by all the physicians present, and reported to the King. When the blood was expressed, and the lungs were wiped, their substance was beheld of a white and almost milky hue.

The heart was large, and thick, and fibrous, and contained a considerable quantity of adhering fat, both in its circumference and over its septum. The blood in the heart, of a black colour, was dilute, and scarcely coagulated; in the right ventricle alone some small clots were discovered.

In raising the sternum, the cartilages of the ribs were not found harder or converted into bone in any greater degree than they are in ordinary men; on the contrary, they were soft and flexible.

The intestines were perfectly sound, fleshy, and strong, and so was the stomach: the small intestines presented several constrictions, like rings, and were muscular. Whence it came that, by day or night, observing no rules or regular times for eating, he was ready to discuss any kind of eatable that was at hand; his ordinary diet consisting of sub-rancid cheese, and milk in every form, coarse and hard bread, and small drink, generally sour whey. On this sorry fare, but living in his home, free from care, did this poor man attain to such length of days. He even ate something about midnight shortly before his death.

The kidneys were bedded in fat, and in themselves sufficiently healthy; on their anterior aspects, however, they contained several small watery abscesses or serous collections, one of which, the size of a hen's egg, containing a yellow fluid in a proper cyst, had made a rounded depression in the substance of the kidney. To this some were disposed to ascribe the suppression of urine under which the old man had laboured shortly before his death; whilst others, and with greater show of likelihood, ascribed it to the great regurgitation of serum upon the lungs.

There was no appearance of stone either in the kidneys or bladder.

The mesentery was loaded with fat, and the colon, with the omentum, which was likewise fat, was attached to the liver, near the fundus of the gall-bladder; in like manner the colon was adherent from this point posteriorly with the peritoneum.

The viscera were healthy; they only looked somewhat white externally, as they would have done had they been parboiled; internally they were (like the blood,) of the colour of dark gore.

The spleen was very small, scarcely equalling one of the kidneys in size.

All the internal parts, in a word, appeared so healthy, that had nothing happened to interfere with the old man's habits of life, he might perhaps have escaped paying the debt due to nature for some little time longer.

The cause of death seemed fairly referrible to a sudden change in the non-naturals, the chief mischief being connected with the change of air, which through the whole course of life had been inhaled of perfect purity,—light, cool, and mobile, whereby the præcordia and lungs were more freely ventilated and cooled; but in this great advantage, in this grand cherisher of life this city is especially destitute; a city whose grand characteristic is an immense concourse of men and animals, and where ditches abound, and filth and offal lie scattered about, to say nothing of the smoke engendered by the general use of sulphureous coal as fuel, whereby the air is at all times rendered heavy, but much more so in the autumn than at any other season. Such an atmosphere could not have been found otherwise than insalubrious to one coming from the open, sunny and healthy region of Salop; it must have been especially so to one already aged and infirm.

And then for one hitherto used to live on food unvaried in kind, and very simple in its nature, to be set at a table loaded with variety of viands, and tempted not only to eat more than wont, but to partake of strong drink, it must needs fall out that the functions of all the natural organs would become deranged. Whence the stomach at length failing, and the excretions long retained, the work of concoction proceeding languidly, the liver getting loaded, the blood stagnating in the veins, the spirits frozen, the heart, the source of life, oppressed, the lungs infarcted, and made impervious to the ambient air, the general habit rendered more compact, so that it could no longer exhale or perspire—no wonder that the soul, little content with such a prison, took its flight.

The brain was healthy, very firm and hard to the touch; hence, shortly before his death, although he had been blind for twenty years, he heard extremely well, understood all that was said to him, answered immediately to questions, and had perfect apprehension of any matter in hand; he was also accustomed to walk about, slightly supported between two persons. His memory, however, was greatly impaired, so that he scarcely recollected anything of what had happened to him when he was a young man, nothing of public incidents, or of the kings or nobles who had made a figure, or of the wars or troubles of his earlier life, or of the manners of society, or of the prices of things—in a word, of any of the ordinary incidents which men are wont to retain in their memories. He only recollected the events of the last few years. Nevertheless, he was accustomed, even in his hundred and thirtieth year, to engage lustily in every kind of agricultural labour, whereby he earned his bread, and he had even then the strength required to thrash the corn.

LETTERS.

LETTERS.

To Caspar Hofmann, M.D.   Published at Nurenberg, in the
' Spicilegium Illustrium Epistolarum ad Casp. Hofmannum.'

YOUR opinion of me, my most learned Hofmann, so candidly
given, and of the motion and circulation of the blood, is extremely gratifying to me; and I rejoice that I have been
permitted to see and to converse with a man so learned as
yourself, whose friendship I as readily embrace as I cordially
return it.   But I find that you have been pleased first elaborately to inculpate me, and then to make me pay the
penalty, as having seemed to you " to have impeached and
condemned Nature of folly and error ; and to have imputed
to her the character of a most clumsy and inefficient artificer,
in suffering the blood to become recrudescent, and making it
return again and again to the heart in order to be recon-
cocted, to grow effete as often in the general system ; thus
uselessly spoiling the perfectly-made blood, merely to find her
in something to do."   But where or when anything of the
kind was ever said, or even imagined by me—by me, who, on
the contrary, have never lost an opportunity of expressing
my admiration of the wisdom and aptness and industry of
Nature,—as you do not say, I am not a little disturbed to
find such things charged upon me by a man of sober judgment like yourself.   In my printed book, I do, indeed,
assert that the blood is incessantly moving out from the heart
by the arteries to the general system, and returning from this

by the veins back to the heart, and with such an ebb and flow, in such mass and quantity that it must necessarily move in some way in a circuit. But if you will be kind enough to refer to my eighth and ninth chapters you will find it stated in so many words that I have purposely omitted to speak of the concoction of the blood, and of the causes of this motion and circulation, especially of the final cause. So much I have been anxious to say, that I might purge myself in the eyes of a learned and much respected man,—that I might feel absolved of the infamy of meriting such censure. And I beg you to observe, my learned, my impartial friend, if you would see with your own eyes the things I affirm in respect of the circulation,—and this is the course which most beseems an anatomist,—that I engage to comply with your wishes, whenever a fit opportunity is afforded; but if you either decline this, or care not by dissection to investigate the subject for yourself, let me beseech you, I say, not to vilipend the industry of others, nor charge it to them as a crime; do not derogate from the faith of an honest man, not altogether foolish nor insane, who has had experience in such matters for a long series of years.

Farewell, and beware! and act by me, as I have done by you; for what you have written I receive as uttered in all candour and kindness. Be sure, in writing to me in return, that you are animated by the same sentiments.

Nürnberg, May 20th, 1636.

LETTER II.

To Paul Marquard Slegel, of Hamburg.

I congratulate you much, most learned sir, on your excellent commentary, in which you have replied in a very admirable manner to Riolanus, the distinguished anatomist, and, as you say, formerly your teacher: invincible truth has, indeed, taught the scholar to vanquish the master. I was myself preparing a sponge for his most recent arguments; but intent upon my work 'On the Generation of Animals' (which, but just come forth, I send to you), I have not had leisure to produce it. And now I rather rejoice in the silence, as from your supplement I perceive that it has led you to come forward with your excellent reflections, to the common advantage of the world of letters. For I see that in your most ornate book (I speak without flattery), you have skilfully and nervously confuted all his machinations against the circulation, and successfully thrown down the scaffolding of his more recent opinions. I am, therefore, but little solicitous about labouring at any ulterior answer. Many things might, indeed, be adduced in confirmation of the truth, and several calculated to shed clearer light on the art of medicine; but of these we shall perhaps see further by and by.

Meantime, as Riolanus uses his utmost efforts to oppose the passage of the blood into the left ventricle through the lungs, and brings it all hither through the septum, and so vaunts himself on having upset the very foundations of the Harveian circulation (although I have nowhere assumed such a basis for my doctrine; for there is a circulation in many red-blooded animals that have no lungs), it may be well here to relate an experiment which I lately tried in the presence of several of my colleagues, and from the cogency of which there is no means of escape for him. Having tied the pulmonary artery, the pulmonary veins, and the aorta, in the body of a man who had been hanged, and then opened the left ventricle of the heart, we passed a tube through the vena cava into the right ventricle of the heart, and having, at the same time, attached an ox's bladder to the tube, in the same way as a clyster-bag is usually made, we filled it nearly full of warm water, and forcibly injected the fluid into the heart, so that the greater part of a pound of water was thrown into the right auricle and ventricle. The result was, that the right ventricle and auricle were enormously distended, but not a drop of water or of blood made its escape through the orifice in the left ventricle. The ligatures having been undone, the same tube was passed into the pulmonary artery, and a tight ligature having been put round it to prevent any reflux into the right ventricle, the water in the bladder was now pushed towards the lungs, upon which a torrent of the fluid, mixed with a quantity of blood, immediately gushed forth from the perforation in the left ventricle; so that a quantity of water, equal to that which was pressed from the bladder into the lungs at each effort, instantly escaped by the perforation mentioned. You may try this experiment as often as you please; the result you will still find to be as I have stated it.

With this one experiment you may easily put an end to all Riolanus's altercations on the matter, to which he, nevertheless, so entirely trusts, that, without adducing so much as a single experiment in support of his views, he has been led to invent a new circulation, and even so far to commit himself as to say that, unless the old doctrine of the circulation[1] be overturned, his own is inadmissible. We may pardon this distinguished individual for not having sooner discovered a hidden truth; but that he, so well skilled in anatomy as he is, should obstinately contend against a truth illustrated by the clearest light of reason, this surely is argument of his envy—let me not call it by any worse name. But, perhaps, we are still to find an excuse for Riolanus, and to say, that what he has written is not so much of his own motion, as in discharge of the duties of his office, and with a view to stand well with his colleagues. As Dean of the College of Paris, he was bound to see the physic of Galen kept in good repair, and to admit no novelty into the school, without the most careful winnowing, lest, as he says, the precepts and dogmata of physic should be disturbed, and the pathology which has for so many years obtained the sanction of all the learned in assigning the causes of disease, be overthrown. He has been playing the part of the advocate, therefore, rather than of the practised anatomist. But, as Aristotle tells us, it is not less absurd to expect demonstrative arguments from the advocate, than it is to look for persuasive arguments from the demonstrator or teacher. For the sake of the old friendship subsisting between us, moreover, and the high praise which he has lavished on the doctrine of the circulation, I cannot find it in my heart to say anything severe of Riolanus.

I therefore return to you, most learned Slegel, and say, that I wish greatly I had been so full and explicit in what I have said on the subject of anastomosis in my disquisition to Riolanus, as would have left you with no doubts or scruples

---

[1] Harvey's Doctrine.—ED.

on the matter. I could wish, also, that you had taken into account not only what I have there denied, but likewise what I have asserted on the transference of the blood from the arteries into the veins; especially as I there seem to have pointed out some cause both for my inquiry and for my negation, to hint at a certain cause. I confess, I say, nay, I even pointedly assert, that I have never found any visible anastomoses. But this was particularly said against Riolanus, who limited the circulation of the blood to the larger vessels only, with which, there-fore, these anastomoses, if any such there were, must have been made conformable, viz. of ample size, and distinctly visible. Although it be true, therefore, that I totally deny all anas-tomoses of this description—anastomoses in the way the word is commonly understood, and as the meaning has come down to us from Galen, viz. a direct conjunction between the ori-fices of the [visible] arteries and veins—I still admit, in the same disquisition, that I have found what is equivalent to this in three places, namely, in the plexus of the brain, in the spermatic or preparing arteries and veins, and in the umbilical arteries and veins. I shall now, therefore, for your sake, my learned friend, enter somewhat more at large into my reasons for rejecting the vulgar notion of the anastomoses, and explain my own conjectures concerning the mode of transition of the blood from the minute arteries into the finest veins.

All reasonable medical men, both of ancient and modern times, have believed in a mutual tranfusion, or accession and recession of the blood between the arteries and the veins; and for the sake of permitting this, they have imagined certain in-conspicuous openings, or obscure foramina, through which the blood flowed hither and thither, moving out of one vessel and returning to it again. Wherefore it is not wonderful that Riolanus should in various places find that in the ancients which is in harmony with the doctrine of a circulation. For a circulation in such sort teaches nothing more than that the blood flows incessantly from the veins into the arteries, and from the arteries back again into the veins. But as the ancients thought that this movement took place indeterminately, by a kind of accident, in one and the same place, and through the same channels, I imagine that they therefore found themselves compelled to adopt a system of anastomoses, or fine mouths mutually conjoined, and serving both systems of vessels indifferently. But the circulation which I discovered teaches clearly that there is a necessary outward and backward flow of the blood, and this at different times and places, and through other and yet other channels and passages; that this flow is determinate also, and for the sake of a certain end, and is accomplished in virtue of parts contrived for the purpose with consummate forecast and most admirable art. So that the doctrine of the motion of the blood from the veins into the arteries, which antiquity only understood in the way of conjecture, and which it also spoke of in confused and indefinite terms, was laid down by me with its assured and necessary causes, and presents itself to the understanding as a thing extremely clear, perfectly well arranged, and of approved verity. And then, when I perceived that the blood was transferred from the veins into the arteries through the medium of the heart with singular art, and with the aid of an admirable apparatus of valves, I imagined that the transference from the extremities of the arteries into those of the veins could not be effected without some other admirable artifice, at least wherever there was no transudation through the pores of the flesh. I therefore held the anastomoses of the ancients as fairly open to suspicion, both as they nowhere presented themselves to our eyes, and as no sufficient reason was alleged for anything of the kind.

Since, then, I find a transit from the arteries into the veins in the three places which I have above mentioned, equivalent to the anastomoses of the ancients, and even affording the farther security against any regurgitation into the arteries of the blood once delivered to the veins, and as a mechanism of such a kind is more elaborate and better suited to the circulation of the blood, I have therefore thought that the anastomoses imagined by the ancients were to be rejected. But you will ask, what is this artifice? what these ducts? viz. the small arteries, which are always much smaller — twice, even three times smaller—than the veins which they accompany, which they approach continually more and more, and within the tunics of which they are finally lost. I have been therefore led to conceive that the blood brought thus between the coats of the veins advanced for a certain way along them, and that the same thing took place here

which we observe in the conjunction between the ureters and
the bladder, and of the biliary duct with the duodenum.
The ureters insinuate themselves obliquely and tortuously between the coats of the bladder, without anything in the nature
of an anastomosis, yet in such a manner as occasionally affords
a passage to blood, to pus, and to calculi; it is easy, moreover,
to fill the bladder through them with air or water; but by no
effort can you force anything from the bladder into them. I
care not, however, to make any question here of the etymo-
logy of words; for I am not of opinion that it is the province
of philosophy to infer aught as to the works of nature from
the signification of words, or to cite anatomical disquisitions
before the grammatical tribunal. Our business is not so much
to inquire what a word properly signifies, as how it is commonly understood; for use and wont, as in so many other
matters, are greatly to be considered in the interpretation of
words. It seems to me, therefore, that we are to take especial
care not to employ any unusual words, or any common ones
already familiarly used, in a sense which is not in accordance
with the meaning we purpose to attach to them. You indeed
counsel well when you say, "only make sure of the thing, call
it what you will." But when we discover that a thing has
hitherto been indifferently or incorrectly explained (as the
sequel will show it to have been in the present case), I do not
think that the old appellation can ever be well applied to the
new fact; by using the old term you are apt to mislead where
you desire to instruct. I acknowledge, then, a transit of the
blood from the arteries into the veins, and that occasionally
immediate, without any intervention of soft parts; but it does
not take place in the manner hitherto believed, and as you
yourself would have it, where you say that anastomoses, correctly speaking, rather than an anastomosis, were required,
namely, that the vessels may be open on either hand, and give
free passage to the blood hither and thither. And hence it comes
that you fail in the right solution of the question, when you
ask how it happens that with the arteries as patent or pervious as the veins, the blood nevertheless flows only from the
former into the latter, never from the latter into the former?
For what you say of the impulse of the blood through the
arteries does not fully solve the difficulty in the present in-

stance. For if the aorta be tied near the left ventricle of the heart in a living animal, and all the blood removed from the arteries, the veins are still seen full of blood; so that it neither moves back spontaneously into the arteries, nor can it be repelled into these by any force, whilst even in a dead animal it nevertheless falls of its own accord through the finest pores of the flesh and skin from superior into inferior parts. The passage of the blood into the veins is, indeed, effected by the impulse in question, and not by any dilatation of these in the manner of bellows, by which the blood is drawn towards them; but there are no anastomoses of the vessels by conjunction (per copulam), in the way you mention, none where two vessels meeting are conjoined by equal mouths. There is only an opening of the artery into the vein, exactly in the same manner as the ureter opens into the bladder (and the biliary duct opens into the jejunum), by which, whilst the flow of urine is perfectly free towards the bladder, all reflux into the smaller conduits is effectually prevented; the fuller the bladder is, indeed, the more are the sides of the ureters compressed, and the more effectual is all ascent of urine in them prevented. Now, on this hypothesis, it is easy to render a reason for the experiment which I have already mentioned. I add further, that I can in nowise admit such anastomoses as are commonly imagined, inasmuch as the arteries being always much smaller than the veins, it is impossible that their sides can mutually conjoin in such a way as will allow of their forming a common meatus; it seems matter of necessity that things which join in this way should be of equal size. Lastly, these vessels having made a certain circuit, must, at their terminations, encounter one another; they would not, as it happens, proceed straight to the extremities of the body. And the veins, on their part, if they were conjoined with the arteries by mutual inosculations, would necessarily, and by reason of the continuity of parts, pulsate like the arteries.

And now, that I may make an end of my writing, I say, that whilst I think the industry of every one deserving of commendation, I do not remember that I have anywhere be-praised mine own. You, however, most excellent sir, I conceive have deserved high commendation, both for the care you have bestowed on your disquisition on the liver of the ox, and for the judgment you display in your observations. Go on, therefore, as you are doing, and grace the republic of letters with the fruits of your genius, for thus will you render a grateful service to all the learned, and especially to

Your loving

WILLIAM HARVEY.

Written in London, this 26th of March, 1651.

LETTER III.

To the very excellent John Nardi, of Florence.

I should have sent letters to you sooner, but our public troubles in part, and in part the labour of putting to press my work ' On the Generation of Animals,' have hindered me from writing. And indeed I, who receive your works—on the signal success of which I congratulate you from my heart—and along with them most kind letters, do but very little to one so distinguished as yourself in replying by a very short epistle. I only write at this time that I may tell you how constantly I think of you, and how truly I store up in my memory the grateful remembrance of all your kindnesses and good offices to myself and to my nephew, when we were each of us severally in Florence. I would wish, illustrious sir, to have your news as soon as convenient:—what you are about yourself, and what you think of this work of mine; for I make no case of the opinions and criticisms of our pretenders to scholarship, who have nothing but levity in their judgments, and indeed are wont to praise none but their own productions. As soon as I know that you are well, however, and that you live not unmindful of us here, I propose to myself frequently to enjoy this intercourse by letter, and I shall take care to transmit other books to you. I pray for many and prosperous years to your Duke ; and for yourself a long εὐημερία. Farewell, most learned sir, and love in return.

Yours, most truly,

WILLIAM HARVEY.

The 15th of July, 1651.

LETTER IV.

In reply to R. Morison, M.D., of Paris.

ILLUSTRIOUS SIR,—The reason why your most kind letter has remained up to this time unanswered is simply this, that the book of M. Pecquet, upon which you ask my opinion, did not come into my hands until towards the end of the past month. It stuck by the way, I imagine, with some one, who, either through negligence, or desiring himself to see what was newest, has for so long a time hindered me of the pleasure I have had in the perusal. That you may, therefore, at once and clearly know my opinion of this work, I say that I greatly commend the author for his assiduity in dissection, for his dexterity in contriving new experiments, and for the shrewdness which he still evinces in his remarks upon them. With what labour do we attain to the hidden things of truth when we take the averments of our senses as the guide which God has given us for attaining to a knowledge of his works; avoiding that specious path on which the eyesight is dazzled with the brilliancy of mere reasoning, and so many are led to wrong conclusions, to probabilities only, and too frequently to sophistical conjectures on things!

I further congratulate myself on his confirmation of my views of the circulation of the blood by such lucid experiments and clear reasons. I only wish he had observed that the heart has three kinds of motion, namely, the systole, in which the organ contracts and expels the blood contained in its cavities, and next, a movement, the opposite of the former one, in which the fibres of the heart appropriated to motion are relaxed. Now these two motions inhere in the substance of the heart itself, just as they do in all other muscles. The remaining motion is the diastole, in which the heart is distended by the blood impelled from the auricles into the ventricles; and the ventricles, thus replete and distended, are stimulated to contraction, and this motion always precedes the systole, which follows immediately afterwards.

With regard to the lacteal veins discovered by Aselli, and

by the further diligence of Pecquet, who discovered the receptacle or reservoir of the chyle, and traced the canals thence to
the subclavian veins, I shall tell you freely, since you ask me
what I think of them. I had already, in the course of my
dissections, I venture to say even before Aselli had published
his book,[1] observed these white canals, and plenty of milk in
various parts of the body, especially in the glands of younger
animals, as in the mesentery, where glands abound; and thence
I thought came the pleasant taste of the thymus in the calf
and lamb, which, as you know, is called the sweetbread in our
vernacular tongue. But for various reasons, and led by several
experiments, I could never be brought to believe that that milky
fluid was chyle conducted hither from the intestines, and distributed to all parts of the body for their nourishment; but that
it was rather met with occasionally and by accident, and proceeded from too ample a supply of nourishment and a peculiar
vigour of concoction; in virtue of the same law of nature, in
short, as that by which fat, marrow, semen, hair, &c., are produced; even as in the due digestion of ulcers pus is formed,
which the nearer it approaches to the consistency of milk, viz.
as it is whiter, smoother, and more homogeneous, is held more
laudable, so that some of the ancients thought pus and milk
were of the same nature, or nearly allied. Wherefore, although
there can be no question of the existence of the vessels themselves, still I can by no means agree with Aselli in considering
them as chyliferous vessels, and this especially for the reasons
about to be given, which lead me to a different conclusion.
For the fluid contained in the lacteal veins appears to me to be
pure milk, such as is found in the lacteal veins [the milk ducts]
of the mammæ. Now it does not seem to me very probable
(any more than it does to Auzotius in his letter to Pecquet)
that the milk is chyle, and thus that the whole body is nourished by means of milk. The reasons which lead to a contrary
conclusion, viz. that it is chyle, are not of such force as to
compel my assent. I should first desire to have it demonstrated to me by the clearest reasonings, and the guarantee of
experiments, that the fluid contained in these vessels was chyle,
which, brought hither from the intestines, supplies nourish-

---

[1] Published at Milan in 1622.—Ed.

ment to the whole body. For unless we are agreed upon the first point, any ulterior, any more operose, discussion of their nature, is in vain. But how can these vessels serve as conduits for the whole of the chyle, or the nourishment of the body, when we see that they are different in different animals? In some they proceed to the liver, in others to the porta only, and in others still to neither of these. In some creatures they are seen to be extremely numerous in the pancreas; in others the thymus is crowded with them; in a third class, again, nothing can be seen of them in either of these organs. In some animals, indeed, such chyliferous canals are nowhere to be discovered (vide Liceti Epist. xiii, tit. ii, p. 83, et Sennerti Praxeos, lib. v, tit. 2, par. 3, cap. 1); neither do they exist in any at all times. But the vessels which serve for nutrition must necessarily both exist in all animals, and present themselves at all times; inasmuch as the waste incurred by the ceaseless efflux of the spirits, and the wear and tear of the parts of the body, can only be supplied by as ceaseless a restoration or nutrition. And then, their very slender calibre seems to render them not less inadequate to this duty than their structure seems to unfit them for its performance: the smaller channels ought plainly to end in larger ones, these in their turn in channels larger still, and the whole to concentrate in one great trunk, which should correspond in its dimensions to the aggregate capacity of all the branches; just such an arrangement as may be seen to exist in the vena portæ and its tributaries, and farther in the trunk of the tree, which is equal to its roots. Wherefore, if the efferent canals of a fluid must be equal in dimensions to the afferent canals of the same fluid, the chyliferous ducts which Pecquet discovers in the thorax, ought at least to equal the two ureters in dimensions; otherwise they who drink a gallon or more of one of the acidulous waters could not pass off all this fluid in so short a space of time by these vessels into the bladder. And truly, when we see the matter of the urine passing thus copiously through the appropriate channels, I do not see how these veins could preserve their milky colour, and the urine all the while remain without a tinge of whiteness.

I add, too, that the chyle is neither in all animals, nor at all times, of the consistency and colour of milk; and therefore did these vessels carry chyle, they could not always (which nevertheless they do) contain a white fluid in their interior, but would sometimes be coloured yellow, green, or of some other hue (in the same way as the urine is affected, and acquires different colours from eating rhubarb, asparagus, figs, &c.) ; or otherwise, when large quantities of mineral water were drunk, they would be deprived of almost all colour. Besides, did that white matter pass from the intestines into those canals, or were it attracted from the intestines, the same fluid ought certainly to be discovered somewhere within the intestines themselves, or in their spongy tunics; for it does not seem probable that any fluid by bare and rapid percolation of the intestines could assume a new nature, and be changed into milk. Moreover, were the chyle only filtered through the tunics of the intestines, it ought surely to retain some traces of its original nature, and resemble in colour and smell the fluid contained in the intestines; it ought to smell offensively at least; for whatever is contained in the intestines is tinged with bile, and smells unpleasantly. Some have consequently thought that the body was nourished by means of chyle raised into attenuated vapour, because vapours exhaling in the alembic, even from fœtid matters, often do not smell amiss.

The learned Pecquet ascribes the motion of this milky fluid to respiration. For my own part, though strongly tempted to do otherwise, I shall say nothing upon this topic until we are agreed as to what the fluid is. But were we to concede the point (which Pecquet takes for granted without any sufficient reason in the shape of argument), that chyle was continually transported by the canals in question from the intestines to the subclavian veins, in which the vessels he has lately discovered terminate, we should have to say that the chyle before reaching the heart was mixed with the blood which is about to enter the right side of the organ, and that it there obtains a further concoction. But what, some one might with as good reason ask, should hinder it from passing into the porta, then into the liver, and thence into the cava, in conformity with the arrangement which Aselli and others are said to have found? Why, indeed, should we not as well believe that the chyle enters the mouths of the mesenteric veins, and in this way becomes immediately mingled with the blood, where it might receive digestion and perfection from the heat, and serve for the nutrition of all the parts? For the heart itself can be accounted of higher importance than other parts; can be termed the source of heat and of life, upon no other grounds than as it contains a larger quantity of blood in its cavities, where, as Aristotle says, the blood is not contained in veins as it is in other parts, but in an ample sinus and cistern, as it were. And that the thing is so in fact, I find an argument in the distribution of innumerable arteries and veins to the intestines, more than to any other part of the body, in the same way as the uterus abounds with blood-vessels during the period of pregnancy. For nature never acts inconsiderately. In all the red-blooded animals, consequently, which require [abundant] nourishment, we find a copious distribution of mesenteric vessels; but lacteal veins we discover in but a few, and even in these not constantly. Wherefore, if we are to judge of the uses of parts as we meet with them in general and in the greater number of animals, beyond all doubt those filaments of a white colour, and very like the fibres of a spider's web, are not instituted for the purpose of transporting nourishment, neither is the fluid they contain to be designated by the name of chyle; the mesenteric vessels are rather destined to the duty in question. Because, of that whence an animal is constituted, by that must it necessarily grow, and by that consequently be nourished; for the nutritive and augmentative faculties, or nutrition and growth, are essentially the same. An animal, therefore, naturally grows in the same manner as it receives immediate nutriment from the first. Now it is a most certain fact (as I have shown elsewhere) that the embryos of all red-blooded animals are nourished by means of the umbilical vessels from the mother, and this in virtue of the circulation of the blood. They are not nourished, however, immediately by the blood, as many have imagined, but after the manner of the chick in ovo, which is first nourished by the albumen, and then by the vitellus, which is finally drawn into and included within the abdomen of the chick. All the umbilical vessels, however, are inserted into the liver, or at all events pass through it, even in those animals whose umbilical vessels enter the vena portæ, as in the chick, in which the vessels proceeding from the yelk always so terminate. In the selfsame way, therefore, as the chick is nourished from a nutriment, (viz. the albumen and vitellus,) previously prepared, even so does it continue to be nourished through the whole course of its independent existence. And the same thing, as I have elsewhere shown, is common to all embryos whatsoever : the nourishment mingled with the blood, is transmitted through their veins to the heart, whence moving on by the arteries, it is carried to every part of the body. The fœtus when born, when thrown upon its own resources, and no longer immediately nourished by the mother, makes use of its stomach and intestines just as the chick makes use of the contents of the egg, and vegetables make use of the ground whence they derive concocted nutriment. For even as the chick at the commencement obtained its nourishment from the egg, by means of the umbilical vessels (arteries and veins) and the circulation of the blood, so does it subsequently, and when it has escaped from the shell, receive nourishment by the mesenteric veins ; so that in either way the chyle passes through the same channels, and takes its route by the same path through the liver. Nor do I see any reason why the route by which the chyle is carried in one animal should not be that by which it is carried in all animals whatsoever; nor indeed, if a circulation of the blood be necessary in this matter, as it really is, that there is any need for inventing another way.

I must say that I greatly prize the industry of the learned Pecquet, and make much of the receptacle which he has discovered ; still it does not present itself to me as of such importance as to force me from the opinion I have already given ; for I have myself found several receptacles of milk in young animals ; and in the human embryo I have found the thymus so distended with milk, that suspicions of an imposthume were at first sight excited, and I was disposed to believe that the lungs were in a state of suppuration, for the mass of the thymus looked actually larger than the lungs themselves. Frequently, too, I have found a quantity of milk in the nipples of new-born infants, as also in the breasts of young men who were very lusty. I have also met with a receptacle full of milk in the body of a fat and large deer, in the situation

39

where Pecquet indicates his receptacle, of such a size that it might readily have been compared to the abomasus, or read of the animal.

These observations, learned sir, have I made at this time in answer to your letter, that I might show my readiness to comply with your wishes.

Pray present my most kind wishes to Dr. Pecquet and to Dr. Gayant. Farewell, and believe me to be, very affectionately and respectfully,   Yours,

WILLIAM HARVEY.

London, the 28th April, 1652.

LETTER V.

To the most excellent and learned John Nardi, of Florence.

DISTINGUISHED AND ACCOMPLISHED SIR,—The arrival of your letter lately gave me the liveliest pleasure, and the receipt at the same time of your learned comments upon Lucretius satisfied me that you are not only living and well, but that you are at work among the sacred things of Apollo. I do indeed rejoice to see truly learned men everywhere illustrating the republic of letters, even in the present age, in which the crowd of foolish scribblers is scarcely less than the swarms of flies in the height of summer, and threatens with their crude and flimsy productions to stifle us as with smoke. Among other things that delighted me greatly in your book was that part where I see you ascribe plague almost to the same efficient cause as I do animal generation. Still it must be confessed that it is difficult to explain how the idea, or form, or vital principle should be transfused from the genitor to the gene-trix, and from her transmitted to the conception or ovum, and thence to the fœtus, and in this produce not only an image of the genitor, or an external species, but also various peculiarities or accidents, such as disposition, vices, hereditary diseases, nævi or mother-marks, &c. All of these accidents must inhere in the geniture and semen, and accompany that specific thing, bywhatever name you call it, from which an animal is not only produced, but by which it is afterwards governed, and to the end of its life preserved. As all this, I say, is not readily accounted for, so do I hold it scarcely less difficult to conceive how pestilence or leprosy should be communicated to a distance by contagion, by a zymotic element contained in woollen or linen things, household furniture, even the walls of a house, cement, rubbish, &c., as we find it stated in the fourteenth chapter of Leviticus. How, I ask, can contagion, long lurking in such things, leave them in fine, and after a long lapse of time produce its like in another body? Nor in one or two only, but in many, without respect of strength, sex, age, temperament, or mode of life, and with such violence that the evil can by no art be stayed or mitigated. Truly it does not seem less likely that form, or soul, or idea, whether this be held substantive or accidental, should be transferred to something else, whence an animal at length emerges, all as if it had been produced on purpose, and to a certain end, with foresight, intelligence, and divine art.

These are among the number of more abstruse matters, and demand your ingenuity, most learned Nardi. Nor need you plead in excuse your advanced life; I myself, although verging on my eightieth year, and sorely failed in bodily strength, nevertheless feel my mind still vigorous, so that I continue to give myself up with the greatest pleasure to studies of this kind. I send you along with these, three books upon the subject you name.[1] If you will mention my name to his Serene Highness the Duke of Tuscany, with thankfulness for the distinguished honour he did me when I was formerly in Florence, and add my wishes for his safety and prosperity, you will do a very kind thing to

Your devoted and very attached friend,

WILLIAM HARVEY.

30th Nov. 1653.

[1] [Nardi had written to Harvey requesting him to select a few of the publications which should give a faithful narrative of the distractions that had but lately agitated England.—ED.]

To John Daniel Horst, principal Physician of Hesse-Darmstadt.

EXCELLENT SIR,—I am much pleased to find, that in spite
of the long time that has passed, and the distance that separates us, you have not yet lost me from your memory, and I
could wish that it lay in my power to answer all your inquiries. But, indeed, my age does not permit me to have this
pleasure, for I am not only far stricken in years, but am afflicted
with more and more indifferent health. With regard to the
opinions of Riolanus, and his decision as to the circulation of
the blood, it is very obvious that he makes vast throes in the
production of vast trifles; nor do I see that he has as yet
satisfied a single individual with his figments. Slegel wrote
well and modestly, and, had the fates allowed, would undoubtedly have answered his arguments and reproaches also. But
Slegel as I learn, and grieve to learn, died some months ago.
As to what you ask of me, in reference to the so-called lacteal
veins and thoracic ducts, I reply, that it requires good eyes,
and a mind free from other anxieties, to come to any definite
conclusion in regard to these extremely minute vessels; to me,
however, as I have just said, neither of these requisites is
given. About two years ago, when asked my opinion on the
same subject, I replied at length, and to the effect that it was
not sufficiently determined whether it was chyle or one of the
thicker constituents of milk, destined speedily to pass into fat,
which flowed in these white vessels; and further that the vessels
themselves are wanting in several animals, namely, birds and
fishes, though it seems most probable that these creatures are
nourished upon the same principles as quadrupeds; nor can any
sufficient reason be rendered why in the embryo all nutriment,
carried by the umbilical vein, should pass through the liver,
but that this should not happen when the fœtus is freed from
the prison of the womb, and made independent. Besides, the
thoracic duct itself, and the orifice by which it communicates
with the subclavian vein, appear too small and narrow to suffice

for the transmission of all the supplies required by the body. And I have asked myself farther, why such numbers of blood-vessels, arteries, and veins should be sent to the intestines if there were nothing to be brought back from thence? especially as these are mere membraneous parts, and on this account require a smaller supply of blood.

These and other observations of the same tenor I have already made,—not as being obstinately wedded to my own opinion, but that I might find out what could reasonably be urged to the contrary by the advocates of the new views. I am ready to award the highest praise to Pecquet and others for their singular industry in searching out the truth ; nor do I doubt but that many things still lie hidden in Democritus's well that are destined to be drawn up into the light by the indefatigable diligence of coming ages. So much do I say at this time, which, I trust, with your known kindness, you will take in good part. Farewell, learned friend ; live happily, and hold me always

Yours, most affectionately,

WILLIAM HARVEY.

London, 1st February, 1654-5.

LETTER VII.

To the distinguished and learned John Dan. Horst, principal Physician at the Court of Hesse-Darmstadt.

MOST EXCELLENT SIR,—Advanced age, which unfits us for the investigation of novel subtleties, and the mind which inclines to repose after the fatigues of lengthened labours, prevent me from mixing myself up with the investigation of these new and difficult questions : so far am I from court-ing the office of umpire in this dispute ! I was anxious to do you a pleasure lately, when, in reply to your request, I sent you the substance of what I had formerly written to a Parisian physician as my ideas on the lacteal veins and thoracic ducts.[1] Not, indeed, that I was certain of the opinion then delivered, but that I might place these objections such as they were before those who fancy that when they have made a certain progress in discovery all is revealed by them.

With reference to your letters in reply, however, and in so far as the collection of milky fluid in the vessels of Aselli is concerned, I have not ascribed it to accident, and as if there were not certain assignable causes for its existence; but I have denied that it was found at all times in all animals, as the constant tenor of nutrition would seem to require. Nor is it requisite that a matter, already thin and much diluted, and which is to become fat after the ulterior concoction, should concrete in the dead animal. The instance of pus, I have adduced · only incidentally and collaterally. The hinge upon which our whole discussion turns is the assumption that the fluid contained in the lacteal vessels of Aselli is chyle. This position I certainly do not think you demonstrate satisfactorily, when you say that chyle must be educed from the intestines, and that it can by no means be carried off by the arteries, veins, or nerves; and thence conclude that this function must be performed by the lacteals. I, however, can see no reason wherefore the innumerable veins which traverse the intestines at every point, and return to the heart the blood which they have received from the arteries, should not, at the same time, also suck up the chyle which penetrates the parts, and so transmit it to the heart; and this the rather, as it seems probable that some chyle passes immediately from the stomach before its contents have escaped into the intestines, (or how account for the rapid recovery of the spirits and strength in cases of fainting?) although no lacteals are distributed to the stomach.

With regard to the letter which you inform me you have addressed to Bartholin, I do not doubt of his replying to you as you desire; nor is there any occasion wherefore I should trouble you farther on that topic. I only say (keeping silence as to any other channels), that the nutritive juice might be as readily transported by the uterine arteries, and distilled into the uterus, as watery fluid is carried by the emulgent arteries

---

[1] [Pecquet described the duct as dividing into two branches, one for each subclavian vein.—ED.]

to the kidneys. Nor can this juice be spoken of as preternatural; neither ought it to be compared to the vagitus uterinus, seeing that in pregnant women the fluid is always present, the vagitus an incident of very rare occurrence. What you say of the excrements of new-born infants differing from those of the child that has once tasted milk I do not admit; for, except in the particular of colour, I scarcely perceive any difference between them, and conceive that the black hue may fairly be ascribed to the long stay of the fæces in the bowels.

Your proposal that I should attempt a solution of the true use of these newly-discovered ducts, is an undertaking of greater difficulty than comports with the old man far advanced in years, and occupied with other cares: nor can such a task be well entrusted to several hands, were even such assistance as you indicate at my command;[1] but it is not; Highmore does not live in our neighbourhood, and I have not seen him for a period of some seven years. So much I write at present, most learned sir, trusting it will be taken in good part as coming from yours,

Very sincerely and respectfully,
WILLIAM HARVEY.

London, 13th July 1655 (old style).

LETTER VIII.

To the very learned John Nardi, of Florence, a man distinguished alike for his virtues, life, and erudition.

MOST EXCELLENT SIR,—I lately received your most agreeable letter, from which I am equally delighted to learn that you are well, that you go on prosperously, and labour strenuously in our chosen studies. But I am not informed whether my letter in reply to yours, along with a few

---

[1] [Horst, in the letter to which the above is an answer, had said, "Nobilissime Harveie, &c. Most noble Harvey, I only wish you could snatch the leisure to explain to the world the true use of these lymphatic and thoracic ducts. You have many illustrious scholars, particularly Highmore, with whose assistance it were each to solve all doubts."—ED.]

books forwarded at the same time, have come to hand or not. I should be happy to have news on this head at your earliest convenience, and also to be made acquainted with the progress you make in your ' Noctes Geniales,' and other contemplated works.   For I am used to solace my declining years, and to refresh my understanding, jaded with the trifles of every-day life, by reading the best works of this description.   I have again to return you my best thanks for your friendly offices to my nephew when at Florence in former years; and on the arrival in Italy of another of my nephews (who is the bearer of this letter), I entreat you very earnestly that you will be pleased most kindly to favour him with any assistance or advice of which he may stand in need.   For thus will you indeed do that which will be very gratifying to me.   Farewell, most accomplished sir, and deign to cherish the memory of our friendship, as does most truly the admirer of all your virtues,

WILLIAM HARVEY.

London, Oct. 25th, in the year of the Christian era 1655.

LETTER IX.

To the distinguished and accomplished John Vlackveld,
Physician at Harlem.

LEARNED SIR,—Your much esteemed letter reached me safely, in which you not only exhibit your kind consideration of me, but display a singular zeal in the cultivation of our art.

It is even so.   Nature is nowhere accustomed more openly to display her secret mysteries than in cases where she shows traces of her workings apart from the beaten path; nor is there any better way to advance the proper practice of medicine than to give our minds to the discovery of the usual law of nature, by the careful investigation of cases of rarer forms of disease.   For it has been found in almost all things, that what they contain of useful or of applicable, is hardly perceived unless we are deprived of them, or they become deranged in some way. The case of the plasterer[1] to which you refer is indeed a curious one, and might supply a text for a lengthened commentary by way of illustration. But it is in vain that you apply the spur to urge me, at my present age, not mature merely but declining, to gird myself for any new investigation. For I now consider myself entitled to my discharge from duty. It will, however, always be a pleasant sight for me to see distinguished men like yourself engaged in this honorable arena. Farewell, most learned sir, and whatever you do, still love

Yours, most respectfully,

WILLIAM HARVEY.

London, 24th April 1657.

---

[1] [Vlackveld had sent to Harvey the particulars of a case of diseased bladder, in which that viscus was found after death not larger than "a walnut with the husk," its walls as thick as the thickness of the little finger, and its inner surface ulcerated. —ED.]

GENERAL INDEX.

THE END.